Pharmacy Practice in Developing Countries

Pharmacy Practice in Developing Countries

Achievements and Challenges

Edited by

Ahmed Ibrahim Fathelrahman
Mohamed Izham Mohamed Ibrahim
Albert I. Wertheimer

AMSTERDAM • BOSTON • HEIDELBERG • LONDON
NEW YORK • OXFORD • PARIS • SAN DIEGO
SAN FRANCISCO • SINGAPORE • SYDNEY • TOKYO

Academic Press is an imprint of Elsevier

Academic Press is an imprint of Elsevier
125 London Wall, London EC2Y 5AS, UK
525 B Street, Suite 1800, San Diego, CA 92101-4495, USA
50 Hampshire Street, Cambridge, MA 02139, USA
The Boulevard, Langford Lane, Kidlington, Oxford OX5 1GB, UK

Notices
Knowledge and best practice in this field are constantly changing. As new research and experience broaden our understanding, changes in research methods, professional practices, or medical treatment may become necessary.

Practitioners and researchers must always rely on their own experience and knowledge in evaluating and using any information, methods, compounds, or experiments described herein. In using such information or methods they should be mindful of their own safety and the safety of others, including parties for whom they have a professional responsibility.

To the fullest extent of the law, neither the Publisher nor the authors, contributors, or editors, assume any liability for any injury and/or damage to persons or property as a matter of products liability, negligence or otherwise, or from any use or operation of any methods, products, instructions, or ideas contained in the material herein.

ISBN: 978-0-12-801714-2

Library of Congress Cataloging-in-Publication Data
A catalog record for this book is available from the Library of Congress

British Library Cataloguing-in-Publication Data
A catalogue record for this book is available from the British Library

For information on all Academic Press publications
visit our website at www.elsevier.com

  Working together
to grow libraries in
developing countries

www.elsevier.com • www.bookaid.org

Acquisition Editor: Kristine Jones
Editorial Project Manager: Molly McLaughlin
Production Project Manager: Karen East and Kirsty Halterman
Designer: Greg Harris

Typeset by TNQ Books and Journals
www.tnq.co.in

Printed and bound in the United States of America

Dedication

I dedicate this work to my big family, my mother Suad Eltohami, my wife Khadeja, and my children Huzaifa, Muaz, Ans, Sarrah, and Ibrahim, for their support and sacrifice and to the soul of my father Ibrahim Fathelrahman who left our life just one year ago.

I dedicate this work to Mr. Mohamed Osman Ibrahim Altahir, my English teacher at Eldium secondary school, Khartoum (1983–1984), from whom I learned the basics of the English language.

I also dedicate this work to all those who taught me the ABCs of pharmacy, those who supported and encouraged me throughout my life in the study of pharmacy, and those who played significant roles regarding my knowledge, skills, and professional orientation. Writing this book is not the outcome of the three years it took to be completed. It was enriched, inspired, and fueled by more than 20 years of exposure and learning from others. I specifically dedicate my work to those who occupy a special place in my heart: Professor Zedan Zeid Ibraheim (Egypt), Professor Atef Abdel-Monem (Egypt), Professor Ab Fatah Ab Rahman (Malaysia), Professor Rahmat Awang (Malaysia), Dr. Maizurah Omar (Malaysia), Professor Ron Borland (Australia), and Professor Mohamed Izham M. Ibrahim, who is a coeditor of this book.

—Ahmed Fathelrahman

This book is sincerely dedicated to my beloved wife, Norlela, who has made my writing of this book energizing; not to forget my six lovely children, Syazwan, Fatin, Daniel, Najihah, Imran, and Aiman, as well as my compassionate parents. All of them have been my inspiration and an ongoing motivation in life and I truly hope that one day they can understand the reason behind the countless hours spent in front of my computer.

I would also like to devote this book to the neglected population worldwide, with high aspiration that pharmacists around the world will continue to serve them better. Thank you to the health care environment, which has encouraged me to continue writing for the past 20 years.

Last, it was indeed a pleasure to be working since 1995 alongside my professor, Albert I. Wertheimer, especially on this book.

—Mohamed Izham MI

To Joaquima with thanks for permitting me the time to work on the book and spend less time with the family.
I hope the final product makes that seem like a good decision.

—Albert Wertheimer

Contents

Contributors

Patricia Acuna   Faculty of Pharmacy, Universidad de Valparaiso, Valparaiso, Chile

Muhammad Adnan   College of Pharmacy and Dentistry, Buraydah Private Colleges, Buraydah, Al-Qassim, Saudi Arabia

Mohammed Fadlalla Ahmed Babekir   Department of Clinical Pharmacy, Buraydah Colleges, Buraydah, Al-Qassim, Saudi Arabia

Kadir Alam   Manipal College of Medical Sciences, Pokhara, Nepal

Qais Alefan   Department of Clinical Pharmacy, Faculty of Pharmacy, Jordan University of Science & Technology, Irbid, Jordan

Abubakr Abdelraouf Alfadl   Department of Pharmacy Practice, Uniazah College of Pharmacy, Qassim University, Uniazah, Al-Qassim, Saudi Arabia

Mahmoud S. Al-Haddad   Department of Clinical Pharmacy, Faculty of Pharmacy, Taif University, Taif, Kingdom of Saudi Arabia

Ahmed Al-Jedai   College of Medicine, Alfaisal University, Riyadh, Saudi Arabia; King Faisal Specialist Hospital & Research Centre, Riyadh, Saudi Arabia

Ahmad Almeman   School of Medicine, College of Medicine, Qassim University, Buraydah, Saudi Arabia; Prince Sultan Cardiac Center, Buraydah, Saudi Arabia

Yaser Mohammed Ali Al-Worafi   College of Pharmacy, University of Science and Technology, Yemen; College of Pharmacy-Unizah, Qassim University, Buraydah, Saudi Arabia

Sybil Nana Ama Ossei-Agyeman-Yeboah   Walden University, Minneapolis, MN, United States; West African Health Organisation, Bobo-Dioulasso, Burkina Faso

Tri Murti Andayani   Department of Pharmacology and Clinical Pharmacy, Faculty of Pharmacy, Gadjah Mada University, Yogyakarta, Indonesia

Mukhtar Ansari   College of Pharmacy, University of Hail, Saudi Arabia

Ahmed Awaisu   College of Pharmacy, Qatar University, Doha, Qatar

Nathorn Chaiyakunapruk   School of Pharmacy, Monash University Malaysia, Bandar Sunway, Selangor, Malaysia; Department of Pharmacy Practice, Naresuan University, Phitsanulok, Thailand; School of Population Health, University of Queensland, Brisbane, QLD, Australia; School of Pharmacy, University of Wisconsin-Madison, Madison, WI, USA

Teerapon Dhippayom   Faculty of Pharmaceutical Sciences, Naresuan University, Phitsanulok, Thailand

Mahmoud Elmahdawy   Central Administration for Pharmaceutical Affairs (CAPA), Ministry of Health, Cairo, Egypt

Tarek Mohamed Elsayed   International Islamic University Malaysia, Kuantan, Malaysia

Gihan H. Elsisi   Central Administration for Pharmaceutical Affairs (CAPA), Ministry of Health, Cairo, Egypt

Yu Fang   Department of Pharmacy Administration, School of Pharmacy, Health Science Center, Xi'an Jiaotong University, Shaanxi, China

Ahmed Ibrahim Fathelrahman   Department of Pharmacy Practice, College of Pharmacy, Qassim University, Buraidah, Saudi Arabia

Abdulsalam Halboup   Department of Clinical Pharmacy, Faculty of Pharmacy, Jordan University of Science & Technology, Irbid, Jordan

Mohamed Azmi Ahmad Hassali   Discipline of Social and Administrative Pharmacy, School of Pharmaceutical Sciences, Universiti Sains Malaysia, Pulau Pinang, Malaysia

Azhar Hussain   Hamdard University, Islamabad Campus, Islamabad, Pakistan

Inas Rifaat Ibrahim   Department of Pharmacy, Alyarmouk University College, Baghdad, Iraq

Mohamed Izham Mohamed Ibrahim   College of Pharmacy, Qatar University, Doha, Qatar

Shazia Jamshed   Kulliyyah of Pharmacy, International Islamic University Malaysia, Kuantan Campus, Pahang, Malaysia

Sirada M. Jones   Department of Pharmacy Practice, Naresuan University, Phitsanulok, Thailand

Shahid Karim   College of Pharmacy and Dentistry, Buraydah Private Colleges, Buraydah, Al-Qassim, Saudi Arabia

Nadir Kheir   College of Pharmacy, Qatar University, Doha, Qatar

Nadeesha Lakmali   National Drug Quality Assurance Laboratory, Ministry of Health, Colombo, Sri Lanka

Shafiu Mohammed   Faculty of Pharmaceutical Sciences, Ahmadu Bello University, Zaria, Nigeria

Gamal Khalafalla Mohamed Ali   Central Medical Supplies Public Corporation, Khartoum, Sudan

Dhakshila Niyangoda   Department of Pharmacy, Faculty of Allied Health Sciences, University of Peradeniya, Peradeniya, Sri Lanka; Postgraduate Institute of Science, University of Peradeniya, Peradeniya, Sri Lanka

Satibi Satibi   Faculty of Pharmacy, Universitas Gadjah Mada, Yogyakarta, Indonesia

Ooi Guat See   Discipline of Social and Administrative Pharmacy, School of Pharmaceutical Sciences, Universiti Sains Malaysia, Pulau Pinang, Malaysia

Asrul Akmal Shafie   Discipline of Social and Administrative Pharmacy, School of Pharmaceutical Sciences, Universiti Sains Malaysia, Pulau Pinang, Malaysia

Nithima Sumpradit   Bureau of Drug Control, Food and Drug Administration, Ministry of Public Health, Nonthaburi, Thailand

Waleed M. Sweileh   Department of Pharmacology and Toxicology, College of Medicine and Health Sciences, An-Najah National University, Nablus, Palestine

Abdul Rasoul Wayyes   King's College, London, United Kingdom; Alrafidain University College, Baghdad, Iraq

Albert I. Wertheimer   Department of Pharmacy Practice, School of Pharmacy, Temple University, Philadelphia, PA, USA

Rabiu Yakubu   Jigawa Medicare Supply Organization, State Ministry of Health, Dutse, Nigeria

Mirghani A. Yousif   Department of Clinical Pharmacy, Taif University, Taif, Saudi Arabia

Shukry Zawahir   Faculty of Medicine, University of Ruhuna, Galle, Sri Lanka

Zhi Yen Wong   Discipline of Social and Administrative Pharmacy, School of Pharmaceutical Sciences, Universiti Sains Malaysia, Pulau Pinang, Malaysia

Sa'ed H. Zyoud   Department of Clinical and Community Pharmacy, College of Medicine and Health Sciences, An-Najah National University, Nablus, Palestine

Foreword by Joseph T. DiPiro, PharmD*

The new book by Drs. Fathelrahman, Ibrahim and Wertheimer, *Pharmacy Practice in Developing Countries: Achievements and Challenges,* explores the current state of pharmacy practice in 19 countries in Asia, the Middle East, Africa, and Latin America. This is not an easy task given the dynamic changes that are occurring in disease, health care and pharmacy throughout the world. Our societies are changing and experiencing more burden from chronic diseases such as diabetes and hypertension, and people in many societies have greater expectations from their health care systems. In addition to addressing acute health needs, health care systems are changing to address chronic diseases and promote wellness, and people are becoming more knowledgeable about their health through education and global communication. There are many reasons for changes in the practice of pharmacy, including the process and regulation of drug distribution with greater accessibility to medicines, the increasing prevalence of chronic diseases and the greater reliance on medications to treat chronic diseases.

As pharmacists from around the world communicate, in developed and developing countries, we find that there are many similarities in our practice that focus on and include:

- Assuring effective delivery of medications to patients
- Minimizing potential adverse effects from the medications or drug interactions
- Assisting health care providers and patients to become more knowledgeable about medications.
- Promoting medication adherence
- Assuring the quality of medicines
- Assuring access to medications under conditions of inadequate financial resources.

The culture and traditions in different countries can determine the place of pharmacists in society and the reliance that health care consumers place on pharmacists. In many countries pharmacists are the most accessible health care professional and have great opportunity to recommend and implement wellness and treatment strategies. What pharmacists can

---

*Dean and Archie O. McCalley Chair, School of Pharmacy, Virginia Commonwealth University, Richmond, Virginia, USA.

contribute to health care is determined by the nature of their training and the legal authority within their country. However, in many countries the number of pharmacists is not sufficient to provide the type of care that is needed. Knowing how care by pharmacists is provided in different countries will assist all pharmacists in identifying the best practices and striving to use them in their own country.

While pharmacy practice varies considerably among countries, there is a consistent and growing interest in progressive pharmacy practice that goes by different terms, such as clinical pharmacy or pharmaceutical care. It is patient-focused practice where the pharmacist has a responsibility to the patient. As a part of this transformation in practice other aspects of progressive practice are developing, such as the pharmacists role in a health care team, personalized medicine, and population health. In the final chapter of this book the authors provide a well thought out summary of the issues that account for the gap in practice between countries: professionalism, decision making, the healthcare team, access to patient information, quality of the academic programs, continuing education, country standards of practice, and scholarly activity to advance practice.

An important factor that will surely advance practice in all countries is the quality of pharmacy education, both for students entering the profession and for practitioners advancing their knowledge. Pharmacy education is becoming more standardized at a higher level than in the past. As education improves, so will practice. Progress in pharmacy education and practice is coming from many different countries throughout the world. All countries have something to offer and all countries have something to learn from what others are doing to improve practice.

By promoting cross-country understanding about our profession, this book will be very helpful for anyone with an interest in advancing pharmacy practice across the world and for anyone who is committed to improving practice in their own country.

Foreword by Thony Björk, MSc Pharm*

Pharmacy practice, wherever it is performed, aims to optimize health outcomes to patients and add value for health systems across the world. To achieve this, access to medicines and medicine safety must be in focus, as well as to improve treatment outcomes of individual patients.

This can be done in many different ways, depending on variations in national or local needs, in national or international policy and regulations and of course in available resources. You cannot say that one model to practice pharmacy is better than the other. You have to consider also the culture and the environment the pharmacy has to operate in, not least the political environment.

But of course it is possible to develop and improve the pharmacy practice by learning from each other and to find out some elements of best practice. The most important is to always look at the outcome for the patient. The correct treatment and use of medicines for each individual is the goal. Although we cannot forget that good pharmacy practice also aims to improve all public health and to contribute to the efficiency and quality of the health system.

Calculations indicate that the cost of problems with the use of medicines is equal to or greater than the cost of the medicines themselves. New medicines are also more and more expensive and not always affordable for health care. Managing the costs of medicines is critical to making the best use of limited resources to maximize health care for as many people as possible.

Falsified medicines, expired medicines and unlicensed medicines are a growing problem in many countries, and it is essential that pharmacies have developed standards for how to handle these matters.

* Senior Vice President and Senior Advisor Pharmaceutical Affairs, Apoteket AB (Sweden). Vice President, International Pharmaceutical Federation. Member of the board of the Swedish Medical Agency. Former President of the Swedish Pharmacists Association, the Nordic Pharmacy Association and the Pharmaceutical Group of European Union.

Supplying consumers with medicines alone is not sufficient to achieve the goals of the treatment. Pharmacists have a greater responsibility to handle all the medication-related needs that the patient has to improve the outcomes of medicines use.

In 1992 the International Pharmaceutical Federation (FIP) developed standards for pharmacy practice; "Good pharmacy practice in community and hospital pharmacy settings". Following recommendations from the WHO Expert Committee and the endorsement of the FIP Council in 1997, the FIP/WHO joint document on good pharmacy practice (GPP) was published in 1999. In 2011 the FIP/WHO Joint Guidelines on Good Pharmacy Practice - Standards for Quality Services was revised.

In collaboration with WHO, a first edition of a practical handbook "Developing pharmacy practice — a focus on patient care" was published in 2006. This handbook gives advice on how to meet the changing needs of pharmacists, setting out a new model for pharmacy practice and also presenting a step-by-step approach to pharmaceutical care.

The "Bangkok declaration on good pharmacy practice in the community pharmacy settings" (2007) in the South-East Asia Region was adopted by the FIP South-East Asia Pharmaceutical Forum and set out the commitment of its Member Associations towards raising standards of pharmacy services and professional practice.

The FIP sets out six components to achieve a good pharmacy service:

- being readily available to patients with or without an appointment;
- identifying and managing or triaging health-related problems;
- health promotion;
- assuring effectiveness of medicines;
- preventing harm from medicines; and
- making responsible use of limited health-care resources.

The FIP defines the mission of pharmacy practice as contributing to health improvement and helping patients with health problems to make the best use of their medicines.

To improve the use of medicines, pharmacists have responsibilities for many aspects of the process of medicines use, each of which is important to achieve good outcomes of treatment, prescribed or self-care.

This book offers an excellent overview of the history and development of pharmacy practice in 19 different countries across Africa, Asia and South America. The authors focus on the problems and the possibilities they have identified in each analyzed country but also they offer solutions for the future.

Preface

The pharmaceutical sector and its overall conditions in developing countries are under-researched. There is a scarcity of studies and information on pharmaceutical health services systems. When we were planning for the current book and during the writing and the editing processes, we were thinking of how best the book should be used by readers, such as practicing pharmacists, pharmacy students, pharmacy educators, regulators, pharmaceutical industry professionals, researchers and policy makers. Several chains of communication occurred between the editors and the chapter contributors during the preparation of this book to ensure the contents discussed and presented are as much as possible consistent and useful for everyone dealing with the pharmaceutical sector. This book covers most of the aspects in the pharmaceutical sectors of 19 countries in Asia, Africa and Latin America. It will be a good resource to secure needed statistics and information related to pharmaceutical consumption and expenditure, regulatory aspects, pharmaceutical education, pharmaceutical industry, hospital pharmacy services, and community pharmacy services. This book also focuses on each country's strengths and achievements, as well as areas of weakness, barriers to improvement, and challenges. We do hope the contents will encourage and generate more researchers in developing countries in order to put the pharmaceutical sector in each country in the right order.

-The Editors

Introduction

Ahmed Ibrahim Fathelrahman, Mohamed Izham Mohamed Ibrahim,
Albert I. Wertheimer

Understanding how pharmacy is practiced around the developing world would be interesting and useful. Pharmacy is practiced in many different ways. In many parts of the world, pharmacists have played a significant role in the provision of pharmaceutical care services. In addition, it is also widely believed that pharmacists can make a great contribution to the provision of health care, especially in developing countries.

1. What is pharmacy practice?

What is "pharmacy practice" in general terms? If we asked any pharmacist in the world, "What does the term 'pharmacy practice' mean to you," although everyone may use different words, they will explain: "it is a description of what pharmacists normally do while acting in a professional context and it represents also the essential components and basic requirements for performing every job or action related to pharmacy, including where and how pharmacists do it."

As a field of study that is taught to pharmacy students, however, what does the term pharmacy practice mean? Surprisingly, in the context of pharmaceutical sciences, we searched for a concise and precise definition of the term pharmacy practice and found difficulty in coming out with a reasonable result. Even most of the textbooks of pharmacy practice do not provide a specific definition of it. These sources describe in much detail everything required to perform any sort of practice as a pharmacist in various areas and settings, such as hospitals and community pharmacies, including basic needs and required knowledge and skills. The only written definition we found was by Ben J. Whalley, in his chapter entitled "What is pharmacy practice" in the book *Foundation in Pharmacy Practice* published by the Pharmaceutical Press in 2008.[1] He defined the term pharmacy practice as a discipline within pharmacy that involves developing the professional roles of the pharmacist.

Nevertheless, the book in your hands is not primarily aimed at coming out with a universal definition of pharmacy practice, as this is supposed to be addressed somewhere else. In addition, the definitions of pharmacy and pharmacists have been subjected to numerous changes throughout the history of the pharmacy profession and historically many names have been used to describe those who practice pharmacy or who are involved in certain aspects related to pharmacy. Such information can be sought in any book concerned with the history of pharmacy. Raising the issue of the terminology is just an introductory link that leads us to appreciate the controversy in the conception and the development of pharmacy practice as has been highlighted by Professor A.T. Florence, when he wrote a preface for the book *Pharmacy Practice* by Kevin Taylor and Geoffrey Harding.[2] Florence said "The development of pharmacy practice as an academic discipline has been relatively slow and not without controversy." This is true if we revisit the article written by Donald C. Brodie in 1981, "Pharmacy's societal purpose," in which he emphasized the importance of the core function and societal purpose of pharmacy in making pharmaceuticals available for the people, but the purpose of the pharmacy profession has evolved with advancements in the healthcare system.[3] Pharmacists are expected to provide services beyond the traditional role of dispensing medications, but unfortunately, this is not happening in many developing countries.

2. The dilemma of pharmacy education and practice in developing countries

Pharmacy colleges in developing countries strive to produce a qualified pharmacy graduate prepared with essential knowledge, skills, competencies, and the positive attitude required for practice. As a result students are overloaded with heavy subjects, such as analytical and organic chemistry, pharmacognosy, pharmaceutics, and other courses taught as didactic and practical parts. However, pharmacy graduates in many developing countries are the only graduates among other professions who do not actually apply what they have been taught in colleges. The International Pharmaceutical Federation (FIP), in its policy document on Good Pharmacy Education Practice, recommended that "Basic (first degree) education programs should provide pharmacy students and graduates with a sound and balanced grounding in the natural, pharmaceutical and healthcare sciences that provide the essential foundation for pharmacy practice in a multi-professional healthcare delivery environment." According to Waterfield,[4] it is important for the colleges to have a comprehensive curriculum on pharmaceutical sciences and practice-related courses and for educators to prepare the future knowledge-based pharmacists. According to Waterfield,[4] "the use of tacit skill and knowledge by pharmacists is well documented through terms such as reflective practice." When coming to practice, pharmacy graduates discover that very small proportions of the overwhelming knowledge and skills that they have been given are actually needed for practice as pharmacists.

On the other hand, in many developing countries and in many situations, pharmacists' jobs are occupied by nonpharmacists, such as traditional drug sellers or pharmacy assistants in community pharmacy, veterinary doctors, and non-health-related individuals in the field of marketing and promotion of pharmaceutical products, and chemists and chemical engineers in the pharmaceutical industry (both as production managers and as quality-control analysts). We are not holding a discrimination philosophy against those professions. However, we would like to highlight that there is a great concern for the possibility of a substantial mismatch between the practice of pharmacists and the pharmacy education provided to them. Basically, if the pharmacy practice and the pharmacy education match each other properly, for example, the right knowledge and skills provided to practice, there would be no room for others to compete with pharmacists. Those competitors practice in a manner similar to how pharmacists are supposed to practice and with qualifications absolutely not related to the qualifications normally received by pharmacy graduates.

These issues represent part of the challenges that faced pharmacists 10–20 years ago in most of the developing countries and may be still present in some. Thus, we may say that pharmacy education in some if not most developing countries is lagging far behind and not up to date with current practice needs and consumer demand.

In this context, learning about what shapes the pharmacy profession and what is expected from pharmacists to keep their status, enhance their image, and gain the respect of their community would be essential. Pharmacy educators in most of developing countries have realized the need for preparing future pharmacists for practice in the most suitable way and newly established colleges have started opening departments or programs that focus primarily on pharmacy practice.

3. The gap between pharmacy education and practice worldwide

There has always been a gap between pharmacy education and actual practice of pharmacists worldwide. This is to be expected and is the situation with nearly all of the professions and technical logical occupations. For example, since the 1940s, pharmaceutical manufacturers have prepared the final dosage forms of most drugs in large, efficient, and FDA-approved facilities. Nevertheless, pharmacy faculties around the world have continued emphasis in pharmacy education on chemistry, formulation, and industry-oriented subject matter. A more recent example is the development of clinical pharmacy, beginning in the mid-1970s, which changed the focus of pharmacy practice from manufacturing and the product to an emphasis on the patient. Nevertheless, pharmacy education remained essentially unchanged, with its focus on the product, through the mid-1990s. Today, clinical pharmacy dominates as the principal practice mode around the world and yet many pharmacy schools continue to only pay lip service to the clinical pharmacy subjects. Now, in the second decade of the twenty-first century, we still have almost no education in nuclear pharmacy, in preparing pharmacists to answer consumer/patient questions about complementary products or to provide thorough information about over-the-counter drug products, nutraceuticals, supplements, and other healing systems such as homeopathy, acupuncture, and reflexology, among others.

It is difficult to look into the future at any significant distance, but future practice modalities are in development now; therefore it is possible for us to look slightly into the future regarding the practice of community or ambulatory pharmacy. It is very likely that the current trends that focus on cognitive services by the pharmacist will catch on,[5] be appreciated by patients, and be paid for by insurers and other payers. This would include medication therapy management and other counseling and educational services. Pharmacists in the United States can be licensed to provide immunizations and this has become a common practice in the community.

In the hospital, there is a linear trend in which the pharmacist joins in the medical rounds with the physician caring for patients on a specific service, and when there is a drug problem, or a need for additional therapies is recognized, the health care team turns to the pharmacist to suggest the most appropriate therapeutic strategy in which the least likely opportunities for interactions and adverse events can be expected for that particular patient's known genotype.

Perhaps, sometime in the future, pharmacy education and practice might be more closely aligned, but the current situation is not bad or negative. Usually, it is the educators who show that a new, higher level practice structure or organization may be superior to or more cost-effective compared to the existing system. It is necessary then for pharmacy students to be exposed to what the educators believe will be the practice setting and environment during the next 30 or 40 years of the students' practice careers, knowing that some of the material being taught will not have relevance in the coming several years or perhaps even longer in some situations and cases.

4. The emergence of pharmacy practice as a field of specialty

Can we consider pharmacy practice a field of science or a specialty or merely a description used to depict what pharmacists actually do in various fields of practice, including hospitals, community pharmacy, primary care services, pharmaceutical industry, and others?

Pharmacy practice in developed countries such as the United Kingdom and the United States is led and guided by pharmacy education and research. This is because pharmacy education is responsible for the production of the new generations of practicing pharmacists, and pharmacy research provides guidance by identifying gaps and pitfalls and areas for improvement. For example, in England, pharmacy practice research, which was established primarily in colleges of pharmacy (of course established as a result of a collaboration between professional bodies, officials in health services departments, and academia) and enriched with postgraduation studies in the fields of wellness and health promotion programs, contributed to the development and improvement of pharmacy practice during the 1980s and 1990s.

The situation in developing countries, although varying widely, was different from that of the developed countries until the end of the twentieth century, in that pharmacy education and research were lagging behind the actual practice of pharmacists. This can be seen from the orientation, scope, and contents of pharmacy curricula, which were focused merely on the classic and basic pharmaceutical sciences such as chemistry, pharmacognosy, and pharmaceutics. Of course, this book is not against such core and historically dominant pharmaceutical sciences. However, we are discussing how much is enough from each field of science to prepare future pharmacists for practice in the most suitable way.

On the other hand, pharmacy practice research in developing countries is still lagging behind the scene and what has been published on this area is limited. The establishment of pharmacy practice departments in pharmacy colleges would be the primary solution for the above problems since such departments, via teaching and research, would be responsible for shaping practice, highlighting the emerging community needs and issues, identifying barriers, and recommending policies and other suggestions. In the United States, nearly all of the 130 faculties have two departments: pharmacy practice and pharmaceutical sciences. The latter includes chemistry, pharmaceutics, etc.

5. *The available worldwide literature on pharmacy practice*

Worldwide literature on pharmacy practice as general represents varied resources in terms of presentation, scope, and focus, including books, book chapters, Web-based resources, specialized journals, and journal articles.

The purpose of the following overview is not to provide a comprehensive list of pharmacy practice publications but to establish a baseline awareness of the nature of this literature and to put emphasis on the gaps in the literature that the current book is intended to fill.

Examples from the international journals that focus on pharmacy practice in a broad context are the *Journal of Pharmacy Practice*, which is affiliated with the New York State Council of Health System Pharmacists and published by Sage Journals, and the *International Journal of Pharmacy Practice*, which is affiliated with the Royal Pharmaceutical Society and published by John Wiley & Sons (Wiley-Blackwell).

An example of a reference on pharmacy practice in general is the book entitled *Pharmaceutical Practice*.[6] Other examples are the book *Foundation in Pharmacy Practice*, by Whalley et al.[1] and the book *Pharmacy Practice*, by Kevin Taylor and Geoffrey Harding.[2]

On the other hand, there are several books focusing on specific aspects in pharmacy practice, such as pharmaceutical care, hospital pharmacy, public health in pharmacy, evidence-based pharmacy, community pharmacy, ethics in pharmacy, communication skills in pharmacy, drug information guide for pharmacists, introduction to the profession, and pharmacy practice research.

To our knowledge there is no book on the market documenting or evaluating pharmacy practice in developing countries. There are only published journal articles covering the issues of pharmacy practice in developing countries in general or focusing on certain countries. However, there may be some textbooks about pharmacy practice in particular countries. An example of this is the book entitled *Pharmacy Practice*.[7] This book is about pharmacy practice in India (Source: Patel I, Chang J, Balkrishnan R. A textbook of Pharmacy Practice. Indian J Pharmacol 2011; 43:619-620). On the other hand, some textbooks on pharmacy practice may include a chapter or a section about pharmacy practice in developing countries. Examples of this are *Pharmacy Practice*[8] and *Pharmacy and the US Health Care System*.[9]

In view of the above information and given that the present book is about pharmacy practice in developing countries, it will fill a huge gap in knowledge and provide essential information for academics, researchers, practitioners, policy makers, and pharmacy students as well as those want to establish a pharmacy-related business in a developing country. This book compiles information about pharmacy practice in developing countries that might be found scattered throughout many sources, including histories, features of practice, and strengths and weaknesses. Such book would help in reflecting, redirecting, and guiding pharmacy practice in developing countries toward what is suitable for every country, according to its available resources, communities' needs, supportive environments, and barriers and challenges, instead of merely copying the practice established in the developed countries.

An advantage of this book as a source for information is that it has been written by many authors representing those countries, who have come from various backgrounds and who hold qualifications and have had experiences that represent the broad array of pharmacy practice.

6. Why do we need a special book about pharmacy practice in developing countries?

Even many people might argue that in this advanced era of Information Communication Technology (ICT), a textbook is not necessary. People argue that most of the information could be obtained through the Internet, through Web sites, or scientific databases.

The authors and the publisher have agreed that the valuable information compiled from 19 developing counties will be presented as an e-book and in paper form. It is organized and planned by recognized experts in the field and the country chapters are contributed by invited reputable individuals in the respective focus areas. Information is critically peer reviewed before being presented to provide the best sourced information. This book will remain a beacon of light in the grayness of the information overload. In addition, many countries in the developing world are not totally digital yet, owing to resource constraints. It is not feasible to expect every student in every corner of the developing world to have access to the Internet or to an electronic book reader. For those people, having a bound paper with facts in hand is very satisfactory. For people who have access to digital books, it will be handy. Textbooks are still an essential part of an educational curriculum. Not all colleges can afford to use tablets or iPads to replace books.

One of the main aims of good pharmacy practice is to promote the appropriate use of medicines. Compared to the developed countries, the health care systems and pharmaceutical sectors of developing countries are still unstable and in some countries they are backward. This might be due to several reasons and among them are a lack of effective health and pharmaceutical policies, lack of trained personnel, and lack of financial support and resources. It is important to learn about these drawbacks and the strategies taken by the country's authorities to improve the situation. This textbook is designed to provide valuable information about pharmacy practice in the country, past, present, and future. Many of the strengths and weaknesses of a developing country's health care system and pharmacy practice are not documented. History, the past, is always forgotten and not appreciated. There can be no future direction without understanding the past.

7. What do we mean by "developing countries"?

Developing countries are defined differently by different organizations. According to the International Statistical Institute (http://www.isi-web.org/component/content/article/5-root/root/81-developing), developing countries are defined according to their gross national income (GNI) per capita per year. Countries with a GNI of US $11,905 and less are defined as developing (specified by the World Bank).[10] There are around 137 countries under this category. Developing country is a term generally used to describe a nation with a low level of material well-being. According to the World Bank (http://web.worldbank.org), a developing country is one in which the majority lives on far less money—with far fewer basic public services—than the population in highly industrialized countries. Five million of the world's 6 billion people live in developing countries in which incomes are usually under $2 per day and a significant portion of the population lives in extreme poverty (under $1.25 per day). The World Bank[10] further explains that a developing country may be one:

"…that is largely rural or with a population that is migrating to poorly equipped cities, with a low-performing economy that is based primarily on agriculture and where non-agricultural jobs are scarce and low-paying; Where the populace is often hungry and sorely lacks education, where there is a large knowledge gap and technological innovation is scarce; Where health and education systems are poor and/or lacking and where transportation, potable water, power and communications infrastructure is also scarce; Where the amount of government debt is unsustainable; Where the land mass, population, and domestic markets are small and far disbursed, often on remote islands or in island groups, susceptible to natural disasters, with limited institutional capacity, limited economic diversification; and/or Where government has collapsed and armed conflict has left a fragile state with weak institutions and policies, either unwilling or unable to provide basic social services, especially for the poor. It is estimated that a third of people living in absolute poverty around the world live in fragile states in a vicious cycle of poverty and conflict."

According to the World Trade Organization (WTO), about two-thirds of the WTO's around 150 members are developing countries. Developing countries are a highly diverse group, often with very different views and concerns (http://www.wto.org/english/thewto_e/whatis_e/tif_e/dev1_e.htm). According to the International Monetary Fund[11], developing countries have seen robust growth, reaching more than 7% in 2010, and low employment rates, with very severe unemployment especially among the youth.

The United Nations Development Program rates countries' development annually according to its Human Development Index, which includes measurements of citizens' access to health care, educational attainment, and standard of living, among other factors. In fact, 37 of the 46 states ranked as having low human development are located in Africa. In contrast, 32 of the 47 states considered to have very high human development are found in Europe.[12]

8. What shapes the practice of pharmacists?

The practice of pharmacists is shaped by many factors, such as policies, regulations, and political, economic, and educational structures. In addition, the country's available opportunities and resources, epidemiological and demographical aspects, communities' needs and expectations, and history and culture could also influence the practice of pharmacists. These factors could be barriers or opportunities to practice for the pharmacist. It is recognized that the conditions vary from country to country, and in some countries, even within a country, the practice might differ. The approach taken by countries to set a plan of actions and strategies in facing these challenges would be different.

The FIP has taken the initiative to improve the practice of pharmacy in developing countries. Since the declaration of the World Health Organization's (WHO) Alma-Ata on Primary Health Care in 1978, a lot of changes have happened. Some countries have been quite successful in achieving this mission, but some are still struggling to ensure the right to health and the highest possible level of health to each individual in the country. The FIP and WHO have produced a set of recommendations for developing countries to have a good practice of pharmacy and to improve the existing conditions.[13]

9. Pharmacy practice in developed countries: variability in practice

There can be no denial that there are major differences between pharmacy practice in developed countries and pharmacy practice in some of the lesser developed countries; nevertheless there is not uniformity in the developed countries either. For example, in the United States, there is legal advertising of prescription drugs directly to patients/consumers. The only other country where this practice is permitted is New Zealand. Many persons in government, the insurance industry, and academia believe that the advertising of prescription products to patients unnecessarily increases demand, as patients often imagine that they may have the problem for which the drug is being advertised in magazines or on television. Moreover the United States and Canada are among only a very small number of countries where pharmaceutical products are sold in stock bottles of 90 or 100 or 500 or 1000 tablets or capsules. In those environments, the pharmacist counts out the 36 tablets or 55 tablets required for a specific physician's prescription. In the remainder of developed countries, as well as in the vast majority of lesser developed countries, medications come packaged from the manufacturer in unit-of-use containers, which generally reflect the number of tablets or capsules required for one episode of care. For example, a once-a-day tablet for a chronic condition would be packaged in a box of 30 tablets to cover the need for 1 month.

Other differences throughout the developed world include the nature of pricing, approval of advertising rules for the location of pharmacies, policies for required continuing pharmacy professional education, and licensure requirements. In most of Europe, a license to open a community pharmacy is granted only when the pharmacist applicant can prove either that there are 5000 unserved patients or that there is a distance of approximately 500 m before encountering the next pharmacy. This provides an opportunity for pharmacists to avoid undue competition, which could lead to cutting corners and other potentially unprofessional activities. In the United States, Canada, Mexico, and some other nations the free enterprise system rules and a pharmacist is free to open in any location where he or she believes a profitable practice can be established.

In the United States the government plays no role in the pricing of pharmaceutical products. The marketplace determines pricing and if a product is seen as being priced too high, it will have only very limited sales, so that the manufacturer may eventually lower the price to make it more competitive. Also if a product appears extremely successful, it is not uncommon for the manufacturer to raise the price once or twice a year. All of this can be done without the need for governmental permission or government involvement whatsoever. This is contrasted with the environment in most other countries, where the manufacturer must petition the government to raise prices by demonstrating that its costs have escalated and that the originally expected profit is no longer attainable. Even when permission is granted, this may take many months or in some countries even several years. In about half of the countries of the world, the law requires that a licensed, registered pharmacist be present in the pharmacy during all of its opening hours. This is not the case in most of Africa and major portions of Eastern Europe, the Middle East, and a number of areas in Central America, where a pharmacist, often employed in the pharmaceutical industry, will rent his or her license to be displayed in the pharmacy and will only periodically visit the pharmacy to collect its fees.

Prescribing by physicians for off-label uses is considered illegal in the vast majority of countries and in much of Scandinavia, and an informed consent form must be signed by the patient; this makes little sense, especially for the use of placebos, in which case you are telling the patient that he or she is receiving a drug with no pharmacological value. In the United States and Canada it is typical to see pharmacies that sell, in addition to medications, toys, greeting cards, photo supplies, school supplies, and various other health and beauty aids, cosmetics, and fragrances. In Europe, pharmacies are restricted to medications and other closely related health care products. Related to that regulation is the fact that nonpharmacies are not permitted to sell the items that are normally found in a pharmacy.

Pharmacists in some countries must attend continuing education lectures and programs and complete approximately 15 hours of continuing professional education per year to be able to renew their pharmacy license. There is no continuing pharmaceutical education (CPE) requirement in more than half of the countries today, although the trend toward required CPE is growing and expanding. The number of categories of pharmaceutical products differs greatly among the developed countries. In the United States, there are two categories of drugs: those requiring a doctor's prescription and those sold over the counter for self-medication purposes. Within the prescription category, there are regulations regarding controlled substances that have an addictive or habituating characteristic. Some countries have a third class of drugs that can be obtained only in a pharmacy and others have a fourth category of drugs that must be obtained within a pharmacy and sold only by the pharmacist, and it is not clear which of these is most effective in seeing that appropriate therapeutics are used by patients or which strategy is most cost beneficial. Even the decision as to whether drug should be sold over the counter or require a physician's prescription is not uniformly seen and varies in many countries.

It would be safe to say that there probably is a most efficient and optimal pharmacy system that mixes and matches from among the various policies, traditions, and regulations of the various developed countries. However, at the moment it does not appear that there is one country that has a monopoly on the finest pharmaceutical services provision characteristics.

10. The scope of the present textbook

There is a lack of books that discuss and evaluate pharmacy practice issues in developing countries. All pharmacy practice textbooks in the libraries are based on the experiences of developed countries such as the United States and the United Kingdom. Knowing the huge gap in practice between developed and developing countries and that pharmacy practice in developing countries varies substantially from country to country according to the variations in needs, cultures, challenges, and resources, we assume that a book based on the U.S. or U.K. experience might not be relevant in all aspects or for all situations.

The objective is to provide a book that documents and guides pharmacy practice by highlighting achievements, challenges, and learned lessons. The book is designed for pharmacists, pharmacy students, and other health care professionals as well as for stakeholders in a health care system in both the developing and the developed countries.

Specifically, this book will try to achieve the following:
1. Document the history and the development of pharmacy practice in developing countries.
2. Describe, in general, the current practices of pharmacists in various fields of pharmacy profession.
3. Highlight areas of achievements, strength, uniqueness, and future opportunities.
4. Critique practice by discussing areas of weakness, reasons, barriers, and solutions.
5. Try to establish a consensus on what is supposed to be a best practice (this may vary from country to country and from region to region based on resources, opportunities, policies and regulations, and communities' needs and expectation).

There are altogether 19 country chapters on pharmacy practice:
  Asia: China, India, Indonesia, Malaysia, Nepal, Pakistan, Sri Lanka, and Thailand
  Middle East: Jordan, Iraq, Palestine, Qatar, Saudi Arabia, and Yemen

Africa: Burkina Faso, Egypt, Nigeria, and Sudan
Latin America: Chile

It is hoped that this book will give the various categories of readers an excellent insight into pharmacy practice in developing countries. The uniqueness of the current book is that it represents the first comprehensive reference about pharmacy practice in the developing countries. However, we are not assuming that it is going to be absolutely perfect. Perhaps no book on the market would be immune from limitation conceptually, style-wise, or regarding the information it provides or because of typographical mistakes. Constructive criticism and feedback from readers will be used to enhance the book in its future editions in terms of its presentation style or the contents. In the coming editions, we will try first to increase the coverage of the countries, particularly from the regions that are not represented at all, which is Eastern Europe, or not represented adequately, such as Latin America and Africa.

References

1. Whalley BJ, Fletcher KE, Weston SE, Howard RL, Rawlinson CF. *Foundation in pharmacy practice*. London, UK: The Pharmaceutical Press; 2008. ISBN 978 0 85369 747 3.
2. Taylor KMG, Harding G. *Pharmacy practice*. London, UK: Taylor & Francis; 2001. ISBN 0-415-27158-4.
3. Brodie DC. Pharmacy's societal purpose. *Am J Hosp Pharm* 1981;**38**:1983–6.
4. Waterfield J. Is pharmacy a knowledge-based profession? *Am J Pharm Educ* 2010;**74**(3). Article 50.
5. Albanese NP, Rouse MJ. Scope of contemporary pharmacy practice: roles, responsibilities, and functions of pharmacists and pharmacy technicians. *J Am Pharm Assoc* 2010;**50**:e35–69.
6. Winfield AJ, Richards RME, editors. *Pharmaceutical practice*. 3rd ed. New York, USA: Churchill Livingstone; 2004.
7. Revikumar KG, Miglani BD. *Pharmacy practice*. 1st ed. Career Publications; 2009. ISBN 978-81-88739-50-9. [Source Patel I, Chang J, Balkrishnan R. A textbook of Pharmacy Practice. Indian J Pharmacol 2011; 43:619–20].
8. Taylor KMG, Harding G, editors. *Pharmacy practice*. London, UK: CRC Press, Taylor & Francis Group; 2015.
9. Smith MI, Wertheimer A, Fincham J, editors. *Pharmacy and the US health care system*. London, UK: Pharmaceutical Press; 2013.
10. World Bank. http://web.worldbank.org; 2013 [accessed 23.02.15].
11. International Monetary Fund (IMF). http://www.imf.org/external/country/index.htm; [accessed 30.01.15].
12. United Nations Development Program (UNDP). *Human development report*. 2013.
13. International Pharmacy Federation (FIP). Good pharmacy practice (GPP) in developing countries: recommendations for step-wise implementation. https://www.fip.org/files/fip/Statements/latest/Dossier%20003%20total.PDF; [accessed 30.01.15].

Further reading

1. American Association of Colleges of Pharmacy (AACP). *CAPE, educational outcomes, 2013*. 2014. Alexandria, VA.
2. International Pharmacy Federation (FIP). *FIP statement of policy on good pharmacy education practice*. 2000. The Hague, The Netherlands.
3. International Statistical Institute. http://www.isi-web.org/component/content/article/5- root/root/81-developing [accessed 30.01.15].
4. WTO. http://www.wto.org/english/thewto_e/whatis_e/tif_e/dev1_e.htm [accessed 30.01.15].

Pharmacy Practice in Asia

CHAPTER 1

Pharmacy Practice in Thailand

Nathorn Chaiyakunapruk, Sirada M. Jones, Teerapon Dhippayom,
Nithima Sumpradit

Chapter Outline

1. Country background and vital health statistics

Thailand, a democratic country with a constitutional monarchy, is located at the center of the Indochina peninsula in Southeast Asia and covers an area of approximately 514,000 km^2. The country has 77 provinces with a population of around 65 million people; 96% are Thais, 51% are females, and 44% live in the municipal area.[1] Most Thai people are Buddhists (93%), with a small percentage of Muslims, Christians and others. The official language is Thai. Free education is provided up to grade 12, and the country's literacy rate was 97% in 2010.[2]

Thailand has experienced rapid changes in its demographics in the past half-century, with an increasing proportion of the elderly population.[3,4] This is due to a decline in the total fertility rate and an increase in life expectancy at birth.[2] In 2010, life expectancies at birth for males

Pharmacy Practice in Developing Countries. http://dx.doi.org/10.1016/B978-0-12-801714-2.00001-0
3

and females were 69.5 and 76.3 years, respectively.[5] Chronic and behavior-related diseases, as well as virulent infectious diseases such as human immunodeficiency virus (HIV)/AIDS and tuberculosis, have become health problems for the Thai population.[3] Cancer, accidents, hypertension, cerebrovascular disease, and heart disease are the leading causes of death in 2010.[2] Total healthcare expenditure has been shown to increase over time; in 2010, it accounted for approximately US\$13,000 million (exchange rate: 32 Thai baht per US\$) and represented approximately 3.9% of the gross domestic product (GDP).[6]

2. Overview of the healthcare system

Thailand's healthcare services are delivered by private and public sectors. The majority of the healthcare service system is delivered by the public sector, especially by the Ministry of Public Health (MOPH). The MOPH healthcare services system has been organized as a multilevel structure to ensure geographical equity and delivery system efficiency. It consists of 93 regional/general hospitals covering all provinces in Thailand, 731 district hospitals, and more than 9700 Tumbon Health Promoting Hospitals (THPHs) or subdistrict health centers.[2] A network of urban and rural community primary healthcare centers and the health volunteer systems in villages also play an important role in primary healthcare services.[3,7] The private healthcare services are also abundantly available. There are approximately 320 private hospitals and 7000 medical clinics across the country.

Drugstores are divided into four groups: drugstores for modern medicines, traditional medicines, veterinary medicines, and wholesale drugstores. Drugstores for modern medicines are the most common drugstores in Thailand, which are further classified into two types: type 1, which are licensed to sell modern medicines and are operated by registered pharmacists; and type 2, which are licensed to sell only ready-packed modern medicines that are not dangerous drugs or specially controlled drugs and are operated by other health professionals such as nurses (see the drug classification system in Section 5).[8] Because a registered pharmacist is legally required in the type 1 modern drugstore, this chapter uses the term *community pharmacy* or *pharmacy* when referring to a type 1 modern drugstore. In 2011, there were 11,603 community pharmacies in Thailand.[9] About one-third (33.8%; 3923/11,603) of pharmacies are located in Bangkok (1 pharmacy per 2116 population); the remaining pharmacies are found in regional areas across the country (1 pharmacy per 7500 population), as calculated based on the 2010 census.[1]

The overall situation of the health care workforce, especially the ratio of citizens to healthcare providers, has been improving steadily (Figure 1). This is due to an increasing and continuous production of health care personnel. However, the distribution of personnel remains one of the major challenges, with health personnel being highly concentrated in cities and the Bangkok area.[10]

There are three main public health insurance schemes in Thailand (Table 1): the Civil Servant Medical Benefit Scheme (CSMBS), Social Security Scheme (SSS), and Universal

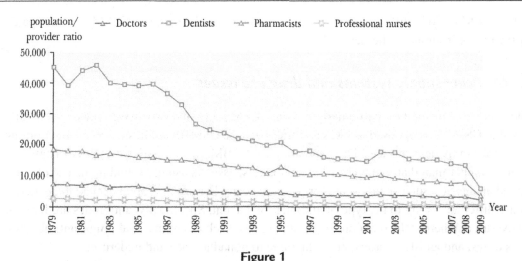

Figure 1

Ratios of citizens to healthcare providers, 1979–2009. *From Thailand's health profile 2008–2010.*[10]

Table 1: Public health insurance schemes in Thailand

Type	Operated Organization	Population Coverage
Civil Servant Medical Benefit Scheme (CSMBS)	Controller General's Department of the Ministry of Finance (CGD)	5 million (7.5%) civil servants, public employees, and their dependents
Social Security Scheme (SSS)	Social Security Office, Ministry of Labor	9 million (16.6%) private employees and temporary public employees
Universal Coverage Scheme (UCS)	National Health Security Office (NHSO)	47 million (75%) Thai nationals who are not covered under CSMBS and SSS

Coverage Scheme (UCS). The CSMBS, operated by the Comptroller General's Department of the Ministry of Finance, covers approximately 5 million civil servants, public employees, and their dependents. It is fully funded by a general tax using a prospective payment with a diagnosis-related group (DRG) approach for inpatient services and a fee-for-service (FFS) payment method for outpatient services. The SSS is operated by the Social Security Office at the Ministry of Labor and covers approximately 9 million private employees and temporary public employees. Its funding source is from employees, employers, and the government. The UCS, operated by the National Health Security Office (NHSO), covers approximately 47 million Thai nationals who are not covered under the CSMBS and the SSS. Remuneration in the UCS applies DRGs for inpatient services, while capitation is applied for outpatient services. Funding for CSMBS comes from general taxes. Presently, almost all of the Thai population (97%) has healthcare coverage.[2] Private health insurance is also available for personal options to increase their choices of benefit packages. The National List of Essential Medicines (NLEM) serves as a reference source for medicine benefit package. The current

2013 NLEM has 676 different drug items. The medicines listed in the NLEM are fully paid by the public insurance schemes.[11,12]

3. Medicine supply systems and drug use issues

The overuse of medicines, particularly of non-NLEM items and expensive drugs, is generally found in CSMBS as opposed to UCS and SSS because CSMBS applies the FFS direct billing system for outpatient services. Drug spending for CSBMS beneficiaries is approximately fivefold higher than that in the UCS.[13] The underuse issue is usually found in the use of opioid analgesics, such as morphine for palliative care. For antimicrobial agents, the patterns of use differ according to the type of antimicrobial agent. Specifically, antibiotics are likely to be overused, whereas the other antimicrobial agents, such as antimalarial drugs, antituberculosis drugs, and anti-HIV drugs, are vulnerable to nonadherence and underuse.

Pharmaceutical expenditure in Thailand accounted for approximately 43% of the total health expenditure, or 2.6% of national GDP, in 2005.[14] In 2010, the total drug expenditure in Thailand (at consumer price) was approximately US \$4517 million.[15] Anti-infectives for systemic use (including antibiotics), drugs for diseases of the cardiovascular system and alimentary tract, and metabolism drugs were the top three groups with the highest consumption.[15,16]

Self-medication is a common practice among Thais. At a community level, Thai people can access medicine via private clinics and pharmacies. They can purchase most medicines, including antibiotics, contraceptives, and antihypertensive drugs from pharmacies. Some dangerous drugs (drugs that need to be dispensed by a pharmacist), such as antibiotics and nonsteroidal anti-inflammatory drugs, are illegally available in groceries in villages.[17,18]

Problems regarding access to medication in Thailand generally involve issues of availability of medicines for rare diseases (or orphan drugs) and affordability of costly medicines. To support access to orphan drugs, Thailand applies measures such as the establishment of orphan drug list, fast-track registration, and tax exceptions. Public hospitals and the public health sector are allowed to import certain orphan drugs without a license or registration. Research and development of drugs and vaccines for neglected diseases are promoted.[19] To increase access to expensive (yet important) drugs, Thailand applies several measures, such as the use of centralized purchasing, the use of compulsory licensing to produce or import generic version of selective patent drugs,[20] and development of a vendor-managed inventory system for essential vaccines.[21] The selection of medicines is based on cost-effectiveness analyses and total budget implications.[12]

There is no legal measure on pharmaceutical price control for hospital settings. Retail x prices of drugs in public hospitals are normally no greater than 15% of hospital purchase prices, whereas those in private clinics and hospitals have higher markups. Charges in pharmacies are subject to price control by the Ministry of Commerce. However, in practice, the manufacturer or wholesale price depends largely on market segmentation and differential classes of trade, whereas the retail price depends on the competitiveness of the market.[11,22]

In Thailand, the National Drug Policy was developed to ensure the availability, affordability, and rational use of medicines and the safety, effectiveness, and quality of traditional, complementary, and alternative medicines. The policy was first introduced in 1971, with one of its goals being to develop the NLEM. The current policy is the National Drug Policy B.E. 2554 (2011) containing comprehensive strategies to improve medicine use, accessibility, and sustainability for Thai people. Additionally, a long-term problem relating to overutilization of health services and medicines among CSMBS has been seriously addressed in recent years with the implementation of several national initiatives on cost containment and drug price policy. In 2010, CSMBS spending on health services and medicines first appeared under the budget line.

4. Pharmaceutical industry

The pharmaceutical industry in Thailand consists of production and importation. Local manufacturers are generally a formulation-based industry and almost all are Thai-owned private companies; a few manufacturers are state-owned, such as the Government Pharmaceutical Organization and the Defence Pharmaceutical Factory. The affiliates of multinational pharmaceutical companies generally supply the Thai market by importing finished products from abroad. Some companies have formulation and packing factories, but they have not established local plants for the production of active ingredients in Thailand. Some invest in the Thai pharmaceutical industry in the form of joint ventures. In 2010, the total production and importation value of pharmaceuticals was $4.7 billion, 32% of which was accounted for domestic production.[23] Major channels for drug distribution were hospitals (62.5% of the medicines), pharmacies (26.3%), and ambulatory health settings (6.5%).[15]

5. Drug and pharmacy-related regulations

Drug regulation in Thailand was first introduced in 1909 when the adulteration of drug products and narcotic substances was prohibited.[24] The current law is the Drug Act B.E. 2510 (1967) and its amendments, which regulate the medicinal products for human and animal use.[25] Activities under these acts have been carried out by the Food and Drug Administration (FDA), the central regulatory agency under the supervision of the Drug Committee appointed by the MOPH. The FDA collaborates with other MOPH agencies, such as the Department of Medical Science and Provincial PublicHealth Offices (PPHO), in respective provinces throughout the country as well as non-MOPH agencies to ensure effective regulatory systems on medicines for both human and animal uses. The Drug Act requires that any drug advertisement including its contents, texts, pictures, and scripts must be truthful as well as neither misleading nor exaggerating. All drug advertisements directed to either health professionals or consumers via any means or channels must be pre-approved by the FDA. Direct-to-consumer advertising of dangerous drugs and special control drugs are prohibited.

According to the Drug Act, medicines in Thailand are classified into two major groups: modern and traditional medicines. In terms of distribution control, medicines are classified into four categories; (1) household remedies—the medicines that require no sale license; (2) ready-packed drugs—the medicines that are declared by MOPH neither as dangerous nor as special control drugs and therefore can be sold in drugstores by any health professional; (3) dangerous drugs—the medicines which can be sold without a prescription but must be dispensed by licensed pharmacists; and (4) special control drugs—the medicines that require a prescription to dispense.

Drug regulation system consists of two phases: pre-marketing control and post-marketing surveillance. Pre-marketing control involves regulations on licensing of drug manufacturing, importation and sales, drug registration, and advertising. Manufacturing plants are subject to inspection for compliance with good manufacturing practices and quality assurance. Drug registration is intended to ensure drug quality, safety, and efficacy and to ensure proper labeling. The registration for new drugs and biological products is a very stringent process. New generic drugs and some generic products are subject to bioequivalence requirements to ensure that they have similar therapeutic equivalence to their original products. The regulation of traditional drugs is less stringent than that of the modern drugs. Post-marketing surveillance involves inspection of premises, documents, products, and practice of personnel in charge in plants, companies, and pharmacies to ensure law and regulation compliance; monitoring pharmaceutical products in the market to ensure conformity of the proclaimed quality and safety; surveillance programs to watch for adverse drug reactions, abuse, or any unsafe-for-use cases (called pharmacovigilance); and re-evaluation of the registered pharmaceutical products to ensure if the registered drug profiles still meet with update scientific evidence. Several risk management measures are applied to medicines that fail to pass the postmarketing surveillance requirements. These measures include notifying for corrective actions, drug reclassification, revision of a product's warning and precaution statement, and withdrawal from the market.

Pharmacists may pursue a career in the pharmaceutical industry. Their work involves regulatory affairs, pharmaceutical production and quality assurance, pharmaceutical sales and marketing, health economics and outcomes research, administration, consulting, and advisory roles. Many pharmacists may also pursue a career that allows them to advance the country's drug system as well as health policy to improve the health of people and increase the overall efficiency of the system. They hold positions within government agencies, healthcare provider organizations, national research units, and nongovernmental organizations, such as the FDA, Drug and Medical Supply Information Center at the Bureau of Health Administration, PPHO, the NHSO, the Health Systems Research Institute, the International Health Policy Program, the Health Intervention and Technology Assessment Program, the Pharmacy Council of Thailand, and the Drug System Monitoring Mechanism Development Program (DMC) are funded by the Thai Health Promotion Foundation.

Table 2: Key professional organizations, pharmacy-related organizations, and agencies in Thailand

Name	Description	Websites
Pharmacy Council of Thailand (PCT)	Governs, implements, and issues pharmacist licensures and accredits pharmacy curriculums for all pharmacy schools in the country	http://www.pharmacycouncil.org
The Association of Hospital Pharmacy (Thailand) or ThaiHP	Provides continuing education opportunities to Thai hospital pharmacists, hosting several communities of practice (CoP), such as the Adverse Drug Reaction's Community of Pharmacy Practice (ADCoPT), Pharmacist Initiative for Patients Living with HIV/AIDS (Thailand), PIPHAT, Group of Thai Aseptic Dispensary, Chemotherapy, and Pharmaceutical Care Pharmacists (GTAPP). Thai HP as well as provides standards of hospital pharmacy practice, which is re-enforced in conjunction with HAI	http://thaihp.org http://adr.thaihp.org http://piphat.thaihp.org http://gtopp.thaihp.org
The Healthcare Accreditation Institute (Public Organization) or HAI	Accredits health institutions, hospitals, and health service facilities from both public and private sectors	www.ha.or.th
College of Pharmacotherapy of Thailand (CPhT)	Supervises, implements, and accredits pharmacy residency programs in Thailand	http://thaibcp.pharmacycouncil.org
Community Pharmacy Association (Thailand) or CPA	Supports and promotes professional activities and continuing education for community pharmacists	http://pharcpa.com

Professional pharmacy organization management is another area where pharmacists make a wide impact on pharmacy practice and health system. Pharmacists in these organizations serve the professionals a whole by representing pharmacists with regard to education, practice, accreditation, reimbursement, health policy planning, and future planning for practitioners and graduating students. Examples of professional pharmacy organizations are provided in Table 2 and include the Pharmacy Council of Thailand (PCT), The Association of Hospital Pharmacy (Thailand), and Community Pharmacy Association (Thailand). The College of Pharmacotherapy of Thailand (CPhT) oversees the implementation of pharmacy residency programs in Thailand, under the supervision of PCT. The College of Pharmaceutical and Health Consumer Protection of Thailand was also established with consent from the PCT to strengthen capacity and expand the roles of pharmacists in pharmaceutical and health consumer protection.

It is important to note that Thai drug regulation and policies are now in transition. The new Drug Act is in the final approval process; once it is enacted, it will replace the current one.

Under the new Drug Act, drug classification systems, registration requirements, regulations on drugs for animal use, drug advertisement and promotion control, and other issues are subject to change. Global trends also have forced changes to Thai drug regulations and policies. Recently, pressure from the international trade regarding Trade-Related Aspects of Intellectual Property Rights has increasingly intensified in Thailand as it greatly affects access to medicines for all Thai people.

Becoming a member of the Association of Southeast Asian Nations Economic Community in 2015 and Thailand's medical hub policy have posted both opportunities and challenges. Major challenges include, but are not limited to, an increased flow of pharmaceutical and other health products, information and technology, human resources, emerging diseases and others. Thai pharmacists in academic, government agencies, healthcare provider organizations, national research units, healthcare facilities, nongovernment organizations, industry and other areas need to prepare and adjust for such upcoming changes.

6. Pharmacy education

Pharmacy education has been established in Thailand for over a century. The first Thai pharmacy school, named the Drug Compounding School, was found in 1913.[26] The first degree originally offered was a certificate for the 3-year program in pharmaceutical production (1913–1937). The program subsequently expanded to the 4-year and 5-year program with the Bachelor of Sciences (B.S.) or the Bachelor of Pharmacy (B.Pharm.) degree. Thai pharmacy education recently underwent another drastic transition when the PCT announced that all schools must offer only a 6-year program by the year 2014.[27,28] The PCT is the governing body that issues pharmacy licensure and accredits pharmacy curriculums. The 6-year programs are required to comply with the core curricular structure guideline for the accreditation. All pharmacy graduates must complete experiential professional clerkships of no less than 2000 h (versus 500 h in the 5-year program) to be candidates for pharmacy licensure. Naresuan University was the first university in Thailand launching the inaugural Doctor of Pharmacy (PharmD) degree. The PharmD program was originally offered as a 2-year post-baccalaureate program, then transitioned to then entry-level or 6-year program in 1997. The program initially focuses on institutional clinical pharmacy practice, with the last year devoted to experiential professional clerkships. The program has been built upon the principles of pharmaceutical care and the evolution of the profession toward clinical pharmacy practice. In addition, a number of clinical residency programs in pharmacotherapy have recently been established and approved by the PCT.

Another drastic change in Thai pharmacy education is the increased number of universities that offer pharmacy degrees. In early 1990s, only six publicly funded universities offered the 5-year pharmacy degree. Currently, there are a total of 19 pharmacy schools in Thailand (14 publicly funded and five privately owned universities) offering both 5-year program and

Table 3: List of pharmacy schools in Thailand

No	University	Founded	Websites
1	Faculty of Pharmaceutical Sciences, Chulalongkorn University	1913	www.pharm.chula.ac.th
2	Faculty of Pharmacy, Chiangmai University	1966	www.pharmacy.cmu.ac.th
3	Faculty of Pharmacy, Mahidol University	1968	www.pharmacy.mahidol.ac.th
4	Faculty of Pharmaceutical Sciences, Prince of Songkla University	1980	www.pharmacy.psu.ac.th
5	Faculty of Pharmaceutical Sciences, Khon Kaen University	1983	www.pharm.kku.ac.th
6	Faculty of Pharmacy, Silapakorn University	1985	www.pharm.su.ac.th
7	Faculty of Pharmacy, Rangsit University	1987	www.rangsitpharmacy.com
8	Faculty of Pharmaceutical Sciences, Huachiew Chalermprakiet University	1993	www.pharmacy.hcu.ac.th
9	Faculty of Pharmaceutical Sciences, Naresuan University	1994	www.pha.nu.ac.th
10	Faculty of Pharmaceutical Sciences, Ubon Rachathani University	1994	www.phar.ubu.ac.th
11	Faculty of Pharmacy, Srinakharinwirot University	1996	www.pharmacy.swu.ac.th
12	Faculty of Pharmacy, Mahasarakham University	1999	www.pharmacy.msu.ac.th
13	Faculty of Pharmacy, Siam University	2006	www.pharmacy.siam.edu
14	Faculty of Pharmacy, Payap University	2006	www.pharmacy.payap.ac.th
15	School of Pharmacy, Walailak University	2007	www.pharmacy.wu.ac.th
16	School of Pharmacy, Eastern Asia University	2008	www.pharmacy.eau.ac.th
17	Faculty of Pharmaceutical Sciences, Burapha University	2009	www.pharm.buu.ac.th
18	School of Pharmaceutical Sciences, University of Phayao	2010	www.pharmacy.up.ac.th
19	Faculty of Pharmacy, Thammasat University	2012	www.pharm.tu.ac.th

6-year PharmD degree (Table 3). The numbers of pharmacy graduates and registered pharmacists have also increased dramatically from 10,503 registered pharmacists in 1995 to 29,987 pharmacists in 2012.[29]

The paradigm shift from bachelor to PharmD program has tremendously influenced pharmacy practice in Thailand, especially hospital pharmacy practice. Hospital pharmacists in university hospitals and large hospitals have been more involved in pharmacy education through preceptorships. Required rotations for sixth-year pharmacy students include internal medicine, drug information, ambulatory care, and community pharmacy. To fulfill the increasing demand in experiential training experiences for pharmacy students, pharmacy schools have sought out partnerships with all levels of practice sites by developing memorandum of agreements, especially with university, regional, and provincial hospitals throughout the country. Preceptor development program have been an area of focus in all pharmacy schools. Research in pharmacy education has been conducted to ensure high-quality pharmacy education and enhance the competency of pharmacy graduates.[27,30] In addition, the concept of health promotion has also been integrated into the PharmD curriculum, particularly smoking cessation.[31,32]

7. Hospital pharmacy practice

Before 1990, hospital pharmacy practice in Thailand was mainly responsible for drug procurement, distribution, and dispensing of pharmaceutical products to hospital inpatients and outpatients. The concept of clinical pharmacy and pharmaceutical care were introduced to Thai hospital pharmacists in the early 1990s. Hospital pharmacy practice has subsequently shifted the focus of their service from the product to patient care in response to the PCT vision that "The philosophy of pharmaceutical care is the ultimate goal of professional achievement."[33] During the initial period, the MOPH and schools of pharmacy of the four regional universities found a collaborative project to engage Thai hospital pharmacists to the pharmaceutical care concept and expand their practice to involve more patient care. Hospital pharmacists who chose to participate in the program needed to attend a 5-day series of workshops to gain pharmacotherapy knowledge and pharmaceutical care skills to apply at their workplaces. The workshop content included pharmacokinetics, therapeutic drug monitoring, adverse drug reactions, medication use evaluation, and research methodology. Attendances of the programs also gained pharmacy continuing education credits approved by PCT.

At present, Thai hospital pharmacy services are generally classified into four categories: outpatient pharmacy service, inpatient pharmacy service, drug information service, and other services (e.g., sterile products and chemotherapy, therapeutic drug monitoring, and quality management), depending on the hospital size and resources. Prior to 1990, the main services for outpatients and inpatient units were drug dispensing and distribution. After the concept of pharmaceutical care was adopted, the services for inpatient care focus more on clinical pharmacy activities such as ward-rounding, medication reconciliation, and various types of drug therapy monitoring. With the limited human and financial resources, daily dose distribution system is the most common hospital drug distribution system in Thailand. Pharmaceutical care services for special populations or specialties (e.g., cardiovascular diseases, cancer, other chronic diseases) have also become more prevalent in hospital pharmacy practice.

DIS is one of the main services that hospital pharmacists have provided. The main responsibilities of the DIS unit include answering drug-related questions, preparing drug information monographs and presenting to the hospital Pharmacy and Therapeutic Committee (PTC), and monitoring and reporting adverse drug reactions. Assessment of drug-related skin reactions or allergies has been the cornerstone for hospital pharmacists and is often included in the DIS unit. Most hospitals have implemented their own allergy alert system to prevent re-exposing their patients to known allergies.

In the era of patient safety, hospital pharmacists play a major role in hospital quality improvement process. Most hospitals have appointed a medication safety committee, in which a pharmacist's participation is required. A number of large hospitals may also have a quality improvement department to oversee the safety and quality process of the entire hospital, and pharmacists are generally employed in this department. To date, there are three major hospital accreditation organizations in Thailand: the Healthcare Accreditation Institute (Public Organization) (HAI), the Joint Commission International (JCI), and the International Organization for Standardization (ISO). The accreditation organization for government hospitals is mainly HAI, while JCI is more common among large private hospitals in Bangkok. HAI collaborates with major professional organizations for the assessment of specific professional standards. For example, hospital pharmacy practice would be assessed and accredited by the Association of Hospital Pharmacy (ThaiHP) to ensure safe and effective medication use system as part of the hospital accreditation.[34] The standards declared by ThaiHP for hospital pharmacies to accomplish are as follows: (1) leadership and practice management, (2) drug information and education, (3) optimizing medication therapy, (4) medication distribution and control, (5) facilities, equipment and information resources, and (6) research.[35] In addition to the above services, pharmacists in district hospitals, who serve populations at the district level, are also responsible for the supervision of healthcare facilities at the subdistrict level (THPH), primary healthcare services including primary care pharmacy practice, herbal drugs and Thai traditional medicines, and consumer health protection. In selected hospitals, the provision of herbal drugs and Thai traditional medicines by pharmacy department is very well recognized and have become a service model for other hospitals in the country.

8. Community pharmacy practice

The major role of community pharmacists is to provide direct patient care for people in the community. One of the most common activities is to supply over-the-counter (OTC) drugs (household remedies and ready-packed drugs) to the patient. In addition to the provision of OTC drugs for self-medication, community pharmacists also perform triage and dispense nonprescription medicines for the treatment of minor ailments. Based on a survey in 2009, the most common minor ailments encountered at community pharmacies are those related to the following systems: respiratory (53.8%), musculoskeletal (11.8%), and digestive systems (8.5%).[36] Several medicines considered as prescription-only medicines in most developed countries are classified as "dangerous drugs" in Thailand, which means pharmacists can dispense them without prescription. These include most medicines for self-limited minor ailments, such as selected antibiotics, nonsteroidal anti-inflammatory drugs, oral hormonal contraceptives, antidepressants, and topical high potency corticosteroids. The wide range of dangerous drug list gives pharmacists a great opportunity to deliver an extensive service for the treatment of common minor ailments in Thailand.[37]

Community pharmacy provides dispensing service for prescription medicines. However, only small fraction of prescriptions is filled at a community pharmacy. This is because drug prescribing and dispensing services are not formally separated in Thailand. As a result, physicians in private clinics can both prescribe and dispense medicines. Every hospital also has a pharmacy department to dispense medicines to their outpatients. In some occasional circumstances when prescriptions are to be dispensed in a community pharmacy, there is no dispensing fee. All prescriptions of controlled substances and narcotic drugs need to be kept on file and the report of purchasing and selling must be submitted to the FDA.

Most extended services outside of the conventional practices of community pharmacies were initiated as pilot or research projects led by academia and some proactive community pharmacists. Currently, four community pharmacy services have been successfully integrated into the healthcare delivery system and are now reimbursable from a number of funding bodies such as the Thai Health Promotion Foundation,[38] certain branch/region of the NHSO,[39,40] and the Bangkok Metropolitan Administration (BMA).[41] These four community pharmacy services are prescription refilling services, screening services for chronic diseases, smoking cessation services, and medication therapy management (MTM).

Only few community pharmacies have successfully performed a prescription refilling service for patients with chronic diseases under an established linkage with public hospitals under the UCS.[40,42] Practice guidelines for prescription refilling depend on specific agreements between pharmacies and public hospitals. Generally, patients with stable control of their conditions are eligible to have their prescription refilled at community pharmacies. Patients need to have their prescriptions refilled at pharmacy on a monthly basis and see medical practitioners every 3–6 months. Compensation for the provision of refilling services are made by the contracted healthcare facilities.

The community pharmacist is one of the most accessible health professionals and is located in an ideal position to provide public health services. Some community pharmacies have provided screening services for diseases such as diabetes, hypertension, and cardiovascular diseases. However, there is no agreement on types of screening tools; therefore, different pharmacies may use different tools. For example, community pharmacies in KhonKaen provided a self-checked random or fasting capillary blood sugar (FBS) to all eligible clients to identify individuals at risk of diabetes.[43] This is different from the sequential screening provided by seven pharmacies in Bangkok as they employed a diabetes risk assessment tool and subsequent self-checked FBS only to those with a high diabetes risk score.[44]

Smoking cessation service is a well-recognized health promotion practice in community pharmacies in Thailand.[45] This service has been promoted by the Thai Pharmacy Network for Tobacco Control (TPNTC), which obtained financial support from the Thai Health Promotion Foundation. As of 2007, more than 1000 community pharmacists have been trained in a comprehensive 2-day smoking cessation training program.[38] Results from a national survey conducted in 2007 showed that over two-thirds of the survey respondents (71.1%) performed smoking cessation services at least once and had at least one cessation aid available in their pharmacies (74.1%).[46] Community pharmacists also receive compensation from TPNTC for providing smoking cessation services or referring patients to TPNTC for further proper care.

Medication therapy management has been provided by some community pharmacists. This service is reimbursable under the contractual agreement with the Health Department of the BMA.[41] Eligible patients are identified by nurse practitioners at the primary care units (PCUs). Pharmacists have access to a patient's medical record through the nurse practitioner before conducting MTM at a patient's home for a maximum of three times (2–4 weeks interval), with two further monthly follow-up visits.[47]

Recently, a contractual agreement at a national level between NHSO and the Community Pharmacy Association (Thailand) was established.[48] The services covered in this agreement were screening services for diabetes, hypertension, abdominal obesity, and depression as well as smoking cessation service. The operation of these services began in January 2014, with 200 community pharmacies in Bangkok participating in the initial phase. There is an attempt by the PCT and the Community Pharmacy Association (Thailand) to achieve a compensation contractual agreement with the existing health benefit schemes, such as the UCS[49] and the SSS.[50] However, one of the main obstacles for the NHSO is concern over the varying practices of community pharmacies nationwide.[51] To ensure the high quality of services in community pharmacies, the Community Pharmacy Accreditation Project was introduced in a collaboration between the Pharmacy Council and the FDA.[52] The number of accredited community pharmacies is gradually increasing, with 547 pharmacies at present.[53] Accredited community pharmacies have been approved by the Pharmacy Council for accomplishing the following standards: (1) premises, equipment, and supporting facilities; (2) quality management; (3) good pharmacy practice; (4) regulation compliance and ethics; and (5) services and participation in community.

Good Pharmacy Practice (GPP) provided by accredited community pharmacies includes the following: (1) promoting the rational use of medicine; (2) identifying the patient; (3) reviewing prescription and consulting prescribers if needed; (4) dispensing medication with suitable information; (5) recording patient drug profiles; (6) monitoring therapeutic outcomes; (7) referring patients for appropriate treatment; (8) conducting a sequential counseling for those who need it; (9) reporting adverse outcomes of drugs and health-related products; and (10) collaborating with physicians and other healthcare professionals.[54]

9. Achievements of pharmacy practice

Pharmacy practice and education in Thailand has evolved tremendously in recent decades. The roles of pharmacists in all practice settings have advanced to focus more on patient care. These achievements were the result of several factors, ranging from leadership in the profession, a growing number of dedicated pharmacists with advanced clinical skills, a changing environment and healthcare system that both challenges and facilitates the development of pharmacy practice, and strong professional organizations and support toward the arena of paradigm changes.

9.1 Advancing roles of hospital pharmacists

Hospital pharmacists have become an integral part of the patient care team for both inpatient and outpatient care. The model for providing pharmaceutical care was initially developed only in a few hospitals but has expanded to all hospital levels, ranging from district, regional/ general hospitals, and university-affiliated hospitals. A number of specialties (e.g., infection disease, cardiology, oncology, pediatrics, nephrology, critical care, drug information services) have been developed and recognized nationwide. Pharmacists have become involved in medication management in a number of outpatient clinics, such as anticoagulation management, asthma and chronic obstructive pulmonary disease, HIV, and tuberculosis clinics. The pharmacist's role as a drug expert involves medication reconciliation, management of drug-related problems, and patient education. These pharmacy services have been evaluated for clinical, humanistic, and economic outcomes and have demonstrated a high value to other healthcare professionals.

The success of hospital pharmacy practice can be attributed to a number of reasons. One of them is the strong hospital pharmacy organization. Many professional organizations and communities of practice (COPs) have also been formed to support these changes. These include Adverse Drug Reaction's Community of Pharmacy Practice (AdCoPT), Group of Thai Oncology Pharmacy Practitioner, and Pharmacist Initiative for Patients Living with HIV/AIDS [Thailand] (PIPHAT) under the support of ThaiHP. Another reason is the development of PharmD program in Thailand, as previously mentioned, because many pharmacists in secondary and tertiary care hospitals have become greatly involved in the clinical experience clerkships of the program. This has encouraged hospital pharmacy practice changes toward more advanced knowledge and skills of pharmacotherapy and pharmaceutical care specialties.

9.2 Expanding roles of pharmacists in community settings

Community pharmacists have provided a number of innovative services ranging from advanced professional practice (e.g., medication use review) to public health practices such as health prevention (e.g., risk assessment,[55] screening for chronic diseases)[44] and health promotion (e.g., smoking cessation services).[45] The role of pharmacists for home healthcare visits has also been highly recognized, especially in the metropolitan area.[47] These extended services have been accepted by local and national funding bodies as part of health benefit packages for the Thai population.

Pharmacists in settings other than the community pharmacy have also expanded their roles toward people in the community by delivering primary healthcare services. Over the past few years, there has been an increasing number of district hospital pharmacists who engaged in several collaborative works with other primary healthcare professionals. These include public health services to the community (e.g., chronic disease screening and community education), and holistic care to individual patients outside hospitals, such as multidisciplinary home healthcare.

Consumer protection is another successful story of the expanding role of pharmacists and is worth documenting. It is the primary duty of pharmacists who are the only healthcare professionals employed in the Consumer Protection and Public Health Pharmacy Department of all PPHOs. They are appointed as competent officers under several acts of consumer protection and thus are responsible for the provision of various controlling approaches to ensure the safety of drug, food, and health-related products. These approaches include periodical inspections of the existing products and business settings in the area as well as law enforcement. A number of proactive methods have also been introduced. Among these, the most well-recognized innovation of consumer protection pharmacists is the training of junior-high and high school students to become consumer product inspectors in the community.

9.3 System changes facilitating the advancement of pharmacy practice

The quality assurance system plays a major role in supporting the advanced and expanding roles of pharmacists in Thailand. The HAI has a strong influence on the quality of care in Thai hospitals. This allows pharmacists to work as an integral part of the health system, providing pharmacy services and ensuring optimal medication use system. The development of quality pharmacy brands, through the initiation of the Community Pharmacy Accreditation Project endorsed by the Pharmacy Council and the FDA, supports community pharmacists to adhere to good pharmacy practice and provide more innovative services.

Almost all hospitals in Thailand have implemented electronic medical records to support and ensure the quality and continuity of their patient care. Although the comprehensive system of electronic medical records and computerized physician orders is not complete, the dispensing information is now computerized in most hospital pharmacy departments. This development has allowed pharmacists to readily access and utilize pharmacy data to support the provision of pharmaceutical care efficiently and effectively. These databases have also served as valuable assets for utilization review and research work that aimed to enhance the quality use of medicine policies within hospitals and at a national level.[56,57]

The success of pharmacy practice in Thailand would never have come this far without strong support from the academic sector. It has been clear that putting a greater emphasis on patient-oriented education and the development of the PharmD program have advanced the roles of pharmacists in Thailand. This paradigm shift has taken the pharmacy profession into a new level of practice and should be recognized as another achievement of pharmacy practice in Thailand.

10. Challenges

As practice continues to evolve, the Thai pharmacy care system has faced a number of challenges. The distribution of registered pharmacists has not yet met the workforce demands. Despite the continuing production of pharmacy graduates each year, the number of pharmacists in hospitals and community pharmacies is still insufficient. Hospital pharmacies are growing in size, demanding a higher quality of services to comply with HAI requirements. However, with the limitation in financial support in human resource development and newer technology such as pharmacy automation, Thai hospital pharmacy practice has yet to reach its best practice standards.

The number of registered pharmacists who have entered the community pharmacy workforce is also suboptimal, despite a growing number of community pharmacies throughout the country. This could contribute to the low participation of community pharmacies in the Community Pharmacy Accreditation Project. The situation impeded the possibility of considering the community pharmacy to be integrated into the universal health coverage scheme at a national level.

The changes in professional practice and the mandatory 6-year curriculum have generated ongoing intense discussion among pharmacy faculties and professional organizations on how to reconcile pharmaceutical care and pharmaceutical science doctrines. The uncertainty is associated with the potential separation of pharmacist licenses with limitations in practice, which could worsen the current workforce situation. As the number of pharmacy schools and pharmacy graduates increases, the job market for pharmacists is not aligned. There is a strong need for streamlining between the education sector and the practice sector to improve manpower and human resource development, as well as a great deal of leadership to guide the direction of pharmacy professionals within the healthcare system.

The current Thai pharmaceutical manufacturing system could also pose some challenges to pharmacy practice in the country. Local pharmaceutical industries in Thailand may become vulnerable because they are lacking capacity in research and development, as well as the high technology required to produce raw materials.[58] This issue becomes more challenging when the proportion of pro-biological products increases without the infrastructure of local industries being prepared for the change.

11. Recommendations and way forward

We believe that there is a strong need for pharmacists to extend their roles beyond focusing only on drug-specific issues to embarking upon what is needed as a primary care provider with expertise in drugs. There is a strong need to have a strategic approach to embed the community pharmacy setting within the healthcare system; currently, there is a lack of seamless linkage between community pharmacy service and other services in the healthcare system. In addition, the opportunity for expanding the role of pharmacists in the PCU setting is tremendous but still requires further exploration of potential roles. The idea of the family pharmacist model was explored and implemented in some areas, but it is still in its infancy stage. The exploration and development of pharmacist roles suggested in this chapter require the concerted effort of all sectors, including academics, professional organizations such as pharmacy councils, and healthcare payers in the system. Because a number of challenges in pharmacy practice will be encountered in the future, we believe that there is a need to have evidence synthesized to guide implementation, or even create best practices of Thai pharmacy professionals in this current circumstance, in order to move pharmacy practice in the right direction.

12. Lessons learned

The main lesson learned from pharmacy practice in Thailand is that the advancement of pharmacy practice strongly depends upon professional leaders and their dedication to society. Leadership in the education sector has been one of the key success factors in changes to pharmacy practice in Thailand. Successful implementation also requires a great deal of planning and leadership. The pharmacy profession in Thailand has advanced its role to a new level and still continues to evolve. We believe that the experience of Thai pharmacists can offer a unique perspective and can be valuable lessons to other countries.

13. Points to remember

- Pharmacy education in Thailand is now a 6-year PharmD program.
- The paradigm shift from a bachelor to PharmD program has tremendously influenced pharmacy practice in Thailand, especially hospital pharmacy practice.
- Several extended community pharmacy services have been accepted by local and national funding bodies as part of health benefit packages for Thai population.
- Despite the continuing production of pharmacy graduates each year, the numbers of pharmacists in hospitals and community pharmacy sectors are still insufficient.
- The next era of pharmacy practice should move toward the establishment of a primary care provider role for pharmacists within the context of the current healthcare system.

Acknowledgments

We would like to thank Dr. Sripen Tantives and Dr. Rungpetch Sakulbumrungsil for their critical comments of this manuscript.

References

1. National Statistical Office. *Executive summary: the 2010 population and housing census.* 2011. Available at: http://popcensus.nso.go.th/file/popcensus-20-12-54.pdf. [last accessed 17.10.12].
2. Bureau of Policy and Strategy, Ministry of Public Health. *Public health statistics.* 2010. Available at: http://bps.ops.moph.go.th/index.php?mod=bps&doc=5. [last accessed 04.10.12].

3. Pagaiya N, Noree T. *Thailand's health workforce: a review of challenges and experiences.* Washington (DC): The International Bank for Reconstruction and Development/The World Bank; 2009.

4. Wibulpolprasert S, editor. *Thailand health profile 2005–2007.* Nonthaburi: The War Veterans Organization of Thailand; 2007.

5. National Statistical Office. *Statist year book 2011 Thailand.* Bangkok; 2011.

6. Tangcharoensathien V, Patcharanarumol W, Vasavid C, Prakongsai P, Jongudomsuk P, Srithamrongsawat S, et al. *Thailand health financing review 2010.* 2010. Available at: http://papers.ssrn.com/sol3/papers.cfm?abstract_id=1623260. [last accessed 05.10.12].

7. Wibulpolprasert S, editor. *Thailand health profile 2001–2004.* Bangkok: Express Transportation Organization; 2005.

8. Drug Act B.E. 2510 as amended by Drug Act (No. 5) B.E. 2530. Available at: http://drug.fda.moph.go.th/zone_law/files/lawHeadPDF.pdf [last accessed 18.10.12].

9. Bureau of Drug Control. *The 2011 national statistics of pharmaceutical business licensing.* 2012. Available at: http://drug.fda.moph.go.th/zone_search/files/sea001_d16.asp. [last accessed 13.10.12].

10. Wibulpolprasert S, editor. *Thailand health profile 2008–2010.* Nonthaburi: The War Veterans Organization of Thailand; 2010.

11. Tarn YH, Hu S, Kamae I, Yang BM, Li SC, Tangcharoensathien V, et al. Health-care systems and pharmaco-economic research in Asia-Pacific region. *Value Health* 2008;**11**(Suppl. 1):S137–55.

12. Yoongthong W, Hu S, Whitty JA, Wibulpolprasert S, Sukantho K, Thienthawee W, et al. National drug policies to local formulary decisions in Thailand, China, and Australia: drug listing changes and opportunities. *Value Health* 2012;**15**(Suppl. 1):S126–31.

13. Limwattananon C, Limwattananon S, Cheawchanwattana A. *Analyzing and forecasting drug Expenditure for outpatients in provincial hospitals under civil servant medical benefit scheme and universal health coverage scheme.* Nonthaburi: Health Systems Research Institute; 2009.

14. Faramnuayphol P, Ekachampaka P, Taverat R, Wattanamano N. Health service systems in Thailand. In: Wibulpolprasert S, editor. *Thailand health profile 2005–2007.* Nonthaburi: The War Veterans Organization of Thailand; 2007. p. 294–308.

15. Kedsomboon N, Sakulbumrungsil R, Kanchanaphibool I, Udomaksorn S, Jitraknati A. *Research and systems development for national drug account.* Nonthaburi: Health Systems Research Institute; 2012.

16. Jitraknatee A. Antibiotic values. In: Kiatying-Angsulee N, Kedsomboon N, Maleewong U, editors. *Situation report on drug system 2010: antimicrobial resistance.* Bangkok: Drug System Monitoring and Development Center; 2011. p. 21–5.

17. Arpasrithongsakul S. Situation of antibiotics in groceries. In: Kiatying-Angsulee N, Kedsomboon N, Maleewong U, editors. *Situation report on drug system 2010: antimicrobial resistance and antibiotic use.* Bangkok: Usa; 2011.

18. Sringernyuang L. *Availability and use of medicines in rural Thailand* [doctoral dissertation]. University of Amsterdam; 2000.

19. Olliaro P, Vijayan R, Inbasegaran K, Lang C, Looareesuwan S. Drug studies in developing countries. *Bull World Health Organ* 2001;**79**.

20. Wibulpolprasert S, Chokevivat V, Oh C, Yamabhai I. Government use licenses in Thailand: the power of evidence, civil movement and political leadership. *Global Health* 2011;**7**:32.

21. PATH, World Health Organization. *An assessment of vaccine supply chain and logistics systems in Thailand.* Seattle: Health Systems Research Institute, Mahidol University; 2011.

22. Supakankunti S, Janjaroen W, Tangphao O, Ratanawijitrasin S, Kraipornsak P, Pradithavanij P. Impact of the World Trade Organization TRIPS agreement on the pharmaceutical industry in Thailand. *Bull World Health Organ* 2001;**79**:461–70.

23. Bureau of Drug Control FaDA. *Values of modern drug production and importation year 1987–2010.* 2011. Available at: http://wwwapp1.fda.moph.go.th/drug/zone_search/files/sea001_001.asp. [last accessed 10.06.12].

24. Food and Drug Administration. *Drug control division: introduction.* Ministry of Public Health; 2004. Available at: http://www.fda.moph.go.th/eng/drug/intro.stm. [last accessed 10.09.12].

25. Food and Drug Administration. *Narcotics control division*. 2004. Available at: http://www.fda.moph.go.th/eng/narcotics/intro.stm. [last accessed 12.09.12].

26. Nawanopparatsakul S, Keokitichai S, Wiyakarn S, Chantaraskul C. Challenges of pharmacy education in Thailand. *Silpakorn Univ Int J* 2009–2010;**9–10**:19–39.

27. Kapol N, Maitreemit P, Pongcharoensuk P, Armstrong EP. Evaluation of curricula content based on Thai pharmacy competency standards. *Am J Pharm Educ* 2008;**72**. Article 09.

28. Chan RC, Ching PL. Pharmacy practice in Thailand. *Am J Health Syst Pharm* 2005;**62**:1408–11.

29. The Pharmacy Council. Number of registered pharmacists from 1995 to 2011. http://www.pharmacycouncil.org/main/member.php [accessed 15.07.12].

30. Sonthisombat P. Pharmacy student and preceptor perceptions of preceptor teaching behaviors. *Am J Pharm Educ* 2008;**72**. Article 110.

31. Nimpitakpong P, Chaiyakunapruk N, Dhippayom T. Smoking cessation education in Thai schools of pharmacy. *Pharm Educ* 2011;**11**:8–11.

32. Sookaneknun P, Suttajit S, Ploylearmsang C, Kanjanasilp J, Maleewong U. Health promotion integrated into a Thai PharmD curriculum to improve pharmacy practice skills. *Am J Pharm Educ* 2009;**73**. Article 78.

33. Hepler CD, Strand LM, Tromp D, Sakolchai S. Critically examining pharmaceutical care. *J Am Pharm Assoc (Wash)* 2002;**42**:S18–9.

34. The Healthcare Accreditation Institute (Public Organization). *Hospital accreditation process*. 2012. Available at: http://www.ha.or.th/ha2010/th/process/index.php?key=process&GroupID=76. [last accessed 19.10.12].

35. The Association of Hospital Pharmacy (Thailand). Hospital pharmacy standard. Available at: http://www.thaihp.org/index.php?option=contentpage&sub=29&lang=th [last accessed 19.10.12].

36. Thomudtha P, Waleekhachonloet O, Sakolchai S, Limwattananon S, Limwattananon C. Drug expenditure and economic impact of community pharmacy visits by poor households. *Isan J Pharm Sci* 2012;**8**:15–26.

37. Order of the Ministry of Public Health: dangerous drugs. Available at: http://drug.fda.moph.go.th/zone_law/files/ประกาศกระทรวงสาธารณสุข%20เรื่อง%20ยาอันตราย%201.pdf [last accessed 18.10.12].

38. Thai Pharmacy Network for Tobacco Control. *The 2007 annual report to the thai health promotion foundation*. Bangkok; 2008.

39. Chalongsuk R, Lochid-amnuay S. Client satisfaction in pharmacy under the Thai universal coverage scheme: a case study at the community pharmacy of Sawang Dan Din crown prince hospital. *Thai J Health Res* 2006;**20**:41–57.

40. Chalongsuk R, Lochid-amnuay S, Suntimaleewolagun W. A study of a refill prescription service system comparing a hospital pharmacy and an accredited pharmacy. *J Health Syst Res* 2007;**1**:249–61.

41. Tunpichart S. Community pharmacy under health department of the Bangkok metropolitan administration. *J Com Pharm* 2008;**7**:8–12.

42. Chiratan P. A collaboration between accredited community pharmacy and primacy care unit under the universal health coverage scheme to enhance health promotion services. In: *The community health fairs and drug usage; 2012 June 26–27; Mahasarakham*. 2012. p. 45–6.

43. Khumsikiew J, Arkaravichien W, Honsamoot D, Sangkar P. Diabetes and hypertension screening by accredited community pharmacy in Khon Kaen under a pilot project with the National Health Security Scheme. *Srinagarind Med J* 2009;**24**:215–23.

44. Dhippayom T, Fuangchan A, Tunpichart S, Chaiyakunapruk N. Opportunistic screening and health promotion for type 2 diabetes: an expanding public health role for the community pharmacist. *J Public Health (Oxf)* 2012.

45. Thananithisak C, Nimpitakpong P, Chaiyakunapruk N. Activities and perceptions of pharmacists providing tobacco control services in community pharmacy in Thailand. *Nicotine Tob Res* 2008;**10**:921–5.

46. Nimpitakpong P, Chaiyakunapruk N, Dhippayom T. A national survey of training and smoking cessation services provided in community pharmacies in Thailand. *J Community Health* 2010;**35**:554–9.

47. Tunpichart S, Sakulbumrungsil R, Somrongthong R, Hongsamoot D. Chronic care model for diabetics by pharmacist home health in Bangkok Metropolitan: a community based study. *Int J Med Med Sci* 2012;**4**:90–6.

48. Community Pharmacy Association (Thailand). *Guideline for community pharmacy in the National Health Security system*. 2013. Available at: http://www.pharcpa.com/files/2556/1013_0101.pdf. [last accessed 10.02.14].

49. Lochid-amnuay S, Kassomboon N, Putthasri W, Puangkantha W. Recommendations on incorporating accredited community pharmacy into universal coverage in Thailand. *Thai J Hosp Pharm* 2011;**21**:189–202.
50. Chalongsuk R, Pongcharoensuk P, Lochid-amnuay S. A survey of utilization of pharmacy services by Social Security Beneficiaries in Bangkok and the Vicinity. *J Health Sci* 2008;**17**:48–58.
51. Lochid-amnuay S, Waiyakarn S, Pongcharoensuk P, Koh-Knox CP, Keokitichai S. Community pharmacy model under the universal coverage scheme in Thailand. *Thai J Hosp Pharm* 2009;**19**:110–22.
52. Putthasri W, Kessomboon N, Lochid-amnuay S, Puangkantha W. *Development of contractual agreement between accredited community pharmacy and the universal coverage scheme: a final report Bangkok*; 2010.
53. Community Pharmacy Development and Accreditation Office. *Search for accredited community pharmacy.* 2012. Available at: http://newsser.fda.moph.go.th/advancepharmacy/2009/search.php. [last accessed 17.10.12].
54. Community Pharmacy Development and Accreditation Office. *Standard of accredited pharmacy.* 2012. Available at: http://newsser.fda.moph.go.th/advancepharmacy/2009/way.php. [last accessed 15.10.12].
55. Chaiyakunapruk N, Laowakul A, Pikulthong N, Karnchanarat S, Ongphiphadhanakul B. Implementation and evaluation of osteoporosis screening services in community pharmacy, using the osteoporosis self-assessment tool for Asians (OSTA). *J Am Pharm Assoc* 2006;**46**:6.
56. Chaiyakunapruk N, Asuphol O, Dhippayom T, Poowaruttanawiwit P, Jeanpeerapong N. A retrospective evaluation of statins utilization pattern in a tertiary care hospital in Thailand. *Int J Pharm Pract* 2011;**19**:7.
57. Chaiyakunapruk N, Thanarungroj A, Cheewasithirungrueng N, Srisupha-olarn W, Nimpitakpong P, Dilokthornsakul P, et al. Estimation of financial burden due to oversupply of chronic diseases medications. *Asia Pac J Public Health* 2012;**24**:8.
58. Tantivess S. *Review of situation and research on Thailand's drug system: conference paper for brainstroming on developing drug system research programs*. Health Systems Research Institute; 2007.

CHAPTER 2

Pharmacy Practice in Malaysia

Mohamed Azmi Ahmad Hassali, Asrul Akmal Shafie, Ooi Guat See, Zhi Yen Wong

Chapter Outline

1. Introduction

1.1 Background of Malaysia healthcare system

The history and background of Malaysia's healthcare system started before the independence of the country. Hospitals were built for tin mining workers, and each of them were charged 50 cents a year for treatment. The tin mining industry has led to the constructions of most hospitals by the end of the nineteenth century in the state of Perak and Taiping Hospital, which was built in 1880 and is considered to be the oldest hospital in Malaysia.[1]

Pharmacy Practice in Developing Countries. http://dx.doi.org/10.1016/B978-0-12-801714-2.00002-2

After the independence of Malaysia, the government focuses very much on improving the socio-economic development of the rural population. With a total of 65 hospitals during independence in 1957, the Ministry of Health (MOH) started to develop and upgrade the existing healthcare services and had shown an excellent achievement in providing healthcare services in 20 years.[1]

The development of pharmaceutical services started with the establishment of the Medical Store in Petaling Jaya in 1964 and the Pharmaceutical Services Division in 1974 to deliver more comprehensive pharmacy services to the Malaysian population. The National Laboratory, which was renamed as the National Pharmaceutical Control Bureau in 1992, functioned as a pharmaceutical regulatory agency and also as the Secretariat to the Drug Control Authority.[1]

The vision of the MoH is for Malaysia to be a nation working together for better health. Meanwhile, the MOH has mission to lead and work in partnership for the people to fully attain their potential in health and appreciate health as a valuable asset, as well as to ensure a high-quality health system, with an emphasis on professionalism, caring, teamwork value, respect for human dignity, and community participation.[1,2]

The focus of the Ministry is now more extensive, especially in providing equitable, accessible, and quality health facilities. This development is consistent with the shifting patterns in environmental health and health technology development globally and is pursuant to the changes in diseases, health, environment, and technological development in the world.[1]

2. Health sector and system

Malaysia's healthcare system is a two-tier system consisting of the public and private sectors. The public healthcare system established in the early 1960s is funded by the government and financed mainly from taxes on earned income; it provides service to everyone through a network of general hospitals, district hospitals, and health clinics.[3,4] As of 2011, there were 138 public hospitals, 985 health clinics (including child health clinics), and 1864 rural/community clinics nationwide.[2]

The privatization of healthcare services in the 1980s was an effort to reduce the government's financial burden and has resulted in an increase of private hospitals and clinics. The private sector provides healthcare services on a nonsubsidized, fee-for-service basis through a large network of private clinics and hospitals. As of 2011, there were 220 private hospitals and 6589 registered private clinics nationwide.[5] The private healthcare sector mainly caters to the urban population or those who can afford to pay. Private sector health expenditure is funded by private health insurance, managed care organizations, out-of-pocket spending by individuals, private corporations, and nonprofit institutions.[3]

3. Vital health statistics

According to the Ministry of Health Malaysia, the total population in Malaysia was approximately 28,964,300 in the year 2011, with an annual population growth rate of 1.3%.[2] The mortality rate in 2011 was reported as 4.6 per 1000 populations, with total of 133,415 deaths.[6]

In terms of morbidity, for the period of 2000–2011, the number of admissions in MoH Hospitals had increased to 38.4% from that of 1,555,133 in 2000 to 2,151,666 in 2010.[7] The total expenditure on health, including both public and private sectors, was reported to be RM33.691 million in 2009.[2]

4. Medicines use issues

Table 1 shows the most commonly used medicines in Malaysia according to the National Medicines Use Survey 2006–2008.[8] Gliclazide was reported as the most used drug in 2008. Drugs for cardiovascular diseases dominated the rankings, with amlodipine ranking second among the top 20 drugs used in 2008. Lovastatin, a lipid-modifying drug, was ranked 9th in 2008. A policy change in the public sector to replace chlorothiazide in 2007 caused a significant

Table 1: Top 20 medicines by utilization in defined daily dose (DDD)/1000 population/day, 2006–2008

Rank	Drugs (2006)	Drugs (2007)	Drugs (2008)
1	Glibenclamide	Metformin	Gliclazide
2	Metformin	Glibenclamide	Amlodipine
3	Metoprolol	Atenolol	Metformin
4	Atenolol	Metoprolol	Perindopril
5	Nifedipine	Nifedipine	Metoprolol
6	Acetylsalycylic acid	Amlodipine	Atenolol
7	Chlorothiazide	Perindopril	Nifedipine
8	Gliclazide	Gliclazide	Glibenclamide
9	Amlodipine	Acetylsalycylic acid	Lovastatin
10	Frusemide	Enalapril	Acetylsalycylic acid
11	Perindopril	Chlorothiazide	Enalapril
12	Enalapril	Salbutamol	Hydrochlorothiazide
13	Salbutamol	Lovastatin	Furosemide
14	Captopril	Furosemide	Simvastatin
15	Diclofenac	Captopril	Captopril
16	Chlorphenamine	Simvastatin	Salbutamol
17	Simvastatin	Chlorphenamine	Mefenamic acid
18	Lovastatin	Diclofenac	Diclofenac
19	Mefenamic acid	Mefenamic acid	Chlorphenamine
20	Prednisolone	Prednisolone	Prednisolone

Table 2: Top 20 drugs by expenditure in 2006–2008

Rank	Drugs (2006)	Drugs (2007)	Drugs (2008)
1	Atorvastatin	Amlodipine	Amlodipine
2	Amlodipine	Olanzapine	Atorvastatin
3	Simvastatin	Atorvastatin	Omeprazole
4	Clopidogrel	Diclofenac	Gliclazide
5	Diclofenac	Amoxicillin and enzyme inhibitor	Metformin
6	Atenolol	Clopidogrel	Erythropoietin
7	Amoxicillin and enzyme inhibitor	Gliclazide	Diclofenac
8	Cefuroxime	Resperidone	Clopidogrel
9	Erythropoietin	Simvastatin	Ciprofloxacin
10	Gliclazide	Cefuroxime	Cefuroxime
11	Metformin	Metformin	Diphtheria-Hemophilus influenzae B-pertussis-poliomyelitis-tetanus
12	Ciprofloxacin	Pseudoephedrine, combinations	Pantoprazole
13	Metoprolol	Metoprolol	Olanzapine
14	Risperidone	Omeprazole	Amoxicillin and enzyme inhibitor
15	Pseudoephedrine, combinations	Ceterizine	Atenolol
16	Ceftriaxone	Ciprofloxacin	Pseudoephedrine, combinations
17	Aciclovir	Enalapril	Simvastatin
18	Insulin and analogs, intermediate-acting combined with fast-acting (human)	Rosiglitazone	Esomeprazole
19	Propranolol	Quetiapine	Amoxicillin
20	Felodipine	Erythropoietin	Perindopril

increase in the use of hydrochlorothiazide in 2008. The most used drugs in other therapeutic groups were salbutamol (ranked 16th) for respiratory drugs, mefenamic acid and diclofenac (ranked 17th and 18th, respectively) for nonsteroidal anti-inflammatory drugs, chlorphenamine (ranked 19th) for antihistamines, and prednisolone (ranked 20th) for systemic corticosteroids.

Table 2 shows the expenditure on medicines in Malaysia according to the National Medicines Use Survey 2006–2008.[8] There was a 9.7% increase in the drug expenditure in 2008 as compared to 2007. Based on the analysis and report, amlodipine has been recorded the highest expenditure among the individual drugs. This may be due to the high prevalence of hypertension and high usage of this drug. The drugs that appeared at the top 10 lists of drug expenditure in both 2007 and 2008 were amlodipine, atorvastatin, diclofenac, clopidogrel, gliclazide, cefuroxime, and metformin.

5. Pharmacy practice in Malaysia

Pharmacy service in Malaysia came into existence in 1951 with the enactment of three main legislations governing its profession: the Registration of Pharmacist Act 1951, Poison Act 1952, and Dangerous Drug Act 1952. The establishment of the basic structure of pharmacy service within the public healthcare system in Malaysia can be explained in part by the history of the country. During the British colonization, pharmacy service in Malaysia was restricted primarily to the procurement, storage, and distribution of drugs from the United Kingdom through the Crown Agents.[9]

Following independence, pharmaceutical service in Malaysia has grown from simply supplying the nation's pharmaceuticals to regulating and ensuring the quality, safety, and efficacy of pharmaceutical products. The establishment of a Drug Control Authority (DCA) and its executive arm, National Pharmaceutical Control Bureau (NPCB), under the Control of Drugs and Cosmetics Regulations 1984 gave rise to a more systematic pharmaceutical regulatory system in Malaysia.[9]

In the 1990s, further expansion of pharmacy service was hampered by the shortage of pharmacists in the public workforce. Hence, in order to raise the number of pharmacists in the country to the World Health Organization's recommended pharmacist-to-general population ratio of 1:2000 by the year 2020, governments have taken measures to increase the number of local academic institutions offering undergraduate pharmacy courses. In addition, the Ministry of Health and Pharmacy Board amended the pharmacist registration process in 2005 to require a period of 4 years (which was then shortened to 2 years in 2011) of mandatory government service in order to retain sufficient manpower in the public sector. The increase in the number of pharmacists in the public sector had allowed the establishment and expansion of clinical pharmacy service within the MoH.

The private sector is an important component in Malaysia's healthcare system as a health service provider, through private hospitals and clinics, laboratories, and community pharmacies. There were 10,762 registered private doctors throughout the country in the year 2011.[2] Consultation, treatment, and medicine costs are charged separately in private hospitals and clinics. There are approximately 1700 community pharmacies in the whole country.[10] Patients pay only the medication costs when they visit to a community pharmacy; pharmacist consultation and dispensing services are free of charge. Dispensing separation is not practiced in Malaysia, whereby private doctors are allowed to dispense their medications.

6. The healthcare funding system and health insurance system

In the public health sector, the MoH is the major provider and source of funding. The government highly subsidizes the services to ensure that Malaysians have equitable access to quality health services at affordable rates. The fee for an outpatient visit is RM1 per visit and RM5 for a specialist. The charge includes the consultation fee, pathological tests, and medicines prescribed. As mentioned previously, in the private health sector (including private hospitals and clinics, laboratories, and community pharmacies), consultation, treatment, and medicines costs are charged separately. In the community pharmacy setting, patients pay only the medication costs when they visit a community pharmacy; the pharmacist consultation and dispensing services are free of charged. Dispensing separation is not practiced in private clinics and community pharmacies in Malaysia.

Financing for the private health sector is mostly from out-of-pocket expenditures or/and reimbursements from third-party payers, such as employers and private health insurance. Under the Employee's Social Security Act, both employer and employee contribute monthly to the Social Security Organization to administer the social security insurance scheme, which covers death, injury, invalidity, or disease related to occupation. In addition, Employee Provident Fund members are entitled to withdraw 30% of their contributions for reimbursement of healthcare expenditures, such as critical illness insurance.[11] In addition, various private insurance companies provide personal insurance coverage for hospitalization, specialist consultation fees, and prescribed medicines.

7. Pharmaceutical industry

The pharmaceutical industry in Malaysia involves manufacturing, importation, and distribution. The multinational pharmaceutical companies dominate the importation and distribution sector, while the manufacturing sector consists of local and foreign generic pharmaceutical manufacturers.[12]

Pharmaceutical products manufactured can be classified as prescription medicine, over-the-counter (OTC) medicine, herbal and health supplements, and traditional medicines.[13] Local generic manufacturers produce almost all dosage forms, including sterile preparations such as eye preparations and injections, soft gelatin capsules, controlled-release medications, and granules for reconstitution.[12]

In 1986, drug registration was introduced in Malaysia and the DCA was established. Therefore, all drugs/medicines in pharmaceutical dosage forms and cosmetics have to be registered before sale and marketing is permitted in the country.[13] Currently, there are about 40 local generic manufacturers in Malaysia, producing about 30% of the domestic demand according to the MIDA[12]. They export the product to countries in South East Asia, Africa, and the Middle East, with new markets being explored beyond these countries; the growth in exports is 10–12% annually.[13]

In terms of regulations, as in most of the developed countries, the manufacture and marketing of pharmaceutical products in Malaysia are strongly regulated. Malaysia was admitted a member of The Pharmaceutical Inspection Convention and Pharmaceutical Inspection Co-operation Scheme (PIC)/S in 2002 and manufacturers are required to be in compliance with the Current Good Manufacturing Practice (CGMP) of PIC/S. The regulations are enforced and monitored closely by the NPCB.[14]

8. Pharmaceutical market

Malaysia's pharmaceuticals market is posting strong growth. Pharmaceutical expenditures were reported to be MYR6.06 billion (US$1.96 billion) in 2012 and MYR6.66 billion (US$2.18 billion) in 2013.[15] Malaysia's market for drugs is growing at the average annual rates of 10–12%.[16] In 2013, the 29 million Malaysian spent an average of $375 per year on healthcare, with about $75 of that going to pharmaceuticals, which is more than double the amount compared to that before 10 years.[16]

The pharmaceutical market in Malaysia is dominated by prescription drugs, which contribute approximately 70% of the market; this is expected to continue in the future. Prescription drugs in Malaysia are classified into three categories: imported proprietary drugs, imported generic drugs and generics manufactured locally by Malaysian companies. Over the years, proprietary drugs, as the innovator, have had the strongest demand in the Malaysian market. They hold about 70% of the market share. Nevertheless, the usage and acceptance of generics have been steadily increasing.[12]

Malaysia has been importing many proprietary drugs because foreign pharmaceutical companies do not manufacture their products here in Malaysia. Most foreign companies distribute their products through their own sales representative and/or through local distributors.[16]

In 2009, it was estimated that the total market size for prescription and OTC medicine was about RM4.5 billion, while the traditional medicine and health supplement market was estimated at RM3 billion. Market growth is consistent between 8% and 10% annually for the past several years.[13]

In 2012, there were 234 local drug companies licensed under Malaysia's DCA. The major companies include Pharmaniaga Manufacturing Berhad, Hovid Berhad, and CCM Duopharma Biotech Sdn Bhd. They primarily produce generic drugs, especially antibiotics, painkillers, injectables, and health supplements.[16]

To attract and encourage foreign pharmaceutical manufacturers to set up operations in Malaysia, the government offers a number of tax incentives. These duty exemptions and multiyear tax holidays have successfully attracted about six major Indian companies since 2011, including Ranbaxy, Strides Arcolab, Cipla, Biocon, and Dr Reddy's Labs.[16] These generic manufacturers are using Malaysia as a manufacturing center to target both the Malaysian market and other Southeast Asian countries.[16]

9. Hospital pharmacy practice

Over the years, the traditional dispensing role of pharmacists has been transformed to the provision of patient-centered pharmaceutical care. Pharmacy services in MoH hospitals have been expanded to various services (Table 3). Pharmacies in private hospitals offer some or all of the same pharmacy services as MoH Hospitals.

10. Clinical pharmacy, drug information specialists, and centers

The development and improvement of clinical pharmacy services at hospitals have expanded the traditional dispensing role of the pharmacist to a profession that provides pharmaceutical care to patients. Over the years, clinical pharmacy services have been expanded to include

Table 3: Pharmacy services offered in MOH hospitals/clinics

Pharmacy Services in Hospitals	Description
Inpatient pharmacy	Inpatient pharmacy provides medications to the wards and clinic in the hospital by using the unit of dose and unit of use system. Dispensing and counseling services are also provided for patients who are discharged.[17]
Clinical pharmacy service	Pharmacists in wards provide therapeutic drug monitoring, medication counseling, and dispensing of medications to discharged patients.[18] They are also involved in ward rounds and provide counseling to promote the proper and effective use of drugs.[18]
Medication therapy adherence clinic (MTAC)	MTAC pharmacists provide monitoring of patients' medication therapy and provide information about medication and therapy with the aim of improving adherence.[19] They are also involved in clinical discussions with doctors and dosage adjustment for some medications, such as warfarin and insulin.[19] Currently, there are 11 types of MTAC provided in MOH hospitals: diabetes, warfarin, respiratory, nephrology, neurology, retroviral disease, hemophilia, geriatric, heart failure, psoriasis, and rheumatology.[19]
Home medication review (HMR)	Pharmacists in hospitals also offer home visits to assess patients' medication usage, with the aim of increasing patients' understanding of treatment and optimizing the therapeutic effect of medications, in addition to reducing the medication utilization problem.[20] However, currently only a few services are provided under the HMR program—namely for neurology, psychiatry, and geriatrics.[20]
Nonsterile pharmacy	For syrup medicines which are not available in market, nonsterile pharmacies prepare extemporaneous preparations for patients who cannot tolerate oral forms and for children.[21]
Clinical pharmacokinetic services	These pharmacists are involved in patient monitoring and consult with doctors on therapeutic drug monitoring.
Oncology pharmacy service	Hospital pharmacists in cytotoxic drug reconstitution (CDR) are involved in the preparation and reconstitution of cytotoxic drugs according to patients' need. Currently, there are 58 public hospitals that offer CDR services.[22]
Parenteral nutrition service	These pharmacists are involved in the preparation of parenteral nutrition for patients who cannot tolerate oral intake.
Methadone replacement therapy	To prevent bloodborne viral infections (e.g., HIV, hepatitis B, hepatitis C) due to needle sharing, hospital pharmacies offer methadone replacement therapy. Pharmacists are involved in preparation and supervision of patients' consumption after the doctors prescribe methadone syrup for patients.[23] As of 2010, there were 172 methadone dispensing facilities in MoH (38 hospitals and 134 health clinics) that were managed by pharmacists.[24]
Drug information enquiry service	Pharmacists provide answers for healthcare professionals and public enquiries about drugs.
Nuclear pharmacy service	Pharmacists provide services in the preparation of radiopharmaceuticals for patients. Currently, there are only five MoH hospitals offering this service.[25]
Procurement and supply services	Pharmacists are involved in pharmaceutical procurement and stock management.

medication counseling, medication therapy adherence clinics, methadone dispensing and counseling, ward pharmacy service, drug information service, clinical pharmacokinetics service, parenteral nutrition service, oncology pharmacy service, and nuclear pharmacy service.[24]

In addition, pharmacists in the major hospitals provide drug and poison information to healthcare professionals and the public. Two major drug information centers in Malaysia are the National Poison Center at the Universiti Sains Malaysia and the National Drug Information Center at Hospital Kuala Lumpur.[26] The National Poison Center plays an important role in the treatment of poisoning cases by providing information on poisons, giving advice on managing poisoning cases, and carrying out supportive analytical tests to identify poisons to assist in the diagnosis, management, and prognosis of poisoning cases and interpretations of laboratory results for poisoning cases.[27] The National Poison Center is also involved in organizing poison awareness and prevention education among healthcare professionals and the public, in addition to conducting research and documentation of poisoning incidence.[27]

11. Community pharmacy practice

In Malaysia. there are 10,077 registered pharmacists and approximately 3300 pharmacies in the private sector, including community pharmacies.[28] Community pharmacy benchmarking guidelines have been introduced and are revised from time to time by the MoH to provide an overview of the requirements that community pharmacies are expected to fulfill in the areas of infrastructure, equipment, personnel, and practice.[29] Community pharmacies are premises with at least one pharmacist holding a Type A license issued under the Poison Act 1952, who can supply poison (controlled medicines) either by retail only or both retail and wholesale. For all community pharmacies, the executive board and share equity are represented by pharmacists.[29] Other requirements and guidelines are shown in Table 4.

In Malaysia, general practitioners are legally allowed to dispense medications. The absence of dispensing rights has limited the community pharmacist's professional roles, including dispensing, pharmaceutical care, and quality use of medicines.[30]

The primary role of pharmacists in primary care is supplying Poison Group C, which according to the Poison Act 1952, this group of poisons (controlled medicines) can be dispensed by a registered pharmacist in a licensed pharmacy premise without a prescription.[31] The limited role in dispensing prescription medicines (Poison Group B) has diverted the pharmacists' role ito supplying health supplements and foods, homecare, personal hygiene products, and beauty products.[30] Medical care now requires teamwork and collaborative practice, in which all healthcare professionals have equally important yet specific roles for the betterment of public health.[32] Therefore, there is definitely a need to transform the community pharmacy practice in Malaysia.

Table 4: Community pharmacy benchmarking guidelines[33]

Premises	• Area: a minimum of 200 sq. ft.
	• Designated area for counseling, waiting area
	• Designated area for wet and dry compounding/dispensing
	• Exterior display:
	Signboard: pharmacy/advertisement ratio
	Logo
	• Display of types of services available, for example, blood glucose, cholesterol, pregnancy, blood grouping tests, or electronic blood pressure monitoring
	• Security
	Locks on main door/gate
	Lock on psychotropic drugs
	Poison products under lock and key
	• Insurance
	Professional indemnity
	Public liability
	Fire and burglary
	• Level of cleanliness and hygiene
	Pest control
	• General environment for clients
	Conform to occupational and safety health requirements:
	escape way
	Noise level
	Arrangement/display of OTC products; ease of selection of products
	Temperature, lighting, and ventilation
	• Availability of refrigerator
	• Method of pharmaceutical waste disposal
Equipment	• Inventory control: computerization/stock cards
	• Availability of mortar and pestle, weighing balance, counting tray, and measuring cylinders
Personnel	• Professional image presented, with staff dress code
	• Training for staff
Dispensing of medicines	• Dispensing must be under the supervision of the pharmacist
	Dangerous drugs and psychotropics
	Prescription and pharmacy only medicines (group C)
	OTC medicines
	Cases of referral to pharmacists by pharmacy/sales assistants
	• Screening of prescription by the pharmacist, who must ensure that the patient receives sufficient information and advice to enable the safe and effective use of the medicines
	• Interventions
	• Records
	• Dispensing container: use of amber bottle
	• Labeling (printed and handwritten) bears the proprietary/generic names, strength, quantity, manufacturer's name, batch number, and expiration dates
	• Maintenance of patient medication record (by means of card, a record book, computer)
Dispensing errors	• Steps to minimize (e.g., incorrect selection, incorrect interpretation)
	• Checking procedures and cautions

Table 4: Community pharmacy benchmarking guidelines[33]—cont'd

Inventory management	• External use: preferably to store separately from internal use items • Control of expired and expiring stocks • Storage space/compartments
Reference library	• Martindale: The Complete Drug Reference • British National Formulary (BNF) • Drug Information Management System (DIMS) • Other reference books and relevant legislation references
Professional standards	• Pharmacist's ethics • The accountability of the pharmacist • Professional competence: Involvement in continuing education • Observance of relevant laws • Ensure confidentiality of patient information • Extent of interaction with colleagues and other health professionals • Participation in Malaysian Pharmaceutical Society (MPS) activities
Participation in health promotion activities	Participation in community activities.

12. Public health practice and health promotion

In Malaysia, health promotion has been adopted as part of the national health agenda.[34] Malaysian Health Promotion Board (MySihat) is a body formed under the MoH in June 2006. It is operated as an independent body consisting of representatives from various related Ministries, nongovernmental organizations, and professionals who possess expertise relevant to health promotion, with the objectives to set and develop the health promotion agenda across different sectors and settings, as well as to promote the adoption of healthy lifestyles and healthy environment through various settings and sectors.[35]

One of the greatest challenges in promoting and executing an effective health promotion programs is often the lack of manpower support from volunteers and partnerships from private sectors. A survey was done in 2011 at the Jelutong district in the state of Penang to investigate the perceptions of the public toward health promotion activities (diabetes and hypertension screenings and health seminars), which were carried out by pharmacists. The results showed that the participants seem satisfied with the health promotional activities. The survey concluded that the general public must be educated about the benefits of joining health promotion activities so that the ultimate goal of health promotion campaigns, which is to improve health outcomes for communities—including improvements in quality of life, function, independence, equity, mortality, and morbidity—can be achieved.[34]

13. The position of traditional and herbal medicines

Traditional and complementary medicine is widely used throughout the world. Approximately 80% of the population in some Asian and African countries depend on traditional medicine for primary healthcare purposes. In Malaysia, traditional medicine has contributed significantly to the health care of the community. People use traditional and complementary medicines for the purpose of healing diseases and maintaining health.[36] A study carried out in November 2009 showed that the prevalence rates of using traditional and complementary medicines among Malaysians in their lifetime were 69.4% (67.6–71.2%) and 55.6% (53.8–57.4%) within 12 months of the study.[37] Besides that, Malaysians are estimated to spend US$500 million annually on traditional therapies, compared to only US$300 million on conventional therapies.[38]

Malaysia, with forests still covering about 59.5% of the total land area today,[39] has an abundance of natural resources that can be developed into health products. Malaysian traditional medicines are considered as one of the most valuable and rich cultural heritages of Malaysia as they reflect a diverse culture and tradition.[38] Therefore, the MOH Malaysia has taken this positive advantage to produce high quality and safe traditional and complementary medicine to be used by the consumers.[40]

In Malaysia, traditional and complementary medicine are generally classified into six major groups, including traditional Malay medicine, traditional Indian medicine, homeopathy, complementary medicine and Islamic medical practice.[36] Up to 2011, there are 11 integrated hospitals in the MOH equipped with traditional and complementary medicine units, providing various services, for example acupuncture, Malay massage, herbal therapy as an adjunct treatment for cancer patients and Malay post-natal treatment.[36]

14. Pharmacy education on various levels and Continuing Professional Development (CPD)

All pharmacy degree offered in public universities in Malaysia consists of 4 years curriculum whereas private universities and colleges offer range from three and half year to 4 years courses. As of 31 October 2013, there are 19 universities/institutions in Malaysia that offers pharmacy degree program in which 5 of them are public universities.[41] Immediately upon graduation from universities, pharmacy graduates in Malaysia must engage as a provisional registered pharmacist (PRP) in any premises accredited and approved by Pharmacy Board Malaysia. According to The Registration of Pharmacists Act 1951, PRPs need to obtain experience to the satisfaction of the Pharmacy Board for a period not less than one year.[42] The certificate of satisfactory experience will be granted if the Pharmacy Board is satisfied that a person has gained experience.[42] The Pharmacy Board may extend for not more than one year the period of training of a PRP if the Board is not satisfied with the performance of that person as a pharmacist.[42] Besides, PRPs are required to pass the Pharmacy Jurisprudence Examination which conducted by the Pharmacy Board three times annually.[42]

Pharmacy graduates with degree obtained from other countries (i.e., as listed in First Schedule of Registration of Pharmacist Act 1951) must undergo provisional training before he or she can be fully registered in Malaysia.[42] However, a person can apply for exemption if he or she holds qualifications referred in the First Schedule and had been registered by any registration body responsible for registration of pharmacists recognized y the Pharmacy Board.[42] The certificate of exemption will be granted if the Board is satisfied that such person has gained experience which is not less both in character and scope and in length of time in an institution or hospital approved by the Board.[42] Any person is entitled for full registration of pharmacist if he or she had obtained certificate of satisfactory experience or certificate of exemption.[42]

For postgraduate degree in Pharmacy, universities in Malaysia offer postgraduate degree (i.e., by research or coursework) in six major disciplines namely Clinical Pharmacy, Pharmaceutical Chemistry, Pharmaceutical Technology, Pharmacology, Physiology, and Social and Administrative Pharmacy.[43]

In addition, in order to maintain professionalism, pharmacists practicing in Malaysia need to continuously update themselves with latest drug information through participation in the Continuing Professional Development (CPD) program. Compulsory CPD is being practiced by pharmacist working in MOH since the year 1988. CPD is needed for their performance evaluation, promotion, and career advancement in MOH.[44]

In the private sector, a minimum of 30 CPD points within two years is compulsory for renewal of the Annual Retention Certificate.[45]

Pharmacists can update themselves by attending organized seminars and lectures or through online learning. CPD points will be granted for each activity performed through CPD grading system.[45]

15. Pharmacy practice in pharmacy curricula

Pharmacy practice is one of the main streams in pharmacy degree. It provides pharmacy students with the skills necessary to practice pharmaceutical care. It also explores the role of the pharmacist, professionalism, dispensing, health and the individual, health care in society, the psychosocial aspects of medicine treatment, communicative skills, patient counseling, and legal aspects of practice.[46] In the last two decades, little attention has been paid to social-behavioral factors involved in illness and health and other factors that are affected by the delivery of health services since most pharmacy education programs in Malaysia had focused on basic pharmaceutical sciences and pharmaceutical technology.[46] Today, most pharmacy degree program in Malaysia had incorporated pharmacy practice as part of their curriculum. In fact, pharmacy practice is one of the core areas that need to be incorporated into the pharmacy degree program before it can get recognition from Pharmacy Board Malaysia and National Accreditation Board.[47]

16. Research on pharmacy practice

The Malaysia's government focuses a lot in research and development (R&D) activities and in order to attract more investments in this area, the government offers a wide range of incentives and financial assistance. The Promotion of Investments Act, 1986 defines research and development (R&D) as "any systematic or intensive study carried out in the field of science or technology with the objective of using the results of the study for the production or improvement of materials, devices, products, produce or processes".[48]

The Pharmacy Practice and Development Division is a division formed under Pharmaceutical Services Divisions, Ministry of Health Malaysia, and it is responsible to ensure the quality of drug procurement and usage through effective pharmacy practice in order to improve pharmacy services in Malaysia to be on par with other developed countries. In the area of R&D, it improves and monitors the quality of studies and research done at the Pharmaceutical Services Division level.[10]

To further support the development of the pharmaceutical industry in Malaysia, the Government has taken the effort to develop the clinical trial services sector. A Clinical Research Center (CRC) under the National Institute of Health of the Ministry of Health (MOH) has been established to conduct clinical trials, clinical epidemiology and economic research, and manage complex medical databases. The CRC comprising a network of 27 centers around the country acts as the one-stop-center by providing a single point of contact to access all MOH hospitals and clinics to conduct clinical trials in Malaysia. These clinical trial centers have linkages to more than 50 general and district hospitals, and more than 100 health clinics as potential sites for clinical trials with access to 550 clinical investigators and 17 million patients from diverse therapeutic areas in the public healthcare system in Malaysia.[48]

Malaysia has nine international contract research organizations (CROs) operating in its shores and four local CROs. The country has 138 secondary and tertiary MOH hospitals that service over 15 million patients in various therapeutic areas, which has generated about 175 active investigators. This is merely a fraction of the approximately 2800 specialists at MOH facilities (in total there are 5000 specialists from both the public and private sectors). (*Source: Contract Research at MOH Hospitals. Berita MMA* 2011 (*January*):17–18).[48]

17. Challenges

In Malaysia, the scenario is that the general practitioners can prescribe as well as dispense medications from their clinics. The absence of dispensing right has limited the community pharmacist's professional roles, especially in the delivery of pharmaceutical care.[49] Under the Malaysian Poison Act 1952 (Section 7) and Poison Regulation 1952 (Regulation 3), private GPs' clinics are given the right to perform dispensing.[48] The limited chance to dispense prescription medicines has also driven the pharmacists to diverse their role in supplying health supplements and foods, homecare, personal hygiene products, and beauty products.[50–51]

The community pharmacies in Malaysia have limited opportunity to optimize their clinical knowledge and role. Community pharmacies are functioning much like a personal store while community pharmacists seldom involve in primary health care, but instead, as drug sellers or typical "assistant" providing advices on the medication.[52] This rising of "price war" phenomenon brings a negative impact on the pharmacy profession Malaysia, through the unhealthy business competition among community pharmacies by price undercutting of the pharmaceutical products.[53] The Malaysian community pharmacists are facing challenges from the professional services and economic perspectives. In 2007, the National Medicines Policy in which one of the component mentioned that quality use of medicines, prescribing and dispensing functions must be separated.[54] Nevertheless, strong oppositions of the implementation of dispensing separation have been constantly received from MMA and consumers.[12] The shortage of community pharmacists and the possibility of increasing patients' health expenditure were the common reasons for the parties to object the separation of prescribing and dispensing in Malaysia.[51]

Another issue that has been raised up recently among the community pharmacists is the distribution of pharmacy in the country. There are definitely sufficient community pharmacies in the city but insufficient community pharmacies in small towns and rural places. Profit-minded businessmen have already started to over-crowd the city area. There are community pharmacies being controlled by non-pharmacists, or even general practitioners, where the main motive is to earn money, rather than to serve the community.

18. Recommendations: way forward

The Ministry of Health Malaysia is currently reviewing all the possible models for the healthcare reformation with a technical working group comprised of various stakeholders in healthcare. While the exact scheme of the universal healthcare model has yet to be finalized as of 2012, the pharmacy profession in Malaysia is positively anticipating a shift in practice specifically in the separation of prescribing and dispensing of medications. Recently, the Pharmaceutical Services Division, Ministry of Health Malaysia had proposed a new Pharmacy Bill to replace the pre-independence legislations (namely the Registration of Pharmacists Act 1951, Poisons Act 1952, and Sale of Drugs Act 1952). Some of the important transformation that is set in the proposed bill include reclassification of medicines, liberalization of pharmacists' practice license to more than one premises and more deterrent penalties to ensure better quality and safer medicines for the public.[55]

Meanwhile, while awaiting this cornerstone legislative change on dispensing separation, community pharmacists in Malaysia are shifting their professional responsibilities from merely dispensing to providing extended services. While at present these services are provided free of charge, community pharmacists are now calling for some compensation in the form of professional fee. However, there remained several issues regarding the provision of non-dispensing pharmacy services that have yet to be systematically evaluated.

19. Conclusions

Transformation of the healthcare system is essential in Malaysia in order to bring about improvement in pharmaceutical care provided by the community pharmacies to the population; as dispensing will be totally entrust to pharmacists in the reformed system. The community pharmacies have to transform their current practice to a more comprehensive, clinically inclined and quality practice. There is definitely a need for the transformed healthcare system to optimize patient safely and therefore, serving as the most accessible healthcare professional, community pharmacists play a pivotal role in the main stream of primary healthcare system. Thus, it is crucial to developing and implementing critical strategies to optimize the current and extended pharmacy services provided to the general public.

20. Lessons learned

- "Malaysia's 29 million people now spend an average of $375 per year on healthcare..."
- Despite the challenges, the pharmacy profession in Malaysia has the responsibility to successfully bring transformation to the healthcare system.
- Every practicing pharmacist plays important professional roles to meet the needs of the society and individual patients in the primary healthcare system.

References

1. Ministry of Health Malaysia. MOH Background. [cited February 13, 2014]. Available from: http://www.moh.gov.my/english.php; 2013.
2. Minitry of Health Malaysia. *Health fact 2012*. Health Informatics Centre PaDD; 2012.
3. Chee HL, Barraclaugh S, editors. *Healthcare in Malaysia. The dynamics of provision, financing and access*. New York: Routledge; 2007.
4. Healy J, editor. *Malaysia health system review*. Geneva: WHO Press; 2012.
5. Thomas S, Loo SB, Nordin R. Health care delivery in Malaysia: changes, challenges and champions. *J Public Health Afr* 2011;2:e23.
6. Ministry of Health Malaysia. *Health indicators 2012*. Health Informatics Centre, Ministry of Health; 2012.
7. Ministry of Health Malaysia. *Annual report 2011*. Ministry of Health; 2011.
8. Ministry of Health Malaysia. *Malaysian statistics on medicines (MSOM) 2008*. 2013.
9. Pharmaceutical Sevice Division, Ministry of Health Malaysia. [December 13, 2012]. Available from: http://pharmacy.gov.my/index.cfm?&menuid=137&lang=EN; 2012.
10. Ministry of Health Malaysia. Official Portal of Pharmaceutical Services Division. [cited February 13, 2014]. Available from: http://www.pharmacy.gov.my/v2/en; 2014.
11. Employee Provident Fund. *EPF savings and your retirement*. [cited February 13, 2014]. Available from: http://www.kwsp.gov.my/portal/documents/10180/449171/Risalah_Eng.pdf; 2012.

12. Hassali MA, Yuen KH, Mohamed Izham MI, Wong JW, Ng BH, David HSS. Malaysian pharmaceutical industry: opportunities and challenges. *J Generic Med* 2009;**6**:246–52.

13. The Malaysian Organisation of Pharmaceutical Industries (MOPI). The Malaysian Pharmaceutical Industry. [cited February 15, 2014]. Available from: http://mopi.org.my/; 2014.

14. Ministry of Health Malaysia. Official Portal of National Pharmaceutical Control Bureau (NPCB); Industry. [cited February 15, 2014]. Available from: http://portal.bpfk.gov.my/index.cfm?&menuid=21; 2014.

15. Business Monitor International. *Malaysia pharmaceuticals and healthcare report Q1 2014*. 2013.

16. Gross A. *Malaysia pharmaceutical market update*. [Pharmaphorum: Pacific Bridge Medical 2013; Pharma article]. Available from: http://www.pharmaphorum.com/articles/malaysia-pharmaceutical-market-update-2013; 2013.

17. Pharmaceutical Services Division Ministry of Health Malaysia. *Inpatient pharmacy (Ward pharmacy)*. [updated November 19, 2013]. Available from: http://www.pharmacy.gov.my/v2/en/content/inpatient-pharmacy-ward-pharmacy.html; 2013.

18. Pharmaceutical Services Division Ministry of Health Malaysia. *Clinical Pharmacy Service*. [updated November 30, 2013]. Available from: http://www.pharmacy.gov.my/v2/en/content/clinical-pharmacy-service.html; 2013.

19. Pharmaceutical Services Division Ministry of Health Malaysia. *Perkhidmatan medication therapy Adherance clinic (MTAC)*. [updated November 19, 2013]; Available from: http://www.pharmacy.gov.my/v2/ms/entri/perkhidmatan-medication-therapy-adherance-clinic-mtac.html; 2013.

20. Pharmaceutical Services Division Ministry of Health Malaysia. *Perkhidmatan "Home medication Review" (HMR)*. [updated March 19, 2013]; Available from: http://www.pharmacy.gov.my/v2/ms/entri/perkhidmatan-home-medication-review-hmr.html; 2013.

21. Pharmaceutical Services Division Ministry of Health Malaysia. *Non-sterile pharmacy*. [updated November 19, 2013]. Available from: http://www.pharmacy.gov.my/v2/en/content/non-sterile-pharmacy.html; 2013.

22. Pharmaceutical Services Division Ministry of Health Malaysia. *Cytotoxic drug reconstitution (CDR)*. [updated November 25, 2013]. Available from: http://www.pharmacy.gov.my/v2/en/content/cytotoxic-drug-reconstitution-cdr.html; 2013.

23. Pharmaceutical Services Division Ministry of Health Malaysia. *Methadone replacement therapy*. [updated November 18, 2013]. Available from: http://www.pharmacy.gov.my/v2/en/content/methadone-replacement-therapy.html; 2013.

24. Pharmaceutical Services Division Ministry of Health Malaysia. *Annual report* 2010. Petaling Jaya (Malaysia); 2010.

25. Pharmaceutical Services Division Ministry of Health Malaysia. *Nuclear pharmacy*. [updated July 11, 2013]. Available from: http://www.pharmacy.gov.my/v2/en/content/nuclear-pharmacy.html; 2013.

26. Jaafar S, Noh KM, Muttalib KA, Othman NH, Healy J, Maskon K, et al. Malaysia health system review. *Health Syst Transit* 2013;**3**(1):103.

27. National Poison Centre Universiti Sains Malaysia. About Us. Available from: http://www.prn.usm.my/about_prn.html; 2014.

28. Ministry of Health Malaysia. *Health facts 2014*; 2014.

29. Ministry of Health Malaysia. *Community pharmacy benchmarking guideline 2011*. Pharmaceutical Services Division; 2011.

30. Che Awang MZ. *Pilot study is the best prescription*. The Star Online; [cited October 28, 2008]. Retrieved from: http://www.thestar.com.my; April 24, 2008.

31. Poisons Act 1952 Sect. 18.

32. Shafie AA, Hassali MA, Azhar S, Ooi GS. Separation of prescribing and dispensing in Malaysia: a summary of arguments. *Res Soc Adm Pharm* 2012;**8**(3):258–62.

33. Malaysia Pharmaceutical Society. *Community pharmacy*. [cited February 17, 2014]. Available from: http://www.mps.org.my/; 2014.

34. Hassali MA, Saleem F, Shafie AA, Aljadhey H, Chua GN, Masood I, et al. Perception towards health promotion activities: findings from a community survey in the state of Penang. *Malays J Public Health Med* 2012;**12**(2):6–14.

35. Ministry of Health Malaysia. Official website of Malaysian Health Promotion Board. [cited February 16, 2014]. Available from: http://www.mysihat.gov.my/; 2014.

36. *Traditional and complementary medicine programme in Malaysia*. Traditional & complementary medicine division, Ministry of Health Malaysia; 2011. p. 58.

37. Siti ZM, Tahir A, Ida Farah A, Ami Fazlin SM, Sondi S, Maimunah AH, et al. Use of traditional and complementary medicine in Malaysia: a baseline study. *Complement Ther Med* 2009;**17**(5):292–9.

38. Farooqu M. The current situation and future direction of traditional and complementary medicine (T&CM) in malaysian health care system. *Altern Integr Med* 2013;**1**(1).

39. WWF-Malaysia. [cited February 16, 2014]. Available from: http://www.wwf.org.my/about_wwf/what_we_do/forests_main/; 2014.

40. Ministry of Health Malaysia. Official Portal of Traditional and Complementary Medicine Division. [cited February 15, 2014]. Available from: http://tcm.moh.gov.my/v4/; 2014.

41. Pharmaceutical Services Division Ministry of Health Malaysia. *List of authorized local universities offering pharmacy course*. [updated October 31, 2013]. Available from: http://www.pharmacy.gov.my/v2/en/content/list-authorized-local-universities-offering-pharmacy-course.html; 2013.

42. Legal Research Board. *Malaysian laws on poisons and sale of drugs*. Selangor, Malaysia: International Law Book Services; 2010.

43. Ministry of Higher Education Malaysia. *Postgraduates programmes by public universities*. Available from: http://jpt.mohe.gov.my/PEMASARAN/booklet Education Malaysia/MOHE booklet - IPTA Postgraduate Programme Edition 1_2010.pdf; 2010.

44. Malaysian Pharmaceutical Society. *CPD for renewal of annual retention certificate (questions & qnswers)*. [updated April 4, 2013]. Available from: http://www.mps.org.my/newsmaster.cfm?&menuid=37&action=view&retrieveid=3565; 2013.

45. Pharmacy Board Malaysia. *Continuing professional development for pharmacist*. [cited February 24, 2014]. Available from: http://www.pharmacy.gov.my/v2/sites/default/files/document-upload/cpd-brochure.pdf; 2013.

46. Monash University Malaysia. Bachelor of Pharmacy. Available from: http://www.monash.edu.my/study/under graduate/pharmacy/bachelor-pharmacy; 2014.

47. Pharmacy Board Malaysia. *Guidelines on approval and recognition of a pharmacy programme*. [cited February 25, 2014]; 2007.

48. (MIDA) MIDA. Official Website of Malaysian Investment Development Authority (MIDA); Pharmaceuticals Industry. [cited February 17, 2014]. Available from: http://www.mida.gov.my/env3/index.php?page=pharmac euticals; 2014.

49. Tarn YH, Hu S, Kamae I, Yang BM, Li SC, Tangcharoensathien V, et al. Healt-care systems and pharmaco-economic research in Asia-pacific region. *Value Health* 2008;**11**(Suppl. 1):S137–55.

50. Wong SS. Pharmacy practice in Malaysia. *Malays J Pharm* 2001;**1**(1):2–8.

51. Hassali MA, Awaisu A, Shafie AA, Saeed MS. Professional training and roles of community pharmacists in Malaysia: views from general medical practitioners. *Malays Fam Physician* 2009;**4**(2&3):71–6.

52. Anonymous. *Dispensing role of pharmacists limited*. Malaysia: The Star Online. [cited October 28, 2008]. Retrieved from: http://www.thestar.com.my; July 18, 2008.

53. Hassali MA, Shafie AA, Al-Haddad M, Balamurugan T, Awaisu A, Siow YL. A qualitative study exploring the impact of the pharmaceutical Price war among community pharmacies in the state of penang, Malaysia. *J Clin Diagn Res* 2010;**4**(5):3161–9.

54. Ministry of Health Malaysia. *National medicines policy of Malaysia*. Putrajaya: Ministry of Health Malaysia; 2007.

55. Pharmaceutical Services Division MOH. *Online public Engagement on pharmacy bill*. [December 13, 2012]; Available from: http://pharmacy.gov.my/newsmaster.cfm?&menuid=132&action=view&retrieveid=401&lang=EN; 2012.

CHAPTER 3

Pharmacy Practice in Indonesia

Tri Murti Andayani, Satibi Satibi

Chapter Outline

1. Country background

The population of Indonesia according to the 2014 national census is 247 million, with 58% living on the island of Java, the world's most populous island. Despite a fairly effective family planning program that has been in place since the 1960s, the population is expected to grow to around 264 million by 2020 and 308 million by 2050, falling to sixth, behind Pakistan and Brazil, sometime before 2050.

2. Vital health statistics

The crude death rate (per 1000 people) in Indonesia was last reported at 7.01 in 2010, according to a World Bank report published in 2012.[1] Data from the Ministry of Health's

Pharmacy Practice in Developing Countries. http://dx.doi.org/10.1016/B978-0-12-801714-2.00003-4

Basic Health Research collected in 2007–2008 indicate that the main causes of child deaths are diarrheal disease (25.2%) and pneumonia (15.5%). Dengue hemorrhagic fever is the main cause of death among children between the ages of 5 and 15 in urban areas, responsible for 30.4% of deaths in this age group, while diarrhea at 11.3% is the main cause of death among the same age group in rural areas. The main causes of death across all ages of the population over 5 years are stroke (15.4%), tuberculosis (7.5%), and injuries (6.5%). According to the World Health Organization (WHO), ischemic heart disease, lower respiratory infections, malaria, HIV/AIDS, and nutritional deficiencies also contribute to mortality rates.[2]

3. Overview of the health care system

The World Bank estimates that Indonesia spends less than 3% of its gross domestic product on health (of which less than 1% is public spending). This is less than the average for countries in the East Asia and Pacific region (6.1%) and the lower middle income group of countries (5.9%). Despite the government's recent increases in health spending, public health expenditure remains quite low. As a result, Indonesia has relatively few hospital beds per 10,000 population compared to its neighbors in the region. Many public health facilities reportedly suffer from weak infrastructure and a lack of equipment. The country as a whole suffers from a lack of doctors, nurses, and to some extent midwives, particularly in rural and remote areas. Private expenditure as a percentage of total health spending is 50% in Indonesia, a smaller percentage than what is spent in most neighboring countries.[3]

The human resource situation in health has major deficiencies in numbers and quality of the health workforce. Decentralization is one of many factors exacerbating long-standing problems with maldistribution and reportedly low productivity and quality of health workers. This in turn influences the quality, efficiency, and equity of health care provision. A limited number of health workers affects the health service in Indonesia. In 2006, the ratio of general practitioners was 19.9 per 100,000 population, while the ratio of midwives per 100,000 population was 35.4. Most general practitioners and midwives work in urban areas, and a limited number are in remote areas.[4]

Since 2005, the public finance and supply systems for pharmaceuticals have faced some major changes. These include the decentralization of most public health services to district governments in 2001, establishment of the Askeskin/Jamkesmas SHI scheme for the poor, the creation of Badan Pengawas Obat dan Makanan (BPOM, the National Agency for Drug and Food Control) as an independent therapeutic goods regulatory agency, and the introduction of competitive tendering for public procurement of medicines. There have been changes to the regulations covering unbranded generic drug prices and the participation of foreign manufacturers in the national pharmaceutical market, while state-owned pharmaceutical manufacturers have been corporatized and partially privatized.

4. Medicine supply systems and drug use issues

Pharmaceutical products are very sensitive and susceptible to the environment, and the slightest change in the quality of a product can have a negative impact on its efficacy or safety and even may turn it into a "poison." Therefore the WHO agency issued a drug distribution standard set for good distribution practice (GDP) (WHO Technical Series 937 Annex 5 of 2006). Ideally, the entire distribution system of the company that serves the pharmaceutical drug is required to meet those standards. In Indonesia, implementation of the standards began only in 2008, and many companies are now starting to use the standard distribution. In addition to GDP, drug distribution rules were set in the right way. These drug distribution rules (CDOB) were issued by BPOM and they became a reference for pharmaceutical distribution among companies in Indonesia.

At this time BPOM has been improving and implementing the drug distribution system based on the concepts of responsiveness, efficiency, and quality.[5] However, to improve the affordability and efficiency of drug distribution, there are two types of drugs, namely generic drugs and branded drugs, so that the practitioner can choose the medication according to the patient's illness.

Drugs are divided into two classifications, namely acute and chronic medication drugs. Acute medication is usually a group of drugs that works for one treatment therapy, such as patients with dengue fever, typhoid, and so on. Chronic medication is intended for continuous therapy, such as for patients with hypertension, cholesterol, or diabetes, who will be taking the drug for the long term. Usually for the chronic category the transfer of product brands tends to be minimal, because it depends on the doctor's recommendation and suitability factor. In other words, the chronic drug category tends to be easier than the expected demand for acute medicine. Along the distribution chain, an interesting phenomenon has also occurred in Indonesia. Drugs with a popular brand are found not only through the official channels such as pharmacies and hospitals, but also in drugstores that incidentally do not have a pharmacist. It is illegal and, if caught, means an offense. But the market in Indonesia seems far from the word "clean." As a result, the term "gray market" is used to describe the situation (i.e., prescription drugs found in drugstores, sold directly by doctors (dispensing), and so on). The gray market is likely to offer prices that are usually lower, but with a variety of sources.

Drug manufacturers typically designate a national distributor to reach pharmacies and hospitals. Before 2000, the manufacturers, who are often referred to as the principals, tended to assign a single distributor, unlike for consumer products, which have led to multiple distributors. Appointment of a sole distributor identified by the principal needs only a simple form of cooperation and thus the principal does not have to take care of several distributors. In addition, the number of distribution points that must be reached by the distributor is still small. National distributors can sell directly to retailers or through the PBFs (Pedagang Besar Farmasi; pharmaceutical wholesalers), with limited area coverage. The need for local PBFs is due to the limited coverage, for example, the need to reach certain areas that do not have National Distributor branches/representative offices. But these local PBFs also have another role, to distribute the product to the gray market mentioned earlier. They are rarely touched by BPOM or the national distributor tighter supervision. In addition to the gray market, local PBFs finally also take the distribution point of the national distribution.

At the retail level, for example, in some pharmacies, the same drug can be obtained from more than one distributor. Even the prices obtained from local PBFs are often lower. National distributors usually provide discounts to local PBFs, so prices in local PBFs become lower. This is a difficult area to control.[5]

Currently there are approximately 12,000 pharmacies, 1300 hospitals, and 2300 PBFs. Pharmacies also have led the way to the modernization of the business, forming groups and franchises, offering 24-h service, and so on. In short the pharmaceutical market in Indonesia has grown increasingly competitive and the least participation was from the service provider. In terms of demand, the government continues to promote the national insurance program, and demand continues to grow. Knowingly or not the drug market will grow from the insurance sector, which makes sense because of the current relatively high cost of treatment. So in addition to infrastructure and demand, the industry is also constantly being educated by private insurance companies and national insurance companies.

The demand for drugs in Indonesia has been redefined by market mechanisms and has had an impact on the promotion of drugs. This condition is caused by the pharmaceutical industry marketing its products with certain sales targets, so that at the end of a particular month or year the pharmaceutical industry or PBFs give massive discounts to achieve the target sales of their products.

5. Overview of pharmacy practice and key pharmaceutical sectors

Since 1975, there has been a shift in the practice of pharmacy, initially being product-oriented, to patient care. Changes in health care and pharmacy practice provided good opportunities for pharmacists to indicate their function and show their important role in the health sector. The mission of the pharmacy profession must address the needs of society and individual patients. At one time, the acts of deciding on drug therapy and implementing it were relatively simple, safe, and inexpensive. The physician prescribed and the pharmacist dispensed. However, there is substantial evidence to show that the traditional method of prescribing and dispensing medication is no longer appropriate to ensure safety, effectiveness, and adherence to drug therapy. Public health interventions, pharmaceutical care, rational drug use, and effective management of pharmaceuticals are key components of a health care system that is accessible, sustainable, affordable, and fair, to ensure efficacy, safety, and quality of treatment.

Pharmacists in Indonesia have begun to engage in health promotion and public health practice. One program in which pharmacists in hospitals participate is the Hospital Community Health

Education program (PKMRS/Penyuluhan Kesehatan Masyarakat Rumah Sakit). This activity is an extension activity, or the provision of information about the health of the community hospital (patient, family, and hospital staff). Pharmacist Dr Sardjito Yogyakarta periodically participates in activities of the PKMRS.

In addition to the PKMRS, pharmacists and students run community health promotions through drug information centers in their respective institutions. Activities undertaken may include health promotion, through Web sites, leaflets, etc., and through outreach to the community. There is also a pharmacist (lecturer) who wrote a book aimed at warning the public about the dangers of alcohol, how to choose a drug, and a variety of tips on healthy living.

6. Drug- and pharmacy-related regulations, policies, and ethics

Indonesia's domestic pharmaceutical industry is mainly engaged in the production and marketing of branded generics (drugs that are off patent), generics, and licensed drugs from pharmaceutical companies abroad. Indonesia's domestic pharmaceutical industry is based on formulation, not research. Research and development (R&D) activities are very limited, with financial support averaging below 2% of total sales. Research conducted is limited to product formulation and not the development of new drug molecules. Future implications are that Indonesia's domestic pharmaceutical companies will never compete in the market segment of patented drugs/innovative medicines. The competition area of the domestic pharmaceutical companies in Indonesia is in the market of branded generics and generic drugs. Development of the over-the-counter (OTC) market in Indonesia is also quite high from year to year. The OTC drug market share is dominated by domestic pharmaceutical companies. Indonesian pharmaceutical market competition is very tight. Companies that are not consistent in maintaining and improving their competitiveness will lose their market share in a relatively short time. The Indonesian pharmaceutical industry should have the preparation and readiness to exploit the potential of the ASEAN pharmaceutical market.

The highest retail prices of generic drugs are set in two decrees of the Ministry of Health. The first one was set on February 23, 2012 by the Decree of the Minister of Health of the Republic of Indonesia (No. 092/Menkes/SK/II/2012 on Generic Drug Retail Price 2012).[8] The second was set also on February 23, 2012 in the form of Decree of the Minister of Health of the Republic of Indonesia (No. 094/Menkes/SK/II/2012 on Drug Price for Government Procurement 2012).[9] In this decree, it is stated that the HET is the highest selling price of generic drugs at pharmacies, hospitals, and other health care facilities for the whole of Indonesia. Kepmenkes (Decree of the Minister of Health) 92/2012 was set to ensure the availability and distribution of drugs to meet the needs of health care, thereby rationalizing the HET needed for generic drugs specified in the Decree of the Ministry of Health No. 632/Menkes/SK/III/2011. The HET is valid throughout the generic pharmacy, hospital, and pharmaceutical services facilities in Indonesia. Therefore, the maximum price for any sale of generic drugs can be no higher than the HET contained in the Kepmenkes.

Indonesia is a country rich in natural ingredients. Natural ingredients are used in traditional medicine. Indonesia pays great attention to traditional medicine in the making of regulations. The classification of natural medicine in Indonesia is organized by the National Agency of Drug and Food Control by Decree No. HK.00.05.4.2411 BPOM. Based on the process for filing a claim and the type and level of efficacy evidenced, in accordance with the decree, Indonesia natural medicines are grouped into three categories, namely herb, standardized herbal medicine, and fitofarmaka. Herbs are the Indonesian natural remedies that are known empirically or based on studies to have efficacy as a drug. Standardized herbal medicine is a natural medicine that Indonesia claims proven in preclinical efficacy, and standardization has been made for the raw materials used in the finished product. Fitofarmaka is a natural medicine with claims of efficacy proven by/based on clinical trials and standardization of the raw materials used in the finished product. As of 2011, there are five new traditional medicines including fitofarmaka.

The Health Ministry through Permenkes (Regulation of the Ministry of Health) No. 6/2012 regulates the industry and the business of traditional medicine to provide a conducive business climate for manufacturers of traditional medicine with attention to safety, efficacy/benefit, and quality of traditional medicines. Under these regulations, traditional medicines are made by the industry and the business of traditional medicine. The industries in question are the IOT (Industri Obat Tradisional; traditional medicine industry) and IEBA (Industri Ekstrak Bahan Alam; extract industry for natural materials), while the businesses in question are UKOT (Usaha Kecil Obat Tradisional; small and traditional medicine), Usaha Menengah Obat Tradisional (medium traditional medicine), herbal concoction effort, and effort carrying herbs. Each IOT and IEBA required to have at least one pharmacist, while UKOT has at least one pharmaceutical technical personnel (TTK). A responsible pharmacist is required to ensure that traditional medicines are manufactured in accordance with CPOTB (Traditional Medicine Making the Good) as well as to guarantee quality and usefulness. Traditional medicine to be distributed shall comply with the requirements of Permenkes 007/20 122 on the registration of traditional medicine. Indonesia is also familiar with the Indonesian Herbal Pharmacopoeia (first edition) established by the Ministry of Health of Indonesia through Decree No. 261/2009. This herbal pharmacopoeia sets standards intended for the raw herbal ingredients used as raw materials and products of traditional medicine and treatment so that safety, quality, benefits, and usefulness are ensured. The Indonesian herbal pharmacopoeia contains general provisions and 70 monographs on botanicals and extracts. In addition it contains information on and explanations of analytical methods and general testing procedures, microbiology, biology, chemistry, and physics.[10]

At the college level, the Faculty of Pharmacy at the University of Gadjah Mada (UGM) in Yogyakarta and other schools of pharmacy in Indonesia have responded to interest in pharmaceutical natural products and expect very understanding and competent graduates in the field of natural medicine. Dr Sardjito Yogyakarta in 2010 opened an herbal clinic for the treatment of several diseases.

7. Core pharmacy practices

7.1 Hospital pharmacy

According to management, hospitals are classified as public hospitals and private hospitals. Public hospitals are run by the government, local government, and legal entities that are nonprofit. Based on the level of care, hospitals are classified into general hospitals and specialized hospitals (primary care to one area or one particular type of disease). General hospitals and specialized hospitals are classified by the facilities and capabilities of hospital services. Public hospitals are classified into four classes, namely the classes A–D, of which a class A hospital is a hospital that has the facilities and capabilities of leading high service, while hospitals with minimum facilities and poor service delivery capabilities are classified in class D (Departemen Kesehatan RI, 2009). Hospital classification established a hospital referral system in the transfer of knowledge, transfer of documents, transfer of specimens, and transfer of patients.[11]

Entering the era of the free market, Indonesia has had to face the challenges of improving the quality of all health services, including improving hospital health care to a world class hospital service. The hospital carries three main roles, namely health service, education, and research. The third harmonization has a key role in achieving the best quality hospital. Comprehensive health services are health services that include promotion and prevention in addition to curative and rehabilitative services.

The number of private hospitals in Indonesia is quite large, about 50% of hospitals in 2008, and the majority (82%) are managed by nonprofit organizations. In Indonesia, ambulatory care/primary care is largely done by the private sector, with 30% of patients receiving outpatient services from the private sector, whereas in Java and Bali, the private sector serves more than 50% of outpatients.

Pharmacists in hospitals, in implementing their functions, are incorporated in the IFRS (Instalasi Farmasi Rumah Sakit; The Hospital Pharmacy). The IFRS is a unit in the hospital and is a facility of pharmacy administration under the leadership of a competent pharmacist. The IFRS is responsible for the conduct, provision, and management of all aspects of medical supplies in the hospital, which can be nonclinical pharmaceutical care and clinical pharmacy services. The responsibility of the pharmacist in pharmaceutical care services includes nonclinical aspects, namely planning, procurement, receipt, storage, and distribution of drugs needed in the hospital, and the clinical pharmacy services, which are performed directly and in their implementation require interaction with patients, doctors, and nurses; distribution of medicines and pharmaceutical products for patients and caregivers; and counseling and drug information. The responsibility and authority of pharmacists are further regulated in the law, by government regulation and the Ministry of Health. Along with the development of health, pharmacy service orientation has now shifted more toward clinical pharmacy services (pharmaceutical care), which is a form of service and direct responsibility for the pharmacist profession in pharmacy work to improve the quality of life of patients.[6]

The role of clinical pharmacy itself has a good impact on various outcomes of therapy for these patients, on the humanistic (quality of life, satisfaction), the clinical (for better control of chronic disease), and the economic (reduction of health care costs) levels. However, as mentioned above, the role of the pharmacist apparently has not been much recognized or felt by the people of Indonesia, in contrast to what happens in the international community, including for clinical pharmacists in the United States, in terms of popularity, responsibility, and even salary. England is the country with Europe's longest implemented clinical pharmacy. Most of the research on the crucial role of clinical pharmacy in health care is largely derived from experience in the United States and the United Kingdom. In Australia, 90% of private hospitals and 100% of government hospitals provide clinical pharmacy services. Indeed, many factors that lead to clinical pharmacy services and the role of the pharmacist profession in Indonesia are not at the same level as in other countries.[7]

7.2 Industry pharmacy

The age of the pharmaceutical industry in Indonesia is still relatively young compared to developed countries. In the Dutch colonial period until the war of independence the number of pharmaceutical factories in Indonesia was still very small, such as a drug manufacturers in Jakarta Manggarai, a quinine factory, and the Institut Pasteur, which produces serum and vaccines. Similarly, pharmaceutical distribution facilities and pharmacies were still very limited. At that time the pharmaceutical companies were producing drugs as well as distributing drugs. This situation did not change much until the beginning of independence. As of 1983, there has been significant progress since 90% of the drug needs have been met by the pharmaceutical industry in the country, although most of the raw materials still have to be imported. The number of pharmaceutical manufacturers in 1983 was 286 plants consisting of 37 companies of domestic investment, 40 Foreign Direct Investment (FDI) companies, and 209 private companies nationwide. The number of Indonesian pharmaceutical manufacturing companies that exist today is relatively not much changed compared to 1983. At this time the number of pharmaceutical factories of 202 consists of 4 state-owned, 30 foreign, and 168 national private companies. The value of drug sales has increased; in 1980 drug circulation in Indonesia was worth US $483 million and in 2004 it was approximately US $2 billion.[12] The market share of the Indonesian pharmaceutical market (2004) compared to the global pharmaceutical market is relatively small, namely 0.25%. The pharmaceutical market share in Indonesia is dominated by 60 companies by as much as 84%, while 139 companies have a market share of only 16%. This means that most of the Indonesian pharmaceutical manufacturing companies are operating on a small scale. Nonetheless the Indonesian pharmaceutical market growth is still relatively high (around 15% in 2004) and it is the largest pharmaceutical market in ASEAN. Future pharmaceutical market growth in Indonesia is predicted to still be fairly high considering that Indonesia's per capita drug consumption is the lowest among ASEAN countries. In 2001, drug expenditure per capita in Indonesia was US $4.5, while in Malaysia and Thailand it was US $12.9 and US $12.7, respectively. With further improvements in per capita income and health insurance systems in Indonesia in the future, the value of drugs in Indonesia could be great. This situation will certainly have a positive correlation with the growth of the pharmaceutical industry in the future.[12] Indonesian exports of drugs have increased from year to year, comprising about 5% of the total sales of the pharmaceutical industry in Indonesia. With the implementation of the ASEAN harmonization of pharmaceutical regulations in 2008, a single ASEAN market in pharmaceuticals was created, in the sense that there are no tariff or nontariff barriers in the trade of pharmaceuticals in the ASEAN region. This means opportunities for the pharmaceutical industry to develop exports for the ASEAN market, but at the same time the Indonesian domestic market will be threatened by the freer entry of ASEAN pharmaceutical products into Indonesia.

7.3 Community pharmacy

So that pharmacists can implement pharmaceutical care in the community well, DirJen Yanfar and Medical Devices and the Health Department, in collaboration with the Indonesian Pharmacist Association (ISFI), are now known as the IAI (Ikatan Apoteker Indonesia) and set standards to improve the quality of pharmacy services to the community.[6] In addition, there is also Government Regulation No. 51 of 2009 on the work of pharmacy to regulate pharmacy employment service facilities. The pharmacist's services in pharmacies are prescription service (the screening process, drug compounding, labeling, packaging, delivery, provision of drug information, counseling, and monitoring of drug use), promotional activities, and education of the community in self-medication for disease in regard to choosing the appropriate medication, home care services particularly for the elderly, and patients needing treatment for chronic diseases. For these activities the pharmacist shall keep notes in the form of records of treatment (medication record). With the functions of promoting and education, pharmacists in the community pharmacy can be put in a position to promote healthy behavior. Pharmacists in community pharmacy can play a role in smoking cessation programs, alcohol consumption, healthy nutrition, and increased physical activity for prevention against disease and disability. But there are still barriers to pharmacists conducting health promotion, including the lack of confidence of pharmacists and the public perception that pharmacists only provide drug services.

7.4 Medicine marketing and promotion

In modern marketing, advertising has a very important role that cannot be ignored by marketers. Advertising is a form of nonpersonal communication addressed to the target audience through a variety of media to promote a product, service, or idea.[5] Direct-to-customer advertising was intended to increase patient awareness of the disease and the proper use of drugs and medicines and provide a choice to the customer according to the needed medication. Unlike in the United States and New Zealand, where direct-to-customer advertising can be done for ethical and OTC drugs, in Indonesia, according to the POM Regulation of Drug Promotion in 2002, ethical drugs cannot be promoted to the general public but can be promoted only to health professionals. In the promotion of drugs audiovisual and electronic media are allowed only to drug-free and nonfinite. According to Government Regulation on the Security of Pharmaceuticals and Medical Devices No. 72 of 1998, ethical drugs may be advertised only in the print media or print media for medical scientific pharmaceutical science. Thus, the selection of prescription drugs is entirely dependent on doctors and key information about the drug obtained from the patient's verbal communication with pharmacists and doctors. Drug advertisements should contain information about the pharmaceutical that is objective (must provide information in accordance with reality and should not deviate from the nature of the benefit and safety of drugs that have been approved), complete (must include not only information about drug efficacy, but also information about the things that must be considered, such as the existence of contraindications and side effects), and not misleading (the drug information must be truthful, accurate, and responsible and shall not use public fears of a health problem).[13]

Per the Regulation of the Health Ministry of the Republic of Indonesia No. 2406/Menkes/per/XII/2011, general guidelines on the use of antibiotics, the use of antibiotics in health care is often not precise so that it causes less effective treatment, increased risk to patient safety, spread of resistance, and high cost of treatment and that increases in the accuracy of the use of antibiotics in health care should be made in the general guidance of antibiotic use. Disease infection is still one important public health problem, particularly in developing countries. One of the mainstay drugs to overcome the problem comprises the antimicrobials, including antibacterial/antibiotic, antifungal, antiviral, and antiprotozoal medicines. Antibiotics are the drugs most widely used in infections caused by bacteria. Various studies have found that about 40–62% of antibiotics are used inappropriately. Several studies that evaluated the use of antibiotics in various parts of the hospital found that 30–80% is not based on the indication. The intensity of the relatively high use of antibiotics causes a variety of problems and is a global threat to health, especially bacterial resistance to antibiotics, the impact on morbidity and mortality, and the negative impacts on the economy and society.

8. Special pharmacy-related services and activities

Pharmacists are responsible not only for the drug as a product, with all its implications, but also for the therapeutic effects and safety of the drug in order to achieve an optimal effect. Pharmacists who are specialized in medical communications/drug information provide educational services about pharmaceutical products for health care professionals and consumers.

One aspect of pharmacy services is drug information services provided by pharmacists to patients and other concerned parties. Drug information is an aid for physicians in making decisions about treatment options about the most appropriate medication for a patient. Drug information services provided certainly must be complete, objective, continuous, and always up to date. Drug information services are aimed to support the rational use of medicines.

The practice of clinical pharmacy services is relatively new in Indonesia, arriving around the beginning of the twenty-first century. The concept of clinical pharmacy itself has not been fully accepted by health workers in hospitals, so that clinical pharmacy services in Indonesia is growing quite slowly. Paradigm pharmacists who provide patient care on the ward, monitor the treatment of patients, provide information and counseling on a regular basis, and provide treatment recommendations are still not common, because it is considered that the function of the pharmacist in the IFRS is only to serve to prepare the medicine. Pharmacists themselves have seemed less convinced that they can play a role in treatment. In addition, pharmacists are not yet fully implementing their functions so that the public and patients are less familiar with the pharmacist's profession, especially in hospitals, because in most hospitals, the number of hospital pharmacists is still small.[14]

9. Pharmacy education

Pharmacy education in Indonesia at this time varies, starting from pharmacy school, three diploma programs, graduate programs, professional programs, master programs, program specialists, and doctoral programs. Three diploma programs in the field of pharmaceuticals today can be divided into two pharmaceutical DIII and a DIII pharmaceutical analyst. A 110–120 credit study load program is scheduled in six semesters (3 years). Some universities have a specialization for the graduate program. The Faculty of Pharmacy at the UGM in 2011 divided students into four interests, which were pharmaceutical sciences, pharmaceutical industry, clinical and community pharmacy, and pharmacy natural materials, while the School of Pharmacy at Bandung Institute of Technology (ITB) is divided into two degree programs including pharmaceutical science and technology, as well as pharmaceutical clinics and community.

A master's program has a study load of 36–50 credits to be completed in four semesters. Some universities in Indonesia have opened several pharmaceutical master programs, which include pharmaceutical sciences, clinical pharmacy, and pharmacy management. Airlangga University is the only university in Indonesia to offer a pharmacy specialist pharmacy program. The program consists of one semester of college and three semesters of deeper specialization/field. Fields/current specializations are geriatric stroke, hematology–oncology, pediatrics, infectious diseases, and cardiovascular diseases. The doctoral program can be taken for 4–10 semesters with a minimum study load of 40 credits to graduate with a master's degree.

To get a degree in pharmacy, students should be studying for 5 years consisting of undergraduate pharmacy and pharmacist professional programs. Undergraduate education in Indonesia (including pharmaceuticals), in accordance with the decree of the Ministry of Education No. 232/U/2000, has loads of 144–160 credits scheduled in eight semesters (4 years), while the pharmacist professional education, in accordance with the decree of the APTFI (Asosiasi Perguruan Tinggi Farmasi Indonesia) and IAI (formerly ISFI), is held for at least two semesters with a load of 28–40 credits. The Association of Colleges of Pharmacy Indonesia has set the standard minimum curriculum (core curriculum) for undergraduate and professional pharmacy programs to generate pharmacists that actually have competence in carrying out the work and pharmacy services. However, each pharmacy college is given the freedom to develop and add institutional curriculum. Pharmacist profession curriculum programs can be evaluated and revised if necessary, at least once every 3 years. Previously, the practice of pharmacy in the professional education in Indonesia was very small compared to the lecture portion of the class. However, at this time, practice has a greater proportion. The PKPA (Praktek Kerja Profesi Apoteker) is implemented when students are in the pharmacy profession program. The PKPA itself in the core curriculum APTFI and IAI has loads of 8 credits. The PKPA credits are equivalent to 8 h/day for 5 days or 40 h/week. In fact the Faculty of Pharmacy at the University of Gadjah Mada determines PKPA loads of 13 credits, and ITB 16 credits.

Research on pharmacy services in Indonesia today is relatively increased. A recently published journal also focuses on pharmacy services. The Faculty of Pharmacy, Gadjah Mada University, in Yogyakarta in 2011 began publishing the *Journal of Management and Pharmacy Services* (JMPF). As of this writing, JMPF has published Volumes 1 (Nos. 1–4) and 2 (No. 1). The publication of research journals is expected in terms of pharmacy services to continue to grow and become a driving force in the implementation of pharmacy services as a whole.

Several research themes within the scope of pharmacy services that have been published in the journal include medication safety, drug-related problems of various diseases, evaluation of the quality of life of patients with degenerative diseases, evaluation of drug therapy in various diseases, evaluation of the implementation of standards of pharmaceutical care, the role of standards in the implementation of IAI pharmacy services in the pharmacy, the influence of counseling, etc. The diverse themes showed interest in research to explore the implementation of pharmaceutical services in Indonesia.

10. Challenges

In the past four decades there has been a shift in the practice of pharmacy, from initially being product-oriented to patient care. The role of pharmacists has shifted from the manufacturing and supply of medicinal products to providing service and information and primarily service to the patients. Pharmacists are responsible for ensuring that the drug therapy given to patients is according to proper indications, the most effective, safe, and comfortable for the patient. Responsibility is directly for the patient's medicine-related needs, giving pharmacists an important role in the outcome of therapy and quality of life of patients. Another challenge for pharmacists is to ensure that medicines are used rationally and patients receive medication according to clinical needs, with individual doses required in the appropriate time period, and that is most cost-effective.[15]

Community pharmacists play a role in monitoring the population database and pharmacy services through direct intervention with the patient. Clinical and economic outcomes should be considered in making the right decisions for the population. Pharmacists in managed-care organizations are responsible for widespread clinical services and medication management-oriented quality. Patient management is based on the interaction between health care professionals covering all aspects of individual patient care.

Call-center pharmacists need to be developed to educate both the patient and the prescriber and to provide patient counseling, drug information, customer service, drug utilization review, medical management, and formulary management. Pharmacists in the call center can interact with patients to support effective and optimal drug therapy. In recent years, drug information services is growing in some areas, both in hospital and in community pharmacy services. Pharmacists can access the databases separately to help the prescriber, community health services, and the public by providing information on drug–drug interactions, drugs and food, drugs and disease, drugs and test diagnostics, side effects, the use of drugs in specific populations (e.g., elderly, pediatric, immunosuppressed), parenteral nutrition calculations, chemotherapeutic dosing regimens, toxicology and poisoning, and evidence-based medical literature reviews.

Rapid technological developments and the impact of technology require a pharmacist or pharmacy information technology specialist in "informatics." Pharmacists here play a role in the development of software dispensing, automated medication-dispensing machines, programmed infusion devices, and system maintenance, clinical and technical knowledge needed to effectively implement and reduce errors.

Pharmacists who work well in practice and academics are responsible for model development for practice, research, and teaching in health care. The required curriculum is that integrated with the practice of pharmacy so they can contribute to the development of sustainable practices. Associated with clinical pharmacy services, pharmacists have the opportunity to be preceptors for a pharmacy faculty or school to assist in preparing future pharmacists. Pharmaceutical industry also provides a variety of land for pharmacists, in drug development research, postapproval drug marketing, pharmaceutical sales, drug information, quality control, administration, consulting, and advisory roles. Therefore, there is a need for a supported curriculum that includes advances in clinical pharmacotherapeutics and pharmacoeconomics.

11. Recommendations

Economic and political circumstances may affect the health care system and also influence the practice of pharmacy. Therefore, we need a change in pharmacy education. The role and functions of pharmacists should be evaluated and the outcomes of teaching pharmacy curriculum should be clearly defined. Outcomes of pharmacy education can be used as a framework for integrating science, professional skills, interprofessional practices, and professionalism in pharmacy services, systems management, and public health. Educational change not only requires revision and restructuring of the curriculum, but also requires a commitment to faculty development to prepare teachers to educate pharmacists in various patterns. The pharmacy school or faculty must create, assign, and evaluate pharmacy practice models to be used in health services in the community.

The problems and challenges faced by the pharmaceutical industry of Indonesia in the next 5 years will be very different from 5 years ago. Competition is changing the landscape because it requires new strategies and new paradigms. Similarly, the government is expected to have a broad knowledge and understanding of the competitiveness of the pharmaceutical industry so that regulations and policies are made to create value for the advancement of the pharmaceutical industry in Indonesia.

In the era of the single ASEAN pharmaceutical market, the government can no longer act in a "domestic inward-looking" manner in making regulations in the pharmaceutical field, but should also consider the "regional regulation," which has been harmonized by ASEAN.

It should be highlighted that regulations and government policies that do not "match" with the dynamics and development of the regional and global pharmaceutical industry will have negative implications for the competitiveness of the pharmaceutical industry.

Going forward, the government's policies in the pharmaceutical industry need to be research-based and not ad hoc and partial.

Faced with an increasingly tight competition in the era of the single ASEAN pharmaceutical market, the government should have a vision, scenarios, and a clear policy on increasing the competitive advantage in the pharmaceutical industry of Indonesia (that is sustainable). Similarly, in R&D, the government should be able to play more roles. Government can be an effective mediator to garner mutual cooperation between the pharmaceutical industry and the research centers at various universities. Pharmaceutical companies conducting research collaboration with universities should be given meaningful incentives, including tax deductions. The pharmaceutical industry is a knowledge-based industry in which the role of intangible assets is very large in the competitiveness and performance of the company. Intangible assets of Indonesian pharmaceutical industries covering human capital, structural capital, customer capital, and general partner capital are relatively weak. Of about 170 Indonesian domestic pharmaceutical companies, only 30 have the potential to develop export markets, particularly the Southeast Asian market. The rest of the pharmaceutical companies will face tough challenges as the players in the domestic market will be growing with the entry of the ASEAN pharmaceutical company based outside Indonesia. In this context, there should be a new orientation of the Indonesia pharmaceutical industry to maintain control of the domestic market and export market development. At the same time, Indonesian intangible assets to the pharmaceutical industry need to be strengthened to increase competitive advantage and industry performance. The pharmaceutical industry needs to strengthen the competence of Indonesia in addition to marketing, and also needs to strengthen the lines of R&D, including research materials to be developed as herbal Indonesia fitofarmaka for modern medicine and marketed widely, including export to many countries. It needs to be emphasized that Indonesia is a mega-biodiversity center of the world. Now pharmaceutical companies in Indonesia are building ASEAN networks and strategic alliances with domestic companies in each ASEAN member country. In line with this, the government needs to make reciprocal negotiations bilaterally with ASEAN member countries. In this context, the authorities in the field of pharmacy must be proactive in such a way that the pharmaceutical industry in Indonesia does not miss the opportunity of the single ASEAN pharmaceutical market.

12. Conclusions

Changes in health care and pharmacy practice provide many new opportunities for pharmacists to indicate their functions. Providing high-quality health care to patients requires that education, training, and licensing be based on building competencies of pharmacists. Public health interventions, pharmaceutical care, rational drug use, and effective management of pharmaceuticals are key components of a health care system that is accessible, sustainable, affordable, and fair, which in turns ensures the efficacy, safety, and quality of treatment. Pharmacists have an important role in the health sector. Pharmacists occupy a position at the forefront of the health care system to improve treatment outcomes and quality of life of patients.

13. Lessons learned

13.1   Pharmacy education in Indonesia at this time varies as pharmacy school, three diploma programs, graduate programs, professional programs, master programs, program specialists, and doctoral programs. The Association of Colleges of Pharmacy Indonesia has set the standard minimum curriculum (core curriculum) for undergraduate and professional pharmacy programs that generates pharmacists who actually have competencies in carrying out the work and pharmacy services.

13.2   The responsibilities of the pharmacist in pharmaceutical care services include nonclinical forms of products, namely planning, procurement, receipt, storage, and distribution of drugs needed in the hospital, while the clinical pharmacy services are performed directly and in their implementation require interaction with patients and doctors and nurses, among others; physician drug order services; distribution of medicines and pharmaceutical products for patients and caregivers; and counseling and drug information.

13.3   Indonesia is a country rich in natural ingredients, one use of which is as traditional medicines. The Health Ministry through Permenkes No. 6/2012 regulates the industry and the business of traditional medicine to provide a conducive business climate for manufacturers of traditional medicines with attention to safety, efficacy/benefit, and quality.

13.4   Intangible assets of Indonesian pharmaceutical industries covering human capital, structural capital, customer capital, and general partner capital are relatively weak. Of about 170 Indonesian domestic pharmaceutical companies, only 30 have the potential to develop export markets, particularly the Southeast Asian market.

References

1. The World Bank. *Indonesia health review*. 2012.
2. World Health Organization. *Statistics: countries—Indonesia*. 2014.
3. World Bank. *Giving more weight to health: assessing fiscal space for health in Indonesia*. 2009.
4. Policy Note Series. Pharmaceuticals: Why Reform is Needed. Indonesian Health Sector Review; 2009.
5. Sampurno. *Manajemen Pemasaran Farmasi*. Yogyakarta: Gadjah Mada University Press; 2009.
6. Departemen Kesehatan RI. Keputusan Menteri Kesehatan Republik Indonesia Tentang Standar Pelayanan Farmasi Di Rumah Sakit Dan Apotek. Jakarta; 2004.
7. Carter J, Slack M. *Pharmacy in public health basic and beyond*. USA: American Society of Health System Pharmacist Inc.; 2010.
8. Kementrian Kesehatan. Keputusan Menteri Kesehatan No 092/2012 tentang Harga eceran tertinggi obat generik di Indonesia tahun 2012. Jakarta (Indonesia); 2012.
9. Kementrian Kesehatan. Keputusan Menteri Kesehatan No 094/2012 tentang harga obat untuk pengadaan pemerintah. Jakarta (Indonesia); 2012.
10. Departemen Kesehatan RI. Kebijakan Obat Nasional. Jakarta; 2005.
11. Departemen Kesehatan RI. Undang Undang no 44 tahun 2009 tentang Rumah Sakit. Jakarta; 2009.
12. Sampurno. *Memperkuat Kapasitas dan Kompetensi Industri Farmasi Indonesia*. Jakarta: Badan POM; 2005.
13. Departemen Kesehatan RI. Pedoman Supervisi dan Evaluasi Obat Publik dan Perbekalan Farmasi. Jakarta; 2002.
14. Hermansyah A, Sukorini AI, Setiawan CD, Priyandani Y. The conflicts between professional and non professional work of community pharmacists in Indonesia. *Pharm Pract* January–March 2012;**10**(1):33–9.
15. The Council on Credentialing in Pharmacy. Scope of Contemporary Pharmacy Practice: Roles, Responsibilities, and Functions of Pharmacists and Pharmacy Technicians Approved for distribution. Washington (DC); 2009.

CHAPTER 4

Pharmacy Practice in China

Yu Fang

Chapter Outline

1. Country background

The People's Republic of China (PRC), commonly known as China, is a sovereign state located in East Asia. It is the most populated country in the world, with a population of more than 1.35 billion. Its capital is Beijing. The Communist Party of China has led the PRC under a single-party system since the state's establishment in 1949. It exercises jurisdiction over 22 provinces (including Taiwan), five autonomous regions, four direct-controlled municipalities (Beijing, Shanghai, Tianjin, Chongqing), and two mostly self-governing special administrative regions (Hong Kong, Macau). China covers an area of 9.6 million square kilometers and is the world's second-largest country by land area. China officially recognizes 56 distinct ethnic groups, the largest of which are the Han Chinese, who constitute about 91.5% of the total population.

As one of the Four Great Ancient Civilizations, China has a recorded history of more than 5000 years. Since 221 BCE, when the Qin Dynasty first conquered several states to form a Chinese empire, the country has expanded, fractured, and reformed numerous times. The Republic of China overthrew the last dynasty in 1911 and ruled the Chinese mainland until 1949. After the defeat of the Empire of Japan during World War II, the Communist Party defeated the nationalist Kuomintang on mainland China and established the People's Republic of China in Beijing on October 1, 1949.

The economic history of China stretches over thousands of years and has undergone alternating cycles of prosperity and decline. For a large part of the last two millennia, China was the world's largest and most advanced economy. Since the introduction of economic reforms in 1978, China has become one of the world's fastest-growing major economies. As of 2013, it is the world's second-largest economy by both nominal total gross domestic product (GDP) and purchasing power parity. It is also the world's largest exporter and importer of goods.[1]

2. Vital health statistics

China has undergone rapid demographic and epidemiological changes during the past few decades, including striking declines in fertility and child mortality and increased life expectancy at birth.[2] Judging from important indicators that reflect national health, the Chinese people are now among the healthiest in developing countries. Life expectancy at birth in China has increased by more than 50 years since 1960, reaching 74.99 years in 2013, although it remains lower than the Organisation for Economic Cooperation and Development average (80.1 years). Maternal mortality rate decreased from 51.3 per 100,000 in 2002 to 24.5 per 100,000 in 2012. The infant mortality rate in China has fallen greatly over the past two decades, decreasing from 42 deaths per 1000 live births in 1990 to 12 deaths in 2012.[3]

According to a survey conducted in 2003, a decline in infectious diseases was seen between 1998 and 2008, although the incidence of noncommunicable diseases (NCDs) rose continually over the same period. China faces a severe threat from NCDs. An estimated 82% of China's disease burden is due to NCDs—a number that is expected to increase over time.[4]

Causes of death in China have changed in recent decades. The main causes of death during 1982–2010 included malignant neoplasms, cerebrovascular disease, heart disease, respiratory disease, injury and poisoning, endocrine and metabolic disease, digestive disease, genitourinary disease, nervous system disease, mental disorders, perinatal disease, tuberculosis, and nontuberculosis infectious diseases. Since 1987, endocrine and metabolic diseases have been among the top 10 causes of death in urban residents, increasing steadily. This increase has been seen in the rural population as well since 1997. Tuberculosis has been excluded from the top 10 causes of death in urban residents since 1992 and in rural residents since 2005. Deaths due to mental disorders became a problem beginning in 1992 in urban residents and 13 years later in rural residents. A similar trend was found for nervous system diseases. Between 1982 and 2010, malignant neoplasms, cerebrovascular disease, heart disease, respiratory disease, and injury and poisoning were the five leading causes of death in both urban and rural populations.[5]

3. Overview of the health care system

Medical and health care systems covering both urban and rural residents have been established in China. Among these systems, the first is the public health service system, which covers disease prevention and control, health education, maternity and childcare, mental health, health emergency response, blood collection and supply, health supervision, family planning, and some other specialized public health services. A medical and health care system based on community-level health care networks provides public health services.

The second area of coverage is the medical care system. In rural areas, there is a three-level medical service network that includes the county hospital, township hospitals, and village clinics. The county hospital plays the leading role, and township hospitals and village clinics offer service at the base. In contrast, cities and towns offer a new type of urban health service system that features division of responsibilities as well as cooperation among hospitals at all levels and community health care centers.

The third leg of the health care system is medical care assurance. This system comprises mainly basic medical care assurance supported by many forms of supplementary medical insurance and commercial health insurance. The basic medical security system covers basic medical insurance for working and nonworking urban residents, a new type of rural cooperative medical care, and urban–rural medical aid. This system covers, respectively, employed and unemployed urban populations, rural populations, and people suffering from economic difficulties.

The fourth leg is the pharmaceutical supply system, which covers the production, circulation, price control, procurement, dispatch, and use of pharmaceuticals. Recent work has focused on establishing a national system that addresses essential medicines.[3] By the end of 2012, the essential medicine system had provided full coverage, with all grassroots government-run medical and health institutions supplying essential medicines with zero markup (under which essential medicines are sold to patients for procurement price plus a fixed distribution cost, with no profit to the health facility for the sale). This system is now being extended to village clinics and nongovernmental medical and health institutions.[6]

By the end of 2012, there were 950,297 medical and health care institutions around the country, an increase of 144,297 since 2003. The number of licensed doctors (assistants) reached 2,616,000, or 1.94 per 1000 people (compared with 1.5 per 1000 in 2002). Registered nurses totaled 2,497,000, or 1.85 per 1000 people (compared with 1 per 1000 in 2002). The number of hospital beds reached 5,725,000, or 4.2 per 1000 people (compared with 2.5 per 1000 in 2002).[3]

China's health expenditure comes primarily from the government's general tax revenue, social medical insurance, commercial health insurance, and residents' out-of-pocket spending. In 2011, the total health expenditure in China reached 2434.591 billion yuan, or 1806.95 yuan per capita. The total expenditure accounted for 5.1% of the country's GDP. Between 1978 and 2011, the health expenditure grew by an average annual rate of 11.32%. Individual "out-of-pocket" spending declined from 57.7% in 2002 to 34.8% in 2011, showing that health financing is working increasingly better in the areas of risk protection and redistribution.[6]

The aging Chinese population and an increase in chronic medical conditions have escalated the demand for pharmaceutical services.[7] Two streams of medical practice exist in China: traditional Chinese medicine (TCM) and western medicine. They have been practiced alongside each other at every level of the health care system since the late 1800s.[8,9] TCM is a separate department at the Ministry of Health (MoH) and at provincial and county bureaus of health. It has its own medical schools, hospitals, and research institutes. Overall, it is estimated that 40% of health care in China is based on TCM, with a higher proportions in rural areas. The collaboration between the two systems is well illustrated by the fact that approximately 40% of the medicines prescribed in hospitals practicing western medicine are traditional. Similarly, in hospitals practicing traditional medicine, 40% of all prescribed drugs are western medicines.[10] The central government continues to have a policy for the expansion of TCM. An increase in the number of traditional Chinese pharmacists is one of the priorities for manpower development. Their number continues to increase, currently reaching nearly 100,000.[6] Hospital and community pharmacies are responsible for dispensing medicines that are used in both streams,[11] and western and Chinese over-the-counter medications are equally popular in China.[12]

4. Medicine supply systems and drug use issues

Because of the changing economic system, the Chinese government has revised its pharmaceutical distribution network. It has been changed from a centrally controlled supply system to a market-oriented system. A competitive mechanism has been introduced into the pharmaceutical market, which improves the availability of pharmaceuticals. Figure 1 shows the new pharmaceutical supply chain in China.[13]

Under this supply chain, not only has domestic pharmaceutical production grown dramatically, but numerous imported drugs have begun to enter the Chinese market. The current supply chain is different from the drug supply mechanism under a central planned economy. Whereas earlier pharmaceutical manufacturing firms could sell drugs only to wholesalers, now they are able to sell their products to drug wholesale stations and drug stores, as well as

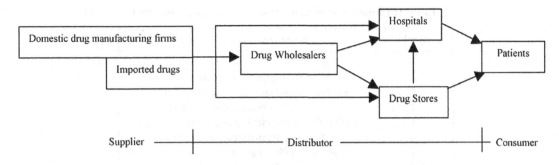

Figure 1
Pharmaceutical supply chain in China. *Source: Ref. 13.*

directly to hospitals. Also, large distributors can sell drugs to smaller ones. The wholesale prices are thus different because of the different purchasing volumes. There is a considerable imbalance of retail market sales within the supply chain, with hospital pharmacies accounting for roughly four-fifths of all retail pharmaceutical sales.[14] The rest of the retail drugs are dispensed by drug stores, including retail enterprises and rural drug supply outlets. Patients can buy drugs from hospitals and drug stores. Because of information asymmetry regarding knowledge of drugs, it is physicians—the agents of patients (the consumer)—who decide which drug is required and thus purchased.[13]

Pharmaceuticals are divided into three pricing classes: government fixed, government guided, and market regulated. Government-fixed and government-guided pricing applies to pharmaceuticals listed in the pharmaceutical directory of the national basic medical insurance and some special pharmaceuticals (e.g., narcotics, psychotropic drugs, immunomodulators, contraceptives).

Pricing policies differ among brand-name drugs and generic drugs, new drugs, high-quality drugs, and ordinary drugs. The government recently introduced strict price controls on a wide range of pharmaceutical products, an action that is putting pressure on the profit margins of domestic producers. The government intervened and set prices on 32 occasions between 1998 and 2013. Each time, the average price reduction across therapeutic categories was 20%. These cuts have had a significant impact on the Chinese pharmaceutical industry. From 2003 to 2006, the average profit percentage in the pharmaceutical industry decreased from 9.7% to 6.3%.[15] Also, the number of drugs subject to price controls rose from roughly 1500 to 2700 during this decade (1900 products were regulated by central government and 800 by local governments). By 2013, these drugs represented only about 20% of all medicines, but 60% of the value of all drugs sold. On May 4, 2015, Chinese National Development and Reform Commission (NDRC) announced that the government will abandon price controls on most (about 2700) drugs, instead the prices will be decided by the market starting from June 1, 2015.

According to the 2013 Annual China Pharmaceutical Industry Hundred List released by the China Food and Drug Administration (CFDA), the Guangzhou Pharmaceutical Group Co. Ltd., Tianjin

Table 1: China's top pharmaceutical companies in 2013

Rank	Pharmaceutical Companies
1	Guangzhou Pharmaceutical Holdings Co. Ltd
2	Tianjin Pharmaceutical Holdings Co. Ltd
3	Shanghai Pharmaceutical Holdings Co. Ltd
4	North China Pharmaceutical Group Co. Ltd
5	Harbin Pharmaceutical Group Holding Co. Ltd
6	Xiuzheng Pharmaceutical Co. Ltd
7	Shijiazhuang Pharmaceutical Group Co. Ltd
8	Buchang Pharmaceutical Co. Ltd
9	Kangmei Pharmaceutical Co. Ltd
10	Tianjin Tianshili Group Co. Ltd

Pharmaceutical Group Co. Ltd., and Shanghai Pharmaceutical Group Co. Ltd. were the three most profitable pharmaceutical companies (Table 1). The market concentration of the top 100 enterprises reached 45.1%. In January 2013, the Ministry of Finance, the National Development and Reform Commission (NDRC), and 12 other departments jointly issued guidelines for accelerating mergers and reorganization of enterprises in key industries. Thus, by 2015, the top 100 companies in pharmaceutical industry sales will account for more than 50% of all of the industry's sales.[16]

TCM has more than 2000 years of history and is well known as the quintessence of Chinese culture. It has made indelible contributions to the well-being of the Chinese people. Since 1949, the development of TCM has consistently been a health policy priority in China. During the 1990s, the government issued one of its most important health care reform policies. It stressed that high-quality health services should be based on the integration of TCM and western medicine. During the last six decades, TCM has experienced unprecedented growth—from only four TCM hospitals nationwide with an average of 30 beds per hospital in 1950 to 3590 TCM hospitals with a total of 686,793 beds in 2013.[17]

5. Overview of pharmacy practice and key pharmaceutical sectors

Significant changes have occurred in the Chinese pharmaceutical profession during the past few decades.[18] The philosophy of pharmaceutical care was first introduced in China during the mid-1990s. It stated that patient-centered services should be provided by pharmacists for the purpose of improving the rational use of medications and ultimately enhancing the quality of patients' lives.[14]

China has two pharmacist qualification systems. The first is a professional qualification system. Here, only pharmaceutical professionals who pass the national pharmacist licensing examination can obtain a Licensed Pharmacist Certificate, register with a provincial regulatory authority, and work in institutions where medicines are manufactured, distributed, or used. The minimum qualifications required to apply for the licensed pharmacist qualification examination are a secondary technical school diploma and a major in pharmacy or a related discipline (e.g., medicine, chemistry, biology, nursing). The current minimum qualifications for registration as a pharmacist are low, and future adjustment is anticipated.[19] Meanwhile, depending on the academic background, a certain amount of work experience is also needed. Currently, people with secondary, tertiary, bachelor's, or master's degrees can apply for the examination after 7, 5, 3, or 1 year(s) of experience, respectively. No work experience is required for candidates with doctorate degrees.[20] The CFDA and the Ministry of Human Resources and Social Security are the governing bodies charged with overseeing the licensing examinations. They are also responsible for registration and mandatory continuing education of licensed pharmacists.

The second pharmacist qualification system is a specialized system under which a pharmaceutical specialist is assigned a specific title (e.g., chief pharmacist, associate chief pharmacist, pharmacist in-charge, pharmacist, assistant pharmacist) according to his or her educational background, work experience, and professional skills. These pharmacists work mainly in medical institutions and are overseen by China's MoH. At present, passing the licensure examination is not mandatory for pharmacists in medical institutions. As a result, the vast majority of these pharmacists (unlike licensed pharmacists) have specialized qualifications. For example, 345,000 pharmacists worked in Chinese medical institutions at the end of 2010. Among them, only 48,000 were licensed.[21] There are also more than 4-million pharmacy technicians working in China's community pharmacies.[22] The role of the pharmacy technician requires a high school diploma or equivalent and some training and certification at the college level, which takes 3–6 months to complete. Under the direct supervision of a pharmacist, pharmacy technicians help dispense prescription medications and perform other administrative duties in community pharmacies.

6. Drug-related and pharmacy-related regulations, policies, and ethics

China attaches great importance to the building of a legal system for drug safety supervision. The Drug Administration Law was issued by the National People's Congress in 1984. For the first time, the research, production, selling, and use of drugs were covered by legal stipulations, and the legal responsibility for the production and sale of counterfeit and inferior drugs was defined. Later, a revised version of the legislation came into effect—the 2001 Drug Administration Law. The law aimed to "strengthen drug regulation, ensure drug quality and safety for human beings, and protect the health of people and their legitimate rights and interests in the use of drugs." Under the 2001 Drug Administration Law, licensing authority is vested in the CFDA. The licensing scheme consists of nine levels,[23] as follows:

1. A prospective pharmaceutical product manufacturer must obtain a manufacturer's license from a provincial-level branch of the CFDA by demonstrating that it has appropriate facilities, levels of staff, and other arrangements for quality control.

2. A prospective new drug cannot be tested clinically in humans until the sponsor has submitted the data and related samples from the laboratory stages of research and convinced the CFDA to grant it a clinical test certificate.

3. A new drug certificate (NDC) may be obtained only after the sponsor has demonstrated that its prospective new drug successfully passed laboratory and clinical tests, according to which safety and efficacy are assumed. The CFDA issues the NDC after verifying this process and the test data.

4. A prospective manufacturer must also obtain a production permit number from the CFDA before beginning to manufacture a new drug or other drugs regulated by national standards.

5. A prospective drug wholesaler must obtain a pharmaceutical trader's license from a branch of the CFDA at the provincial level. A prospective drug retailer must do so at the county level. Among other requirements, licensing is conditioned upon having appropriate staff, facilities, and management systems.

6. Before making medicinal preparations for patients, a medical organization must obtain prior approval from the health authority at the provincial level. It must also obtain a dispensing permit issued by a branch of the CFDA at the same level. To ensure quality, licensing is conditioned on the organization's facilities, management systems, and sanitation, among other requirements.

7. Drugs cannot be imported into China without a Registration Certificate for Imported Drugs (RCID). For an RCID to be issued, prospective importers generally must satisfy the CFDA criteria for safety and efficacy. They may be exempt, however, if the drug is for emergency hospital use or individual use. Also, before each importation, the importer must obtain customs clearance for the imported drug from an affiliate of the CFDA at the port designated for their drugs to enter China. The 2001 Drug Administration Law no longer imposes compulsory testing on imported drugs unless they are entering China for the first time. However, a pharmaceutical testing institution appointed by an affiliate of the CFDA will carry out selective testing on imported drugs after they enter the Chinese market.

8. Three pharmaceutical types—biological products stipulated by the CFDA, drugs being sold for the first time in China, and other drugs stipulated by the State Council—must pass tests conducted by appointed institutions before being imported or marketed. This compulsory testing ("a test pass license") is a de facto licensing requirement.

9. No over-the-counter drug can be advertised in China unless the sponsor obtains an advertising license from a branch of the CFDA at the provincial level and an advertising permit from a branch of the State Industry and Commerce Administration at the county level or above. Only medicinal and pharmaceutical journals, jointly authorized by the Health Authority under the State Council and the CFDA, can carry advertisements for prescription-only drugs.[23]

The Drug Administration Law stipulates that a drug manufacturer or distributor shall have qualified pharmaceutical professionals for drug manufacturing or distribution. The Provisional Regulations on Licensed Pharmacist Qualification System promulgated in 1994 and the

Provisional Regulations on Licensed Pharmacist of Chinese Medicine Qualification System promulgated in 1995 indicated that the Licensed Pharmacist Qualification System should be carried out comprehensively. A series of supporting regulations and regulatory documents addressing examination, registration, and continuing education were published thereafter. The Provisional Regulations on Licensed Pharmacist Qualification System was revised in 1999. The national unified syllabus, examination, registration, and management were enforced accordingly.[20]

7. Core pharmacy practices

7.1 Hospital pharmacy

To improve the level of the rational clinical use of drugs and change the way health care is delivered and paid for in China, the MoH of China has been issuing a series of new policies. They address the accreditation of tertiary hospitals and antimicrobial use in hospitals.[24] They also mandate that clinical pharmacy services be integrated into China's hospitals. Internationally, the development of clinical pharmacy services has expanded the role of the pharmacist from being product focused to being patient focused.[25,26] This new role aimed to provide patient-focused care and promote the high-quality, rational use of medications. In 2011, the MoH issued a policy that all secondary hospitals should have three full-time clinical pharmacists and all tertiary hospitals should have five.[27]

Antimicrobial stewardship has provided a platform for facilitating clinical pharmacy services in China because antimicrobial resistance is of major concern.[28,29] During 1999–2001, the prevalence of resistance among hospital-acquired *Staphylococcus aureus* infections was 77%,[28] and that of *Streptococcus pneumoniae* was more than 80% and was on the rise.[29] Accordingly, the MoH released a series of campaigns and policies stating that all secondary and tertiary hospitals should have clinical pharmacists trained in infectious diseases.[24] These trained pharmacists must be able to give guidance and approval for restricted antimicrobial use.[24,30] This highlights the important contribution of clinical pharmacy services to antimicrobial control as per international practices.[31]

By the end of 2012, China was reported to have 1624 tertiary hospitals and 6566 secondary hospitals, which would require at least 27,818 clinical pharmacists to meet the policy requirements of the MoH. With only 15 clinical pharmacists graduating from one of the country's largest courses in 2007 and new courses introduced only recently, a focus on educating pharmacists and pharmacy support staff seems vital. It therefore seems inevitable that there will be a large lag time before these MoH goals are reached and clinical pharmacy services are a routine part of China's hospital systems.[32]

7.2 Industrial pharmacy

China has established a complete pharmaceutical industry chain and has become one of the largest pharmaceutical producers in the world. The Chinese pharmaceutical industry has grown at an annual rate of 16.72% since 1978. The industry is still small-scale, however, with a scattered geographical layout, duplicated production processes, and outdated manufacturing technology and management structures. The Chinese pharmaceutical industry also has a low market concentration and weak international trading competitiveness coupled with a lack of patented domestically developed pharmaceuticals.[14]

Currently, China is home to 4875 drug companies, decreasing from more than 5000 in 2004 according to government figures. The number is expected to drop further. As of 2013, China was the world's third largest market for medications, and in 2015 it is predicted to become the second largest. The products of China's domestic companies account for 70% of the market, and the top 10 companies account for about 20%, according to Business China. In contrast, the top 10 companies in most developed countries control about half the market. Since June 30, 2004, the CFDA has been closing manufacturers that do not meet the new GMP standards. Foreign players account for 10–20% of overall sales, depending on the types of medicines and ventures included in the count. But sales at the top-tier Chinese companies are growing faster than those at western companies, according to IMS Health, Inc.[33]

The pharmaceutical market in China is dominated by generic drugs. That industry operates with basic technology and simple production methods. Domestic pharmaceuticals are not as technologically advanced as western products but nonetheless occupy approximately 70% of the market in China.[34] Domestic companies are mainly government owned and are fraught with overproduction and losses. The Chinese government has begun consolidating and upgrading the industry in an effort to compete with foreign corporations.

It is estimated that most hospitals derive 25–60% of their revenue from prescription sales. Although hospitals remain the main outlets for distributing pharmaceuticals in China, this situation will change with the separation of hospital pharmacies from health care services and with the growing number of retail pharmacy outlets. These outlets are expected to proliferate once the government introduces its system to classify drugs as "over-the-counter." The government is now encouraging the development of chain drug stores, but the full effect might not be seen for several years.[34]

7.3 Community pharmacies

Community pharmacies are becoming increasingly recognized in many parts of the world as a source of professional medical advice.[35,36] This is also occurring in China, where community pharmacies have emerged as a source of primary health care.[37] To establish and operate a pharmacy in China, the number of permanent residents, terrain, transportation, and practical needs of the locality must be taken into consideration. According to the Provisions for Supervision of Drug Distribution adopted by the CFDA in 2006, ownership of a pharmacy is not restricted to pharmacists,[38] provided that a pharmaceutical professional is present when medications are distributed and pharmaceutical care services are offered.[39] The Drug

Administration Law of the People's Republic of China, revised in 2001, stipulates that community pharmacies must have legally qualified pharmaceutical professionals, including pharmacists and pharmacy technicians. This law is not strictly enforced, however, and most pharmacies sell medications without the presence of a pharmaceutical professional. As a result, rules concerning the operation and ownership of community pharmacies were tightened in early 2012. According to this 12th Five-Year Plan on Drug Safety released by the State Council,[40] newly opened community pharmacies must be staffed by licensed pharmacists during business hours to ensure the quality of medications and services. Also, by 2015, all community pharmacies must be owned by licensed pharmacists.

After the latest round of health care reforms in 2009, community pharmacies have come to play a significantly more important role in China. In 2009, the number of community pharmacies reached nearly 388,000, a 6.1% increase from the previous year. This increase was primarily a result of the establishment of pharmacy chains, which accounted for 35% of pharmacies in 2009, while the number of independent pharmacies decreased.[22] Each community pharmacy in China caters to an average of 3532 people. In contrast, the number of licensed pharmacists was only 185,692 in 2010, equivalent to approximately 7380 people per licensed pharmacist, which is much higher than in the United States, Canada, and other developed countries.[41–43] There is a lack of pharmacists in China. This shortage is worse in rural areas, which suffer from chronic understaffing in both the hospital and community pharmacy sectors. In 2010, a total of 388,000 pharmacists (licensed pharmacists and pharmaceutical specialists) were working in a variety of settings. This number translates to approximately 0.29 pharmacists per 1000 people, lower than that in India and Brazil.[18] A community pharmacist must register in a provincial pharmacists' association to work. Two professional societies represent all Chinese pharmacists in community pharmacies: the Chinese Pharmaceutical Association (CPA; run by the Ministry of Civil Affairs) and the China Licensed Pharmacist Association (run by the CFDA).

Community pharmacies are a profitable business in China. From 1978 until 2009, the average annual medication sales growth in China was 20%, reaching USD 21.8 billion in 2009.[22] Hospitals, however, remain the main outlets for medication distribution in China, with more than 19,000 hospital pharmacies accounting for 74% of the total medication sales in 2009.[14] This situation is changing because the government is encouraging the establishment of community pharmacies that are not associated with hospitals. Unlike many developed countries, no official data on community pharmacist salaries are available because of the lack of a national survey of Chinese pharmacists.

Both prescription and nonprescription medicines can be sold in community pharmacies, with the exception of narcotic drugs, some psychotropic substances, abortion drugs, anabolic steroids, peptide hormones, chemical products used in the production of narcotics, radiopharmaceuticals, and vaccines. These products can be prescribed and dispensed only in designated medical institutions. Current regulations state that prescription medications cannot be sold without a medical prescription.[44] Because of the shortage of pharmacists and the profit-driven behavior of some retailers, the illegal sale of prescription medications (e.g., antibiotics) is common in China, especially in rural areas.[45]

7.4 Medication marketing and promotion

China uses the 2001 Drug Administration Law to regulate medicine promotion, Similar to the Food and Drug Administration and Federal Trade Commission in the United States, on the national level in China, the CFDA and the State Administration for Industry and Commerce (SAIC) have concurrent jurisdiction over drug promotion, although SAIC often defers to CFDA's greater scientific and pharmaceutical expertise. On the provincial level, the regulatory authorities are the provincial food and drug administrations and the local administrations for industry and commerce.[46]

Regulation of drug promotion is currently dichotomous. The government closely oversees drug advertisements with clear rules on form and content and with established penalties for violations. In contrast, it largely ignores nonadvertising drug promotion. There are no regulations or standards for such promotion other than the general consumer protection requirement that the promotion not be false or misleading. Violations are punished with limited administrative penalties.[46]

Drug promotion presents a challenging dilemma for regulatory authorities. On one hand, advertising and promotion are important sources of drug information. Physicians report that they often use promotion as a source of information about new drugs—a reliance that increases as their medical careers progress. In developing countries, drug promotion is particularly crucial. Drug company sales representatives are often the most important source of information about new medicines. Studies have found that physicians rely heavily on industry-based sources of information. On the other hand, there are safety, public health, and economic concerns over inappropriate promotion of drug use. Studies have shown that heavy promotion of new drugs can lead to inappropriate prescribing and overprescribing of drugs, causing serious safety concerns. The promotion of newer, more expensive drugs can also lead to the displacement of older, less costly drugs with no evidence that the newer drugs are more effective.[46]

Medical representatives are salespeople employed by pharmaceutical companies to persuade doctors to prescribe their drugs to patients. A medical representative is, above all, a provider of information to make doctors and other medical professionals more knowledgeable. Medical representatives offer new products, devices, and drugs designed to cure or address a multitude of illnesses and ailments. Without medical representatives, doctors would not become aware of new advancements in treatments, more effective drugs, and devices that provide enhanced treatment opportunities.

Medical representatives are usually assigned a geographical territory in which they operate. This can be as small as a few city blocks and as large as a country. A medical representative's job description may include the following: develop and manage an assigned territory with the goal of maximizing sales; achieve quarterly and annual sales goals, meet target call goals with a focus on top customers, host product presentations to designated customers, understand and address both business and scientific needs of health care professionals, and engage in meaningful dialogue with customers. The representatives are under intense competitive pressure to "out-do" other drug companies with similar products. Beyond meeting at doctors' offices or during leisure time, the symposium circuit allows representatives to discuss doctors' preferences. It also allows a drug researcher to present a novel drug to a new audience.[47]

8. Special pharmacy-related services

Prior to 1990, the roles of pharmacists in hospital and community pharmacies mainly involved supplying and dispensing medications, bulk compounding, administrative functions, and staff supervision and management. Since then, numerous developments have taken place in the various aspects of pharmaceutical education, legislation, and practice that encompass industry, hospitals, and communities.[48] The introduction and acceptance of clinical pharmacy and pharmaceutical patient care in the practice of pharmacy in China during the 1990s led some pharmacists to become involved in related professional activities, such as drug information services and patient medication counseling.[49]

The field of clinical pharmacy has grown rapidly since introduction of the Temporary Regulations of Pharmacy Administration for Medical Institutions in 2002. At that time, the government required all hospitals to develop clinical pharmacy programs to promote appropriate drug use and take responsibility for helping to establish patient care services in community pharmacy settings.[27] In January 2006, the MoH established 1-year clinical pharmacy training programs with both didactic and experiential components for practicing pharmacists.[50] To date, however, no standard working model for clinical pharmacists has been developed in China. This deficiency is because the clinical pharmacist system has only recently been established, and the pilot program for training clinical pharmacists has just been completed.[51]

The implementation of pharmaceutical care in Chinese hospital pharmacies continues to expand. Pharmaceutical care provision as part of routine community pharmacy practice, however, has not been a priority for a sector that is facing many challenges, including a shortage of pharmacists, lack of professional skills, lack of reimbursement systems for health care services, and poor public awareness of pharmacists.[52] The challenge of providing pharmaceutical care has led pharmacists to change their practices in community settings. Pharmacists from Shanghai Changhai Hospital, for example, were the first to extend pharmaceutical care from hospital patients alone to community residents. This expansion resulted in increased medication education across all levels and an expanded scope for pharmaceutical care.[53] The role of the community pharmacist in primary care has undergone significant changes, with a greater emphasis on providing patient-centered care and documenting health care services, including counseling patients, profiling medications, and performing functions other than dispensing medicines.[12]

9. Pharmacy education

Statistics from late 2012 showed that 703 higher education pharmaceutical institutions existed in China (including universities and colleges), with 21 pharmacy-related specialties offering more than 700 programs. Among these institutions, 41 were selected to obtain profile statistics on their undergraduates. The data showed that 49,854 state-plan undergraduate students were enrolled in 162 programs.[54] Currently, 97 universities and colleges offer TCM programs in China, training students in knowledge and experimental skills, including examination of TCM documents and literature, pharmaceutical analysis, Chinese medicine, acupuncture, tuina (a form of massage), Chinese pharmacology, and pharmacognosy.[55]

Traditionally, pharmacy education has focused on drug products and has emphasized chemistry, pharmaceutics, and the control and regulation of drug product delivery systems.[56] The majority of pharmacy programs in China (generally 4 years in length) are basically product-oriented rather than patient-oriented.[9] The dramatically changing health care delivery system and the increasingly prominent role of community pharmacies in primary health care are shifting focus to a broader role for pharmacists.[57] This fundamental paradigm shift is reinforcing the idea that pharmacists can help improve patients' health-related quality of life rather than simply providing products. This idea highlights the importance of shifting the emphasis of pharmacy education from the product to the patient.[58]

The education that pharmacy students currently receive in China encompasses the following three major areas: (1) general education (1 year), including English, mathematics, physics, chemistry, and biological sciences; (2) didactic pharmaceutical education (2.5 years or more), composed of basic pharmaceutical sciences such as pharmacology, pharmaceutics, pharmaceutical analysis, pharmaceutical chemistry, pharmacy administration; and (3) experiential education (less than 6 months), comprising the experience gained by working in a pharmaceutical practice setting, usually a drug-manufacturing enterprise. After graduating, most pharmacy graduates work in hospitals or industry. Of the approximately 300,000 pharmacy school graduates during 1949–1998 in China, a total of 52% worked in hospital pharmacies, 21% in the pharmaceutical industry, and 9% for wholesale distributors or in community pharmacies during their first year after graduation.[59]

The continuous growth of the pharmaceutical profession inevitably requires expansion and modernization, justifying the need for a new pharmacy program and curriculum that can produce a more skilled workforce. Clinical pharmacy education in China was developed only recently, with the West China School of Pharmacy at Sichuan University offering the first 5-year clinical pharmacy BS degree during 1989–1999.[60] Since 2000, the Ministry of

Education has allowed only pharmaceutical sciences as a first-level discipline for BS degrees.[61] Students wishing to study clinical pharmacy at the bachelor's level may select clinical pharmacy—but only as a second level of study under pharmaceutical sciences. Since 2008, some universities, such as China Pharmaceutical University, have been allowed to once again offer BS, MS, and PhD degrees in clinical pharmacy (3–7 years in length).[50] As of 2012, a total of 24 universities were allowed to offer a first-level, 5-year BS degree in clinical pharmacy.[54] Another 14 universities have offered clinical pharmacy MS and PhD programs (3–7 years in length).[60] Unlike the curricula for pharmacy and other medical courses, a standardized curriculum for clinical pharmacy has not yet been established.[50] To establish a uniform, highly qualified model with which to train clinical pharmacists, the MoH is considering a proposal for an entry-level professional degree of Doctor in Clinical Pharmacy, similar to the Doctor of Pharmacy (PharmD) degree in the United States. Introduction of the PharmD program in 2004, pioneered in China by Sichuan University, Chengdu, is a welcome development.[50]

For the 5-year BS in Clinical Pharmacy program at China Pharmaceutical University, students spend the first 2 years studying basic sciences (i.e., biology and chemistry). Beginning at the first semester of the third year, students study core subjects, including diagnostic basics, biostatistics, internal medicine, surgery, gynecology, pediatrics, clinical pharmacology, and clinical therapeutics. During the final (fourth) year of undergraduate study and under the supervision of both a physician and a clinical pharmacist, students become involved in hospital pharmacy practice activities. They go on patient care rounds and learn about medication order reviews, therapeutic drug monitoring, supplying drug information to patients, and the roles of other health care practitioners in the hospital. Upon graduation, students must have completed their core courses, laboratory courses, pharmacy practical examinations, and thesis.[62] The curricula for the postgraduate MS in Clinical Pharmacy vary widely across schools that offer this degree. Students pursuing a Clinical Pharmacy PhD must spend a significant portion of their program engaged in laboratory research.[60]

10. Achievements in pharmacy practice

10.1 Hospital pharmacy services

In 2009, the Chinese government implemented health care reform with the aim to ensure accessible and affordable health services for all people by 2020.[63] This reform focuses on public hospitals, which deliver more than 90% of China's inpatient and outpatient services. Since the economic reform in 1985, the government subsidies to public hospitals gradually dropped. It is estimated that 90% of public hospitals' revenue is currently generated directly from selling prescription medication, medical tests, and equipment.[64,65] Medications alone accounted for more than 50% of this revenue,[66] a finding that led to a perception of inappropriate prescribing. Reynolds and McKee claimed that two financial incentives existed in China to support that perception: "One was created by pharmaceutical companies, who sometimes arrange to split profits with prescribers, illegally and covertly, while the other emanated from all health providers, which are entitled to make a 15% profit on sales to fund services".[67] As a result, overprescribing has become a concern in the context of China's increasing health care expenditures.[63]

China's MoH conducted a pilot program to introduce clinical pharmacists in 50 hospitals during 2005–2008. In 2011, the MoH issued the Regulation of Pharmacy Management in Medical Institutions,[27] according to which all secondary hospitals should have three full-time clinical pharmacists and tertiary hospitals should have five, and pharmacists should make up no less than 8% of the total medical professionals in a hospital.

10.2 Community pharmacy services

Community pharmacists in China typically compound and dispense medications by following the prescriptions issued by clinical physicians, dentists, or other authorized medical practitioners, (e.g., public health physicians, radiologists). In this role, pharmacists act as skilled intermediaries between physicians and patients, ensuring the safe and effective use of medications. The Fourth Chinese National Health Care Survey revealed a high prevalence of self-medication in China that had increased from 36% in 2003 to 70% in 2008. The most common reason for self-medication in China was that the people thought they knew enough to take care of themselves. In particular, self-perceived illness status, economic circumstances, and education had a positive association with the probability of self-medication. These data reinforce the responsibility of community pharmacies and pharmacists to protect patients from drug-related problems when self-medicating.

Chinese pharmacists have indicated a willingness to implement pharmaceutical care. However, they are restricted by limited knowledge and skills in this field and by underdeveloped pharmacy education. In China, patients do not pay fees for the medications dispensed to them, and current insurance programs do not pay pharmacists for health care services. Under such circumstances, some community pharmacies have set fees for professional services delivered outside their usual and customary dispensing activities to generate enough revenue to cover the costs of employing qualified pharmacists. This lack of reimbursement reduces the willingness of pharmacists to offer high-quality dispensing and counseling services.

In 2003, based on the "Guidelines for Good Pharmacy Practice (GPP)" and "GPP in Developing Countries" drafted by the International Pharmaceutical Federation (2014), the China Nonprescription Medicines Association (CNMA) adopted the first edition of GPP in China as a recommended standard for pharmacy practice in community pharmacies.[68] A revised version of this document was approved by the CNMA in 2007.[69] The GPP aimed to promote health, achieve sufficient supplies of medicines and medical devices, monitor patient self-care, and improve prescription and medicine use through the actions of pharmacists in community pharmacy settings. This document details the role of pharmacists in community pharmacy services and describes pharmaceutical care as a set of activities that must be developed by pharmacists. To date, 86 retail pharmacies have achieved GPP certification. The CNMA is planning to consult with the government to institutionalize the GPP system in the near future.[68]

11. Challenges in pharmacy practice

Although the medical care system and the health of Chinese citizens have improved since the economic and political reforms of the late 1970s,[63] the disparity between urban and rural areas and among regions has increased, and health care expenditures have grown.[70] Facing these challenges, in 2009 China unveiled a health care reform plan. With the primary health care system as its foundation and focus,[71] this plan would enable residents to access primary health care for simple health problems instead of seeking help at hospitals. Community pharmacies, with their convenient locations and easy accessibility, were identified as having a critical role in ensuring that more people in China had access to health services. As a result, the health care reform plan highlighted the responsibilities of community pharmacies and pharmacists in providing primary health care.[72]

According to the health care reform blueprint (2009), China was to invest USD 124 billion on health care from 2009 to 2011. The reforms focused on five key issues: (1) facilitating broad coverage of basic medical insurance, (2) setting up a national system for essential medicines covered by the medical insurance system, (3) expanding the network of local-level clinics, (4) improving the basic public health system, and (5) initiating a pilot reform of public hospital operations.[73] Since the announcement of these reforms, a series of regulations and guidelines have been released, including those that addressed the following: (1) construction of county hospitals, health centers, community health service centers, and village clinics; (2) the price of essential medicines; (3) the reform of public hospitals in 16 pilot cities; and (4) China's drug distribution industry (for 2011–2015).[74] These guidelines particularly emphasized pharmacists' responsibilities for providing low-cost medicines and promoting appropriate use of medications in both hospital and community pharmacy settings.

12. Recommendations: the way forward

Following the initial actions, a number of activities must be initiated to further develop pharmacy services in China.

12.1 Enactment of the Chinese pharmacist law

Following introduction of the provisional regulations of the Licensed Pharmacist Qualification System in 1994 and their revision in 1999 by the Ministry of Personnel and State Drug Administration, the number of licensed pharmacists in China has increased sharply from

98,310 in 2003 to 185,692 in 2010. With licensed pharmacists playing an increasingly important role in patient care, the legal and professional obligations of licensed pharmacists should be stipulated in law. To date, no such laws are currently in place in China, thereby hindering the development of pharmacists' skills for providing clinical pharmacy and pharmaceutical care services. Also, there are many types of pharmacists in China, including licensed pharmacists in industry, hospitals, and community pharmacies and pharmacists in medical institutions. Their responsibilities, as defined in the CFDA regulations,[75] do not include the duty to maintain and properly care for patients. Thus, the not-yet-enacted Chinese Pharmacist Law, which clearly specifies the provision of patient care services as one of the principal duties of pharmacists, must be passed to promote appropriate advice on the use of medications by all citizens. The Chinese Pharmacist Law has already been drafted by the MoH and the CFDA. It should be implemented in the near future.

12.2 Development of standards for pharmaceutical care activities

The adoption of standards for conducting pharmaceutical care activities is an important step toward improving patient care throughout the nation. Pharmaceutical organizations, government, universities, and other health care stakeholders should work together in developing nationally mandated standards to ensure quality pharmaceutical care practices in both hospital and community settings. Training programs delivered by health departments are also needed to ensure that the standards are correctly implemented by all pharmacists.

12.3 Development of the pharmacy workforce

Pharmacists are expected to become more involved in pharmaceutical care in the near future. Hence, pharmacist development must be an academic and practical priority to ensure an adequate supply of high-quality pharmacists. In February 2011, the MoH issued the Long-Term Medical and Health Personnel Development Plan (2011–2020),[76] which projects that the number of Chinese pharmacists will reach 550,000 by 2015 and 850,000 by 2020. The training of more pharmacy technicians to perform the traditional duties of pharmacists is also critical for pharmacy education. This step could allow more time for pharmacists to play a caring, advisory role in patient care.

12.4 Increasing public awareness of pharmacists

In line with the CFDA program to increase public awareness of health care issues, the CPA carried out a "Pharmacist on Your Side" campaign.[77] That campaign continued efforts to increase public awareness about the vital role of pharmacists in primary health care teams beyond simply dispensing medications. Through increased awareness of the potential contribution of pharmacists to the Chinese health care system, more opportunities for educating pharmacists would be made available to satisfy the vast needs of the country.

12.5 Pharmacy services reimbursement

The lack of third-party reimbursement for dispensing and advancing patient services provided by pharmacists is a barrier that must be addressed. To foster greater awareness of the value of pharmacist services and to ensure the long-term success of pharmaceutical care, policymakers need to focus more attention on obtaining compensation for community pharmacy services. Ultimately, pharmacists will be able to enhance their revenues by increasing the array of patient care services, exploring innovative markets for pharmaceutical care services, and continuing to improve their reimbursement rates from third-party payers (including private insurance companies, government programs such as the New Cooperative Medical Scheme in rural areas, and basic medical security for urban residents).[78] Introducing patient contributions toward advanced pharmaceutical care services is another potential policy option.

13. Conclusions

Significant progress has been made in the development of various pharmacy settings in China during the past several decades. Despite this achievement, the country faces new challenges in an evolving health care system. A number of developments must be undertaken to continue progress, including enactment of the Chinese Pharmacist Law, development of standards for pharmaceutical patient care services, development of a pharmacy workforce, increased public awareness about the value of pharmacists, encouraging professional organization involvement in advancing the pharmacy profession, and proper remuneration for care provision. In the future, Chinese pharmacists are expected to become an integral part of the health care system. In doing so, they can serve the health care needs of the population, especially in community and hospital pharmacy settings.

14. Lessons learned/points to remember

- A new goal was set in China to prepare pharmacy professionals to provide pharmaceutical care. The clinical pharmacy field thus has grown since 2002, when the government required all hospitals to develop clinical pharmacy programs to address drug-related problems and to promote rational drug use in hospitals, which is the core of pharmaceutical care in China.
- Hospital pharmacy practice is changing from being "drug centered" to "patient centered", and the primary focus for hospital pharmacy is changing from drug supply to pharmaceutical care. Thus, the pharmacist's activities are changing from drug dispensing and compounding to rational drug use and patient care.
- There is a lack of skilled professionals in pharmacy practice to carry out pharmaceutical care services. The social status of pharmacists in China has been given little attention up to now.

References

1. The Bureau of Statistic. Available from: http://www.stats.gov.cn/tjsj/ [accessed 31.05.14].
2. Yang G, Wang Y, Zeng Y, Gao GF, Liang X, Zhou M, et al. Rapid health transition in China, 1990–2010: findings from the Global Burden of Disease Study 2010. *Lancet* 2013;**381**(9882):1987–2015.
3. The State Council. Medical and Health Services in China. Available from: http://news.xinhuanet.com/english/bilingual/2012-12/26/c_132064944.htm [accessed 31.05.14].
4. The CDC. Addressing Noncommunicable Diseases in China. Available from: http://www.cdc.gov/globalhealth/stories/ncd_china.htm [accessed 31.05.14].
5. Lian Z, Xie Y, Lu Y, Huang D, Shi H. Trends in the major causes of death in China, 1982–2010. *Chin Med J* 2014;**127**(4):777–81.
6. The State Council. White paper: medical and health services in China. Available from: http://www.china.org.cn/chinese/2012-12/27/content_27526876.htm [accessed 10.05.14].
7. World Bank. Toward a healthy and harmonious life in China: stemming the rising tide of non-communicable diseases. Available from: http://www.worldbank.org/content/dam/Worldbank/document/NCD_report_en.pdf. [accessed 18.06.14].
8. Chen ZM. The development of higher pharmaceutical education in China's reform. *Am J Pharm Educ* 1998;**62**:72–5.
9. Xu J, Yang Y. Traditional Chinese medicine in the Chinese health care system. *Health Policy* 2009;**90**(2–3):133–9.
10. Hesketh T, Zhu WX. Health in China. Traditional Chinese medicine: one country, two systems. *BMJ* 1997;**315**:115–7.
11. Wang H, Chen L, Lau A. Pharmacy practice and education in the People's Republic of China. *Ann Pharmacother* 1993;**27**:1278–82.
12. China Nonprescription Medicine Association. *Blue paper: the industrial development of Chinese nonprescription medicine*. 1st ed. Beijing: Chemical Industry Press; 2011. ISBN: 9787122109101.
13. Yu X, Li C, Shi Y, Yu M. Pharmaceutical supply chain in China: current issues and implications for health system reform. *Health Policy* 2010;**97**:8–15.
14. Sun Q, Santoro MA, Meng Q, Liu C, Eggleston K. Pharmaceutical policy in China. *Health Aff* 2008;**27**:1042–50.
15. Wang Ziyan. China's pharmaceutical price policies and practices [dissertation], 2007.
16. Medicine economic news. China's top 100 pharmaceutical companies in 2013. Available from: http://web.yyjjb.com:8080/html/2014-05/23/content_209208.htm [accessed 10.05.14].
17. Shen JJ, Wang Y, Lin F, Lu J, Moseley CB, Sun M, et al. Trends of increase in western medical services in traditional medicine hospitals in China. *BMC Health Serv Res* 2011;**11**:212.
18. World Health Organization. WHO human resources for health. Available from: http://apps.who.int/gho/indicatorregistry/App_Main/view_indicator.aspx?iid=320 [accessed 14.06.14].
19. Huang SX. Licensed pharmacist system in China. *Asian J Soc Pharm* 2007;**2**(2):41–4.
20. An FD, Yu BY. The status and prospects of the licensed pharmacist qualification system in China. *Eur J Bus Manage* 2011;**5**:1–4.
21. State Council. *White paper: status quo of drug supervision in China*. 1st ed. Beijing: Foreign Languages Press; 2008. ISBN: 9787119052649.
22. Ministry of Commerce. The "twelfth five" national plan for development of pharmaceutical distribution industry. Available from: http://henan.mofcom.gov.cn/aarticle/sjdixiansw/201106/20110607586364.html [accessed 14.06.14].
23. Zhang Q. The Chinese regulatory licensing regime for pharmaceutical products: a law and economics analysis. *Mich Telecommun Technol Law Rev* 2009;**15**:417–52.
24. Ministry of Health. Policy on the clinical use of antimicrobials. Available from: http://www.moh.gov.cn/mohyzs/s3584/201205/54645.shtml [accessed 03.06.14].
25. Nissen L. Current status of pharmacist influences on prescribing of medicines. *Am J Health Syst Pharm* 2009;**66**:S29–34.

26. Anderson S. The state of the world's pharmacy: a portrait of the pharmacy profession. *J Interprof Care* 2002;**16**:391–404.
27. Ministry of Health. Regulations of pharmacy administration for medical institutions. Available from: http://www.moh.gov.cn/mohyzs/s3585/201103/51113.shtml [accessed 03.06.14].
28. Zhang R, Eggleston K, Rotimi V, Zeckhauser RJ. Antibiotic resistance as a global threat: evidence from China, Kuwait and the United States. *Global Health* 2006;**2**:6.
29. Yao K, Yang Y. Streptococcus pneumoniae diseases in Chinese children: past, present and future. *Vaccine* 2008;**26**:4425–33.
30. Ministry of Health. Introduction to "Policy on the clinical use of antimicrobials" and management on antimicrobial stewardship. Available from: http://www.moh.gov.cn/mohyzs/s3586/201205/54646.shtml [accessed 03.06.14].
31. Paskovaty A, Pflomm JM, Myke N, Seo SK. A multidisciplinary approach to antimicrobial stewardship: evolution into the 21st century. *Int J Antimicrob Agents* 2005;**25**:1–10.
32. Penm J. Development of clinical pharmacy services in China. Available from: http://sydney.edu.au/china_studies_centre/china_express/issue_4/features/Development-of-clinical-pharmacy-services-in-China.shtml [accessed 03.06.14].
33. Chinadaily. Pharmaceutical market to hit 2.3t yuan by 2020. Available from: http://www.chinadaily.com.cn/business/2012-12/29/content_16068017.htm [accessed 03.06.14].
34. The World Bank. A generic drug policy as cornerstone to essential medicines in China.
35. Dugan BD. Enhancing community pharmacy through advanced pharmacy practice experiences. *Am J Pharm Educ* 2006;**70**(1):1–4.
36. Alvarez-Risco A, van Mil JW. Pharmaceutical care in community pharmacies: practice and research in Peru. *Ann Pharmacother* 2007;**41**(12):2032–7.
37. Beach M. Role of pharmacies in Chinese world of health care. *Lancet* 1999;**354**(9177):493.
38. National People's Congress. *Drug administration law of the People's Republic of China*. 1st ed. Beijing: Law Press China; 2001. ISBN: 7503633603.
39. The China Food and Drug Administration. Provisions for Supervision of Drug Distribution. Available from: http://eng.sfda.gov.cn/WS03/CL0768/61650.html [accessed 04.07.14].
40. State Council. National Drug Safety Program (2011–2015). Available from: http://www.gov.cn/ldhd/2011-12/07/content_2014120.htm [accessed 06.07.14].
41. Christensen DB, Farris KB. Pharmaceutical care in community pharmacies: practice and research in the US. *Ann Pharmacother* 2006;**40**(7):1400–6.
42. Jones EJ, Mackinnon NJ, Tsuyuki RT. Pharmaceutical care in community pharmacies: practice and research in Canada. *Ann Pharmacother* 2005;**39**(9):1527–33.
43. Yamamura S, Yamamoto N, Oide S, Kitazawa S. Current state of community pharmacy in Japan: practice, research, and future opportunities or challenges. *Ann Pharmacother* 2006;**40**(11):2008–14.
44. State Council. *The regulations for implementation of the drug administration law of the People's Republic of China*. 1st ed. Beijing: China Legal Publishing House; 2002. ISBN: 780083136.
45. Fang Y, Chen WJ, Yang SM, Hou HJ, Jiang MH. Analysis of antibiotics sales without prescription in pharmacies in West China- taking Xi'an as an example. *Chin Health Serv Manage* 2012;**28**(3):184–6.
46. Ma F, Lou N. *Regulation of drug promotion in China*. 2013. Available from: http://www.cov.com/files/Publication/8f6c9827-8e74-46e3-9ad1-5a06fd38fdc5/Presentation/PublicationAttachment/553e7d55-9a39-4075-8ac8-8419e132e9db/Regulation_of_Drug_Promotion.pdf. [accessed 09.07.14].
47. Medical Representative. What is a Medical Representative? Available from: http://www.medicalrepresentative.net/ [accessed 18.07.14].
48. Liu XY, Zhu Z. Reshaping the role of the pharmacist. *Chin Pharm J* 2010;**45**(7):556–7.
49. Hu JH. *Integrated pharmaceutical care*. 1st ed. Shanghai: The Second Military Medical University Press; 2001. ISBN: 7810600214.
50. Jiang JH, Liu Y, Wang YJ, Liu X, Yang M, Zeng Y, et al. Clinical pharmacy education in China. *Am J Pharm Educ* 2011;**75**(3):2–3.

51. Zhu M, Guo DH, Liu GY, Pei F, Wang B, Wang DX, et al. Exploration of clinical pharmacist management system and working model in China. *Pharm World Sci* 2010;**32**(4):411–5.

52. Fang Y, Yang SM, Feng BL, Ni YF, Zhang KH. Pharmacists' perception of pharmaceutical care in community pharmacy: a questionnaire survey in Northwest China. *Health Soc Care Community* 2011;**19**(1):189–97.

53. Yao C. *Practice and experience in integrated pharmaceutical care.* Seoul: The 4th Asian Conference on Clinical Pharmacy; July 24–26, 2004.

54. Peng SX. *Chinese pharmaceutical yearbook.* 1st ed. Shanghai: The Second Military Medical University Press; 2012. ISBN: 978-7-5481-0375-2.

55. Qiao WZ. The education of Traditional Chinese Medicine in China. Available from: http://www.gfmer.ch/TMCAM/Hypertension/Education_Traditional_Chinese_Medicine_China.htm [accessed 20.05.14].

56. Graber DR, Bellack JP, Lancaster C, Musham C. Curriculum topics in pharmacy education: current and ideal emphasis. *Am J Pharm Educ* 1999;**63**(2):145–51.

57. Kennie-Kaulbach N, Farrell B, Ward N, Johnston S, Gubbels A, Eguale T, et al. Pharmacist provision of primary health care: a modified Delphi validation of pharmacists' competencies. *BMC Fam Pract* 2012;**13**:27.

58. Bugnon O, Hugentobler-Hampaï D, Berger J, Schneider MP. New roles for community pharmacists in modern health care systems: a challenge for pharmacy education and research. *Chim (Aarau)* 2012;**66**(5):304–7.

59. Peng SX. *Chinese pharmaceutical yearbook.* 1st ed. Beijing: Chinese Medical Science and Technology Press; 1999. ISBN: 7-5304-2558-7.

60. Ryan M, Shao H, Yang L, Nie XY, Zhai SD, Shi LW, et al. Clinical pharmacy education in China. *Am J Pharm Educ* 2008;**72**(6):1–7.

61. Peng SX. *Chinese pharmaceutical yearbook.* 1st ed. Beijing: Chinese Medical Science and Technology Press; 2001. ISBN: 7-5304-2679-6.

62. China Pharmaceutical University. Clinical Pharmacy Program. Available from: http://school.cucas.edu.cn/HomePage/179/2010-01-22/Program_20348.shtml [accessed 20.05.14].

63. Yip W, Hsiao WC. The Chinese health system at a crossroads. *Health Aff* 2008;**27**(2):460–8.

64. Alcorn T, Bao B. China progresses with health reform but challenges remain. *Lancet* 2011;**377**:1557–8.

65. Hsiao WC. When incentives and professionalism collide. *Health Aff* 2008;**27**:949–51.

66. The Lancet. Chinese doctors are under threat. *Lancet* 2010;**376**:657.

67. Reynolds L, McKee M. Factors influencing antibiotic prescribing in China: an exploratory analysis. *Health Policy* 2009;**90**:32–6.

68. Yang SM. *Chinese pharmaceutical law and regulations.* 1st ed. Beijing: Chemical Industry Press; 2005. ISBN: 7502566570.

69. Yang SM. *Chinese pharmaceutical law and regulations.* 2nd ed. Beijing: Chemical Industry Press; 2007. ISBN: 9787122011916.

70. Chen Z. Launch of the health-care reform plan in China. *Lancet* 2009;**373**:1322–4.

71. Liu Q, Wang B, Kong Y, Cheng KK. China's primary health-care reform. *Lancet* 2011;**377**(9783):2064–6.

72. Bhattacharyya O, Delu Y, Wong ST, Bowen C. Evolution of primary care in China 1997–2009. *Health Policy* 2011;**100**(2–3):174–80.

73. China Chemical Reporter. China to spend RMB850 BLN on health-care reforms in next three years. Available from: http://www.ccr.com.cn/online_about.aspx?id=22005 [accessed 11.06.14].

74. Wang GQ. China issues guideline to strengthen drug distribution. Available from: http://news.xinhuanet.com/english2010/china/2011-05/05/c_13860308.htm [accessed 12.06.14].

75. The China Food and Drug Administration. Provisional Regulations on Licensed Pharmacist Qualification System. Available from: http://www.sfda.gov.cn/WS01/CL0001/ [accessed 10.05.14].

76. Ministry of Health. The long-term medical and health personnel development plan (2011–2020). Available from: http://www.jkb.com.cn/document.jsp?docid=210519&cat=0I./ [accessed 15.05.14].

77. China Pharmaceutical Association. "Pharmacist on Your Side" campaign. Available from: http://www.cpa.org.cn/Index.html [accessed 18.05.14].

78. Yip W, Hsiao WC, Chen W, Hu S, Ma J, Maynard A. Early appraisal of China's huge and complex health-care reforms. *Lancet* 2012;**379**:833–42.

CHAPTER 5

Pharmacy Practice in Sri Lanka

Shukry Zawahir, Dhakshila Niyangoda, Nadeesha Lakmali

Chapter Outline

1. Country background

Sri Lanka, an island in the Indian Ocean (previously called the Isle of Serendipity and Ceylon), is known for its pristine beaches, nature reserves, and ancient cultural sites that date back 2500 years. The island's climate, landscape, and rich cultural heritage have attracted millions of travelers from all over the world, despite its small size (65,000 km²).[1] The first signs of human inhabitants in Sri Lanka date back to the Stone Age, about 1.75 million years ago.

These people are said to have come from South India and reached the island through Adams Bridge, as told in the epic Hindu book of Ramayana.[2]

Sri Lanka's population is about 20.33 million (per the 2012 World Bank estimate), with the population growth of approximately 1.2% per year. The biggest ethnic group in Sri Lanka is the Sinhalese, who accounts for 72% of the total population of the country. There are three main languages in Sri Lanka: Sinhala, Tamil, and English. Buddhism is the dominant creed of the largest ethnic group, the Sinhalese; other minority ethnic groups include Hindus, Muslims, and Christians.[3]

Sri Lanka is mainly an agrarian country. The chief crop is rice, with which the country is almost self-sufficient. Tea, rubber, and coconut are also important agricultural crops, with tea being a major foreign exchange earner. In addition, other crops of importance are cocoa and spices, such as cinnamon, cardamom, nutmeg, pepper, and cloves. Fruit and vegetables, native to both tropical and temperate regions, grow well in Sri Lanka. Sri Lanka is also a major exporter of precious and semi-precious stones. Tourism has emerged as an important industry. There has also been a rapid growth in manufacturing industries, which offer a wide range of export goods such as petroleum products, leather goods, ready-made garments, and electronic equipment.

Gross national income per capita (PPP international $, 2012) was 6030. The total expenditure on health (TEH) per capita (international $, 2012) was 189 and the total expenditure on health as a percentage of gross domestic product (GDP, 2012) was 3.2.[4]

2. Vital health statistics

The mortality rate among Sri Lankans has declined since 1946. This is mainly due to the eradication of malaria, extension of health services in the rural areas and improved nutrition, which reflects the life expectancy of the population. The life expectancy for both males and females has increased for the past decades. According to the Annual Health Bulletin 2012, life expectancy is 70.5 years for men and 79.8 years for women.[5] Noncommunicable diseases, which include heart disease, stroke, cancer, diabetes, and respiratory disease, now account for 65% of all deaths in Sri Lanka and are a significant factor in escalating healthcare costs.[6]

In Sri Lanka, registration of vital events commenced in 1867 with the enactment of civil registration laws. Under the Births and Deaths Registration Act, the registration of both births and deaths was compulsory in Sri Lanka from 1897. According to the law, every live birth has to be registered within 42 days and a death within 5 days from the date of occurrence. Still births are registered in areas where there is a Medical Registrar. According to 2012 statistics from the Registrar General Department, the crude birth rate was 17.5/1000 population, and the crude death rate was 6/1000 population.[5] Based on 2006 data, the maternal mortality ratio per 100,000 live births was 22.3.[5]

In Sri Lanka, hospital mortality information is collected using the Indoor Morbidity and Mortality Return in each government hospital and is processed by the Medical Statistics Unit. This system has been collecting morbidity and mortality data since 1985. Morbidity data is available only for patients seeking treatment as inpatients in government hospitals in Sri Lanka. Morbidity data of patients attending the outpatient departments of government hospitals, ayurvedic institutions, and the private sector are not routinely collected. However, based on the limited information collected from government hospitals through surveys, registers are maintained and necessary action has been taken through special campaigns and programs for control of diseases such as tuberculosis (TB), cancer, and leprosy and from notifications.

3. Overview of the healthcare system

Since enacting the free healthcare policy, Sri Lanka's healthcare arena continues to be dominated by the government sector. The private sector, although still relatively insignificant in size compared to its public counterpart, has increasingly contributed toward serving the healthcare needs of the country.

Sri Lanka provides cost-effective healthcare at no direct cost to the patient. The country's maternal mortality ratio, neonatal mortality rate, life expectancy at birth, and many other health indicators are comparable with those of the developed world. Although these Sri Lankan indicators are the best in the region, much has to be done to ensure quality and safety in the delivery of healthcare, especially in hospitals.

As of December 2012, there were 621 medical institutions with inpatient facilities. There were 487 primary health care units and 337 medical officers of health areas in Sri Lanka. The number of beds in the hospitals increased to 76,087 in 2012, with 3.7 hospital beds per 1000 population.

The hospitals in Sri Lanka are categorized as follows: teaching hospital, provincial general hospital, district general hospital, base hospital type A, base hospital type B, divisional hospital type A, divisional hospital type B, and divisional hospital type C. In addition to these types of hospitals, there are primary care units and maternity homes with inpatient beds. This is the smallest type of hospital. There are two provincial general hospitals and 17 district general hospitals in the country. There are a few specialized hospitals for the treatment of chronic diseases such as TB, leprosy, mental illnesses, cancer, chronic rheumatologic diseases, and infectious diseases. These hospitals are included in the "other" category and have about 5000 beds. In 2012, Sri Lanka had 22 base hospitals type A with a total of 7759 patient beds, as well as 46 base hospitals type B, with a total of 9151 patient beds. The average number of beds in a type A hospital was 352 and 198 in type B.[5]

The presence of private sector is seen most prominently in outpatient care, catering to an estimated share of 50% of total outpatient volumes. On the other hand, the private sector caters to 5–10% of the country's inpatients.[7] Generally, the private healthcare sector is the choice of higher-income earners and individuals with access to medical insurance. As such, the demand for private healthcare has stemmed mainly from urban areas, with a significant concentration in the capital where disposable incomes are high.

Private hospitals have recorded steady compound annual growth rates in revenue over the last 5 years, in the range of 13–25%.[7] Private hospitals are essentially dependent on visiting specialists to attract patients, given the doctor-centric nature of the country's healthcare industry. The bulk of the graduates from local medical facilities are absorbed by the government sector, and these doctors practice a limited number of hours in the private sector subsequent to completing the required number of hours at public hospitals.

Private sector expenditure stems from several sources, including out-of-pocket (OOP) expenditure, which consists of household medical expenditure, health insurance, not-for-profit organizations, and employer arrangements. In Sri Lanka, OOP expenditure dominates private healthcare spending, accounting for more than 80%, and relatively low health insurance penetration levels in the country (as low as 6%).[7]

The total government health expenditure for 2012 was Rs 89,291 million. Total expenditure on health (TEH) is defined to include all expenditure on personal health services, community (public health and preventive) health services and gross capital formation in healthcare providers. TEH was estimated to be Rs 238,613 million in 2012 and 3.1% of the GDP.[5]

Each year, the Ministry of Health receives foreign aid in the form of money, materials, drugs, medical equipment, and technical input. During 2012, the foreign component of the health expenditure was Rs 7510 million (national), which accounted for 8.41% of the TEH.[5]

The total number of medical officers was 15,910 in 2012. Accordingly, the number of medical officers per 100,000 population was 78. The total number of nurses was 36,486 in 2012, or 180 nurses per 100,000 population. A shortage of qualified paramedical staff, such as pharmacists, medical laboratory technicians, radiographers, physiotherapists, and electrocardiogram technicians still exists. The total number of pharmacists employed at public hospitals throughout the island in 2012 was 1365, which is 6.7 pharmacists per 100,000 population.[5] Almost all of them have a diploma in pharmacy qualification.

4. Medicine supply systems and drug use issues

The government of the Democratic Socialist Republic of Sri Lanka provides free healthcare services to every citizen in the country. Primary healthcare is the key approach to attaining this goal. The supply of essential drugs is a major element in this approach.

Drug expenditures have been increasing each year because of the increased demand for better service, the escalating unit cost of medicines, changing patterns of morbidity etc. At the same time, the efficient use of the available drugs has received some setbacks. Some of the reasons are overprescribing, pilferage, and wastage.

Officials in the healthcare system have the responsibility for procuring, distributing, storing, prescribing, and dispensing, whether at national, provincial, regional, or institutional level of the state sector.

To ensure a proper drug management system in the state sector, an organizational framework exists within the Ministry of Health:

1. Cosmetics Devices and Drug Regulatory Authority (CDDRA) for the registration of drugs
2. Medical Supplies Division (MSD) at the central level for estimation, storage, distribution, and monitoring of drugs
3. National Drug Quality Assurance Laboratory (NDQAL) for the quality assurance of drugs
4. The State Pharmaceutical Corporation of Sri Lanka (SPC) for procurement
5. Regional Medical Supplies Divisions (RMSD) for the storage and distribution for provisional council institution

MSD follows a management cycle of pharmaceuticals, the major activities of which are depicted in the following figure (Figure 1).

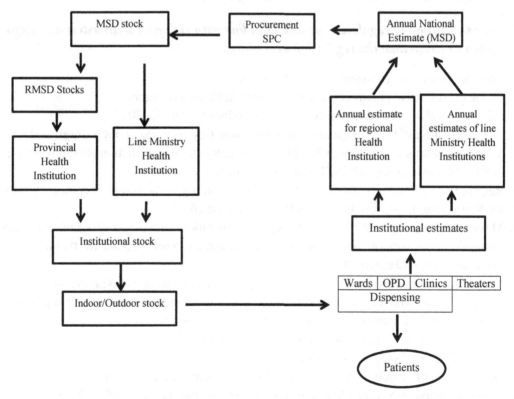

Figure 1
Major activities of MSD.

CDDRA provides the following services regarding the drug supply management:

- Regulation of cosmetics, medical devices, and medicinal drugs used in Sri Lanka through a market authorization scheme and a postmarketing surveillance system
- Inspection of manufacturing premises for compliance of good manufacturing practices (GMP)
- Inspection and licensing of retail and wholesale establishments of pharmaceuticals and vehicles used to transport pharmaceuticals
- Monitoring of suspected adverse drug reactions
- Recall of cosmetics, medical devices, and medicinal drugs from the market on safety grounds
- Control of advertisement on medicinal drugs
- Control of narcotics, psychotropic substances, and precursors used as medicines, as industrial chemicals, or for other scientific purposes
- Regulation of clinical trials
- Development of guidelines and manuals on medicines and related practices
- Training of healthcare professionals and their students with regard to the Cosmetics, Devices, and Drugs Act and its regulations
- Providing awareness programs for the general public

4.1 Harmonization of regulatory processes in line with stringent authorities and steps taken to strengthen the regulation procedures

1. GMP audits of foreign manufacturing facilities
2. Regulation of active pharmaceutical ingredient (API) manufacturers
3. Prior approval for advertisements on cosmetics (since September 2012)
4. Implementation of three-language policy for cosmetics, over-the-counter drugs, and Schedule IIa drugs since March 31, 2013, by which patient information should be given in all three languages (Sinhala, Tamil, and English)
5. Registration of similar biotherapeutic products according to the format recommended by the World Health Organization (WHO) since August 16, 2013
6. Making bioequivalence studies mandatory for registration (oral preparations of antibiotics, slow-release preparations, combination products, and some selected narrow therapeutic index drugs) from January 2014
7. Making lot release certificates mandatory for private sector vaccines (in progress)
8. Making vaccine vial monitors (VVM) mandatory for private sector vaccines (in progress)
9. Standardization of market authorization holder (in progress)
10. Implementation of novel recall procedure (in progress)
11. Prequalification of suppliers (in progress)
12. Development of guidelines on advertisements of cosmetics (in progress)
13. Implementation of National Medicines Regulatory Authority Act No 5 of 2015, certified on 19th March 2015. The new act was come to an operation from 1st July 2015 to repeal the Cosmetics, Devises and Drug Act No: 27 of 1980. Amendments on Regulations under new act is still in progress, hence provisions & procedures on regulatory process will be

changed in future. (Reference: Gazette of the Democratic Socialist Republic of Sri Lanka. National Medicines regulatory Authority Act, No. 5 of 2015, Department of Government Printing, Sri Lanka; 2015)

5. Overview of pharmacy practice and key pharmaceutical sectors

Pharmacy practice has always been and always will be an essential part of the healthcare system. Regrettably, in Sri Lanka, pharmacy practice is decades behind the rest of the world. The major contribution of pharmacists to current pharmacy practices in Sri Lanka is dispensing either at community pharmacies or hospital pharmacies. Almost all the hospital pharmacists have a diploma with a pharmacy qualification, whereas community pharmacists are apprentices pharmacists with external training and are registered with the Sri Lanka Medical Council (SLMC) as a pharmacist. There are many reasons for the current state of pharmacy practice, as will be discussed in the following sections. There are very few pharmaceutical companies based in Sri Lanka, and few graduate pharmacists work in the formulation and production areas.

5.1 Reflections on current pharmacy practices in Sri Lanka

In Sri Lanka, pharmacists have been dispensing medications since the ancient times. However, this may not be done in a professional manner, not only in community pharmacies and hospital pharmacies but also in medical practitioner's dispensaries.

Generally, patients in Sri Lanka receive medicines in printed envelopes, which should include all of the necessary details, such as the name of the patient, name of the drug, dosage, and frequency of administration. However, often no information is filled in except the dosage (e.g., "1 to be taken 2 times daily"). The practice of supplying medicine in envelopes has serious implications, such as the following:

1. Medicine in an envelope is easily accessible to children. There is no cautionary advice, such as "Keep away from children," printed on the envelope. When tablets and syrups are manufactured by pharmaceutical companies, they are expected to apply child-resistant caps. However, when medicines are dispensed in pharmacies, the rule does not seem to apply.
2. If two or more family members visit the doctor at the same time, most of the time the patients will be given several envelopes, with only the dosages written on the envelopes. Thus, there is a very high risk of a mix-up. Such incidents can have fatal consequences.
3. The instructions printed on the bottom of the envelope, "Store the medicine in an airtight container after opening the pack," make the practice even worse. Even if the patient finds an airtight container, there is no label to attach on the container. Therefore, there is no way for the patient to identify dosages and frequencies, and the potential for error again exists.
4. When medicines are supplied in envelopes, the integrity of the product cannot be guaranteed. Most medicines undergo deterioration on exposure to the environment.
5. The patient is not properly counseled and has no knowledge of what the medicines are for.

6. *Drug- and pharmacy-related regulations, policies, and ethics*

In Sri Lanka, drug regulation and monitoring of pharmacy practice are entirely handled by CDDRA, with the vision to achieve a healthier nation by ensuring the provision of safe, quality, and efficacious pharmaceutical products and safe and quality cosmetic products.[8]

1. **Cosmetics, Devices and Drugs (CDD) Act**
   The Cosmetic, Devices and Drugs Act No. 27 of 1980 (as amended by Act No. 38 of 1984, No. 25 of 1987, and No. 12 of 1993) provides the legislative framework to control the use of cosmetics, medical devices, and medicinal drugs in the country. The regulations under the CDD Act were published in Gazette Extraordinary No. 378/3 of December 2, 1985 and further amendments were made from time to time.
   The Act controls the following:
   a. Registration
   b. Manufacture
   c. Importation
   d. Transportation
   e. Sale (retail and wholesale)
   f. Labeling
   g. Advertising
   h. Distribution of drug samples
   i. Testing
   j. Disposal of outdated or spoiled drugs

Steps are being taken to introduce a new act for further strengthening of the entire regulatory process.[8]

2. **Poisons, Opium and Dangerous Drugs (Amended) Act**
   The Poisons, Opium and Dangerous Drugs Ordinance (Chapter 218), as amended by Act No. 13 of 1984, regulates the following for poisons, opium, and dangerous drugs:
   a. Importation
   b. Storage
   c. Distribution
   d. Use
3. The main provisions of the CDD Act with regard to drugs are as follows:
   a. Only drugs that are registered with the Cosmetics, Devices and Drugs Authority (CDDA) can be manufactured, imported, offered for sale, or used in the country
   b. Licenses are required for the importation, manufacture, wholesale trade/retail trade, and transportation of drugs
   c. All drugs registered with the CDDA should conform to specified standards
   d. Labeling on the packs and advertisements regarding drugs, medical devices, and cosmetics should conform to the relevant regulations

7. Core pharmacy practices

7.1 Hospital pharmacy

According to 2012 Ministry of Health data, Sri Lanka has 621 government medical institutions in categories that includes teaching hospitals, provincial general hospitals, district general hospitals, base hospitals, divisional hospitals, primary medical care units, maternity homes, and other medical care facilities. There are approximately 1365 pharmacists working in regional public sectors.[5] Almost all of the hospital pharmacists have diploma in pharmacy qualification proficiency certificate only. The distribution rate of pharmacists in government medical institutions is 6.7 per 100,000 population.

Hospital pharmacists in Sri Lanka are responsible for drug procurement, storage, distribution, and dispensing to both inpatients and outpatients of the hospital. In addition to these services, other services such as sterile products and chemotherapy reconstitution, patient counseling on the rational use of drugs, and local purchasing are also being carried out by pharmacists at tertiary hospitals; however, these additional services are in their early stages, with room to improve in the future. A weekly drug-delivery system is the most common drug distribution format to inpatients or wards. The concept of clinical pharmacy and pharmaceutical care has yet to be introduced to Sri Lankan hospital pharmacy services.

7.2 Industrial pharmacy

The Sri Lankan pharmaceutical industry comprises 15% of the local market,[9] as there are few pharmaceutical manufacturers in Sri Lanka. Some of the local pharmaceutical manufacturers include State Pharmaceutical Manufacturing Corporation (SPMC), Astron Ltd, Interpharm (Pvt) Ltd, J. L. Morison Son and Jones (Ceylon) PLC, GlaxoSmithKline Pharmaceuticals Ltd, Ceylinco Pharmaceuticals Ltd, Gamma Pharmaceuticals (Pvt) Ltd, and Unical (Ceylon) (Pvt) Ltd (Table 1). All of these are members of Sri Lanka Pharmaceutical Manufacturers Association, which was founded in 1963 with the mission of collectively lobbying with its stakeholders for the benefit of local manufacturers of pharmaceuticals in making their ventures successful.[10] Sri Lanka Pharmaceutical Manufacturers Association has partnered with the Ministry of Industries in establishing Sri Lanka Pharmaceutical Laboratory (SLPL) and enhancing human resources capabilities through training.[10] Although more than 200 pharmaceutical products are being locally manufactured,[9] all most all of them are in oral liquid, solid dosage, or topical dosage forms (Table 1).

The State Pharmaceutical Manufacturing Corporation (SPMC), which was established in 1987 by a grant aid received from the Japanese government through the Japan International Cooperation Agency, is the largest manufacturer of oral solid dosage forms (tablets and capsules) in Sri Lanka.[11] SPMC is the only state-owned pharmaceutical manufacturer in the country. It actively produced 40 drugs in 2012 out of its total of 63 products.[12] Every section

Table 1: Top 10 manufacturers in Sri Lanka

Name of the Company	Type	Year of Establishment	Number of Products	Major Dosage Forms	Location
State Pharmaceutical Manufacturing Co-Operation	Local	1987	46	Tablets and capsules	Rathmalana Sri Lanka
M.S.J. Industries (Ceylon) Pvt.	Local	1939	75	Tablets and liquids	Colombo 15
Astron Ltd	Local	1956	43	Tablet, capsules, liquids, powders, semi-solids, creams, and ointments	Rathmalana Sri Lanka
Lina Manufacturing Pvt Ltd	Local	1995	10	Capsules for dry powder inhalers	Rathmalana Sri Lanka
Glaxowelcome Ceylon Ltd	Multinational	2000	5	Tablets and liquids	Rathmalana Sri Lanka
Emergen Life Sciences Pvt Ltd	Local	2012	06	Capsules for dry powder inhalers	Rathmalana Sri Lanka
Gamma Pharmaceuticals (Pvt) Ltd	Local	1962	40	Tablets, capsules, liquids, semi-solids, creams, and ointments	Piliyandala Sri Lanka
Unical Ceylon (Pvt) Ltd	Local	1964	5	Tablets	Rathmalana Sri Lanka
Holychems	Local	2009	1	Ointment	Waththala Sri Lanka
CIC Life Sciences	Local	2013	10	Capsules	Colombo Sri Lanka

of the SPMC conforms to the current GMP (cGMP) requirements under the guidelines of the WHO.[9] SPMC maintains British (BP) and United States (USP) pharmacopeia quality standards.[9] Some of other manufacturing industries are maintaining Indian pharmacopeia quality standards as well. Majority of the medicines are imported and distributed by various pharmaceutical companies in Sri Lanka. Some of the importers details are shown in the (Table 2).

7.3 Community pharmacy

In Sri Lanka, Medical Ordinance No. 26 of 1927 has a provision that pharmacists and persons who fulfill the prescribed requirements should be registered at SLMC.[13] The dispensing of drugs and poisons is restricted only to registered pharmacists. Persons who have a certificate, diploma, or degree in pharmacy can get registered at SLMC as a pharmacist and granted equal right to dispense irrespective of their qualification. The registrar of SLMC keeps a record of persons qualified to act as pharmacists in Sri Lanka.

Table 2: Example of medicine importers in Sri Lanka

Name of the Company	Year of Establishment	Number of Products	Major Dosage Forms	Principal Companies	Location
Emarchemie NB	1999	About 800	Tablets, capsules, parenteral preparations, creams, gels, eye drops, ear drops, suppositories, syrups, suspensions, inhalers, nebulizers	Merck Ltd India, Dr Reddy Laboratories Ltd India, Ranbaxy Laboratories India, Laboratorios Bago SA Argentina, Pharmaniaga Manufacturing Berhad Malaysia, Renata Ltd Bangladesh	Colombo Sri Lanka
Sunshine Healthcare Lanka	1967	About 800	Tablets, capsules, parenteral preparations, creams, gels, eye drops, ear drops, suppositories, syrups, suspensions, inhalers, nebulizers	Abbott Laboratories-USA, Novo Nordisk Denmark, Galderma France, Zydus Calida India, Unison Lab Thailand, Glenmark India, Calida Pharmaceuticals India, Fourrts Labs India	Colombo Sri Lanka
ABC Pharma		About 200	Tablets, capsules, parenteral preparations, creams, gels, eye drops, ear drops, suppositories, syrups, suspensions, inhalers, nebulizers	Teva Pharmaceuticals Israel, PT Bio Pharma Indonesia	Colombo Sri Lanka

Pharmacies should be registered at CDDRA.[8] CDDRA maintains a list of registered pharmacies, which is made available to the public via their official Website (http://www.cdda.gov.lk/). Also, the Website gives a list of what should be looked for when patronizing a pharmacy.

SPC also has wholesale and retail outlets in several cities in the country,[14] and almost all other community pharmacies are private and mostly separate pharmacies. It is prohibited by the Act to keep a pharmacy open without a registered pharmacist.

The dispensing of medicines, except over-the-counter drugs, without a proper prescription is prohibited in Sri Lanka. Prescription of drugs using a brand name is also prohibited by the law. Air conditioning of all pharmacies is a must in Sri Lanka.

7.4 Medicine marketing and promotion

Medicine marketing in Sri Lanka is regulated by the Cosmetics, Devices and Drugs Act, No. 27 of 1980. Medical representatives maintain the link between pharmaceutical companies and the healthcare professionals who will make the decision on whether a product is the best option for a patient. They work strategically in order to increase the use of their company's products. These products are being sold mainly to private hospitals, private practitioners, and pharmacies as the state-governed healthcare institutions are being supplied by the government through the SPC and MSD.

Sri Lankan pharmaceutical companies prefer to recruit males who have passed the General Certificate of Education (G.C.E.) Advanced Level examination in the biostream as medical representatives. In some companies, graduates are also working as medical representatives. In addition, good communication skills, fluency in English, and a license to ride or drive are considered when recruiting.

The medical representatives are then trained, at the company level, on a particular product or medical area while being educated about the latest pharmaceutical innovations, their indications, and the limitations of products they are dealing with. Also, they should have a thorough understanding of doctor-patient requirements and expectations of their customers before they go into the field. In the field, they are usually based in a specific geographical location. They work with contacts on a one-to-one basis in order to maximize the sale of their company's products.

8. Special pharmacy-related services and activities

Sri Lanka introduce a drug policy based on a report prepared by Prof. Senaka Bibile and Dr S. A. Wickremasinghe.[14] Other developing countries have prepared their drug policies based on these ideas to ensure the rational use of pharmaceuticals.

In Sri Lanka, the SPC is the sole supplier of pharmaceuticals, surgical consumable items, laboratory chemicals, and equipment to all institutions administered by the Ministry of Health.[14] SPC pharmacy outlets (Rajya Osu Salas) offer a 5% discount on prescriptions for pregnant mothers, persons over 60 years of age, and children under 5 years.[14] All state-owned healthcare institutions supply medical care and pharmaceuticals free of charge to all patients in wards and clinics, as well as outpatients.

The National Poison and Drug Information Center of Sri Lanka provides information to the public as well as health professionals regarding drugs and poisons.[15] It conducts awareness programs and poison prevention activities, as well as postgraduate courses in toxicology.

State universities, including the University of Colombo, University of Sri Jayewardenepura, University of Peradeniya, University of Jaffna, University of Ruhuna, Kotelawala Defense University, and Open University of Sri Lanka have started to produce graduates in pharmacy (BPharm and BSc Pharmacy). Therefore, many undergraduate research projects are now being carried out in the field of pharmacy.

9. Pharmacy education

Pharmacy training was first introduced in Sri Lanka in the early 1950s. By 1957, a full-time pharmacy certificate course was introduced.[16] Since then, three types of pharmacy certificates have been developed: a certificate of proficiency in pharmacy, a certificate of efficiency in pharmacy, and a diploma of pharmacy. A Bachelor of Science (Special in Pharmacy) degree course commenced at the University of Colombo in 1999. The Bachelor of Pharmacy (BPharm) program was introduced in 2006 at the University of Peradeniya (UP) in the central part of Sri Lanka, the University of Sri Jayewardenepura (USJ) in Colombo, and the University of Jaffna (UJ).[16] The University of Ruhuna (2010) in Galle, Southern province, Open University of Sri Lanka (2013), and Kotelawala Defense University (2014) in Colombo have also started BPharm degree programs at their respective universities (Table 3). To date, no local university has provided a postgraduate program in pharmacy.

Currently, approximately 100 graduate pharmacists have been produced from local public universities. After their advanced-level examination, some students get scholarships and study BPharm or PharmD overseas, especially in South Asian countries.

10. Achievements in pharmacy practice

Since 2006, three universities—University of Peradeniya, University of Sri Jayawardenepura, and University of Jaffna—have recruited about 60–70 students from the G.C.E. (Advanced Level) Examination Bioscience stream to graduate with a Bachelor of Pharmacy degree. This is one of the sound achievements in the pharmacy field.

Table 3: Universities offering pharmacy degree programs

University/Institute	Year of Establishment	Number of Years of Study	Number of Students Enrolled/Year	Degrees Offered	Ownership
University of Colombo	1999	2	10	BSc pharmacy	Government
University of Sri Jayewardenepura	2006	4	10–20	BPharm	Government
University of Peradeniya	2006	4	11–30	BPharm	Government
University of Jaffna	2006	4	3–16	BPharm	Government
University of Ruhuna	2010	4	15–20	BPharm	Government
Kotelawala Defense University	2013	4	25	BPharm	Government
Open University of Sri Lanka	2013	4	100	BPharm	Government

At the beginning of the BPharm programs, there was great resistance for undergraduate pharmacy students to be trained in some of the government teaching hospitals in Sri Lanka. This issue has been overcome by sending the students to some other government hospitals in different regions after a court order.

Later, the course duration was reduced from 4 years to 3 years; some selected students with higher grades in their 3rd year could continue their fourth year as a special degree. The rest of the students graduated with a 3-year general degree. As a result of allied health science students' struggle for nearly 6 months in 2014, it was officially announced that allied health science degree programs, including the Bachelor of Pharmacy program, should be comprised of 120 credits irrespective of their duration.

11. Challenges in the pharmacy practice

In Sri Lanka, the practice of pharmacy is one of the neglected areas of health services and medical practice. Both community and hospital pharmacies are in a deplorable state. Although official reports have made recommendations for their improvement, nothing has been done in this direction.[17]

In many government sectors, including the Ministry of Health, government hospitals, and CCDRA, only few or no graduate pharmacists are employed. At present in Sri Lanka, the clinical pharmacy service is minimal or almost neglected; this is perhaps due to professional isolation, lack of qualified clinical pharmacists, and lack of recognition of the role of clinical pharmacists within the healthcare system. The lack of experience and expertise among practitioners and academics in Sri Lanka has resulted in a relative inability to develop and deliver a rigorous and effective clinical pharmacy teaching program. There are no clinical pharmacy mentors, clinical tutors, or role models. The current BPharm programs are taught predominantly by academics with pharmacy, medical, and science backgrounds, including clinical pharmacologists, but with little or no clinical pharmacy experience. Students had limited exposure to clinical placements during their undergraduate years, which may be due to a lack of understanding about the goal of health professions. Sri Lankan academics were concerned about gaps in clinical pharmacy expertise, so they approached Australian pharmacist academics to collaborate in the development and teaching of the clinical pharmacy subject.

At present, the proper regulation of cosmeceuticals and nutraceuticals is not practiced in Sri Lanka.

The migration of pharmacy professionals also remains high, adding further strain on the industry. On a to separate note, intensifying competitive pressures over the medium to longer term could challenge the existing players.

Community pharmacy practice should be improved in Sri Lanka, and law enforcement regarding dispensing prescription and controlled drugs should be strengthened. In the current practice, almost everyone can get any drug from most private community pharmacies in Sri Lanka.

Pharmacy institutions in the country are facing problems due to a lack of equipment and laboratory facilities to conduct pharmacy-related practical studies during their undergraduate pharmacy training.

There are no categories in the qualified pharmacist registration process to differentiate between external apprentice pharmacists, diploma pharmacists, and graduate pharmacists. There is no separate category for graduate pharmacists in the government sector. Both diploma and graduate pharmacists are recruited on the same salary scale.

12. Recommendations

One way to develop a generation of pharmacists who will be better equipped to engage in contemporary pharmacy practice and deliver better patient care is by introducing comprehensive clinical pharmacy teaching curricula at the university level. The introduction of clinical pharmacy services in healthcare facilities would need to be supported by government resources. Enablers to capacity building, such as the development of clinical pharmacy teachers in academia, the establishment of clinical pharmacy positions in hospitals, and acceptance by the medical profession, are also important.

The number of graduate pharmacists in public sectors should be increased in order to provide better services. There should be postgraduate pharmacy programs offered by Sri Lankan institutions.

Enforcement of policies related to community pharmacy practice should be strengthened. There should be clearly distinguished registration categories for pharmacists with different pharmacy qualifications.

The migration of qualified pharmacists should be suppressed, and they should be given opportunities to serve the country. It is also important to have awareness programs about pharmacy practice for other health professionals, policy makers, school children, and the general public.

A drug information service (DIS) should be implemented within hospital pharmacy departments. The main responsibilities of the DIS should include answering drug-related questions, preparing drug information monographs and presenting them to the Pharmacy and Therapeutic Committee, and monitoring and reporting adverse drug reactions.

Finally, the concept of clinical pharmacy and pharmaceutical care should be introduced in Sri Lankan hospital pharmacy services.

13. Conclusions

Although the healthcare system in Sri Lanka is up to an acceptable level overall, pharmacy practice is decades behind the rest of the world. It is necessary to enhance the image of the pharmacy profession with high-quality services—not only for patients but also doctors, nurses, and other healthcare professionals. This can be achieved if the Ministry of Health, pharmacy academics, all pharmacists (i.e., external, internal, diploma, and graduates), the pharmaceutical society of Sri Lanka, and other stakeholders work together as a one team toward the goal.

This progress could start with the production of highly qualified and competent pharmacists in the country and specialized pharmacy practitioners with postgraduate qualifications and appropriate training. In addition, the establishment of a pharmacy council would upgrade the quality of pharmacy education and services in Sri Lanka, provide more opportunities to graduate pharmacists to practice in various pharmacy fields in the public sector, and allow pharmacists to conduct high-quality research in pharmacy.

14. Lessons learned/points to remember

- Pharmacy practice in Sri Lanka needs much improvement.
- Highly qualified and experienced pharmacists should be produced in order to have better practice and training for future generations.
- Interprofessional understanding is vital to improve pharmacy practice and pharmaceutical care.
- All categories of pharmacists, even if they serve different fields in the country, should unite and work together toward the same goal.

Acknowledgment

Special thanks to Ms. Thilani Dias, lecturer, B.Pharm Program, University of Ruhuna, C.M Chanaka Indrajith, Factory Manager, Farmchemie (Pvt) Ltd, Sri Lanka, Dr B.V.S.H.Beneragama, Former Director, Cosmetics, Devices & Drug Regulatory Authority, Sri Lanka, Dr Sriyani Dissanayake, Deputy Director, Cosmetics, Devices & Drug Regulatory Authority, Sri Lanka, Ms Chinta Abewardena, President, Pharmaceutical Society of Sri Lanka and Ms. Sivasinthujah Paramasivam, Lecturer, Faculty of Medicine, University of Jaffna, Sri Lanka for their valuable contributions toward the success of this book chapter.

References

1. CORI. *CORI Country report Sri Lanka*. Country of origin research and information (CORI) [cited July 10, 2014]. Available from: http://www.refworld.org/; 2010.
2. Ralph TH, Griffith MA. *Rámáyan of Válmíki* [cited July 20, 2014]. Available from: http://www.sacred-texts.com/hin/rama/index.htm; 2003.
3. The World Bank. Sri Lanka. Available from: www.worldbank.org/en/country/srilanka; 2013.
4. WHO. *WHO health statistics _Sri Lanka*. Genewa: World Health Organization; 2012.
5. Ministry of Health. *Annual health bulletin 2012*. Colombo: Medical Statistics Unit, Ministry of Health, Sri Lanka; 2012.
6. WHO. *Sri Lanka's low-cost people-centred approach to health challenges*. Geneva: WHO; 2014.
7. RAM. *Standpoint commentary: the private healthcare sector of Sri Lanka*. Colombo; 2013.

8. CDDRA. *Cosmetics, devices & drug regulatory authority*. Colombo [cited July 20, 2014]. Available from: http://www.cdda.gov.lk/index.php?option=com_content&view=article&id=50&Itemid=92&lang=en; 2014.

9. Pathirana S. *More drugs procurement from local manufacturers – SLPMA*. See more at: http://dailynews.lk/?q=business/more-drugs-procurement-local-manufacturers-slpma#sthash.p5N1AtVR.dpuf. Daily News; 2013 [17.10.13].

10. SLMA. *Sri Lanka pharmaceutical manufacturers association*. Colombo [cited October 12, 2014]. Available from: http://slpmaweb.org/; 2014.

11. SPMC. *SPMC products*. Colombo: SPMC [cited October 15, 2014]. Available from: http://www.spmclanka.lk/index.php; 2014.

12. SPMC. *Annual report, the state pharmaceutical manufacturing corporation of Sri Lanka*; 2012.

13. SLMC. *Sri Lanka medical council*. Colombo [cited July 22, 2014]. Available from: http://www.srilankamedicalcouncil.org/; 2014.

14. SPC. *State pharmaceutical cooperation of Sri Lanka*. Colombo [cited October 10, 2014]; Drug Policy. Available from: http://www.spc.lk/spc.html; 2014.

15. NPDIC. *National poison and drug information centre*. Colombo [cited October 05, 2014]; Poison and Drug Information Services in Sri Lanka. Available from: http://203.94.76.60/NPDIC/index.html; 2014.

16. Coombes ID, Fernando G, Wickramaratne M, Peters NB, Lynch CB, Lum E, et al. Collaborating to develop clinical pharmacy teaching in Sri Lanka. *Int J Pharm Educ* 2013;**13**(1):23–35.

17. Health Action International. *Undergraduate medical and pharmacy education: the need for change and the way forward*. July–September 2005.

CHAPTER 6

Pharmacy Practice in Pakistan

Azhar Hussain, Shazia Jamshed

Chapter Outline

1. Country background

Pakistan is positioned in the South Asian region and is linked to Central Asian republics through Afghanistan (to the northwest) and China (to the North), sharing borders with India to the east and Iran to the west. The land area of Pakistan is 796,096 sq. km.

The country is administratively divided into five provinces: Punjab, Sindh, Khyber

Table 1: Demographic, economic, and health indicators of Pakistan

No	Indictors	Statistics
1	Total population (thousands), 2012	179,160.1
2	Population under 18 years (thousands), 2012	73,844.9
3	Population under 5 years (thousands), 2012	21,995.9
4	Annual number of births (thousands), 2012	4603.8
5	Crude birth rate (%), 2012	25.7
6	Crude death rate (%), 2012	7
7	Life expectancy, 2012	66.4 years
8	Urbanized population (%), 2012	36.5
9	Under-5 mortality rate, 2012	8
10	Low birth weight (%), 2008–2012	32
11	Underweight (%) 2008–2012, moderate, and severe	31.5
12	Gross National Income per capita, 2012 (US$)	1260
13	Total use of improved drinking water sources (%), 2011	91.4
14	Total use of improved sanitation facilities (%), 2011	47.4
15	Survival rate to last primary grade (%), 2008–2012	52.2

Source: http://www.unicef.org/infobycountry/pakistan_pakistan_statistics.html.

Pakhtunkhwa (formerly the North-West Frontier Province), Gilgit Baltistan, and Balochistan. Islamabad is the capital city. Being the sixth most densely inhabited country, Pakistan has an estimated current population of approximately 158 million people; only 34% live in urban areas.[1]

Although the Gross National Income (the gross domestic product (GDP) plus net receipts from abroad of wages and salaries and of property income) per capita in Pakistan is greater than other low-income countries (US$1360 in 2013), 29.2% of the population (approximately 45 million people) still live below the official national poverty line (Table 1). Socioeconomic development in Pakistan is slow overall, with low levels of literacy: the national adult literacy rate was 54.9% in 2005.[1] The literacy rate is predominantly lower for females in rural areas. The majority of the population (61%) has no access to good-quality drinking water; this problem is more severe in rural areas, where only 23% of people have access to tap water. Approximately 19% of the population and 30% of children under the age of 5 years are malnourished. Communicable diseases are the most prevalent and principal causes of sickness and death in Pakistan, including gastroenteritis, respiratory infections, congenital abnormalities, tuberculosis, malaria, and typhoid fever.[2]

2. Health sector and system

The healthcare system is very well structured in Pakistan, but one cannot overlook some of the inherent issues that are typical for developing countries. The public sector, which is responsible for providing healthcare to the masses, is assisted by the government; the private sector functions in parallel with a more commercial approach. Healthcare expenditures by the government are low, at approximately 3.2% of the GDP, which is less than other countries with the same socioeconomic conditions, such as Bangladesh and Sri Lanka.[3] For health expenditures in Pakistan, 78% are out of pocket.[4,5]

In the public sector, the healthcare provision is decentralized and is predominantly the responsibility of the government at the provincial level. The central Ministry of Health looks after the national policy, planning, coordination, and enactment of the six national health programs on immunization, family planning, tuberculosis, HIV/AIDS, malaria, and nutrition.[2]

There is shortage of qualified and trained staff, essential drugs, medical supplies, and other supplies in most of the public health facilities. Therefore, patients periodically seek medical care in the private health sector, which in itself is a reflection that 70% of the healthcare costs are out-of-pocket expenditures in Pakistan.[3] The healthcare system is largely urban oriented, with private sector healthcare facilities mainly concentrated in urban areas, making it difficult for the rural poor to access and afford. Patients have to seek healthcare in the private health sector or alternative sources (herbalists, *hakeems*), as observed in the latest Pakistan Social and Living Standards Measurement Survey.[2]

3. National Health Policy

The National Health Policy was introduced in 2001, which anticipated a vision to provide healthcare to all. The policy embraces a focused approach by recognizing strategies for the health sector. The main features of the policy included health sector investment, which was an element of the government's Poverty Alleviation Plan; priority was given to primary and secondary healthcare facilities to diminish the load on the tertiary-care facilities. The policy also proposed good governance as a milestone to achieve quality in healthcare. The policy identified specific areas to achieve this vision,[6] such as reducing the frequency of transmissible diseases, diminishing cessation of primary and secondary healthcare, reducing administrative inefficiencies at the district level of health system, reassuring improved gender equity, refining the nutrition status of the population, reducing urban prejudice of the health system, applying drug regulation at community pharmacies, crafting consciousness in the masses regarding public health issues, improving the drug sector, and augmenting the capacity to observe the health policy status and implementation.[7]

4. National Drug Policy

A good National Drug Policy (NDP) is a vital part of a national health policy, which safeguards unbiased access to and coherent use of safe and effective drugs. The Ministry of

Health drafted an NDP that is in line with the recommendations of the Drug Action Program of World Health Organization (WHO) from 1997. The eight-point objectives of the policy promised the development and promotion of essential drugs with a regular and uninterrupted supply, promotion of rational drug use to enhance and maintain public health from inappropriate drugs, accomplishment of self-sufficiency in drugs by encouraging local sources of raw material, shielding the public from substandard drugs, cultivating adequately trained manpower in drug management, improvement of the research base in the country, and development of the pharmaceutical industry. The policy has two broader domains: promoting the pharmaceutical industry and promoting and protecting public health, both with an inherent conflict of interest.[8]

5. Statistics on human resources and capital/workforce

The key healthcare players in Pakistan are physicians (149,201 in number), nurses (76,244), dentists (10,958), pharmacists (8102), and pharmacy assistants (31,000), based on the Pakistan economic survey of 2011–2012.[3] The healthcare providers are quite low in number compared with the country's population: 1206 persons per doctor, 16,426 persons per dentist, 2360 persons per nurse, and 22,216 persons per pharmacist. Medical doctors are quite dominant and hold major administrative and decision-making positions in the health sector.[3] There are 8102 pharmacists (A category), as well as 31,000 pharmacy technicians (B and C categories), in the country.[9] There are over 63,000 community pharmacies in the country.[10] If all the pharmacists and pharmacy technicians were employed at these community pharmacies, still an appreciable number of pharmacies are left without a qualified employee. According to the Pharmacy Council of Pakistan (PCP), 70% of pharmacists are employed in the pharmaceutical industry, while only 10% work at community pharmacies in the country.[9] There are more than 30 pharmacy institutions in the country, from which 2587 pharmacists graduate annually. The current number of pharmacists does not meet the growing demands for optimal healthcare delivery to the population. The Pakistan Pharmacists Association is responsible for the growth of the pharmacy profession. The National Association of Pharmacists endorses and magnifies the role of pharmacists in public health and patient care.[11,12]

6. Top 20 medicines based on expenditure and utilization

The current pharmaceutical market is worth Rs 178 billion (1 US$ = 104.91 PKRs) with an annual growth rate of 17.91%.[5] The local pharmaceutical companies have a market share of 43.79%, with an annual growth rate of 15.31%; they are worth Rs 77.99 billion. Multinational companies are worth Rs 100 billion, with a market share of 56.21% and a growth rate of 20%.

Tables 2 and 3 list the top 20 medicines sold on the basis of expenditure and utilization, as well as the value in Pakistani rupees.

Table 2: Top 20 medicines (by expenditure and utilization)

Rank	Brand Name	Generic	Company	Units Sold	Value in Rs
1	Augmentin	Amoxicillin + clavulanic acid	GSK	37.90 million	3.26 billion
2	Pegasys		Roche	0.25 million	1.47 billion
3	Brufen	Ibuprofen	Abbott	37.06 million	1.43 billion
4	Velosef		GSK	12.13 million	1.41 billion
5	Amoxil	Amoxicillin	GSK	11.60 million	1.35 billion
6	CAC 1000 Plus		Novartis	13.20 million	1.29 billion
7	Flagyl	Metronidazole	Sanofi Aventis	19.93 million	1.25 billion
8	Novidat		Sami	7.71 million	1.25 billion
9	Risek		Getz	6.90 million	1.23 billion
10	Lactogen		Nestle	5.77 million	1.19 billion
11	Ponstan	Mefenamic acid	Pfizer	5.46 million	1.12 billion
12	Humulin 70/30		Eli Lilly	2.48 million	1.02 billion
13	Oxidil		Sami	8.63 million	100 billion
14	Panadol	Paracetamol	GSK	21.25 million	988 million
15	Calpol	Paracetamol	GSK	31.13 million	944 million
16	Methycobal	Methycobalamine		1.11 million	929 million
17	Surbex Z	Multi vitamin	Abbott	5.79 million	827,833 million
18	Meiji FM-T		Meiji	1.52 million	787 million
19	Ampiclox		GSK	3.85 million	763 million
20	Ensure		Abbott Nutrition	1.15 million	741 million

Table 3: Top 20 molecules

No	Molecule	Value in Rs
1.	Infant milk	6.79 billion
2.	Ceftriaxone	4.33 billion
3.	Amoxicillin + clavulanic acid	4.23 billion
4.	Diclofenac	4.10 billion
5.	Peg interferon	2.00 billion
6.	Cefixime	3.58 billion
7.	Omeprazole	3.03 billion
8.	Paracetamol	2.50 billion
9.	Mecobalmine	2.00 billion
10.	Ciprofloxacin	4.09 billion
11.	Amoxicillin	2.07 billion
12.	Levofloxacin	1.93 billion
13.	Ibuprofen	1.66 billion
14.	Esomeprazole	1.94 billion
15.	Cefradine	1.98 billion
16.	Clarithromycin	1.76 billion
17.	Metronidazole	1.60 billion
18.	Artemether + lumefantrine	1.49 billion
19.	Glimepiride	1.46 billion
20.	Vitamin C, calcium, vitamin D, vitamin B6	1.44 billion

7. Pharmacy practice

7.1 Country perspective

In developing countries, due to a lack of qualified personnel, direct contact with pharmacists is not possible in all areas. Therefore, the quality of pharmaceutical services in a given region becomes reliant on the accessibility of a pharmacist. It is a well-known fact that the conditions of pharmacy practice differ between countries and also between different areas within the same country, often because there are fewer pharmacists than required. The direct management of pharmaceutical products by the pharmacist can be helpful in safeguarding the delivery of high-quality services to patients.[13]

8. Background of the pharmaceutical sector

In Pakistan, the pharmaceutical sector is determined by requirements. At the time of the establishment of Pakistan in 1947, there was no manufacturing unit and pharmaceutical requirements were achieved mainly through imports. Significant development in this sector was introduced in the 1980s; since then, the pharmaceutical industry never looked back. In 2008, there were 405 registered pharmaceutical units in Pakistan, of which 31 were multinational. After a year, the number of registered pharmaceutical units topped 4400. The government was hopeful that this would be in the best interest of consumers due to the initiation of price competition.[14] Pakistan has a progressively growing pharmaceutical industry, which has a market value of approximately US$1.72 billion.[15] The pharmaceutical sector is somewhat equally shared by locally produced generics and imported branded prescription medicines. The local industry, however, responded to domestic demands; by 2007, it was valued at US$1.2 billion, with a yearly export of 0.22% of the global pharmaceutical market. The current pharmaceutical market segment is composed of 60% multinational companies and 40% local manufacturers; however, the situation is reversed when considering share by volume, which is 60% for local manufacturers and 40% for multinational firms.[15]

The recent pharmaceutical market conditions for OTC medicines, patented drugs, and generic drugs are illustrated in Figure 1.

The combined sales of prescription drugs and over-the-counter medicines continued to grow in 2011, increasing from US$1.79 billion to US$1.98 billion within a year; this is presumably due to the unforeseen effects of the humanitarian assistance program and pricing pressures, with an upsurge in inflation from the previous year.[16] It is expected that Pakistan's drug market expenditure should increase at the local currency compound annual growth rate of 10.13% in terms of local currency and 6.54% in terms of US dollar between 2011 and 2016, reaching a value of PKR 277.34 billion (US$2.72 billion). A detailed pharmaceutical market forecast is illustrated in Figure 2.

The price of medicine plays a vital role in enhancing access to medicine; sadly, pricing has been a challenging issue for quite some time in the country.[17,18] The pharmaceutical

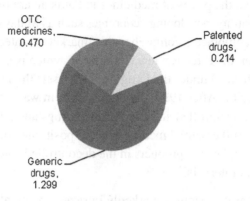

Figure 1
Pharmaceutical market by subsectors. *Source: Pakistan Pharmaceutical Manufactures Association (PPMA), domestic companies, local press, BMI.*

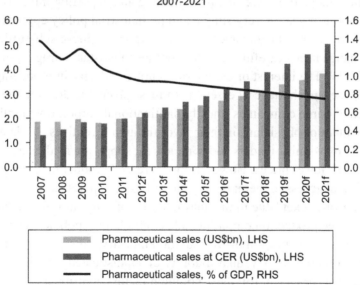

Figure 2
Pakistan pharmaceutical market forecast. f, forecast; CER, constant exchange rate. *Source: Pakistan Pharmaceutical Manufacturers Association (PPMA), domestic companies, local press, BMI.*

market is a brand market; for an individual product, dozens of different brands are registered in the country. For example, ofloxacin, an antibiotic, is available in 34 brands in the market, with inexact effectiveness and safety.[19] To check the prices of medicines in Pakistan, the government highlighted the use of generic medicines; however, there is no ordinance or authoritative rule for generic prescribing or substitution in the public and private sectors.

It is imperative to know that the prices of medicines in Pakistan are in the hands of the government. On the contrary, developing economies such as Malaysia, Thailand, the Philippines, and Indonesia embrace a comprehensive, market-oriented approach to the pricing phenomenon.[20] In Pakistan, the Price Review Committee, which is a subcommittee of the Drug Registration Board formed under the Drug Act 1976, sets the maximum wholesale and retail prices for each medicine. After 1993, the pricing system was altered; all products were divided into categories of uncontrolled and decontrolled drugs and all prices were regulated by the government. About 800 essential medicines were positioned on the controlled list. A more laissez-faire system applies for products in the decontrolled category, with higher price increasing at more frequent intervals.[21,22]

To be precise, the price control system is markedly intricate; in actuality, companies are often able to amplify prices unilaterally due to weak enforcement of regulations.

9. Industrial pharmacy and pharmaceutical technology

The pharmaceutical industry in Pakistan is flourishing and exporting millions of dollars' worth of medicines each year. A very simple and preindustrial policy approach to increase the number of pharmaceutical companies, increase exports, achieve self-sufficiency, and earn foreign exchange needs careful evaluation because Pakistan's drug regulatory structure is not very efficient.[23] The interest of the pharmaceutical industry in producing profitable medicines and the severe shortage of essential and less profitable drugs in the country have been documented.[24] Large companies (mostly multinational corporations) influence the prescribing pattern of physicians in their favor through incentives, while national companies operate by winning tenders and contracts for supplying medicines to government institutes due to their lower prices. However, the increased production of medicines does not guarantee general access to them; the people of Pakistan purchase 77% of their health-care expenses "out-of-pocket" due to the unavailability of drugs at government hospitals. Factors restraining the production output include contradictory policies, lack of funds for upgrading the plants, high duties in the formulation industry, poor policy framework, lack of infrastructure for biotechnology, unavailability of sophisticated machinery, high costs of inputs, and rigorous price control; these common factors contribute to the poor performance of manufacturing in all sectors in Pakistan.[25]

The price of pharmaceuticals is an important factor that can contribute to improved access to medicines. Unfortunately, pricing has been a challenging concern at present in Pakistan, with prices being relatively high when compared with the International Reference Prices. National pharmaceutical companies manufacture low-price medicines and are prospective candidates for increasing the export of medicines in the new free-trade regime.

Unfortunately, the current domestic pharmaceutical industry is operating with low production volumes, obsolete machinery, and low-quality standards that are not comparable with that of multinational corporations; this has eliminated the low-price advantage of national companies.[26] The promotion of generics by physicians, pharmacists, and the government is required for improvements in the quality of generic medicines in Pakistan. A mandatory policy of using generic names to improve access to medicines was initiated in Pakistan, which failed due to the lack of well-established laboratories to conduct bioequivalence studies, the influence of multinational companies, and the protests of doctors. The lack of a health economist or pharmaco-economist on the pricing board of the Ministry of Health highlights the negligence of policy makers in managing medicine policies.[27]

10. Regulatory issues (registration/inspections)

The Drug Control Organization (DCO) at the Ministry of Health is responsible for regulating the pharmaceutical sector in Pakistan. The DCO performs its functions in accordance with the Drugs Act 1976 and its rules. There are three major sections in the DCO headed by drug controllers: Registration, Quality Control, and Research and Development. Drug controllers are the technical heads, while the Director General is the departmental head. The field offices in the provincial headquarters are responsible for monitoring the implementation of the conditions of drug manufacturing licenses and good manufacturing practices. The provincial governments also have inspectors working for postmarketing surveillance. The sale of medicines is the responsibility of provincial governments, who has appointed drug inspectors for this purpose in all provinces at tehsil and district levels.[6]

Under the aegis of the Drug Regulatory Authority of Pakistan (DRAP) Act 2012, there has been an establishment of DRAP that aims to cater to the effective management and implementation of Drugs Act 1976 (XXXI of 1976). This in turn paves the way for synchronization in trade and commercialization of therapeutic goods interprovisionally.

11. Drugs Act

Since the independence of Pakistan, the sale of drugs was controlled under the Drug Act 1940. In 1972, Generic Names Act of 1972 was introduced by the government. According to this act, drugs could be prescribed, dispensed, sold, or distributed by the generic names only. This act was not put into practice because of the pressure of multinational pharmaceutical companies. In 1976, for the first time, a comprehensive drug act was presented, approved, and implemented by the government. It was called the Drug Act of 1976. The manufacturing of pharmaceuticals and its business is regulated through the Drug Act 1976 and its rules. The act controls the registration, manufacturing, marketing, and quality assurance of medicines in the country.[6]

12. Hospital practice

Health care services in hospitals and clinics are usually provided by physicians assisted by nurses; a pharmacist's duties are performed by nurses, mid-wives, female health workers, and other paramedical staff in Pakistan.[12] Hospital pharmacists face significant barriers in providing quality, clinically focused pharmacy services due to the scarcity of pharmacists in hospitals; they are focused on traditional duties instead of patient-oriented pharmaceutical care.[28] Senior physicians are part of committees that formulate health policies; usually, they do not allocate space for the pharmacy profession in healthcare services, which might be due to the physicians' professional fear. There are limited pharmacy services in Pakistan's hospitals due to insufficient numbers of trained personnel, resulting in a lack of patient contact with pharmacists and a lack of recognition of pharmacists as healthcare professionals in Pakistan.[12,29] Limited seats are offered in the public sector hospitals for pharmacists, and their role is confined to drug delivery, procurement, and inventory control. There is an urgent need for implementation of pharmaceutical care services within the nation's healthcare system in order to promote the rational use of drugs in Pakistan.[28]

13. Clinical pharmacy

There are few experts/academicians in the fields of clinical pharmacy, hospital pharmacy, and community pharmacy in Pakistan. Most people in Pakistan are familiar with the concepts of hospital pharmacy and community pharmacy, but are still quite uninformed about the branch of clinical pharmacy.[30] The ideal pharmacist-controlled hospital pharmacy practice is still not implemented in Pakistan. At present, there are only two hospitals in Pakistan where clinical pharmacy services are not mixed with other aspects of hospital pharmacy practice: Shaukat Khanum and Agha Khan; here, pharmacists focus on clinical pharmacy practices along with the distributive and administrative aspects of pharmacy practice. However, practice of the subspecialties of clinical pharmacy (i.e., oncology, infectious diseases, critical care, pediatrics and geriatrics, cardiology, family medicine, pain and palliative care, renal and transplant, drug information, and internal medicine) is still limited in Pakistan.[31] This is mainly due to a lack of trained and skilled mentors to teach the students and residents in a specialized residency program that is not offered in the PharmD program. In addition, there is a lack of communication between pharmacists working in different areas of different hospitals in the country. There is also a shortage of research and documentation of clinical pharmacy services to support the implementation of successful clinical pharmacy practices in Pakistan.[32]

The case study of Ziauddin College of Pharmacy, which is affiliated to a tertiary-care hospital, is worth mentioning here. Despite their academic responsibilities, the pharmacists practice here as preceptors and contribute to knowledge sharing by appraising the students of their day-to-day encounters with patients, thus enhancing the critical reasoning abilities of the students.[33] Keeping in view the paradigm shift from industry to hospital and community, it is now necessary to identify local needs and develop a specific model of pharmacy education.[34]

14. Drug information specialists and centers

Pharmacovigilance is a top priority in healthcare around the world, but unfortunately it is practically nonexistent in Pakistan. All of the officials in the drug delivery system believe that disease-related mortality is sometimes unavoidable, but drug-related death is now unacceptable. The low trust of patients in the healthcare system increases the costs of any adverse drug reaction twice. There is an urgent need to design a pharmacovigilance program for best patient care and implement the concept of pharmaceutical care within the health care system of Pakistan by involving important stakeholders. Pharmacists should take a pharmacovigilance program as an opportunity for best patient care in Pakistan and must play an active role in it.[35,36]

15. Drug companies, medical representatives, and the marketing of pharmaceutical products

Pharmaceutical companies play a vital role in the research, development, and marketing of medicines in the healthcare system through tremendous investments. They provide medications to millions of patients to promote health and improve the quality of life. Healthcare providers and patients can be influenced into prescribing or purchasing of medicines through marketing. These companies hire medical representatives for promoting their products as well as for providing credible and up-to-date information regarding drugs to the prescribers.[23]

The pharmaceutical industry in Pakistan is responsible for influencing the prescribing habits of healthcare providers to a great extent. Items such as journals, calendars, and pens, as well as more expensive ones such as briefcases, laptop computers, air conditioners, and cars, are given as incentives to the prescribers for promotion of a brand.[25] The purpose of these incentives has increased profits rather than the best interest of patients. Patients pay out of their own pockets for drugs in Pakistan due to these unethical promotions by pharmaceutical companies. Still, there is no mechanism to monitor drug promotional campaigns by the pharmaceutical industry in Pakistan, regardless of the evidence for irrational pharmacotherapy due to the unethical practices of pharmaceutical promotion.[25,37] In Pakistan, not only are the educational events the intensive promotional grounds for pharmaceutical products the organization of doctor-led educational events is equally widespread in this regard.[38] The top 10 pharmaceutical companies in 2014 are shown in Table 4.

Table 4: Top 10 pharmaceutical companies

Rank	Pharmaceutical Companies
1	Getz Pharma (Pvt) Ltd
2	Glitz Pharma
3	Global Pharmaceuticals
4	Highnoon Laboratories Ltd
5	Indus Pharmaceuticals
6	Leads Pharma (Pvt) Ltd
7	Werrick Pharmaceuticals (Pvt) Ltd
8	Martin Dow Pharmaceuticals (Pvt) Ltd
9	Zafa Pharmaceuticals (Pvt) Ltd
10	Willsons Pharmaceuticals

16. *Community pharmacy practice*

Health care in Pakistan is predominantly provided by the private sector, with 76% of health care expenditure coming out of the patients' pockets.[39] The distribution of medicines relies heavily on community pharmacies; according to one estimate, 80% of the medicines are being distributed through this channel.

Thus, majority of the population relies on community pharmacies for their health care needs. There are approximately 63,000 community pharmacies in the country.[10] These pharmacies are quite diverse in their geographical distribution and operations; they are located in urban and rural areas, inside hospitals, in general stores and grocery stores, and at market stalls. They often lack adequate facilities, staffing, and equipment, and their compliance with legal requirements also varies.[40,41] In addition, dispensers working in these pharmacies may not be trained, even though they are involved in making diagnoses, recommending therapy to patients, and dispensing medicines.[42,43]

The conditions of community pharmacies in Pakistan have been reported as being unsatisfactory. Inappropriate storage and dispensing of medicines, lack of proper documentation and prescription checks, along with labeling, are the foremost issues to be addressed at these outlets in Pakistan.[44] The lack of qualified personnel at community pharmacies is a common concern. There is shortage of pharmacists who could ensure good pharmacy practices. The dispensers working at community pharmacies generally have minimal formal education, with 10–12 years of schooling, and little or no professional training. They mostly rely on information gathered by the representatives of pharmaceutical companies.[42] Despite their limited qualifications and training, these dispensers are responsible for the functions of a dispenser, store keeper, inventory manager, accountant, prescriber, information provider, and patient counselor.

All kinds of medicines are freely available, irrespective of their status as prescription or over-the-counter drugs. The process of prescription handling is poor, and patients are often treated without a proper prescription. Prescription validation, drug labeling, and patient counseling are the missing components in effective patient management at these community pharmacies. Laws exist, but due to a lack of accountability and weak regulatory framework, these laws are not properly implementated.[45] There is a permission of chain pharmacies in Pakistan; Fazal Din's Pharma Plus was established in 1995 as one of the major pharmacy chains in the city of Lahore. The concept of larger chain pharmacies is now evolving gradually, and their establishment in government hospitals is on the move.

17. Public health practice and health promotion policy

Pakistan was one of the initial signatories to the Alma-Ata Declaration in 1978; however, the first policy dedicated solely to public health and health promotion was launched in 2004. The National Action Plan for Prevention and Control of Noncommunicable Diseases and Health Promotion has acquired a prominent place on the nation's health agenda, which is primarily focused on the community setting through media and female health workers competing for resources with traditional health policies that focus on treatment, cure, and evolving technology in Pakistan. The current public health/health promotion policy gained strength through public–private partnerships, which greatly facilitate the process of policy development, and continues to support research, implementation, and evaluation. The role of pharmacists has been acknowledged in malaria and national HIV/AIDS programs in the country.[46]

18. Traditional and herbal medicines

About 70% of the population, mostly in rural areas in Pakistan, uses traditional, herbal, and homeopathic medicines, finding them to be efficacious, safe, and cost-effective. Approximately 52,600 registered Unani medical practitioners, 16,000 diploma-holding Unani physicians of traditional medicine, and 40,000 registered homeopathic physicians are integrated into the national healthcare system through both public and private sectors in urban and rural areas in Pakistan. The National Institute for Health has established a section on traditional medicine (Tibb). There are 95 dispensaries and 360 Tibb dispensaries and clinics, which provide free medication to the public under the control of the health departments of provincial governments.[47] There are 26 colleges in the private sector and one college in the public sector, which are recognized by the government and under the direct control of the National Council for Tibb, Ministry of Health sector; these schools offer 4-year diploma courses in Pakistani traditional Unani and Ayurvedic systems of medicine.[48]

The Unani, Ayurvedic, and Homeopathic Practitioners Act of 1965 was established in order to arrange for the registration of qualified persons, to maintain adequate standards at recognized institutions, to conduct research, and to perform other activities. Requirements for the registration of practitioners were laid down, and training at recognized institutions was fixed at 4 years. The government thereafter issued the Unani, Ayurvedic, and Homeopathic Systems of Medicine Rules of 1965, which introduced the title of "homeopathic doctor" for registered homeopaths, although the use of analogous titles was forbidden to practitioners of Ayurvedic and Unani medicines.[47]

In Pakistan, research on the utilization of complementary and alternative medicine (CAM) is focused only on small-scale studies that primarily focus on the incidence of use among future healthcare practitioners, patients suffering from noncommunicable diseases, and other special patient populations.[49] Future pharmacy practitioners demonstrated optimistic attitudes about the worth of CAM and most believed that CAM should be included in their curriculum.[50] Thus, it is imperative that CAM modalities be acknowledged and well thought as a vital restorative option.

19. Pharmacy practice in pharmacy curriculum

Pharmacy education has been neglected and has contributed insignificantly to the national healthcare system of Pakistan. The 4-year bachelor of pharmacy (BPharm) degree was upgraded to a 5-year doctor of pharmacy (PharmD) program by the Higher Education Commission (HEC) of Pakistan in 2004, and the pharmacy syllabus was revised (Table 5). Although the number of pharmacy institutions in the country has increased over the years, the change is seen as more quantitative than qualitative. The syllabus has been revised, but still it shows various shortcomings with regard to international standards.[32] The content and the subjects in the final year (fifth year) are just an extension of the first 4 years. The clinical and social aspects of pharmacy, such as drug abuse, geriatric pharmacy, patient counseling, patient compliance, research methods, and evidence-based medicine, have been largely ignored. Other major areas such as pharmacogenomics, pharmacoinformatics (drug information), pharmacoeconomics (economic evaluation of drugs), pharmacoepidemiology (drug utilization studies), public health pharmacy, and drug policy have also been largely neglected.[51] These limitations in the syllabus can largely be explained by the composition of the HEC curriculum

Table 5: Pharmacy curriculum in Pakistan

Year	Curriculum
Year 1	Organic Chemistry, Pharmaceutics I (Physical Pharmacy), Physiology, Anatomy, Biochemistry, English Language, Islamic Culture, Pharmaceutical Mathematics and Biostatistics
Year 2	Pharmaceutics II (Pharmaceutical Preparation), Microbiology, General Pharmacognosy, General Pharmacology, Community Pharmacy, Pakistan Studies
Year 3	Dispensing, Instrumentation Chemistry II, Pathology, Chemical Pharmacognosy, Systemic Pharmacology and Toxicology.
Year 4	Biopharmaceutics, Clinical Pharmacy I, Medical Chemistry I, Industrial Pharmacy I, Quality Control of Drugs, Hospital Pharmacy
Year 5	Medical Chemistry II, Industrial Pharmacy II, Clinical Pharmacy II, Quality Control of Drugs II, Advance Pharmacognosy, Prescription Writing and Community Pharmacy Practice, Advance Clinical Pharmacology, Graduation Research Project

Source: Pharmacy Council of Pakistan, 2014.

committee, in which the majority of the committee members belong to the old school of thought and might not have relevant expertise in making recommendations for a clinical and community-oriented syllabus.[52]

The main challenge that the profession is facing after upgrading the BPharm program to a PharmD program is an inadequate number of experienced and qualified staff, which is one of the reasons for the deficiencies in the clinical content of the PharmD program.[30,53,54] Other important issues are the dual examination system, which is either an annual or a semester system depending on the university, and the lack of uniformity in terms of grading the students. This can deprive capable students of obtaining jobs because candidates are usually short-listed based on their grades in pharmacy school.[55]

20. Challenges in pharmacy practice

The main areas of pharmacy practice in Pakistan are outlined in Table 6.

The limitations in pharmacy education and the role of pharmacists in national health policy have marginalized the pharmacy profession and prevented pharmacists from consolidating their roles in the healthcare system of Pakistan. One of the major challenges faced by the pharmacy profession is the availability of hospital jobs and acceptance of pharmacists in clinical settings by the medical and paramedical personnel.[28] The role of pharmacists is usually played by unqualified and untrained dispensers at hospital pharmacies. If a pharmacist is available, the role is merely that of a storekeeper; the pharmacist is hardly involved in decision-making processes.[12] Most of the clinical and administrative pharmacy services, such as total parenteral nutrition, therapeutic drug monitoring, and ward pharmacy services, are nonexistent at the majority of the public hospitals. Medication errors and adverse drug reactions go unreported because of the lack of pharmacy support services. There are no independent drug information services at public hospitals, which provides opportunities for medical representatives to disseminate biased drug information to doctors.[31]

The Pakistan Pharmacy Council registration policy for category B and C diploma holders in pharmacy needs to be revised. These pharmacy assistant and diploma holders are eligible to

Table 6: Main areas of pharmacy practice in Pakistan

Areas of Pharmacy Practice	Percentage
Community/private pharmacy	10%
Healthcare	10%
Pharmaceutical industry	55%
Sales and marketing	15%
Regulatory affairs and other	5%
Academia and research	5%
Total	100%

register with the PPC and to run a medical store/retail pharmacy in their localities. As a result of this practice, the public is vulnerable to untrained drug traders and quacks.[41] In addition, some of the pharmacists rent their licenses at community pharmacies irrespective of their availability at the pharmacies, which has undermined their role and promoted irrational dispensing practices.[56] Lack of awareness regarding the role of pharmacists in the community is another area of concern, which can be bridged by utilizing the different channels of media, conferences, seminars, and workshops in collaboration with different stakeholders.[57]

Furthermore, the pharmacy curriculum needs drastic revision on a regular basis in order to meet the international requirements of PharmD program. Areas concerning drug policy, rational prescribing, pharmaceutical promotion, pharmacoecnomics, and public health must be incorporated in the current syllabus. The pharmacy institutes need improvement in academic and research facilities qualitatively as well as quantitatively.[32]

The future of the pharmaceutical industry lies with the genetically engineered medicines. But pharmacogenomics, a new key area for improving therapies through biotechnology, is absent in current research and development agenda in Pakistan. There is lack of integration among different disciplines such as pharmacy education, practice, and regulation, namely HEC, the Pharmacy Council of Pakistan, and the Ministry of Health. Along with lack of human resources in Pakistan, the profession also seriously lacks government interest. Although, the pharmacy council is striving to bridge this gap and uplift the profession but the chief criticism on the council is that of corruption in the institute and that of the body structure of not being fully independent which it should have to be.

Apart from all the shortcomings and pitfalls in pharmacy practice research in Pakistan, there are few worth mentioning case studies which are the "Research Milestones" in pharmacy practice arena. Research in the areas of community pharmacy practices and their legal requirements, dispensing practices of drug sellers, generic medicine prescribing and their utilization, recognition of pharmacists in the local healthcare system and drug promotional practices by the pharmaceutical industries are known and recognized globally.[38,56,58,59]

21. Conclusion

The pharmaceutical industry in Pakistan is a pulsating segment which fulfills the majority of local requirements. With its presence in the foreign markets, the industry is amplifying its capacity day by day in terms of manufacturing raw material, inception of bioavailability centers and academic and research partnering with the universities. Moreover, a frail implementation or either a dearth of distinct set of laws and screening system by the national authoritative bodies presumably pave the way for irrational prescribing, dispensing, and promotional practices, escorting to an increased risk to healthcare system in general and patient's health status in particular.

22. Recommendations

It is recommended that the newly created drug regulatory authority could be free from all the biases from the industry and must be managed in a thorough professional manner.

Keeping in view the patient-centered approach evolving globally, the Government of Pakistan should extend health communication messages and endow with guidance of how to increase communication between patients and doctors and pharmacists. It is recommended to revamp the healthcare professionals' curriculum by employing health promotion educators from social and behavioral sciences. They work as collaborators of doctors and pharmacists and in turn build up effective educational tools that inculcate behavioral changes among healthcare practitioners and patients alike.

23. Points to remember

- Pharmacy education is upgraded to 5-years PharmD program but inadequate number of experienced and qualified staff mainly in the area of pharmacy practice is the main hurdle which needs to be overcome in the near future
- Pharmaceutical industry in Pakistan is a vibrantly developing segment which fulfills the majority of local requirements

References

1. Government of Pakistan. *Population census organization everyone counts.* Islamabad 2011. [cited June 26, 2011]. Available from: www.census.gov.pk/.
2. Federal Bureau of Statistics. Pakistan Social & Living Standards Measurement Survey 2005–2006.
3. World Health Organization. *Country profile.* 2010. [cited October 9, 2009]. Available from: http://www.emro.who.int/emrinfo/index.asp?Ctry=pak.
4. Babar TS, Hatcher J. Health seeking behaviour and health services utilization trends in national health survey of Pakistan: what needs to be done? *J Pak Med Assoc* 2007;**57**(8):411–3.
5. BMI. *Pakistan pharmaceutical and healthcare report Q4 2013.* Business Monitor International; 2013.
6. Ministry of Health. *Booklet of drugs control organization.* Available from: http://www.dcomoh.gov.pk/downloads/booklet.pdf; 2010.
7. Ministry of Health. *National health policy 2001. The way forward.* Available from: http://www.nacp.gov.pk/introduction/national_health_policy/NationalHealthPolicy-2001.pdf; 2001.
8. National Drug Policy. National Drug Policy 1997 [November 20, 2009]. Available from: http://www.dcomoh.gov.pk/publications/ndp.php.
9. Ahsan N. Pharmacy education and pharmacy council of Pakistan. *Pak Drug Updates* 2005;**7**:4–5.
10. Babar Z. *Medicalising Pakistan.* CHOWK; 2007. [cited November 20, 2009]. Available from: http://www.chowk.com/articles/11520.
11. Khan DRA. *Pharmacy education and healthcare.* Dawn. [cited September 23, 2007]. Available from: http://www.gcu.edu.pk/Library/NI_Feb07.htm; 2007.
12. Azhar S, Hassali MA, Ibrahim MIM, Ahmad M, Masood I, Shafie AA. The role of pharmacists in developing countries: the current scenario in Pakistan. *Hum Resour Health* 2009;**7**(1):54.
13. Stone L. *Good Pharmacy Practice (GPP) in developing countries International Pharmaceutical Federation.* 1997. [updated 1997]. Available from: http://www.fip.org/files/www2/pdf/gpp/GPP_CPS_Report.pdf.
14. MOH. *Ministry of health booklet of drugs control organization*; 2010.

15. International Marketing Survey. *Pharmaceutical market in Pakistan*; 2008.
16. Pakistan Pharmaceutical and Healthcare Report Q4 2014. BMI Industry Report and Forecast Series Business Monitor International; 2014.
17. Mahmood K. Runaway drug prices in Pakistan. *The Lancet* 1993;**342**(8874):809.
18. Rayyan A. *Pakistan ministry raises prices of 30,000 medicines with a joke*; 2013. http://wwwthenewstribecom/2013/11/28/pakistan-ministry-raises-prices-of-30000-medicines-with-a-joke/. [accessed February 2014].
19. Iqbal M, Hakim ST, Hussain A, Mirza Z, Quereshi F, Abdulla EM. Ofloxacin: laboratory evaluation of the antibacterial activity of 34 brands representing 31 manufacturers available in Pakistan. *Pak J Med Sci* 2004;**20**(4):349–56.
20. Babar ZUD, Ibrahim MIM, Singh H, Bukahri NI, Creese A. Evaluating drug prices, availability, affordability, and price components: implications for access to drugs in Malaysia. *PLoS Med* 2007;**4**(3):e82.
21. DCO. *Drug control authority price review committee government of Pakistan*. Ministry of Health; 2003. Available on: http://www.dcomoh.gov.pk/boards/prc.php. [accessed 08.07.11].
22. DCO. *Drug control authority price review committee government of Pakistan*. Ministry of Health; 2009. Available on: http://www.dcomoh.gov.pk/boards/prc.php. [accessed 08.07.11].
23. Babar ZUD, Ibrahim MIM, Hassali MAA. Pharmaceutical industry, innovation and challenges for public health: case studies from Malaysia and Pakistan. *J Pharm Health Serv Res* 2011;**2**(4):193–204.
24. Khan MM. Murky waters: the pharmaceutical industry and psychiatrists in developing countries. *Psychiatr Bull* 2006;**30**(3):85–8.
25. Gulhati C. Opinion and debate why physicians should not have any contact with pharmaceutical companies? *JPMA* 2007.
26. Asif M, Awan MU. Pakistani pharmaceutical industry in WTO regime-issues and prospects. *J Qual Technol Manage* 2005;**1**(1):21–34.
27. Babar ZUD, Scahill S. Is there a role for pharmacoeconomics in developing countries? *Pharmacoeconomics* 2010;**28**(12):1069.
28. Azhar S, Hassali MA, Ibrahim MMI. Perceptions of hospital pharmacist's role in Pakistan's healthcare system: a cross-sectional survey. *Trop J Pharm Res* 2011;**10**(1).
29. Rathore HA, Wei LS. Archives of pharmacy practice short communication. *Arch Pharm Pract* 2010;**1**(1):5.
30. Khan MU. A new paradigm in clinical pharmacy teaching in Pakistan. *Am J Pharm Educ* 2011;**75**(8).
31. Rabbani F. *Science and practice of balanced scorecard in a hospital in Pakistan*; 2010.
32. Murtaza G, Ahmad M, Iqbal M, Khan SA, Ejaz M, Yasmin T. Pharmacy education and practice in Pakistan: a guide to further development. *Hacettepe University Journal of the Faculty of Pharmacy* 2010;**30**(2):139–56.
33. Khan MU. A new paradigm in clinical pharmacy teaching in Pakistan. *Am J Pharm Educ* 2011;**75**(8):166. 2012/12/11.
34. Anderson C, Futter B. PharmD or needs based education: which comes first?. *Am J Pharm Educ* 2009;**73**(5):92. 2012/12/11.
35. Mahmood KT, Tahir FAM, Haq IU. Pharmacovigilance – a need for best patient care in Pakistan. A review. *J Pharm Sci & Res* 2011;**3**(11):1566–84.
36. Nazir T, Zaidi SMM. Review of the basic components of clinical pharmaceutical care in Pakistan. *T Res J* 2011;**01**(01):01–05.
37. Wazana A. Physicians and the pharmaceutical industry. *JAMA: J Am Med Assoc* 2000;**283**(3):373–80.
38. Masood I, Ibrahim MIM, Hassali MAA, Ahmad M, Mansfield PR. Evaluation of pharmaceutical industry – sponsored educational events attended by physicians in Pakistan. *J Med Mark Device Diagn Pharm Mark* February 1, 2012;**12**(1):22–9.
39. Babar T, Hathcher J. Health seeking behaviour and health services utilization in national health survey of Pakistan: what needs to be done? *J Pak Med Assoc* 2007;**57**(8).
40. Hussain A, Ibrahim MIM, Baber ZD. Compliance with legal requirements at community pharmacies: a cross sectional study from Pakistan. *Int J Pharm Pract* 2011;**20**(3):183–90.
41. Butt ZA, Gilani AH, Nanan D, Sheikh AL, White F. Quality of pharmacies in Pakistan: a cross-sectional survey. *Int J Qual Health Care* 2005;**17**(4):307–13.

42. Hussain A, Ibrahim MIM. Qualification, knowledge and experience of dispensers working at community pharmacies in Pakistan. *Pharm Pract (Internet)* 2011;**9**(2):93–100.
43. Rabbani F, Cheema F, Talati N, Siddiqui S, Syed S, Basir S, et al. Behind the counter: pharmacies and dispensing patterns of pharmacy attendants in Karachi. *J Pak Med Assoc* 2001;**51**(4):149–54.
44. Hussain A, Ibrahim MIM. Medication counselling and dispensing practices at community pharmacies: a comparative cross sectional study from Pakistan. *Int J Clin Pharm* 2011;**33**(1):1–9.
45. Hussain A, Ibrahim MIM. Perceptions of dispensers regarding dispensing practices in Pakistan: a qualitative study. *Trop J Pharm Res* 2011;**10**(2):117–23.
46. Ronis K, Nishtar S. Community health promotion in Pakistan: a policy development perspective. *Promot Educ* 2007;**14**(2):98–9.
47. Shaikh BT, Hatcher J, Shaikh B. Complementary and alternative medicine in Pakistan: prospects and limitations. *Evidence-Based Complementary Altern Med* 2005;**2**(2):139.
48. Shaheen F, Rahman A, Vasisht K, Iqbal Choudhary M. *The status of medicinal and aromatic plants in Pakistan. Medicinal plants and their utilization*. UNIDO; 2003. p. 77–87.
49. Ishaque S, Saleem T, Qidwai W. Knowledge, attitudes and practices regarding gemstone therapeutics in a selected adult population in Pakistan. *BMC Complementary Altern Med* 2009;**9**(1):32.
50. Hussain S, Malik F, Hameed A, Ahmed S, Riaz H, Abbasi N, et al. Pakistani pharmacy students perception about complementary and alternative medicine. *Am J Pharm Educ* 2012;**76**(2):21. 2012/12/11.
51. Khan TM. Challenges to pharmacists and pharmacy practice in Pakistan. *Australas Med J AMJ* 2011;**4**(4).
52. Khan T, Anwar M, Ahmed KKM. A perspective for clinical pharmacy curriculum development and validation in Asian developing nations. *J Young Pharm JYP* 2011;**3**(2):151.
53. Jamshed S, Babar ZUD, Masood I. The PharmD degree in developing countries. *Am J Pharm Educ* 2007;**71**(6).
54. Sa'di Mohammad Al-Haddad M, Hassali MA. Archives of pharmacy practice short communication. *Arch Pharm Pract* 2010;**1**(1):3.
55. Khan MU. Postgraduate courses in clinical pharmacy in Pakistan. *Int J* 2012;**3**(2):281–2.
56. Hussain A, Ibrahim MIM, Baber ZUD. Compliance with legal requirements at community pharmacies: a cross sectional study from Pakistan. *Int J Pharm Pract* 2012;**20**(3):183–90.
57. Hussain A, Ibrahim MIM. Medication counselling and dispensing practices at community pharmacies: a comparative cross sectional study from Pakistan. *Int J Clin Pharm* 2011;**33**(5):859–67.
58. Jamshed SQ, Ibrahim MIM, Hassali MAA, Masood I, Low BY, Shafie AA, et al. Perception and attitude of general practitioners regarding generic medicines in Karachi, Pakistan: a questionnaire based study. *South Med Rev* 2012;**5**(1):22–30.
59. Azhar S, Hassali MA, Ibrahim MIM. A qualitative study evaluating perceptions of hospital pharmacists towards their role in Pakistan's healthcare system. *Int J Pharm Pract* 2010;**17**(Suppl. 1):13. Section 2B The pharmacy profession.

CHAPTER 7

Pharmacy Practice in India

Shahid Karim, Muhammad Adnan

Chapter Outline

1. Background

India is a developing nation located in southern Asia consisting of 29 states and 7 union territories, with 22 nationally recognized languages and a population of 1.2 billion people.[1] India is a rural country with an agriculture-based economy; almost 75% of its population resides in rural areas. In recent decades, India has seen a marked increase in average income levels, leading to rapid urbanization, increased access of the middle class to a better lifestyle, and increased awareness of health insurance. The literacy rate has increased for both males and females to 82% and 65%, respectively. Life expectancy has been reported to be 69.9 years.[2] According to a 2010 World Bank report, around 400 million people in India live on less than 1.25 USD (PPP) per day, and 44% of children are malnourished. The mortality rates of infants and women are still on the higher side, although the government has made efforts to curb them.

Pharmacy had been recognized by ancient Hindus as a complimentary health profession, and they focused vegetables for remedies. Hindu medicine was divided into two periods: Vedic and Brahmanic. The Vedic period was until 800 BC, and it was primitive. Sin was considered to be a main cause for disease in the Vedic period. The Brahmanic period was roughly between 800 BC and 1000 AD; this was considered to be a high-caliber period for Hindu medical education. The three great classics of Brahmanic medicine are the books of Caraka, Susruta, and Vagbhat, which are based on older Vedic contents.[3]

The roots of pharmacy development in India are linked back to Ayurveda in 5000 BC. Ayurveda—the science of life—was first taught by Lord Brahma but was spread by Charaka and Sushruta.[4] The early text on Ayurveda is *Charaka Samhitā*, which focused on vegetable products and some animal and earth products. The classification of drugs in this book was based on the action of drugs on the body parts.[3] Tamilnadu organized a hospital in 900 AD that treated piles, jaundice, hemorrhage, and tuberculosis.[4] Tantrism was a popular philosophical and religious movement that appeared after the decline of Buddhism in India; it brought the art and science of the development of metallic compounds, particularly mercury and sulfur.[3]

Scotch M. Bathgate opened first chemist shop in Kolkata in 1811; this was considered to be the starting point of pharmacy practice in India. Madras Medical School started pharmacy education in December 1860, enrolling students with middle school education; the duration of the pharmacy degree was 2 years. In 1874, the diploma course in pharmacy was introduced by Madras Medical College (MMC), Chennai. The Calcutta Chemists & Druggists Association was found in 1920; it was later renamed as the Bengal Chemists and Druggist association in 1926. The official *Indian Journal of Pharmacy* was first released in 1939. The Indian pharmacopeia was first published under the British Monarchy in 1868. In Bengal, a statutory provision was established for education and examination of compounders in 1881. The Master's degrees in pharmaceutics and applied chemistry were introduced in 1920 and 1940, respectively. In 1943, the first postgraduate pharmacy student to complete the degree was Gorakh Prasad Srivastava.

The standardization of pharmacy education was initiated in 1945. The Indian Pharmaceutical Congress Association had its first annual conference in 1948. The Pharmaceutical Association was the first pharmaceutical society of India; it was started in 1923 and after 2 years was renamed as The Pharmaceutical Society of India. An institute was established in 1949 at west Bengal, which offered a diploma in pharmacy; the Pharmacy Council of India (PCI) in 1953 set the diploma in pharmacy as the minimum requirement to start pharmacy practice. Prof. M.L. Schroff, named as "father of Pharmacy in India," was elected as the president of the PCI in 1954.

In 1932, pharmacy education was started at Banaras Hindu University, as it introduced a Bachelor's of Pharmaceutical Chemistry and was the first university to start a 3-year bachelors program in pharmacy. The school offered pharmaceutical chemistry, pharmacognosy, and pharmaceutical economics. Punjab University was the second institute in India that initiated a Bachelor's in Pharmacy program, in 1944. Andhra University started a Master's in Pharmacy program in 1954, which focused on analysis of food, drugs, and water and manufacturing pharmaceuticals. Furthermore, in 1969, the school offered MPharm in pharmaceutical and food analysis, pharmaceutical chemistry, and pharmaceutical fermentation technology. In 1970, Manipal College of Pharmacy initiated MPharm in pharmacy administration. After 9 years, the MPharm in hospital pharmacy and pharmaceutics was initiated by the College of Pharmacy in New Delhi. Hamdard College of Pharmacy introduced a Master's program in phytochemistry and pharmacognosy in 1982.[4]

According to the PCI, the intake capacity for diploma and Bachelor's of Pharmacy students is 60–120 per year; both programs require animal house, library, auditorium, seminar hall, and herbal garden. These programs further require well-equipped laboratories for analytical chemistry, pharmaceutics, pharmaceutical chemistry, pharmacology, pharmacognosy, and pharmaceutical chemistry. The regulations state that pharmacy institutions running approved BPharm programs under section 12 of the Pharmacy Act are eligible to initiate PharmD programs.[4]

2. Health statistics

The healthcare sector in India faces many challenges, such as the need to reduce mortality rates, physical infrastructure improvements, health insurance, and trained healthcare professionals/personnel. There has been a reported increase in communicable diseases, lifestyle diseases, and noncommunicable diseases. There will be eradication of diseases such as poliomyelitis, leprosy, and neonatal tetanus; however, some infectious diseases that were under control have returned or have developed resistance to drugs, such as dengue fever, viral hepatitis, tuberculosis, malaria, and pneumonia.

Although Indians are more affluent now due to the growth of the middle class, their food habits have changed markedly to unhealthy diets that are high in sugar and fat, leading to an increase in lifestyle diseases such as hypertension, cancer, and diabetes. In addition, the growing elderly population will be a burden to India's healthcare systems and services.

The population does not have access to their medical needs due to a shortage of hospital beds and trained medical staff such as doctors, nurses, and pharmacists. The rural population is further deficient in healthcare services as compared to urban areas. The healthcare workforce showed a negatively skewed representation of females as compared to males. The total healthcare expenditure (combining public funds, private funds and external flows) in the 11th five-year plan equaled 4.1% of the gross domestic product (GDP). The 12th five-year plan (2012–2017) aims to increase the public health investment from 1.1 % to 2–3% of GDP.[5]

3. Overview of the health care system

The healthcare system is the responsibility of the state. Currently, this system is run by both the public and private (for profit as well as nonprofit) organizations. The central government is responsible for policymaking, planning, guiding, assisting, evaluating, and coordinating the work of various provincial health authorities and providing funding to implement national healthcare programs.[6] The service infrastructure of health care in India includes allopathic hospitals, hospital beds, Indian System of Medicine and Homeopathy hospitals, subcenters, Pharmacy Health Care (PHC), Community Health Center (CHC), blood banks, Eye Bank, mental hospitals, and cancer hospitals.[6] The medical and health care facility under Department of Ayurveda, Yoga and Naturopathy, Unani, Siddha and Homeopathy (AYUSH) by management status is shown in Figure 1.

The public sector ownership is divided between central and state governments, municipals, and panchayats (local governments). The facilities include teaching hospitals, secondary-level hospitals, first-level referral hospitals (community health centers/rural hospitals), dispensaries, primary health centers, subcenters, and health posts.

Also included are public facilities for selected occupational groups, such as the organized workforce (Employees State Insurance Scheme), defense, government employees (Central Government Health Scheme), railways, post and telegraph, and mines, among others. The private sector (for-profit/non-profit) is the dominant sector, and services range from >1000-bed to two-bed facilities. The central government healthcare scheme has health-related facilities in 25 cities, which have 246 allopathic dispensaries[6] (Figure 2).

The statewise number of government hospitals and beds in rural and urban areas of India[6] is shown in Figure 3.

Presently, India has been experiencing a growth in private healthcare providers, who currently treat 78% of outpatients and 60% of inpatients. Private healthcare providers include everything from private hospitals that promote medical tourism by offering world-class services to foreign clients and Indians who can afford it, to private doctors with little medical knowledge or formal training at the other end of the spectrum. Furthermore, the strength of the private sector is illustrated by the fact that it controls 80% of doctors, 26% of nurses, 49% of beds,

S. No.	Management	Ayurveda Hospitals	Ayurveda Dispensaries	Unani Hospitals	Unani Dispensaries	Siddha Hospitals	Siddha Dispensaries	Yoga Hospitals	Yoga Dispensaries	Naturopathy Hospitals	Naturopathy Dispensaries	Homoeopathy Hospitals	Homoeopathy Dispensaries	Amchi Hospitals	Amchi Dispensaries	Total Hospitals	Total Dispensaries	% Distribution Hospitals	% Distribution Dispensaries
		2	3	4	5	6	7	8	9	10	11	12	13	14	15	16	17	18	19
1																			
A. Under Jurisdiction of States/Union Territories																			
1	State/Govt./UT Administration	2230	13774	233	941	265	808	6	61	7	62	97	5448	0	5	2838	21069	88.90%	86.80%
2	Local Bodies	11	642	0	45	0	0	0	0	0	0	3	1147	0	0	14	1834	0.40%	7.60%
3	Others	156	383	16	9	1	0	0	75	16	34	110	217	2	129	301	847	9.4	3.50%
	Total (A)	2397	14769	249	995	266	808	6	136	23	96	210	6812	2	134	3153	23750	98.70%	97.80%
B. CGHS & Central Government organizations																			
4	C.G.H.S.	1	33	0	10	0	3	0	4	0	0	0	35	0	0	1	85	0.00%	0.40%
5	Railway Ministry	0	40	0	0	0	0	0	0	0	0	0	129	0	0	0	169	0.00%	0.80%
6	Labour Ministry	0	148	0	0	0	8	0	0	0	0	0	39	0	0	0	195	0.00%	0.00%
7	Ministry of col	0	11	0	0	0	0	0	0	0	0	0	0	0	0	0	11	0.00%	0.70%
8	Research Councils	19	8	8	15	2	2	0	0	0	0	4	32	0	1	33	58	1.00%	0.20%
9	National Institutes	3	8	1	1	1	0	0	0	0	1	1	2	0	0	6	12	0.20%	0.00%
	TOTAL	23	248	9	26	3	13	0	4	0	1	5	237	0	1	40	530	1.30%	2.20%
	All India (A+B)	2420	15017	258	1021	269	821	6	140	23	97	215	7049	2	135	3193	24280	100%	100%

Figure 1

Distribution of AYUSH hospitals and their management. *Source: AYUSH, Ministry of health and family welfare.*

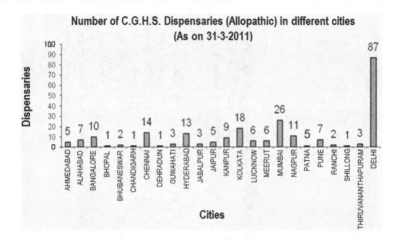

Figure 2

Number of central govt. health scheme dispensaries (allopathic) in different cities. *Source: Central Government Health Scheme, Director General of Health Services (Dte. GHS), Ministry of Health (M/o.) Health and Family Welfare (F.W.), Nirman Bhawan, New Delhi.*

and 78% of ambulatory services. Private actors are now present in all areas of healthcare, including health financing, education, equipment manufacturing, and services. The heavy increase in private healthcare providers can be viewed as a result of the lacking quality care offered by public providers, shortages of doctors, and overcrowding at public healthcare facilities. This subsequently results in about 72% of out-of-pocket expenses that are directed at medicines and put significant pressure on the individual. Some are driven below the poverty line due to the costs they incur in order to access healthcare services.[7]

3.1 Health insurance

Health Insurance in India is in its infancy. In the barely developed health insurance market, the Indian government plays an important role by launching social health insurance and regulating the private health insurance market. Many insurance schemes are operated by the Central and State governments, such as the Rashtriya Swasthya Bima Yojana, which targets families that are below the poverty line, the Employees' State Insurance Scheme, and the Central Government Health Schemes. There are also public and private insurance companies as well as several community-based organizations (Figure 4).[8]

The major public health insurance company in India is the government-run General Insurance Corporation (GIC). The main health insurance product sold in India is the GIC Mediclaim Policy, which was originally offered in 1986. This plan is designed such that the insured is responsible to pay out-of pocket expenses to the doctors and then file a claim to get reimbursed. Thus, such plans are not within the reach of poor because they cannot afford the premium and pay the medical fees upfront, in contrast to the middle class and upper middle

S. No.	State/UT/ Division	Rural Hospitals (Govt.)		Urban Hospitals (Govt.)		Total Hospitals (Govt.)		Provisional /Projected Population as on reference period in (000)	Averege Population Served Per Govt. Hospital	Averege Population Served Per Govt. Hospital Bed	Reference Period
		No.	Beds	No.	Beds	No.	Beds				
	1	2	3	4	5	6	7	8	9	10	11
	India	**7347**	**160862**	**4146**	**618664**	**11993**	**784940**	**1186944**	**98970**	**1512**	
1	Andhra Pradesh	143	3725	332	34325	475	38050	84666	178243	2225	01.01.2011
2	Arunachal Pradesh	146	1356	15	862	161	2218	1184	7354	534	01.01.2009
3	Assam	108	3240	45	4382	153	7622	29814	194863	3912	01.01.2010
4	Bihar	61	1830	169	16686	230	18516	103805	451325	5606	01.01.2012
5	Chattisgarh	119	3270	99	6158	218	9428	22934	105202	2433	01.01.2009
6	Goa	8	1422	9	1187	17	2609	1458	85765	559	01.01.2012
7	Gujarat	318	11099	127	182111	445	193210	60384	135694	313	01.01.2012
8	Haryana	61	1212	93	6667	154	7879	24597	159721	3122	01.01.2010
9	Himachal Pradesh	97	2905	53	5574	150	8479	6856	45707	809	01.01.2012
10	Jammu & Kashmir	61	1820	31	2125	92	3945	11099	120641	2813	01.01.2008
11	Jharkhand	NR	NR	NR	NR	500	5414	29745	59490	5494	01.01.2008
12	Karnataka	468	8010	451	55731	919	63741	58181	63309	913	01.01.2010
13	Kerala	308	12233	138	19727	446	31960	33388	74861	1045	01.01.2012
14	Madhya Pradesh	333	10040	124	18493	457	28533	71050	155470	2490	01.01.2011
15	Maharashtra	523	11672	843	56282	1366	67954	112373	82264	1654	01.01.2012
16	Manipur	217	664	8	721	225	1385	2722	12098	1965	01.01.2012
17	Meghalaya	29	870	10	1967	39	2837	2591	66436	913	01.01.2011
18	Mizoram	20	770	7	660	27	1430	1091	40407	763	01.01.2012
19	Nagaland	23	705	25	1445	48	2150	2197	45771	1022	01.01.2010
20	Odisha	1659	7099	91	8715	1750	15814	41947	23970	2653	01.01.2012
21	Punjab	78	2360	135	8063	213	10423	27704	130066	2658	01.01.2012
22	Rajasthan	380	13754	446	12236	826	25990	68621	83076	2640	01.01.2012
23	Sikkim	30	730	3	830	33	1560	608	18424	390	01.01.2012
24	Tamil Nadu	533	25078	48	22120	581	47198	65629	112959	1391	01.01.2008
25	Tripura	14	950	18	2082	32	3032	3574	111688	1179	01.01.2011
26	Uttar Pradesh	515	15450	346	40934	861	56384	197271	229118	3499	01.01.2011
27	Uttarakhand	666	3746	29	4219	695	7965	9511	13685	1194	01.01.2009
28	West Bengal	364	13693	290	57498	654	71191	91348	139676	1283	01.01.2012
29	A&N Island	31	625	1	450	32	1075	380	11875	353	01.01.2012
30	Chandigarh	1	50	3	570	4	620	1368	342000	2206	01.01.2011
31	D&N Haveli	1	50	1	231	2	281	343	171500	1221	01.01.2012
32	Daman & Diu	0	0	4	200	4	200	243	60750	1215	01.01.2012
33	Delhi	0	0	126	43109	126	43109	16955	134563	393	01.01.2009
34	Lakshadweep	5	160	–	–	5	160	64	12800	400	01.01.2012
35	Puducherry	27	274	26	2304	53	2578	1244	23472	483	01.01.2012

Figure 3
State wise distribution of Govt. Hospitals and beds in rural and urban areas of India. *Source: Directorate General of State Health Service.*

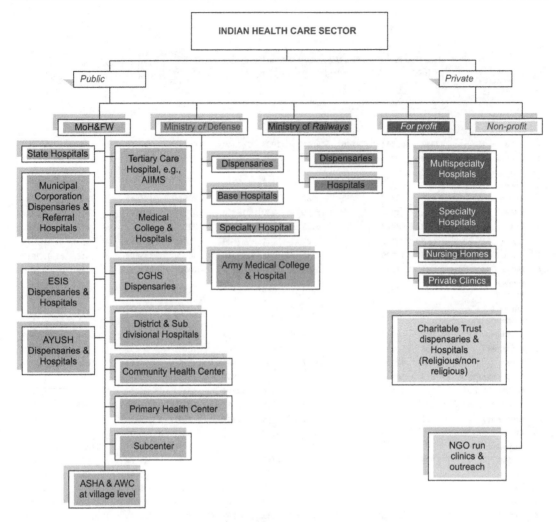

Figure 4

Health care sector in India. *Adapted from:*
http://www.tillvaxtanalys.se/en/home/publications/direct-response/direct-response/2013-05-20-indias-healthcare-system---overview-and-quality-improvements.html.

class. An estimated 300 million people are believed to be covered by health insurance in India. Of these, roughly 243 million are covered by different types of government-sponsored insurance schemes, while approximately 55 million rely on commercial insurers.

After the Insurance Regulatory and Development Authority Act was passed in 1999, a governing body under the name of Insurance Regulatory and Development Authority of India (IRDA) was set up to regulate insurers and protect the insured's interests. IRDA's aim is to set and enforce standards, ensuring speedy settlement, preventing claim frauds, and building information systems. These measures and regulations have accelerated the growth of the insurance industry and the economy in India.[7,8]

4. Medicines supply system and drug use issues

According to a McKinsey & Company report, India's pharma industry is set to quadruple by 2020 to $55 billion. The pharma industry has the potential to reach $70 billion if aggressive growth rates are achieved. Abbott India, Cipla, Sun Pharmaceuticals Industries, and GlaxoSmithKline Pharmaceuticals are the top four drugmakers in terms of market share. The fastest growing companies are Macleods Pharmaceuticals (21.7%), USV (19.9%), and Glenmark Pharmaceuticals (18.6%). The top ranking therapeutic segments in 2013 were anti-infectives, followed by cardiac and gastrointestinal disorders in the second and third positions, respectively. Patented products, consumer healthcare, biologics, vaccines, and public health will capture 45% of the market by 2020. It will ultimately bring loads of responsibilities to pharma logistics, but today there are few big pharma logistic players in India. The delivery of medicines is very critical due to its time- and temperature-sensitive nature, and it is an ultimate challenge for pharma logistics in India.[9]

The pharmaceutical industry in India is practicing high-quality good manufacturing practices (GMP) that ensure strict quality assurance requirements of final products. The transporters are responsible for supplying these finished products to the distributors but transport personnel lack skills for handling medicines during transportation. It is more critical in the case of long distances and it may affect the nature of the drug if the standard requirements during transportation are not followed. The lack of infrastructure, customized packing, and capacity issues are some of the problems affecting the finite life of products. The key problem is the management of pharma logistics by unorganized players.

The pharma industry is rapidly growing in India and pharma business is highly competitive. One key factor for success is the efficiency of supply chain management. Supply chain factors include inventory reduction and reduction of order cycle time. The operational performance depends on logistics cost, while the reduction in the inventory and decreased order cycle time is related to just-in-time deliveries and supply chain speed. The major logistic costs in the pharmaceutical industry include packing and distributions; these logistics comprise 45–55% of the costs in the pharmaceutical value chain.

Radiofrequency and identification devices have benefits such as product integrity, tracking capability, and inventory management, but the use of this technology is minimal in Indian pharmaceutical industries. Some of other major problems facing the pharma logistic sector include infrastructure problems and poor transportation.

The private sector has dominated the Indian cold-chain market, including surface storage and refrigerated transport. Surface storage holds 88% of the cold-chain market, and it is expected to reach 352 billion Indian rupees by 2015. The refrigerated transport section is 12% of the cold-chain market. The services provided by cold-chain pharma market need improvement and require retaining the temperature at transhipment hubs, tracking, qualified persons to handle pharma cargo, special packaging solutions that are cost-effective, immediate customs clearance, and compliance to regulatory requirements at the origin and at the destination. The Indian pharma logistic market in the evolutionary stages, and it requires time to meet the standards of an international market.[10,11]

5. Overview of pharmacy practice and key pharmaceutical sectors

The origin of pharmacy practice in India is rooted to British India, when the pharmacy profession was only business oriented; these professionals were drug sellers or drug dispensers, and there was no restriction on its practice. In early 1930s, Professor M. L. Schroff initiated pharmacy education in India at the Banaras Hindu University. The PCI was inaugurated in 1949 and started working as statutory body under the Pharmacy Act 1948. The formulation of education regulations (ER) was first done in 1953 and was revised in 1972, 1981, and 1991.[11–13] The minimum qualification required to be a pharmacist was fixed by PCI.

Pharmacy Council of India and All India Council of Technical Education monitored pharmacy education and the profession but lacked a solid mechanism for updating curriculum and development in the field of pharmacy. The Bachelor's and Master's in Pharmaceutical Sciences curriculum was highly influenced by evolution of pharmaceutical industries in India. The pharmacy education in the health care system may be lacking due to this reason. The Bachelor's of Pharmacy program in India, with a 3-year pharmaceutical industry-based curriculum, was introduced in 1937.[11.]

India is having 1026 pharmacy schools/faculties, from which 66,243 students (39,853 of which are females) graduate every year. The number of pharmacy graduates per 10,000 populations is 0.6 in India.[14] There is higher percentage of male pharmacists in India (300,000 males, which account for 70% of India's pharmacist workforce). There are 680,482 licensed pharmacists in India.[15] Pharmacists are engaged in diverse areas such as regulatory affairs (1.67%), sales/marketing (5.00%), industrial (2.67%), hospital (20.00%), community (55.00%), academic/research (2.00%), and others (9.00%)/not accounted (2.00%) (Figure 5).[16]

6. Drug- and pharmacy-related regulations, policies, and ethics

The Pharmacy Act of India was introduced in 1948, requiring pharmacists to have a registration certificate issued by their respective states to practice. According to act, the states in India are required to create pharmacy councils and to register pharmacists by keeping information related to their qualification and place of practice. The PCI was established in 1949 under the Ministry of Health. The first ER were framed in 1953, which were subsequently amended in 1972, 1981, and 1991. The minimum qualification required to get the certificate is a diploma in pharmacy issued

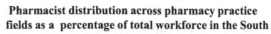

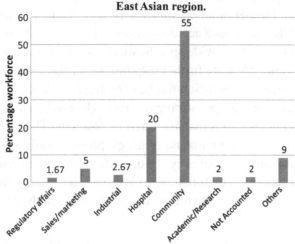

Figure 5

Pharmacist distribution in South East Asian region.

by a recognized institute of the PCI.[11,17] The diploma in pharmacy includes 2 years of study and 500 h of mandatory training at a hospital or community pharmacy. Prior to 1984, registration as a pharmacist was given to those who had 5 years of dispensing experience in hospitals and community pharmacies. It was reported that many registered pharmacists in 1980 misused the Pharmacy Act 32b provision and got registration without proper training and experience. These pharmacists are mostly working at private community pharmacies in India. It was also reported in 2005 that only 50% of pharmacies in India have qualified registered pharmacists.[17]

The retail prices of most medicines in India are set by their states. The competition between the retail chain pharmacies is very high and has a positive impact in reducing medication cost. The All-India organization of Chemists and Druggists in 2007 took an initiative to bridge 500,000 pharmacies and drug sellers in a single corporate entity, named the All Indian Origin Chemists and Distributors Limited. Their purpose is to standardize and share logistics and to obtain a supply through a common system at lower prices.[18]

7. Core pharmacy practices

7.1 Hospital pharmacy

The hospital pharmacy is one of the key departments in hospitals that deals with procurement, storage, compounding, dispensing, manufacturing, testing, packaging, and distribution of drugs. The research in pharmaceutical science and education is also the responsibility of this department; it is carried out under professional and competent pharmacists. The hospital pharmacy has a high impact on the economics of health costs. Today, drug monitoring services and drug information services are integrated in the hospital pharmacy. The hospital pharmacist is capable of purchasing, storing, handling, pricing, and dispensing medications. Furthermore, pharmacists provide drug information to all health care professionals and the public and act as a connection between the patient and the physician. Hospital pharmacists provide specifications for purchasing drugs, chemical and biological medications, etc. They are further responsible for the manufacturing and distributing of medicaments such as transfusion fluids, parenteral products, tablets, capsules, ointments, stock mixtures, and proper storing of drugs. Hospital pharmacists can sterilize and dispense parenteral medications manufactured in hospitals. They fill and label all drug containers and dispense them. The purchase of drugs, proper conditions for drug storage, maintaining records, and supplying of drugs to the outpatient department are the responsibilities of hospital pharmacists. The functions of hospital pharmacists further include medication monitoring services for inpatients and cooperation in the research program of hospitals.[19]

The hospital aspects of a pharmacist's career have always been neglected in India due to low wages; moreover, pharmacists have never been educated for a patient-oriented role. Pharmacists have never been accepted for clinical roles by medical professionals, and pharmacists themselves have been reluctant to accept the clinical responsibilities of their profession. Many hospitals in India have started a clinical-oriented role for pharmacists and have shown positive results, but India is still far behind developed countries in this area. The concept of the hospital pharmacy in India is limited to dispensing drugs at hospital pharmacies.[20] There are 11,993 hospitals with 7,84,940 beds in the country. Out of them, 7347 hospitals with 1,60,862 beds are in rural areas and 4146 hospitals with 6,18,664 beds are in are in urban areas. According to March 2011 data, there are 1,48,124 subcenters, 23,887 primary health centers, and 4809 community health centers in India.[6]

7.1.1 Personnel requirements for hospital pharmacies

The hospital pharmacy is integrated with the dispensing section, manufacturing section, quality assurance section, and clinical pharmacy services. The requirement of personnel for an inpatient pharmacy depends on the nature and quantum of services provided by the department. The requirement of hospital pharmacists in hospitals is based on workload and number of beds in hospital. Generally, small hospitals require a minimum of three pharmacists, but this varies with the number of beds in each hospital. The number of pharmacists required according to beds in a hospital is listed in Table 1.[19]

Table 2 shows number of government hospital beds in rural and urban areas.

Hospital pharmacy departments require competent and professionally trained staff. The director of pharmacy should possess a postgraduate qualification in hospital pharmacy, pharmacology, or pharmaceutics and acts as coordinator between pharmacy and nonpharmacy staff. The following flowchart describes the structure of the hospital pharmacy (Figure 6).

Table 1: Pharmacist requirement in hospitals

Pharmacist Requirement	
Bed Strength	**No. of Pharmacists Required**
Up to 50 beds	3
Up to 100 beds	5
Up to 200 beds	8
Up to 300 beds	10
Up to 500 beds	15

Table 2: State and union territory wise number hospitals and beds in rural and urban areas in India

State	Rural Hospital Beds (Government)	Urban Hospital Beds (Government)	Total Beds (Government)	Proportion of Rural and Urban Beds
Bihar	1830	16,686	18,516	10:90
Chhattisgarh	3270	6158	9428	35:65
Jharkhand	N.A.	N.A.	N.A.	N.A.
Madhya Pradesh	10,040	18,493	28,533	35:65
Odisha	7099	8715	15,814	45:55
Rajasthan	13,754	12,236	25,990	53:47
Uttar Pradesh	15,450	40,934	56,384	27:73
Uttarakhand	3746	4219	7965	47:53
EAG states	55,189	107,477	162,630	34:66
Non-EAG states	114,673	511,187	622,310	18:82
All India	169,862	618,664	784,940	20.5:79.5

N.A., not available.

Source: GOI, Table 6.2.2 State/UT Wise Number of Govt. Hospitals and Beds in Rural and Urban Areas (including CHCs) in India (Provisional), in "Health infrastructure" in "National Health Profile, 2011," Central Bureau of Health Intelligence, Ministry of Health and Family Welfare, 2011.

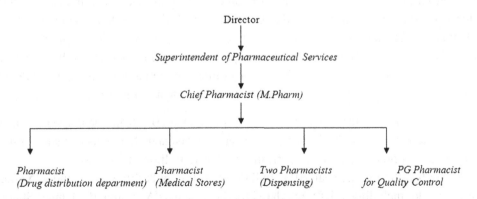

Figure 6

Organization structure of hospital pharmacy. *Source: Nahata MC. Hospital pharmacy practice in India. Drug Intell Clin Pharm June 1984;**18**(6):523–4.*

7.2 Industrial pharmacy

The growth rate of the pharmaceutical industry in India is 15–17% per year.[11] The country is home to 10,500 manufacturing units and over 3000 pharma companies. India exports all forms of pharmaceuticals from active pharmaceutical ingredients (APIs) to formulations, both in modern medicine and traditional Indian medicines. Globally, India ranks among the top exporters of formulations by volume. India's generics exports have been growing at a rate of nearly 24% annually over the last four years. India's pharma exports stood at US$14.7 billion in 2012–13, registering a growth rate of 11%. India plans to increase its total exports to US$25 billion by 2016.[21] India currently has the largest US Food and Drug Administration (FDA)-approved facilities outside the United States and exports to more than 100 countries.

The most important factors that support India are meeting global regulatory expectations and maintaining GMP compliance. The pharma units are following quality systems and risk-based approaches for the implementation of current GMPs. The prices of medicines in India are the lowest around the world; in terms of value, it ranks 14th globally.[11] Because of India's highly competent scientific manpower that is available at a low cost, multinational pharmaceutical companies are attracted to invest in India; for this reason, India is emerging as global outsourcing hub for research and development. Indian pharmaceutical industries engaged in research and development are focused on innovation, with 76.4% and 37.3% of industries producing breakthrough innovations, according to a study by India's National Knowledge Commission.[22]

Today, the size of pharmaceutical industry is greater than 20,000 and it provide 15 different types of job opportunities to pharmacy graduates. Pharmaceutical sales and marketing departments employ 30% of these graduates, with 20% joining production, quality control, and quality assurance departments in the pharmaceutical industry.[23] The pharmaceutical industry is an exciting part of India today, being the third largest manufacturer by volume of sales of pharmaceuticals and 13th in terms of value.[24] The pharmaceutical industry in 2007 had a turnover of around 8.4 billion USD; in addition, 5.8 billion USD have been generated through exports.[2] The compound growth rate in terms of exports was 19.22% in the last decade.[24] The export growth rate for the Indian pharmaceutical industries has been exceeded as compared to imports from 1995 to 2012. The compound annual growth rate (CAGR) of pharmaceuticals versus overall foreign trade in India is shown in Figure 7.

The CAGR of pharmaceuticals exports increased more than 20% from the commencement of the product patent regime to 2012. Drugs, pharmaceuticals, and chemicals account for 4% of the total Indian exports.[25] Exports grew from US$724.15 million in 1995 to US$10,859.696 million in the year 2012. India is exporting bulk drugs to around 175 countries in the world, including strictly regulated markets such as Australia, the United States, Europe, and Japan. The demands for generic drugs are due to their low cost in Europe and the United States, this giving an advantage to Indian pharmaceuticals. Around one-fourth of generic drugs in the world are produced by Indian pharmaceutical industries, and they have a

Compound annual growth rate of Pharmaceuticals vs overall foreign trade in India

Period	India's pharmaceutical exports	India's total exports	India's pharmaceutical imports	India's total imports
1995-1999	9.577	3.451	2.877	2.524
2000-2004	19.318	18.656	15.822	9.572
2005-2009	22.859	15.816	16.626	6.262
2010-2012	23.465	8.178	14.620	9.777

Figure 7

Compound annual growth rate of pharmaceuticals vs overall foreign trade in India. *Source: UNC-TAD, extracted in April 2013.*

significant share in the world pharmaceutical market. Drug intermediates, APIs, finished dosage formulations, and biopharmaceuticals are currently exported by Indian pharmaceutical firms, accounting for 10% of the total world production and 20% of total global generic market.[24] Figure 8 indicates an increase in exports of Indian pharmaceutical products. Medium and large domestic pharmaceutical firms export 90% of the pharmaceutical products. Figure 8 shows an increasing trend in export intensities for Indian pharmaceutical industries, being 45% by 2012, while incredible export growth was seen after 2000. Moreover, it shows stability in import intensities of the Indian pharmaceutical industry, being 10% in 2012.

Germany has the highest market share in total global exports of pharmaceutical products, followed by Switzerland, Belgium, and the United States, as indicated in Figure 9. India's share of the global exports of pharmaceutical products was around 2% by 2011. The magnificent compound annual growth rate of 17.77% was achieved between 1995 and 2011 by Indian medicinal and pharmaceutical exports.[24]

Figure 10 describes the percentage share in sales revenue of the top 10 leading firms, indicating an increase followed by a decrease and another increase from 2000 to 2010. The global share increase of the 10 leading exporters was 61.8% in 2012; however, the share was less than 50% of total exports of pharmaceutical products.

The total export intensity of the top Indian pharmaceutical industry exporters is represented in Figure 11. Matrix Lab Ltd, Sun Pharmaceutical Ltd, and Lupin Ltd have attained the best CAGR and highest trends in export intensity. This could be due to an increased focus on research and development by introducing several new drugs in the regulated market. Overall, a sharp increase in export intensity was observed from 2000 to 2012 by all Indian pharmaceutical industries. A couple of these pharmaceutical industries, such as Orchid Pharma and Cadila Healthcare, are the lowest in exports, probably due to their greater focus on domestic markets and tough regulatory requirements.[24]

The cross-border merger and acquisition activities in the pharmaceutical industries have shown positive impacts in terms of export intensities of Indian pharmaceutical industries. It helped to

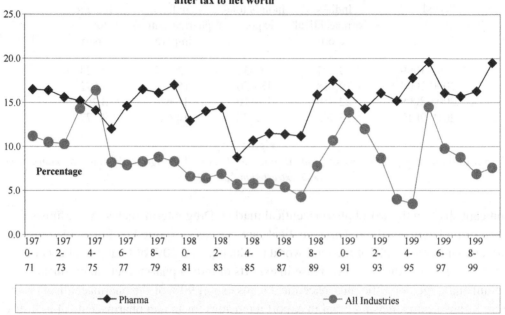

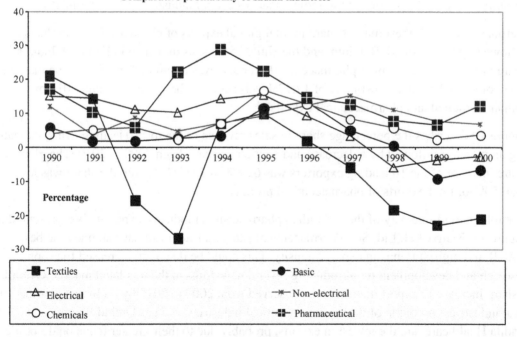

Figure 8
Profitability of pharmaceutical vs nonpharmaceutical industry in India.

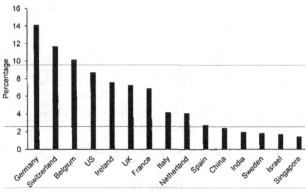

Share of top 15 exporters of pharmaceutical products
in the total global exports (2011)

Figure 9
Share of top 15 exporters of pharmaceutical products in the total global exports (2011).
Source: UNCTAD.

Total exports and share of leading exporters
(US$ million)

Year	Total value of pharmaceutical exports	Value of export by top 10 exporters	Share of top 10 firms (%)
2000	1037.53	453.44	43.70
2001	1146.3	619.95	54.08
2002	1451.56	828.08	57.05
2003	2026.06	1168.76	57.69
2004	2699.88	1551.07	57.45
2005	3066.16	1625.14	53.00
2006	3600.69	1926.66	53.51
2007	5076.79	2807.17	55.29
2008	6515.13	3418.84	52.48
2009	6386.18	3302.77	51.72
2010	7932.96	4061.22	51.19
2011	9072.547	5105.59	56.28
2012	9479.307	5858.794	61.81

Figure 10
Total exports of share of leading exporters. *Source: CMIE Prowess Database.*

expose Indian firms to new technologies and best practices that further lead to high operational efficiency and ease expansion in overseas pharmaceutical markets. The outbound acquisition by Indian firms in 2011 was 6 billion US dollars, which was approximately doubled in 2012 to 11 billion US dollars with 72 outbound acquisitions. The multinational companies in India have also acquired some Indian pharmaceutical firms. The acquisition and mergers have been initiated within pharmaceutical firms in India, such as the merger of Ranbaxy with Sun Pharmaceuticals at a cost of US$ 3.2 billion (approx. Rs. 19,200 crore) by the end of 2014.[24]

Export intensity of top exporters of Indian pharmaceutical industry

Company	2000	2001	2002	2003	2004	2005	2006	2007	2008	2009	2010	2011	2012
Dr Reddy's Lab	26.40	43.10	57.90	57.20	55.90	55.90	56.00	72.80	64.20	68.20	64.00	64.15	72.44
Cipla Ltd	18.60	25.00	35.50	36.40	42.20	45.60	50.10	50.80	52.50	55.80	53.80	53.37	52.58
Ranbaxy Ltd	47.90	42.40	53.30	60.70	62.90	62.20	68.70	72.90	69.20	68.00	60.20	63.41	71.29
Aurobindo Ltd	49.30	54.50	46.90	47.30	47.90	47.70	55.30	55.10	55.60	63.20	66.40	69.24	67.97
Lupin Ltd	18.20	28.60	35.30	40.90	47.50	45.30	44.90	51.20	55.70	53.40	56.60	57.33	58.67
Matrix Lab Ltd	0.90	6.70	9.30	67.60	53.40	50.70	49.50	64.40	62.90	81.40	81.20	80.70	85.97
Orchid Pharma	80.90	85.70	83.20	83.20	74.90	75.70	75.20	78.20	84.00	79.70	79.90	46.80	51.00
Cadila Healthcare	8.60	12.40	15.30	10.50	15.60	12.00	15.50	19.10	24.80	36.10	48.90	26.48	N.A.
Divi's Lab Ltd	87.60	85.70	82.90	84.90	81.60	83.70	85.80	91.00	92.30	91.90	89.10	89.05	86.70
Sun Pharma Ltd	11.60	20.30	19.20	17.80	22.90	26.30	27.00	27.90	33.20	28.70	44.40	44.71	59.01

Figure 11
Export intensity of top. *Source: CMIE Prowess Database.*

7.3 Community pharmacy

The Pharmacy Act 1948 was enacted in India to ensure that every practising Pharmacist in India has a registration certificate.[11,12,26] The educational institutes recognized by the PCI are able to issue this certificate on completion of the minimum diploma of pharmacy. The diploma in pharmacy requires a minimum of 2 years of study and 500 h of practical training, with 3 months in a community or hospital pharmacy.[26] These diploma holder pharmacists are main workforce and manage most of the community pharmacies in India today. A Bachelor's of Pharmacy is designed to fulfill the needs of the pharma industry, with most of these graduates working in pharmaceutical industries and drug regulatory bodies. These BPharm graduates prefer to join the pharma industry due to the high salary scale and other incentives as compared to community pharmacy.

In a practical scenario, these diploma or bachelor's degree holder pharmacists are still unseen in 50% of community pharmacies. Most patients seek advice from community pharmacists related to sexually transmitted diseases, minor illnesses, contraceptive methods, and menstrual problems.[26] Most community pharmacies are run by people who have no understanding of health issues or knowledge of medicine, and they hire pharmacists on low salary scales. Most pharmacists working in community pharmacies lack counseling skills and only dispense drugs. The public perception of pharmacists is poor and pharmacies are considered to be like grocery shops; however, community pharmacies are still the primary source of inexpensive medical care.

7.4 Medicine marketing and promotion

Today, the numbers of prescriptions per medicine have increased in India, and the average cost of a prescription per patient who visited a private clinic is around 600 rupees. The prescribing habits of doctors are highly influenced by the marketing strategies of pharmaceutical industries. Pharmaceutical industries spend less for research and development than marketing. Pharmaceutical industries train medical representatives to promote and sell drugs, using printed product literature, drug samples, and gifts. These medical representatives employed by pharmaceutical industries in India number around 80,000 and they are offered lucrative incentives in addition to their salaries. It was found that general practitioners prescribe new products under the influence of sales representatives. Moreover, medical representatives promote drugs by expressing more indications than registered.

Gifts are one of the major tool uses by pharmaceutical industries to promote their drugs. The variety of gifts include stationery, timepieces, bags, books, folders, office desks, medical supplies, and household items—from clocks to air conditioners, calendars to cars, rubber bands to refrigerators, telephone indexes to television, and office items to overseas trips. Chren and associate indicated that an implicit relationship has been established between doctors and pharmaceutical industries, and it ultimately results in an obligation to respond to gifts.[27]

The promotion of medicine is largely dependent on advertisements. The pharmaceutical industries spend large amounts to advertise in medical and pharmaceutical journals that are widely read by general practitioners and clinical specialists. The survival of medical journals in India is impossible without advertisements by pharmaceutical industries. The advertisement of drugs is closely scrutinized and strict actions are taken in cases of misleading information. The International Federation of Pharmaceutical Manufacturers Associations (IFPMA) and The Association of the British Pharmaceutical Industry (ABPI) codes suggest that drug information should be accurate, current, and balanced. All member companies of the Organization of Pharmaceutical Producers of India (OPPI) have to follow the IFPMA code. The organization of the Pharmaceutical Producers of India requires their internal codes and promotional material to be approved by medical advisors. The critical analysis of these promotional material is also done by a Promotional Quality Improvement and Assurance Committee. Moreover, this committee provides suggestions for improvements in marketing.

Pharmaceutical marketing and promotional services have a high impact on irrational prescribing and their consequences. The Medical Council of India has introduced a new code of conduct for practitioners taking any kind of benefit from pharmaceutical industries. In Rajasthan state of India, a new regulation stated that a doctor must write only the generic name of a drug on the prescription.[27]

8. Special pharmacy-related services and activities

The role of a pharmacist has been enhanced with the emergence of clinical pharmacy, which provides high-quality care and support to patients. Today, pharmacists are providing drug and poison information services, running anticoagulation clinics, and smoking cessation programs, etc.

8.1 Drug information services

The first drug information center (DIC) opened at the University of Kentucky Medical Center in 1962. The World Health Organization (WHO) has recognized the role of DIC to spread the information about rational use of drugs. Today drug information services are provided by pharmacists around the globe. The first independent drug information center in India was established in 1997 by Karnataka State Pharmacy Council. The WHO India Country Office, in collaboration with the Karnataka State Pharmacy Council (KSPC), supported the establishment of five drug information centers. These centers have been established in Haryana (Sirsa), Chhattisgarh (Raipur), Rajasthan (Jaipur), Assam (Dibrugarh), and Goa (Panaji)[28.]

8.1.1 List of drug information centers run at state pharmacy councils in India (regional)

- Drug Information Center, Maharashtra State Pharmacy Council, Maharashtra
- Andhra Pradesh state pharmacy council, Andhra Pradesh
- Drug information center, Jaipur, Rajasthan
- Drug information center, Raipur, Chhattisgarh
- KSPC, Bangalore, Karnataka

8.1.2 DICs set up by Karnataka State Pharmacy Council, CDSCO, and the WHO India Country Office

- Drug information center, Jaipur, Rajasthan
- Drug information center, Raipur, Chhattisgarh
- Drug information center, Panaji, Goa
- Drug information center, Dibrugarh, Assam

8.1.3 Other drug, poison or alcohol information centers in India

- Alcohol and Drug Information Center (ADIC), Trivandrum, Kerala
- Bowring and Lady Curzon Hospital, Bangalore
- Bulletin on Drug and Health Information (BIDI), Kolkata
- CDMU Documentation Center, Calcutta
- Christian Medical College Hospital, Vellore, Tamilnadu
- Department of Pharmacy Practice, Chidambaram, Tamilnadu
- Department of Pharmacy Practice, National Institute of Pharmaceutical Education and Research (NIPER), Chandigarh
- Drug Information Center, Division of Pharmacy Practice, Department of Pharmacy, Annamalai University
- Drug information center (KSPC), Bowring and Lady Curzon Hospital, Bangalore, Karnataka
- Drug information center (KSPC), Victoria Hospital, Bangalore, Karnataka
- Jawaharlal Nehru Medical College Hospital (JNMC), Belgaum, Karnataka
- JIPMER drug information center, Department of Pharmacology, JIPMER hospital Gorimedu, Pondicherry
- JSS, Mysore, Karnataka
- JSS, Ooty
- Kasturba Medical College (KMC), Manipal, Karnataka
- Kempagowda Institute of Medical Sciences (KIMS), Bangalore, Karnataka

- N.R.S. Medical College and Hospital, Calcutta
- National Poison Information Center, All India Institute of Medical Sciences, Ansari Nagar, New Delhi
- Pharma Information Center, Chennai, Tamilnadu
- Poison control center and Department of Analytical Toxicology, Amrita Institute of Medical Sciences and Research, Cochin
- Poison control, training and research center, Government General Hospital, Chennai
- Poison information center, National Institute of Occupational Health, Ahmadabad
- RIPER poison and drug information center, RDT Hospital, Bathalapalli
- Sri Ramachandra Hospital, Porur, Chennai
- Sri Ramakrishna Mission Hospital, Coimbatore, Tamilnadu
- Toxicology and IMCU unit, Government General Hospital, Chennai
- Trivandrum Medical College, Trivandrum, Kerala

8.1.4 Poison information centers in India

The WHO in 2012 reported that 350,000 people died worldwide from unintentional poisoning, and it is the sixth major cause of death in India. The cases of poisoning were found to be more common in children. One retrospective study in India for 10 years reported 42 cases of poisoning in children, most of them with chemical pneumonitis but with low mortality rates. Kerosene oil poisoning is very common between 1 and 3 years of age. Physicians face a major problem due to insufficient drug information services in emergency departments. In 1995, the National Poisons Information Center was established in the Department of Pharmacology at the All India Institute of Medical Sciences, New Delhi with the aim to provide toxicological information and advice on the management of poisoned patients. Furthermore, it has prepared manuals and leaflets for patients and the general public on prevention and management of various poisonings.[29]

8.1.5 Pharmacovigilance program in India

Nationwide adverse reaction monitoring was started in 1982 by the establishment of five centers by the Drug Controller General in India. After a few years, these centers stopped functioning due to insufficient funds and lack of enthusiasm. The Central Drugs Standard Control Organization (CDSCO), Ministry of Health and Family Welfare, launched the National Pharmacovigilance Program (NPP) in November, 2004. According to the WHO, pharmacovigilance is defined as the science and activities related to the detection, assessment, understanding, and prevention of adverse effects or any other possible drug-related problems. The concept of pharmacovigilance is broadened today to include herbal, traditional medicines, biologics, medical devices, and vaccines. It helps in the early detection of unwanted effects and helps to take early action if necessary. The NPP in India is based on recommendation made in the WHO document titled "Safety Monitoring of Medicinal Products – Guidelines for Setting Up and Running a Pharmacovigilance Center."[30,31]

Table 3: SUSARs comparison in INDIA and GLOBAL.

Sr	Drug Name	Reported ADR	SUSARs in INDIA	Global Status
1	Ferrous sulfate	Hematemesis	2	2
2	Ceftriaxone	Neuropathy peripheral	1	4
3	Lohexol	Eosinophilia	1	0
4	Carbimazole	Appetite loss	1	0
5	Efavirenz	Granulomatous lesion	1	1
6	Cisplastin	Micturition Painful	1	18
7	Hydroxychloroquine	Melena	1	2
8	Trihexyphenidyl hydrochloride	Steven-Johnsons syndrome	1	4
9	Neomercazole	Weight increase	1	1
10	Piperacillin sodium + tazobactum sodium	Appetite loss	2	2

The Indian Individual Case Safety Reports Database reported 6300 cases of adverse drug reactions (ADRs) in elderly patients. These cases were reported to the Pharmacovigilance Program of India from July 2011 to March 2014. Among them, 58% of ADRs were reported in females and 42% in male patients. The gastrointestinal system, skin, and appendages disorders are highest, according to the distribution of ADRs in system organ classification.

The Uppsala Monitoring Center (UMC) is an independent foundation and a center for international service and scientific research. The WHO-UMC system has been developed in consultation with the national centers participating in the Program for International Drug Monitoring and is used as a practical tool for the assessment of case reports. There are around 117 countries participating in the WHO program for international drug monitoring; India stands at the seventh position among the top 10 countries contributing to global drug safety database. The comparison of reported suspected unexpected serious adverse drug reactions (SUSARs) in India and globally are shown in Table 3. These SUSARs are related to any medicinal product that is suspected but previously not reported.[31,32]

India is divided into zones and regions for operational efficiency under the pharmacovigilance program in India. The Central Drugs Standard Control Organization, New Delhi is at the top rank, followed by Seth GS Medical College, Mumbai and AIIMS, New Delhi. The pharmaco-vigilance centers in the five regions of India are shown in Table 4.[32]

9. Pharmacy education

To meet the needs of the changing needs of the pharmacy profession, different pharmacy programs are offered in India today: Diploma in Pharmacy (DPharm), Bachelor of Pharmacy (BPharm), Master of Pharmacy (MPharm), the practice-based Doctor of Pharmacy (PharmD), and Doctor of Philosophy in Pharmacy (PhD) (Table 5).[11]

Table 4: Pharmacovigilance centers in five regions of India

Regions of India	Pharmacovigilance Centers
Koltata	IPGMR-SSKM Hospitals
Mumbai	TN Medical College & BYL Nair Charitable Hospital
Nagpur	Indira Gandhi Medical College
New Delhi	Lady Hardinge Medical College
Pondicherry	JIPMER

Table 5: Number of pharmacists who complete pharmacy programs every year in India

Programs	Diploma in Pharmacy	Bachelors in Pharmacy	Masters in Pharmacy	PhD in Pharmacy
Number of pharmacists	20,000	30,000	6000	700

Adapted from: Ref. 11.

Currently, diploma-based pharmacists are the main workforce of pharmacists in the Indian market. These pharmacists are involved in traditional dispensing and other health care services. However, the diploma of pharmacy content is outdated. A vast gap exists between pharmacy education and practice. Overall pharmacy education mainly focuses on biological synthesis, physicochemical studies, analysis, and manufacturing aspects of drugs. The 1940s and 1950s were the decades of developing hospitals and pharmaceutical industries in India. This demanded huge numbers of pharmacists in the market and led to the development of a pharmacy curriculum that satisfied the needs of the pharmaceutical industry and hospital pharmacies. Diploma-based pharmacists have been employed in hospital pharmacies; however, BPharm graduates have fulfilled the needs of pharmaceutical industries. The clinical-based pharmacy practice program was first introduced in 1995 when two institutes (SS Colleges of Pharmacy, Mysore and Ooty) in India initiated a Master's in Pharmacy Practice program. The PCI in 2008 introduced a clinical-based pharmacy program (i.e., PharmD).[11,12] Currently, the pharmacy syllabus has two major divisions: PharmD, which is clinically oriented, and BPharm, which is industry oriented. It has been decided to end diploma in pharmacy programs. These modifications will enhance the competitive skills of pharmacy graduates in the health care system.

The admission criteria[32,33] for DPharm, BPharm, PharmD, and MPharm vary within the states of India and most significantly between private and public sector institutes. A formal application process for admission does not exist in privately funded pharmacy institutes in India. Admission to a DPharm program requires an individual to complete high secondary school education (i.e., 12 years of education). The private institutes have a different admission process to enroll for DPharm in accordance with regulations of the PCI. The curriculum of DPharm is the same throughout India and was framed back in 1991. The outline of the curriculum in India[17] is shown in Figure 12.

Outline of DPharm Degree Curriculum in India

Course Title	Hours of Study	
	Theory	**Laboratory**
Year 1 (Part I)		
Pharmaceutics –I	75	100
Pharmaceutical Chemistry –I	75	75
Pharmacognosy	75	75
Biochemistry and Clinical Pathology	50	75
Human Anatomy and Physiology	75	50
Health Education & Community Pharmacy	50	-
Year 2 (Part II)		
Pharmaceutics –II	75	100
Pharmaceutical Chemistry –II	100	75
Pharmacology and Toxicology	75	50
Pharmaceutical Jurisprudence	50	-
Drug Store and Business Management	75	-
Hospital and Clinical Pharmacy	75	100
Part III (3 months)		
Practical Training	500 in either in a hospital or community pharmacy	

Note: Syllabus framed in 1991

Figure 12

D-Pharmacy curriculum in India. *Adapted from: Basak SC, Sathyanarayana D. Pharmacy education in India.* Am J Pharm Educ *2010;**74**(4):1–8.*

Admission to the BPharm program has been sought by two ways: on the basis of scores on entrance tests or marks obtained in high secondary schools. These entrance requirements are mainly followed by public pharmacy institutes; most of them conduct entry tests as well as consider grades in high secondary school certificates. Some states and institutes specifically focus on entrance test scores for admission; however, a few private pharmacy institutes and Tamilnadu state only consider high secondary school grades for admission in the BPharm program. The majority of states in India conduct entrance examinations for BPharm and Bachelors of Engineering together; the candidates who score lower are placed in the pharmacy program. An overview of the BPharm program degree curriculum[14] at Dr M.G.R. Medical University, Chennai is shown in Figure 13.

The admission criteria for MPharm are based on entrance tests, grades in the Bachelor of Pharmacy program, and a high Graduate Aptitude Test for Engineering score, which entitle a candidate to receive a government scholarship for an MPharm program. The PharmD program allows students holding a DPharm certificate or high secondary school certificate for

Overview of BPharm Degree Curriculum of Dr. M.G.R. Medical University, Chennai

Year	Subjects
1	Pharmaceutical Inorganic Chemistry; Pharmaceutical Organic Chemistry; Anatomy, Physiology, and Health Education; Biochemistry
2	Physical Pharmaceutics; Advanced Pharmaceutical Organic Chemistry; Pharmaceutical Analysis and Physical Chemistry; Pharmaceutical Technology; Pharmacy Practice and Pathphysiology; Biostatistic and Computer Applications
3	Pharmacognosy and Phytochemistry; Medicinal Chemistry I; Pharmaceutical DF and Cosmetic Technology; Pharmacology I; Forensic Pharmacy and Business Management
4	Pharmaceutical Biotechnology; Formulative Pharmacy and Biopharmaceutics; Advanced Pharmacognosy; Pharmacology II; Modern Methods of Pharmaceutical Analysis; Medicinal Chemistry II

Figure 13

Overview of the BPharm degree curriculum of Dr M.G.R. Medical university, Chennai. *Adapted from: Basak SC, Sathyanarayana D. Pharmacy education in India. Am J Pharm Educ 2010;**74**(4):1–8.*

admission; however, BPharm students can pursue the PharmD program in the fourth year. The outline of the PharmD and PharmD (postbaccalaureate) degree program[17] is presented in Figure 14.

The number of pharmacists in India has exceeded 1 million.[11] The areas of the pharmacy profession in India are presented in Figure 15 and the distribution of these pharmacists[12] is presented in Table 6. The healthcare system in India requires changes by providing jobs to pharmacists in government hospitals and primary health care centers.

The 55th Indian Pharmaceutical Congress at Chennai projected the Pharma Vision 2020 Charter, which focuses on practising the highest professional ethical standards of pharmacy, improving the pharmacist image, and intensifying professional issues related to community and government. Pharmaceutical education is also a focus in the Pharma Vision 2020 charter.[11]

10. Achievements

The third largest group of health care professionals in the world is pharmacists. Pharmacists are currently one of the most demanding professionals in India due to the increasing demand of health services and higher expectations of service delivery. Some of the achievements made in the field of pharmacy are listed below:

1. The clinical aspects of the pharmacy profession have always been neglected in India. However, with the introduction of a clinically oriented PharmD curriculum, pharmacists are pursuing their careers in hospitals.
2. Today, India has five regional and 28 peripheral pharmacovigilance centers that contain broad ADR data on the Indian population.
3. The state pharmacy councils in India are currently running many regional drug information centers.

PharmD and PharmD (post baccalaureate) Degree Curriculum Outline[a]

Course Title	Hours of Study[b]		
	Theory	Practical[c]	Tutorial[d]
Year 1			
Human Anatomy and Physiology	99	99	33
Pharmaceutics	66	99	33
Medicinal Biochemistry	99	99	33
Pharmaceutical Organic Chemistry	99	99	33
Pharmaceutical Inorganic Chemistry	66	99	33
Remedial Mathematics/ Biology	99	99	33
Total hours = 1320			
Year 2			
Pathophysiology	99	-	33
Pharmaceutical Microbiology	99	99	33
Pharmacognosy and Phytopharmaceuticals	99	99	33
Pharmacology-I	99	-	33
Community Pharmacy	66	-	33
Pharmacotherapeutics-I	99	99	33
Total hours = 1056			
Year 3			
Pharmacology-II	99	99	33
Pharmaceutical Analysis	99	99	33
Pharmacotherapeutics-II	99	99	33
Pharmaceutical Jurisprudence	66	-	-
Medicinal Chemistry	99	99	33
Pharmaceutical Formulations	66	99	33
Total hours = 1188			
Year 4			
Pharmacotherapeutics-III	99	99	33
Hospital Pharmacy	66	99	33
Clinical Pharmacy	99	99	33
Biostatistics and Research Methodology	66	-	33
Biopharmaceutics and Pharmacokinetics	99	99	33
Clinical Toxicology	66	-	33
Total hours = 1089			
Year 5			
Clinical Research	99	-	33
Pharmacoepidemiology and Pharmacoeconomics	99	-	33
Clinical Pharmacokinetics and Pharmacotherapeutic Drug Monitoring	66	-	33
Clerkship	-	-	33
Project work (Six Months)[e]	-	660	-
Total hours = 1056			
Year 6			
Internship or Residency program			

PharmD (post baccalaureate) – entry directly to the fourth year of the program

[a] Hours of study is based on 33 working weeks.

[b] Practical means Laboratory of the respective subjects; 4th year practical includes work in a Laboratory and in a hospital as well.

[c] Tutorial includes seminar and discussion,

[d] Project work is to be undertaken in a practice site.

Figure 14

PharmD and PharmD (postbaccalaureate) degree curriculum outline. *Adapted from: Basak SC, Sathyanarayana D. Pharmacy education in India. Am J Pharm Educ 2010;74(4):1–8.*

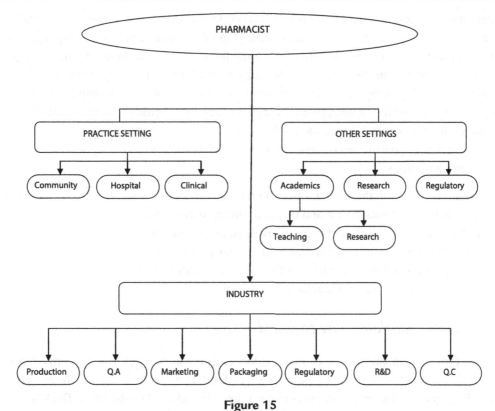

Figure 15
Areas of pharmacy profession. *Source: Pharmacy Council of India.*

Table 6: Distribution of pharmacists according to various pharmacy professions

Pharmacy Profession	Community	Hospital	Industry and regulatory	Academia
Percentage	55%	20%	10%	2%

4. The number of PhDs in pharmacy have reached 700 and MPharm is now 3000.
5. There are over 140 institutes approved by the PCI for the PharmD program as of November 2013.

11. Challenges

The focus of traditional pharmacy practice has now shifted toward patient-oriented care in the developed world, which has shown a positive impact on patient outcomes. The results of clinical pharmacy services reduce medication-related adverse events, decrease the cost of treatment, improve patient outcomes, and decrease readmission rates. In India, the role of clinical pharmacy services has been underestimated in the recent past; however, hospitals have realized the importance of clinical pharmacy and therefore started delivering high-quality clinical pharmacy services. To comply with the international standards of clinical pharmacy practice, the PCI in 2008 started a clinically based 6-year pharmacy program—the PharmD.[11,12,27,33] This program includes mandatory 1-year training for pharmacy graduates at their practice sites, with 6 months to be spent in a general medicine department and the remaining 6 months in other departments. It also includes project work that focuses on pharmacovigilance, pharmacoeconomics, drug utilization studies, and pharmacoepidemiology.

Although development in the field of clinical pharmacy is taking place, the government has not given much consideration to it and there are no regulatory guidelines for a practicing clinical pharmacist. The post of clinical pharmacist at a regulatory level is still not fully recognized. The majority of new pharmacy graduates prefer to join the pharmaceutical industry or academics, but the initiation of the PharmD with 1-year training has resulted in a positive impact toward clinical pharmacy practice in India.

12. Recommendations: way forward

Today, the forms of care are shifting from secondary care providers to primary care providers to patients (Figure 16). This trend has already started in developed countries, such as the behind-the-counter drug option in European countries that was already endorsed by the FDA. The FDA showed positive signs toward boosting the numbers of nonprescription drug statuses to over-the-counter statuses. The health care delivery system is coming closer to the patient due to knowledge and understanding, as well as better diagnostic tools and monitoring devices[34] (Figure 16).

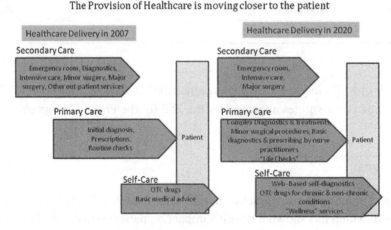

Figure 16
The healthcare delivery status of 2007 and 2020. *Source: PricewaterhouseCoopers.*

13. Conclusions

There is a gradual acceptance of clinically oriented work for pharmacists in India after the introduction of the PharmD curriculum. The results will be more fruitful if there is a modification in the legislative framework for improving the standards of the pharmacy profession in terms of education and clinical practice.

14. Points to remember

- By continually increasing the responsibilities of a pharmacist, a new era of the pharmacy profession has evolved.
- There is a gap in the curriculum, particularly at the DPharm level. This needs to be addressed in future studies and curriculum development actions, as well as in pharmacists' continuing education and professional development programs.
- The elderly population is dramatically increasing in developed countries due to long life expectancies.
- Pharmacy graduates are more inclined to take up jobs in industries rather than working in community pharmacies or as a clinical pharmacist.

References

1. The National Portal of India, New Delhi. *Know India-states and union territories*. http://india.gov.in/knowindia/state_uts.php; 2009 [accessed 01.11.14].
2. Visaria P. Demographics of ageing in India. *Econ Polit Wkly* 2001:1967–75.
3. Rana RD. Pharmacy in ancient India. *Indian J Hist Sci* 1987;**22**(2):119–21.
4. Saha D, Paul S. Glimpse of pharmaceutical education in India: history to advances. *Int J Pharm Teach Pract* 2012;**3**(4):387–404.
5. *Report of the steering committee on health for the 12th five year plan*. Health Division, Planning Commission. p. 7. Available online at: http://planningcommission.nic.in/aboutus/committee/strgrp12/str_health0203.pdf; February 2012.
6. Health infrastructure, National health profile. Available from: http://cbhidghs.nic.in/writereaddata/mainlinkFile/11%20%20Health%20Infrastructure%202011.pdf; 2011 [Retrieved: February 20, 2015].
7. *India's healthcare system – overview and quality improvements*. Retrieved December 2014, from: http://www.tillvaxtanalys.se/en/home/publications/direct-response/direct-response/2013-05-20-indias-health-care-system--overview-and-quality-improvements.html.
8. Rashtriya Swasthya BimaYojana. Rashtriya Swasthya Bima Yojana Web. http://www.rsby.gov.in/; November 25, 2014.
9. Unnikrishnan C. *India sees lowest growth in drug sales in March quarter* [Internet]. [Retrieved January 10, 2015]. Available from: http://www.livemint.com/industry/FQJa39D4bm9oCPfruqzY6N/india-sees-lowest-growth-in-drug-sales-in-march-quarter.html; April 22, 2013.
10. Pharma Bottleneck [Internet]. [January 23, 2015]. Available from: http://www.transreporter.com/detailcontent.php?pro_cat_id=1&pro_id=22; 2015.
11. Desale P. An overview about pharmacy education in India. *Indian J Res Pharm Biotechnol* 2013;**1**(3):329–30.
12. Sachan A, Sachan AK, Gangwar SS. Pharmacy education in India and its neighbouring countries. *Int Curr Pharm J* 2012;**1**(9):294–301.

13. Harappel LJP, et al. Pharmaceutical education in India: past, present and future. *J Pharm Sci Res* 2014;**6**(8):278–81.

14. International Pharmaceutical Federation (FIP). *2013 global pharmacy workforce report*. [cited January 01, 2015]. The Hague (The Netherlands): FIP; 2013. Available from: http://www.fip.org/hr.

15. International Pharmaceutical Federation (FIP). *2012 global pharmacy workforce report*. [cited January 01, 2015]. The Hague (The Netherlands): FIP; 2012. Available from: http://www.fip.org/hr.

16. International Pharmaceutical Federation (FIP). *2006 Global pharmacy workforce report* [cited January 02, 2015]. The Hague (The Netherlands): FIP; 2006. Available from: http://www.fip.org/hr.

17. Basak SC, Sathyanarayana D. Pharmacy education in India. *Am J Pharm Educ* 2010;**74**(4):68.

18. Lowe RF, Montagu D. Legislation, regulation, and consolidation in the retail pharmacy sector in low-income countries. *South Med Rev* 2009;**2**:35–44.

19. Nand P, Khar RK. *Hospital and clinical pharmacy*. 5th ed. Delhi: Birla Publications Pvt Ltd; 2008.

20. Sreelalitha N, Vigneshwaran E, Reddy GNYP, Reddy MR. Review of pharmaceutical care services provided by pharmacists. *IRJP* 2012;**3**(4):78–9.

21. Pharmaceutical sector analysis. Retrieved November 1, 2014, from: http://www.brandindiapharma.in/infographic-on-pharma-sector-business.

22. Innovation in India. *Report of national knowledge commission*. New Delhi: Government of India. http://knowledgecommission.gov.in/downloads/documents/NKC_Innovation.pdf; 2007 [Retrieved March 6, 2015].

23. Burande MD. *Sky is not the limit in pharma industry*. Express Pharma. Retrieved from: %3ca href=http://pharma.financialexpress.com/specials/ipc/3070-sky-is-not-the-limit-in-pharma-industry; December 4, 2013.

24. Tyagi S, Mahajan V, Nauriyal DK. Innovations in Indian drug and pharmaceutical industry: have they impacted exports. *J Intellect Prop Rights* July 2014;**19**:243–52.

25. Annual report 2011–12, Department of Pharmaceuticals, Ministry of Chemicals and Fertilizers. Government of India. http://pharmaceuticals.gov.in/annualreport2012.pdf [Retrieved March 1, 2015].

26. Basak SC, Sathyanarayan D. Community pharmacy practice in India: past, present and future. *South Med Rev* 2009;**2**(1):11.

27. Goyal R, Pareek P. A review article on prescription behaviour of doctors, influenced by the medical representative in Rajasthan, India. *IOSR J Bus Manag* 2013;**8**(1):56–60. Available from: http://www.iosrjournals.org/ccount/click.php?id=5229. [accessed on 15.12.14].

28. Chauhan N, Moin S, Pandey A, Mittal A, Bajaj U. Indian aspects of drug information resources and impact of drug information centre on community. *J Adv Pharm Technol Res* April–June 2013;**4**(2):84–93.

29. Churi S, Harsha CS, Ramesh M. Patterns of poison information queries received by a newly established south Indian poison information center. *Asian J Pharm Clin Res* 2012;**5**:79–82.

30. Bavdekar SB, Karande S. National pharmacovigilance program. *Indian Pediatr* 2006;**43**(1):27.

31. Adithan C. National pharmacovigilance programme. *Indian J Pharmacol* 2005;**37**(6):347.

32. Indian Pharmacopoeia Commission. Occurrence of adverse drug reactions in elderly population in India. *Pharmacovigil Program India* April 2014;**8**(4):1–3.

33. Bhuyan B. Pharmacy education in India: current standard, admission criteria and regulation. *Int J Pharm Biosci* 2013;**4**(2):860–6.

34. *Pharma 2020: challenging business*. Available from: http://www.pwc.com/gx/en/pharma-life-sciences/pharma-2020-business-models/index.jhtml; 2007.

CHAPTER 8

Pharmacy Practice in Nepal

Mukhtar Ansari, Kadir Alam

Chapter Outline

1. Country background

Nepal is a small, land-locked country positioned between China to the north and India to the east, west, and south. Nepal is rectangular in appearance with an elongation of 885 km from east to west and 193 km from north to south.[1] The total land area of Nepal is 147,181 km^2, with a population of 26.6 million. Geographically, Nepal is divided into three ecological regions: mountain, hill, and terai (plains). Only about 7% of the entire population inhabits the mountains due to their high altitude (4877–8848 m above sea level) and lack of basic facilities. The hill area, with an altitude of 610 to 4876 m above sea level, is a densely populated (43% of the total population) region of Nepal. Conversely, Terai constitutes less than one fourth (23%) of the total land area but accommodates about half of the entire population of Nepal.[1,2]

For administrative purposes, Nepal is divided into 14 zones and 75 administrative districts. Districts are further divided into smaller units, such as 3915 village development committees (VDCs) and 58 municipalities. The VDCs are rural areas, whereas municipalities represent urban areas. Each VDC is composed of 9 wards, and the number of wards in each municipality ranges from 9 to 35. Kathmandu is the capital city as well as the principal urban center of Nepal.[3]

2. Health sector and system

The health sector is an important area for the development of a nation. The Ministry of Health and Population (MoHP), Government of Nepal has started various programs to meet the country's health-related challenges. The Nepal Health Sector Program (NHSP) was the first sector-wide program, which was introduced with the aim of increasing people's access to and use of quality essential healthcare services, including maternal and child health services. Later, the MoHP, in collaboration with 11 external development partners, brought the Nepal Health Sector Program Implementation Plan (NHSP-IP, 2004–2009). The goal of NHSP-IP was to achieve health-related Millennium Development Goals, with the aim to improve health outcomes of the poor and those living in remote areas.[4]

In Nepal, MoHP is the regulatory authority of the healthcare system. There are three different departments under the authority of MoHP: the Department of Drug Administration (DDA), the Department of Health Services (DoHS), and the Department of Ayurveda.

The DDA is responsible for regulating and controlling the medicines and related issues within the country. Similarly, activities related to the traditional ayurvedic therapy are under the jurisdiction of the Department of Ayurveda. The DoHS is accountable for delivering preventive, curative, and promotive health services throughout the country. There are six divisions under the functional framework of the DoHS, including a child health division, five centers, and five regional health directorates. Under these regional health directorates, there are 10 zonal hospitals at the zone level. Similarly, there are altogether 15 district public health offices, 65 district hospitals, and 60 district health offices at the district level. Below this hierarchy, there are 214 primary healthcare centers/ health centers (PHCs/HCs), 679 health posts (HPs), and 3134 subhealth posts (SHPs) throughout the country. SHPs located at the VDC level are the first contact point for the general population for seeking healthcare. In the healthcare system, each level above the SHP (e.g., HP, PHC) acts as a referral point. The diagrammatic representation of the healthcare system of Nepal is illustrated in Figure 1.

In developed nations, pharmacists are an integral component of the healthcare delivery system and they significantly contribute toward delivering better healthcare, along with physicians and nurses. However, in Nepal, pharmacists are considered to be professionals who are predominantly concerned with the manufacturing of pharmaceuticals; their status in the healthcare delivery system is not well established yet.[5]

3. Statistics on human capital/workforce

A larger fraction of the people living in rural areas of Nepal are the elderly, children, poor, and unemployed, who have a greater need for healthcare services. However, the persistent shortage of healthcare workers in rural areas remains a major problem. Despite the improvements in the Human Development Index of Nepal in recent decades, there is still a huge shortage of human resources for health, such as doctors, pharmacists, dentists, nurses, and midwives. According to a World Health Organization (WHO) report (2000–2010), the health workforce density per 10,000 population in Nepal is 2.1 for physicians, 4.6 for nursing and midwifery personnel, 0.1 for dentistry personnel, and 0.1 for pharmaceutical personnel.[6]

Although there may be numerous factors for the low health workforce density in the public sector of Nepal, pitfalls during the recruitment of healthcare personnel and their professional development, trainings, rewards, and promotions are more accountable. Furthermore, there is poor retention of healthcare workers in rural areas, probably due to poor infrastructure, lack of opportunities, lower pay and social recognition, and lack of security compared to urban areas. The above factors conjointly result in the preference of qualified healthcare professionals to join private institutions, mainly of urban origin, or migrate to developed nations for better opportunities.[7,8]

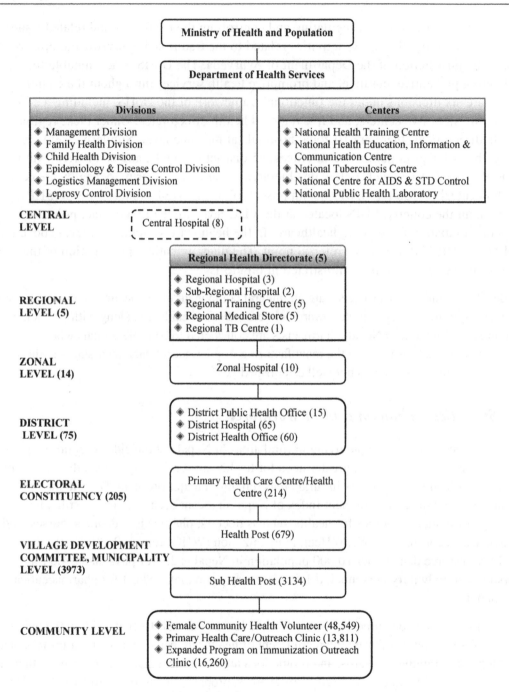

Figure 1
Organizational structure of the Department of Health Services, Nepal.
Glimpse of Annual Report 2008/2009 Kathmandu, Nepal: *Department of Health Services, Ministry of Health and Population. Government of Nepal; 2009 (available on http://nepalpolicynet.com/images/documents/ publichealth/research/DoHS_2065-66-Glimpse%20of%20Annual%20Report-E.pdf).*

Table 1: Distribution of pharmacy assistants and graduates according to their working areas in 2007[5]

Nature/Category of Work	Pharmacy Graduates	Pharmacy Assistants
Industry	215	1
Studying/working abroad	111	–
Education	50	2
Hospital/community pharmacy	35	40
Government service	28	24
Nongovernmental organization	12	2
Information not available	–	39
Total	451	108

Source: NPC News Letter, 2007.

Table 2: Trends in the pharmacy workforce in Nepal within 7 years[5,9]

Pharmacy Workforce	Year 2007	Year 2014	Increase in 7 Years
Pharmacy graduates	451	1798	298.67%
Pharmacy assistants	108	4069	3667.59%

Sources: NPC News Letter, 2007; NPC, 2014; Kafle et al. (available on http://www.dda.gov.np/files/Quantification_2007.pdf).

According to the Act and the regulation of the Nepal Pharmacy Council (NPC), pharmacy assistants or graduates are not authorized to perform professional duties or services unless they are registered with the NPC. According to a conversation with Bijay Yadav, Registrar of NPC (December 3, 2014), there were about 1798 graduate pharmacists (including BPharm, PharmD, MPharm, and PhD) and 4069 assistant pharmacists (diploma in pharmacy) registered with the NPC as of November 9, 2014.[9] Table 1 depicts that the pharmacy graduates are involved mainly in pharmaceutical manufacturing, whereas hospital/community pharmacy is the first choice for the pharmacy assistants in Nepal. From 2007 to 2014, there was a tremendous proliferation in the number of pharmacy assistants as well as pharmacy graduates; however, the latest data on the distribution of their working areas are unavailable. However, the trend in pharmacists' working categories can still be assumed to be the same as that shown in Table 2.

4. Statistics on morbidity and mortality

Not only fertility but also mortality, affect the structure, size, and growth of a population. In the recent past, a faster decline in mortality compared with fertility resulted in a rapid growth in the Nepalese population. The reason for the rapid fall in mortality may be due to increased access to and improved health services. Nepal Demographic and Health Survey (NDHS) data from 2011 show an early childhood mortality rate per 1000 live births for period of 2006–2010 as 33, 13, 46, 9, and 54 for neonatal mortality, postneonatal mortality, infant mortality, child mortality, and under-5 mortality, respectively. The NDHS report further adds that the decline in mortality rates for neonatal, postneonatal, infant, and under-5 mortality over the 15 years preceding the survey were 27%, 48%, 34%, and 38%, respectively. This clearly indicates increased antenatal care and postnatal visits, improved delivery practices, and improved maternal health and newborn care indicators.[1,10]

5. Top 15 medicines based on expenditure and utilization

Health expenditure is increasing day by day. A national health report from Nepal suggests that there was 45.6% increase in health expenditure in fiscal year 2008/9 compared to 2006/7.[11] Similarly, expenditure on medicine also increases day by day. Pharmaceutical quantification carried out by Pharmaceutical Horizon of Nepal (PHON) under DDA found the 15 top-selling allopathic drugs, as listed in Table 3.[12] According to a study conducted about antibiotics utilization in a teaching hospital of central Nepal, beta-lactam (penicillins and cephalosporins) antibiotics (64%) are the highest prescribed and used antibiotics followed by macrolides (16%) and fluoroquinolones (16%).[13]

6. Pharmacy practice: country perspective

In Nepal, there has been a mushrooming of medical and pharmacy schools in recent times. About 18 medical schools are currently recognized by the Nepal Medical Council and few are still in the pipeline. Similarly, about 47 pharmacy colleges are listed by the Nepal Pharmacy

Table 3: Top 15 medicines based on expenditure and utilization

Rank	Drug	Retail sale value (NPR)[a]
1	Amoxicillin	422,566,152.85
2	Vitamin preparations	406,053,246.31
3	Topical skin preparations	395,776,153.28
4	Cough preparations	269,279,359.35
5	Diclofenac	243,524,488.37
6	Ciprofloxacin	242,265,688.31
7	Methyl ergometrine	216,553,784.17
8	Large volume parenteral	206,650,595.61
9	Cefadroxil	189,125,186.40
10	Metronidazole + diloxanide	182,851,819.89
11	Iron preparations	173,425,838.40
12	Ampicillin + cloxacillin	152,970,894.08
13	Ofloxacin	152,440,543.12
14	Ibuprofen + paracetamol	147,327,924.94
15	Vaccines, sera, and toxoids	145,186,405.00

[a]1 USD = 98.977 NPR.

Source: PHON, 2007; Kafle et al. (available on http://www.dda.gov.np/files/Quantification_2007.pdf).

Council.[14,15] Most of the pharmacy colleges in Nepal (mainly those affiliated with other universities) do not have hospitals attached to them, whereas medical colleges have their own functioning teaching hospitals. Despite the availability of such a huge number of medical and pharmacy colleges in Nepal, the area of pharmacy practice has not been well established. About 10 medical colleges or hospitals have pharmacy academic programs. Furthermore, teaching hospitals have pharmacology and pharmacy or related responsibilities. Therefore, medical colleges or hospitals can contribute more toward promoting pharmacy practice services in Nepal.[15,16] Undoubtedly, the pharmacists themselves should struggle and make their own place in the healthcare system. However, the Nepal's Ministry of Health, as a policy maker and regulating authority, plays an influential role toward promoting pharmacy practice in Nepal. Unfortunately, the Ministry of Health underestimates the professional role of pharmacists in the country and is biased, as reflected in its health reform plan, in which there is no room for pharmacists.[17]

7. Background on the pharmaceutical sector

The pharmaceutical sector of Nepal is in growing order. Currently, there are 45 registered pharmaceutical industries manufacturing modern medicines, and 8 industries are concerned with producing veterinary medicines.[18] Nepalese pharmaceutical manufacturers are capable only of producing formulations from pharmaceutical starting materials (imported from India, China, or other countries) and repacking of finished dosage forms. Research and development activities, such as the discovery of new active substances and the production of pharmaceutical starting materials, are beyond its approach.[19] Although a significant number of pharmaceutical industries are available in a small country like Nepal, about 60% of the market share of the pharmaceuticals by value belongs to India.[20]

8. Medicine supply and distribution

Nepal has wide variation in its topography. Hence, the distribution of medicines to the HCs, especially in the public sector, is a great challenge. In addition, the distribution of medicines requires technically competent persons, unlike distributing other commodities. In the public sector, the procurement of medicines can take place through various methods, including tenders, quotations, and direct procurement. Although domestic pharmaceutical production is progressively increasing, it is not enough to fulfill the demands of the public sector's requirements. Therefore, Nepal needs to import more than half of its drugs from neighboring countries, mainly India, to fulfill its pharmaceutical requirements.[21]

In the public sector, the Logistics Management Division (LMD) looks after the procurement, storage, and distribution of logistics, together with essential medicines, to efficiently deliver health services throughout the country. Unfortunately, there is no single specific unit under the Ministry of Health that constitutes experts in the field of pharmaceuticals procurement.

LMD was established in 1993 and fulfills its duties through a network with central stores, five regional medical stores, and district stores. In recent times, LMD has started a web-based inventory management system (LMIS), rural telemedicine program, and e-Post with the aim of providing better health services and information.[21,22]

In Nepal, public sector procurement occurs at both central and peripheral levels. The central body has the authority to decide about all essential medicines for free distribution and about 70% of the total procurement. Apart from this, there is allocation of 10% and 20% of budgets to the regional health directorate and the district, respectively. Procurement of medicines in bulk at the central level results in a reduction of price and greater quality assurance, whereas small-volume procurement at the peripheral level overwhelms the shortage of stocks. For public sector procurement, it is mandatory to abide by the Public Procurement Act, 2007 and the Public Procurement Regulations, 2007.[21,23,24]

A pull system is a demand-based approach for ensuring the reliable availability of health commodities at all service delivery points within the health system. In 2003, Nepal's MoHP started a new system that is an amalgam of a push–pull system. Efficient distribution of commodities, empowerment of field-level health personnel due to decentralized logistical decision-making, reduction in waste and expired medicines, and strengthened community drug programs are the advantages of new pull system. The efficient distribution of commodities under the new pull system is maintained by supplying 50% of the annual estimated consumption of a health facility (HF) directly to the HF and the remaining 50% is stored at the district level for demand-based supply. HFs use the LMIS to forward their demands quarterly to the appropriate district store. Meanwhile, regional medical stores maintain buffer stocks of 20 key essential drugs to supply district stores as needed. All HFs maintain 6 months' maximum stock levels, with regular quarterly resupply.[25] A diagrammatical representation of the new pull system is shown in Figure 2.

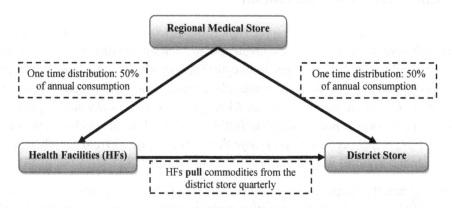

Figure 2
Pull system. *Nepal family health program, pull system (available on http://nfhp.jsi.com/Res/Docs/techbrief13-pull_sys.pdf).*

In the public sector, the major supply of medicines takes place through the national Central Medical Store (LMD) through its five public warehouses. The chain of distribution of medicines in the private sector is from manufacturer to stockists or superstockists to retailers to consumers, but under the legal provisions for each stakeholder. Thus, it seems that procurement and distribution occur simultaneously in the private sector, and there is definite percentage of profit at each level. A diagrammatic sketch of the distribution system in Nepal is shown in Figure 3.

9. Industrial pharmacy and pharmaceutical technology

In Nepal, pharmaceutical industries are the first destination for pharmacy graduates. Industrial pharmacy is probably the oldest pharmacy field and is well established in Nepal. Although there has been remarkable growth in pharmaceutical industries in recent times, there is no proportionate attraction of pharmacists to this field. This is probably due to the weaknesses of Nepalese pharmaceutical industries, including poor research and development efforts, inadequate clinical and regulatory networks, lack of international marketing efforts, low share of the total market,

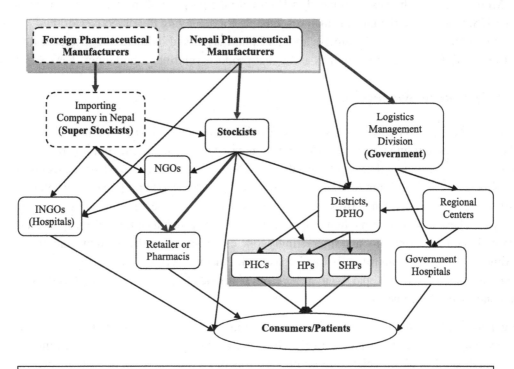

Key: I/NGOs, International/Nongovernmental Organizations; PHCs, Primary Healthcare Centers; HPs, Health Posts; SHPs, Sub Health Posts; **Bold** blue arrow (dark gray in print version), main channels, →, other channels

Figure 3
Distribution pattern of pharmaceuticals in Nepal. *Adapted from Harper et al.*[26]

narrow range of production (tablets, capsules, solutions, and suspensions), no production of injectables, and problems in upgrading. Although Nepalese pharmaceutical industries have easy access to the required technology, equipment, and raw materials from neighboring countries such as India and China, there is no proportionate development in pharmaceutical technologies. Moreover, research and development activities are limited in Nepal.[27]

10. Regulatory issues (registration and inspection)

The Government of Nepal enacted the Drug Act 1978 to control the misuse or abuse of drugs and related pharmaceuticals. Apart from this, the Drug Act 1978 regulates false or misleading information about the efficacy and use of drugs, their production, marketing, distribution, export-import, storage, and utilization. For the active enforcement of the Drug Act 1978, various rules, regulations, and codes have been implemented, such as Regulation on Constitution of Drug Consultative Council and Drug Advisory Committee (2037 BS), Drug Registration Regulation (2038 BS), Interrogation and Inspection Regulation (2040 BS), Codes on Drug Manufacturing (2041 BS), and Drug Standard Regulation (2043 BS).[28] The DDA, under the Ministry of Health, was introduced in 1979 with the purpose of implementing the Drug Act 1978. In addition, the DDA is also responsible for achieving the objectives of the National Drug Policy 1995. There are about 45 pharmaceutical industries registered with DDA that produce modern medicines and 8 that produce veterinary medicines.[18,28]

11. Pharmacy ownership

In Nepal, the DDA is the regulatory body of the Government of Nepal to monitor medicine-related issues, including pricing. DDA can fix the price of any medicine, but it is fixed only for intravenous fluids, oral rehydration salt, and a few others. Drugs are classified as groups Ka, Kha, and Ga. According to clause 5 (17) of the Drug Act 1978, no person can sell or distribute group Ka and Kha drugs without a prescription.[29] However, in actuality, one can easily purchase any type of medicine, including antibiotics such as amoxicillin, from pharmacies without a prescription—and interestingly, one can easily refill the medicine any number of times. Pharmacists can run only one licensed pharmacy at a time. Timing for community pharmacy is not fixed in Nepal, so it varies from pharmacy to pharmacy depending on patient load and their requirements.

In general, only medicinal commodities are sold in pharmacies, but some pharmacies sell general and cosmetic items along with medicines. By law, only professionally trained personnel, such as pharmacists, are authorized to sell medicines from the pharmacies. Therefore, no medicine, including over-the-counter (OTC), can be kept and sold through nonpharmacies. However—mainly in hilly remote areas where there is lack of pharmacies, HCs, healthcare providers, and transportation facilities—nonpharmacies also deal in medicines.

Till recent past (2013), there was no licensure examination for pharmacy professionals (pharmacy assistants and pharmacy graduates) to register with the NPC. Their registrations were performed on the basis of the universities or institutes listed in the NPC directory. Though NPC has started conducting licensure examinations from 2014, amendment in its regulation was made in 2015 to conduct licensure examination officially for the registration of pharmacy professionals. Foreign graduates also need to register with Pharmacy Council of Nepal to practice in Nepal.

The use of generic medicines is limited in Nepal. Prescribing by brand names of the drugs is a common practice, except few hospitals such as Dhulikhel Teaching Hospital, Manipal Teaching Hospital, and Patan Teaching Hospital. It is quite obvious that there are differences in the prices of different brands of the same medicine; however, wide variations in price for the same brand of medicines among different stakeholders (pharmacy outlets) also exist in Nepal.[30] Direct-to-consumer advertising is not common in Nepal, but drug advertising to pharmacists is increasing day by day.

12. Health insurance

As per a directive of the Interim Constitution of Nepal 2007, the Government of Nepal is committed to providing certain healthcare services free of cost to all and some other services to a targeted group of people. The government promotes these latter services through cash or incentives in a safe motherhood program, antenatal care program, uterine prolapse treatment program, and a referral support program (for deprived, helpless, disabled, and underprivileged people; pregnant women; patients with tuberculosis, AIDS, and psychiatric illnesses; citizens with extremes of ages; and victims of the peoples' movement and conflict).[31] In addition, MoHP has also been reinforcing the six community-based health insurance (CBHI) schemes as a trial program in six districts of Nepal. To meet the financial requirements for these services, the Government of Nepal pools fund from various financing sources, such as government funds (tax and non tax revenue), out-of-pocket expenditure (such as user fees from the general public), and institutions and the external donors such as Department for International Development (DfID), AusAid, and the World Bank. However, out-of-pocket expenditures (about one half of the total heath expenditures) predominantly exist but are considered to be the most undesirable way of funding health services in Nepal, where the majority of people reside in rural areas and are poor.[32]

13. Hospital pharmacy practice

Hospital pharmacy practice in Nepal is one of the overlooked areas of pharmacy practice. The concept of hospital pharmacy was started in Patan Hospital in the 1980s. In Nepal, there are more than 100 tertiary care hospitals, but the number of hospitals running their own pharmacies can be counted in your fingertips. The majority of hospitals do not have their own hospital pharmacies.

The concept of a hospital pharmacy is either not clear or intentionally overlooked in hospital management within teaching hospitals. Generally, hospital management rents out space to private vendor, who runs its own private pharmacy. Hence, tertiary care hospitals in Nepal—chiefly teaching hospitals—need to have own hospital pharmacy with pharmacy services.[33,34] The government of Nepal has a mandatory policy that hospitals with more than 25 beds should have at least one pharmacist; however, this law has not been uniformly implemented. Some hospitals of medical colleges have taken the initiative toward developing hospital pharmacy practice.[16] Manipal Teaching Hospital, Patan Teaching Hospital, KIST Teaching Hospital, Dhulikhel Teaching Hospital, Hospital of College of Medical Sciences, and a few others are among the hospitals running hospital pharmacy practices. Furthermore, Manipal Teaching Hospital has a well-developed hospital pharmacy; pharmacists there perform various hospital pharmacy activities, such as good pharmacy practice, drug information, pharmacovigilance, medication counseling, and teaching rational use of medicine to medical and pharmacy students.[35] Hence, this is an area for development in other hospitals, as well as one that provides hidden opportunities for the pharmacists.

14. Clinical pharmacy

Clinical pharmacy is one of the services provided by pharmacists in an attempt to promote rational drug therapy that is safe, appropriate, and cost-effective. Clinical pharmacy is well developed in Western countries,[36] but in Nepal it is in a primitive state. There are many reasons behind the slow growth of clinical pharmacy in Nepal: industry-oriented undergraduate pharmacy education, the lack of established hospital pharmacies, and the undefined role and responsibilities of pharmacists by hospital administration and government. However, in a few hospitals, pharmacists perform clinical pharmacy activities such as medication counseling, drug information, pharmacovigilance, and educating on the rational use of medicines.[16,35] Recently, MPharm in Clinical Pharmacy and PharmD (postbaccalaureate) programs were started at Pokhara University and Kathmandu University (KU), respectively. Some of the clinical pharmacy activities, such as ward rounds, patient medication review, and taking medication histories, are practiced by students in these programs as a part of their coursework.

15. Drug information specialists and centers

Vigorous pharmaceutical promotion from manufacturers may lead to biased information and false claims regarding their products, thus increasing the need for unbiased drug information from healthcare professionals. The concept of drug information started in the early 1960s in developed countries,[37] although it did not start until the 1990s in Nepal. United States Pharmacopoeia (USP) launched the Rational Pharmaceutical Management Project in 1992 in developing countries. One of the prime objectives of the project was to increase the rational use of drugs by disseminating unbiased drug information. Under this project, four drug information centers (DICs)—Tribhuvan University Teaching Hospital, the DDA, the Resource Center for

Primary Healthcare, and Nepal Chemists and Druggists Association—were established in Nepal.[38,39] On September 23, 1996, these centers, along with the Nepal Health Research Council, joined together and formed the Drug Information Network of Nepal (DINoN). Later, four other members—the Nepal Poison Information Center, Britain Nepal Medical Trust, BP Koirala Institute of Health Sciences, and Manipal College of Medical Sciences—joined hands with DINoN. However, this network has been almost inactive in recent years. Meanwhile, a few more hospitals have established their own DICs. Drug information providers in most of the DICs in Nepal are either pharmacists or pharmacologists. Hurdles in running DICs include a lack of trained personnel, lack of financial and drug information resources, poor documentation, and poor dissemination of the limited available information.[39]

16. Medical representatives and the marketing of pharmaceutical products

In Nepal, the manufacture, sale, distribution, export, and import of drugs are regulated through Drug Act 1978 (2035 BS) of Nepal. According to this act, all manufacturers should be registered with the DDA. To date, 45 pharmaceutical industries producing modern medicines and 8 pharmaceutical industries producing veterinary medicines are registered with the DDA.[18] A survey conducted in 2008 suggests that domestic manufacturers make up around 42% of total drug consumption in Nepal.[19]

The WHO in 1998 and the DDA in 2007 published two separate guidelines to facilitate ethical medicine promotion in Nepal.[40,41] In addition, the Drug Act 1978 of Nepal has prohibited the false or misleading advertisement of drugs. Despite this, a study that evaluated drug promotional materials found that essential parameters, such as active ingredients, dosage form or regimen, and major drug interactions, were missing in the promotional materials; in addition, promotional material circulated in hospitals failed to fulfill all of the criteria defined by WHO.[42] Moreover, another study suggests that clinicians accept gift and parties from the medical representatives (MRs) to prescribe their branded medicines.[43]

Pharmaceutical promotion is not regulated strictly by any regulatory authorities. However, few hospitals in Nepal have taken an initiative so that MRs are either not allowed to meet with doctors or only permitted to meet in groups with a prior appointment.[44] Direct-to-consumer advertising is not common in Nepal, but drug advertising to pharmacists is increasing. Clearly there is an urgent need to monitor pharmaceutical promotion.

17. Community pharmacy practice

A community pharmacist is responsible for controlling, dispensing, and distributing medicines. These pharmacists work under legal and ethical guidelines to ensure the correct and safe supply of medical products to the general public. They are involved in maintaining and improving people's health by providing advice and information as well as dispensing prescription medicines. Community pharmacists also sell OTC medical products and instruct patients on the use of medicines and medical appliances. Some pharmacists also offer specialist health checks, such as blood pressure monitoring and diabetes screening, run stop-smoking clinics and weight reduction programs, and are able to prescribe as well as dispense medicines.

In Nepal, there are about 14,899 licensed pharmacies (wholesalers and retailers, as of June 2012).[45] In the past, when there was a shortage of pharmacists in the country, the DDA offered a 45-h orientation training program to persons who had completed basic schooling education.[46] Later, the training period was increased up to 3 months. Those who completed the orientation training were given licenses to open pharmacies in the country. Although these training programs were stopped after 2000 AD, community pharmacies in Nepal are still run by people who have taken such orientation trainings. As orientation training is on hold now, new licenses are issued only to individuals who have completed a diploma in pharmacy (3-year course after schooling/matriculation) or a higher degree in pharmacy. Xeno Pharmacy was the first community pharmacy in Nepal run by registered pharmacists.

There are many challenges in community pharmacy practices, such as the following:

1. **Human resources**: There is acute shortage of pharmacists in this profession. The number of registered pharmacists in Nepal is not enough to replace the oriented pharmacy personnel. Furthermore, the involvement of pharmacists in community pharmacy is minimal.[33]
2. **Education and training**: Pharmacy education in Nepal is more focused on industry. Pharmacists get very minimal exposure to community pharmacy training. Hence, pharmacists lack the professional knowledge required for running community pharmacies. As a result, pharmacists are not willing to work as community pharmacists. Moreover, not enough refresher training programs are offered for people who have taken the orientation. At present, there is no licensing examination for community pharmacists. There is a limited number of drug information sources needed to provide patient counseling.[47] Hence, there is a need for Continuing Pharmacy Education (CPE) programs for pharmacists to enhance their professional knowledge.
3. **Ethical and legal aspects**: The Drug Act 1978 states that no person may sell or distribute group Ka and Kha drugs without a prescription.[29] But, in reality, any drug can be purchased without a prescription and, rarely, one can find some OTC medicines in glossary shops, which is an ethical concern and suggests poor implementation of the Drug Act.[48]
4. **Drug promotion and unhealthy competition**: Pharmaceutical manufacturers promote their products vigorously and provide many bonuses and high profit margins to retailers, which has created unhealthy competition among the retailers.
5. **Others**: There are many other challenges in Nepal, such as the remuneration of community pharmacists, documentation, brand-specific prescriptions that are difficult to honor, patients who do not buy complete courses of their prescriptions, the need for strip cutting and problems in medicine return, shortage of medicines, managing expired medicines, costly software for managing a pharmacy, and documentation.[49]

18. Public health practice and health promotion

Health is a basic human right and is essential for the social and economic development of a nation. The purpose of promoting health is to alleviate the burden of diseases (communicable as well as noncommunicable), as well as the social and economic impacts of such diseases, by integrating activities across sectors and encouraging multisectoral collaboration. The three common approaches often applied for health promotion are the issues-based approach, population-based approach, and setting-based approach.[50]

Nepal is facing several public health problems, such as diarrhea, acute respiratory infections, malaria, visceral leishmaniasis, tuberculosis, leprosy, vaccine-preventable diseases (e.g., Japanese encephalitis and viral hepatitis), encephalitis, meningitis, sexually transmitted diseases including HIV/AIDS, obesity, tobacco use, excessive use of alcohol, diabetes, hypertension and other cardiovascular diseases, malignancies and problems of elderly, malnutrition, vitamin A deficiency, iodine deficiency, anemia, poor environmental conditions, and high population growth. Thus, promoting health is a crucial need of the people of Nepal, so that they can cope with the aforementioned alarming health problems that are still the leading causes of morbidity and mortality.

In Nepal, the National Health Education, Information and Communication Center is responsible for information, education, and communication activities for health promotion. The center disseminates messages and materials using electronic and print media to health institutions, schools, and community groups, among others. WHO also emphasizes the need for an integrated approach to health promotion interventions through a network of communities, schools, and health institutions. However, there are still numerous challenges toward promoting health properly in Nepal, such as a lack of knowledge and awareness about priority health problems, lack of proper approach, inadequate properly trained manpower at all levels, inadequate awareness on community participation, inadequate appropriate multimedia campaign and relevant advocacy materials, security and political instability, technical input, coordination with other partners, and inadequate supervision, monitoring, and evaluation of the programs for further planning and implementation.[51]

19. Position of traditional and herbal medicines

Traditional or herbal medicines are the oldest approaches in Nepalese society to manage diseases. The concept of traditional or herbal medicines is transferred from generation to generation, especially in traditional societies and usually through oral tradition. There are different approaches to traditional and herbal medicines in Nepal, such as Ayurveda, homeopathy, Tibetan medicine, Unani, and faith healing.

1. **Ayurveda**: In Nepalese society, two types of Ayurvedic physicians exists: Vaidya (trained in Ayurvedic colleges or universities) and Kaviraj (learned the knowledge and skill of the profession from their fathers or from the gurus/teachers). Ayurvedic medicines and their

practices are under the jurisdiction of Department of Ayurveda, MoHP, Government of Nepal. There is a 100-bed central Ayurvedic Hospital in Naradevi, Kathmandu, established in 1933, and a 30-bed Mid Western Regional Ayurvedic Hospital in Dang, Western, Nepal. There are 14 zonal Ayurvedic dispensaries and 55 district health centers throughout the country. More than 216 Ayurvedic dispensaries, district, and rural pharmacies supported by the Government of Nepal, as well as numerous private clinics and dispensaries, exist throughout the nation. Apart from this, there is Singh Durbar Vaidya Khana, a government Ayurvedic medicine production industry, the Ayurvedic Medicine Council (1990), and Ayurveda Health Policy (1996).

2. **Homeopathy**: The homeopathy system is recognized by the Government of Nepal, and there is a six-bed Sri Pashupati Homeopathic Hospital in Lalitpur, Kathmandu, under the Government of Nepal. About 200–250 patients are treated free of cost every day. There are several private homeopathic clinics, dispensaries, and homeopathic medical colleges throughout the nation.

3. **Tibetan medicine**: The trend of Tibetan medicine is prevalent in the northern part of Nepal bordering Tibet; this medicine practice was brought over by Tibetan refugees who came to Nepal after the deportation of the Dalai Lama in 1959. Tibetan medicines are practiced in some northern districts of Nepal, such as Dolpa, Mustang, Mugu, Humla, Jumla, Manang, Surkhet, Baglung, Kaski, Gorkha, Rasuwa, Dhading, Kathmandu, Lalitpur, and Solukhumbu.

4. **Unani system**: The Unani system of medicine has its origin in Greece. This system is recognized by the Government of Nepal. There is one government-sponsored Unani dispensary in existence. Hakims (Unani doctors) are trained mainly in India. The practice in Nepal is almost nonexistent.

5. **Faith healing**: Faith healing is a method of treating diseases by prayer and through exercise of faith in God. Faith healing is predominant in the rural, remote, and traditional societies of Nepal. It is of four types: Shaman/Dhami-Jhankri (*tantra-mantra*), Jharphuke (*sweeping and blowing healers*), Pundit-Lama-Pujari-Gubhaju (*priests of different religions*), and Jyotish (*astrologers*).

In recent times, more emphasis is being given to the traditional medicine systems for their institutionalization, industrialization, and commercialization.[52,53]

20. Pharmacy education and professional development

There is an increasing interest in pharmacy education recently, mainly in developing countries. In January 2012, about 19 institutions were registered with the NPC to run graduate or higher-level programs in the field of pharmacy. Similarly, about 29 academic institutions were listed with the NPC for programs offering a diploma in pharmacy, a certificate-level program.[15] Most of these institutions have come in existence in the past few years, which indicates an increasing interest in pharmacy.

Continuing professional development (CPD) is a learning activity for professionals to maintain and develop their professional careers to ensure that they retain their skills to practice safely. CPD activities can be in the form of courses, workshops, conferences, or self-directed activities. In Nepal, CPD is not common. Hiring institutions/organizations and the NPC do not seem to have much interests in promoting professional development. The NPC is planning to initiate a pharmacist licensing examination, but this has yet to be implemented.[54]

21. Pharmacy practice in pharmacy curricula

Currently, four universities in Nepal have pharmacy programs: Tribhuvan University, KU, Pokhara University, and Purbanchal University. The bachelor of pharmacy program (4 years) is the main offering in all four universities. In addition, some universities are also offering a 3-year certificate program, called a diploma in pharmacy (DPharm), and a 2-year master's degree (MPharm). KU introduced the only pharmacy practice course, called Pharmaceutical Care, in its MPharm curriculum. The course was introduced in 2000 but was later replaced by the postbaccalaureate PharmD course in 2010. Furthermore, KU is the only university in Nepal to offer a 3-year Doctor of Philosophy (PhD) program, since 2004. The PhD program is mainly focused on industrial pharmacy and is aimed to the faculty members of KU.[55,56]

The study of pharmacy practice is barely visible in Nepal's pharmacy curricula. However, the pharmacy profession is changing from product oriented to patient oriented. This trend can be seen even in Nepal, with the focus on hospital pharmacy practices (especially in the larger teaching hospitals of Nepal), but pharmacy academic institutions are still lagging behind in this area.[16] Thus, there is a need to introduce and emphasize pharmacy practice and related programs by pharmacy academic institutions in Nepal.

22. Research on pharmacy practice

Although there is not much research on pharmacy practices in Nepal, pharmacists working in this field in different Nepalese institutions are now getting involved in research activities related to pharmacy practice. Examples of institutions that are actively taking part in these activities are Manipal College of Medical Sciences, Kist Medical College, and the School of Medical Sciences.

23. Achievements in pharmacy practice

Pharmacy practice in Nepal is still in its development phase. This section describes some achievements in pharmacy practice in Nepal.

23.1 Upgrades in pharmacy education

One of the biggest achievements in pharmacy practice is the elimination of the orientation training program that was started during 1980s. Since orientation training ended, the minimum qualification required for establishing a new pharmacy is a diploma in pharmacy, which is a 3-year professional pharmacy course completed after one's basic schooling degree (i.e., matriculation). Furthermore, many pharmacy schools emerged in this period to produce new pharmacists, and specialized PharmD (postbaccalaureate) and MPharm in Clinical Pharmacy programs were started in Nepal.

23.2 Pharmacist involvement in hospital and community practices

The number of pharmacists in Nepal has increased drastically in recent years due to the increase in the number of pharmacy colleges. As a result, many pharmacists have chosen the fields of community and hospital pharmacy practice, which were not in existence a decade ago.

23.3 Growth in pharmaceutical production

The real growth in the pharmaceutical sector of Nepal has occurred in the form of production. In 2000 AD, there were very few pharmaceutical manufacturers with a limited number of products. At that time, more than 90% of medicines were imported from neighboring countries, especially from India. At present, more than 40% of Nepal's medicine requirements are fulfilled by domestic manufacturers, which is a big achievement.

23.4 Revision of Nepalese national formulary and national essential drug list

The Nepalese National Formulary (NNF) was first published in 1997. NNF is a good source of drug information. After a period of 14 years, NNF was revised in 2011. Similarly, the National Essential Drug List was first published in 1986 and was revised in 1992, 1997, and 2002. A fourth revision was carried out in 2011, which is a good achievement.

23.5 Establishment of drug information network

Many DICs have been established in the country. Furthermore, they combined together to form the DINoN, which is an excellent achievement.

23.6 Establishment of national pharmacovigilance program

In October 2004, the Government of Nepal announced the DDA as the National Center for Pharmacovigilance. In July 2006, Nepal became a member of the WHO Pharmacovigilance Program. Currently, there are six regional centers that report adverse drug reactions to the national center.

24. Challenges in pharmacy practice

In recent times, there has been more demand for pharmacy and clinical practices in Nepal. Although pharmacy practice is slowly improving, there are several challenges to take pharmacy practice in Nepal to the next level:

- The pharmacy education system is predominantly geared toward industrial pharmacy.
- There are notable numbers of teaching hospitals in Nepal with sophisticated and advanced medical equipment, as well as specialized medical services. However, the hospital management authorities do not promote pharmacy practice services. In general, management teams at teaching hospitals do not want to implement pharmacy-related services in teaching hospitals.
- Despite the availability of rules and regulation in the nation for better pharmacy-related services and patient healthcare, the responsible authorities (e.g., Nepal Medical Council, NPC, and the government) fail to enforce the rules strictly.
- Unethical pharmaceutical promotion and unhealthy competition among pharmaceutical manufacturers is leading to unethical prescribing and medicine utilization.
- Nepotism and bias occur in the recruitment and promotion of healthcare personnel, in both public and private health sectors.
- In the public sector, the purchase and supply of pharmaceuticals require managerially and technically competent professionals. However, this job is being performed by nonprofessionals or those who lack the necessary skills and education.
- There is a lack of training and CPD for pharmacy personnel and, thus, a failure to deliver proper pharmaceutical services to patients.

25. Recommendations: way forward

The quality and intensity of pharmacy practice services delivered to the Nepalese people are not up to the mark. Hence, there is a need for collective efforts by the government, nongovernmental organizations, academic institutions, hospitals (mainly teaching hospitals), and other health-related organizations to realizing the necessity and reinforcement of pharmacy practices in Nepal, so that quality healthcare can be offered to the public. The previously highlighted challenges need to be addressed for better delivery of pharmacy practice and clinical practice services.

26. Conclusions

Despite the numerous pitfalls in pharmacy practices in Nepal, achievements in this field have occurred, such as the upgrades in the pharmacy curricula and education, involvement of pharmacists in hospital and community pharmacy activities, growth in pharmaceutical production, establishment of drug information and pharmacovigilance centers, and their networking. However, these improvements in pharmacy practices are not sufficient to fulfill the country's requirements for quality healthcare delivery to the people of Nepal. Therefore, there is an urgent need to tackle the challenges facing any further upgrades to pharmacy practice services in Nepal.

27. Points to remember

- The concept of industrial pharmacy in Nepal is well-established and growing; however, it is not enough for pharmacists to contribute to healthcare and receive professional recognition from the public.
- The concept of pharmacy practice in Nepal is undefined but gradually improving. However, it will require the great effort of pharmacy professionals toward its development in Nepal. Pharmacists now need to focus on patient-related services rather than product-centered services.
- The Nepal's Ministry of Health undervalues the professional role of pharmacists in Nepal. This biased view about pharmacists is further reflected in the country's health reform plan, in which there is no room for pharmacists.

Acknowledgment

The authors thank Krishna Kumar Limboo, former DGM, HR, and Admin, PBT (PVT) Ltd, Nepal, for his valuable suggestions and copyediting the chapter.

References

1. Nepal. *Nepal demographic & health survey*. Kathmandu: Ministry of Health and Population, New ERA and Macro International Inc.; 2011.
2. Nepal. *Preliminary results of national population census 2011*. Kathmandu: Central Bureau of Statistics; 2011.
3. Nepal. *Nepal in figures*. Kathmandu: Central Bureau of Statistics; 2006.
4. *International health partnership national 'compact' between ministry of health and population and external development partners, government of Nepal* [Internet]. Kathmandu: National Health Development Partnership [cited December 04, 2012]. Available from: http://www.mohp.gov.np/english/projects/nhdp2009_signfinal.pdf; 2009.
5. Pharmacy Human Resource Status in Nepal. *NPC News Lett* 2007;**2**(1):1–8.
6. *WHO. World health statistics*. Geneva: World Health Organization; 2011.
7. *Nepal: strengthening interrelationships between stakeholders* [Internet]. Kathmandu: Global Health Workforce Alliance [cited October 22, 2012]. Available from: http://www.who.int/workforcealliance/knowledge/resources/CCF_CaseStudy_Nepal.pdf; 2011.
8. Shankar PR. Attracting and retaining doctors in rural Nepal. *Rural Remote Health [Internet]* 2010;**10**(1420). [cited 2014 January 20]. Available from: http://www.rrh.org.au/publishedarticles/article_print_1420.pdf.
9. *Pharmacists registered in NPC registration book*. Kathmandu: Nepal Pharmacy Council, Government of Nepal; 2014.
10. *Nepal population report*. Kathmandu: Minstry of Health and Population, Government of Nepal; 2011.
11. Shrestha BR, Gauchan Y, Gautam GS, Baral P. *Nepal national health accounts 2006/07–2008/2009*. Kathmandu: Health Economics and Financing Unit, Minstry of Health and Population, Government of Nepal; 2012.

12. Kafle KK, Karkee SB, Rajbhandari V. *Report on consumption of antibiotics and other medicines.* Kathmandu: Pharmaceutical Horizon of Nepal (PHON); January 2007. 31 p.

13. Ansari M. Evaluation of the most commonly dispensed antibiotics among the pharmacies located in and around National Medical College Teaching Hospital, Birgunj, Nepal. *Indian J Pharm Pract* 2013;**6**(3):62–4.

14. *Recognized institutions: medical colleges* [Internet]. Kathmandu: Nepal Medical Council (NMC) [cited February 11, 2012]. Available from: http://www.nmc.org.np/recognized-institution/medical-college.html; 2012.

15. *List of departments/colleges offering Diploma in Pharmacy (DPharm) & Bachelor in Pharmacy (BPharm)* [Internet]. Kathmandu: Nepal Pharmacy Council (NPC) [cited February 11, 2012]. Available from: http://www.nepalpharmacycouncil.org.np/downloads/List%20of%20departments_colleges.pdf; 2012.

16. Shankar PR, Subish P. Developing pharmacy practice in medical schools in Nepal. *Indian J Pharm Pract* 2010;**3**(4):5–7.

17. Ansari M. *More pharmacists. The Kathmandu Post* [Internet]. [cited January 30, 2014]; Voice of the People. Available from: http://www.ekantipur.com/the-kathmandu-post/2013/01/28/letters/voice-of-the-people/244639.html; January 28, 2013.

18. *List of the Nepalese pharmaceutical industries producing modern and veterinary medicines* [Online]. Kathmandu: Department of Drug Administration, Ministry of Health and Population [cited September 23, 2012]. Available from: http://www.dda.gov.np/industry.php; 2012.

19. *Nepal pharmaceutical country profile.* Kathmandu: Ministry of Health and Population, Government of Nepal; 2011.

20. *National pharmaceutical expenditure survey.* Kathmandu: Ministry of Health and Population, Government of Nepal; 2011.

21. *Central bidding and local purchasing.* Kathmandu: Ministry of Health and Population, Government of Nepal; May 2009. 18 p.

22. *Introduction* [Internet]. Kathmandu: Logistics Management Division, Department of Health Services, Ministry of Health and Population [cited November 06, 2012]. Available from: http://www.dohslmd.gov.np/; 2012.

23. *The public procurement act, (2063 BS) 2007.* Kathmandu: Nepal Law Commission, Government of Nepal; 2007.

24. *The public procurement rules, (2064 BS) 2007.* Kathmandu: Nepal Law Commission, Government of Nepal; 2007.

25. *Nepal family health program, pull system.* Kathmandu: USAID; 2007. 4 p. Technical Brief No. 13.

26. Harper I, Brhlikova P, Subedi MS, Bhattarai S, Basu S, Gupta AD, et al. *Drug procurement in Nepal* [Internet]. UK: The Centre for International Public Health Policy [cited November 09, 2012]. Available from: http://www.csased.ac.uk/__data/assets/pdf_file/0009/38826/DrugProcurementNepal.pdf; 2007.

27. Karmacharya JB. *Nepalese pharmaceutical industries and world health organization recommended good manufacturing practices* [Internet]. Kathmandu: PEXOP [cited January 05, 2013]. Available from: http://www.scribd.com/doc/86532355/Nepalese-Pharmaceutical-Industries-Who-Gmp; 2005.

28. *DDA background.* Kathmandu: Department of Drug Administration, Ministry of Health and Population, Government of Nepal; 2012.

29. *Drug act.* Kathmandu: Department of Drug Administration, Ministry of Health and Population, Government of Nepal; 1978.

30. Ansari M, Thapa S, Day TK, Sinha JR, Khan S. Price variation of essential medicines among different stakeholders of Eastern Nepal: a concern of government's free drug scheme. *J Med Use Dev Ctries* 2009;**1**(4):25–34.

31. Stoermer M, Fuerst F, Rijal K, Bhandari R, Nogier C, Gautam GS, et al. *Review of community-based health insurance initiatives in Nepal.* Kathmandu: Health Sector Support Programme, Department of Health Services, Ministry of Health and Population; 2012.

32. Torres LV, Gautam GS, Fuerst F, Adhikari CM. *Assessment of the government health financing system in Nepal: suggestions for reform.* Kathmandu: Health Sector Support Programme, Department of Health Services, Ministry of Health and Population; 2011.

33. Recounting a hospital pharmacy practice in Nepal. *Nepal Pharm Counc (NPC) News Lett* 2010;**3**(1):1–2.
34. Ansari M. Teaching hospitals of Nepal need to have own hospital pharmacy with pharmacy services. *Int J Pharm Teach Pract* 2013;**4**(3):695–6.
35. Palaian S, Alam K. Activities of the pharmacists in a teaching hospital in Nepal. *South Med Rev* 2008;**1**(1):6–9.
36. LeBlanc JM, Dasta JF. Scope of international hospital pharmacy practice. *Ann Pharmacother* 2005;**39**:183–91. http://dx.doi.org/10.1345/aph.1E317.
37. Evens RP. The state of the art, and future directions of drug information centers. *Pharm Int* 1985;**6**:74–7.
38. Indicators for rapid assessment of pharmaceutical supply system. *Rational pharmaceutical management project update*. Arlington, VA: Management Sciences for Health; 1995. 4 p.
39. Anupa KC, Subish P, Mishra P. Drug information services in Nepal-the changing perspectives. *Kathmandu Univ Med J* 2008;**6**(1):117–21.
40. *Ethical criteria for medicinal drug promotion*. Geneva: World Health Organization; 1988.
41. *Guidelines on ethical promotion of medicine*. Kathmandu: Department of Drug Administration, Ministry of Health and Population; 2007.
42. Alam K, Sah AK, Ojha P, Palaian S, Shankar PR. Evaluation of drug promotional materials in a hospital setting in Nepal. *South Med Rev* 2009;**2**(1):2–6.
43. Giri BR, Shankar PR. Learning how drug companies promote medicine in Nepal. *PLoS Med* 2005;**2**(8):e256.
44. Alam K. *Utilization pattern and controlling system of antibiotics in tertiary care hospital in Nepal* [dissertation]. Bangkok, Thailand: Chulalongkorn University; 2011.
45. Prasad RR. Number of registered pharmacy outlets till June 2012. *Drug Bull Nepal* 2012;**24**(1):7–9.
46. Kafle KK, Gartoulla RP, Pradhan YMS, Karkee SB, Quick JD. Drug retailer training: experiences from Nepal. *Soc Sci Med* 1992;**35**(8):1015–25.
47. Poudel A, Khanal S, Alam K, Palaian S. Perception of Nepalese community pharmacists towards patient counseling and continuing pharmacy education program: a multicentric study. *J Clin Diagn Res* 2009;**3**(2):1408–13.
48. Wachter DA, Joshi MP, Rimal B. Antibiotic dispensing by drug retailers in Kathmandu, Nepal. *Trop Med Int Health* 1999;**4**(11):782–8.
49. *Paradigm shift in pharmacy profession. Proceeding of NPSA-NPSS workshop*. Kathmandu, Nepal; March 12, 2010.
50. *Regional strategy for health promotion for South-East Asia*. New Delhi: World Health Organization, SEARO; 2008. 34 p. Report No.:SEA/HE/194.
51. *Health promotion in Nepal* [Internet]. World Health Organization, SEARO, Country office for Nepal [cited November 20, 2012]. Available from: http://www.nep.searo.who.int/EN/Section4/Section46.htm; 2008.
52. Koirala RR. *Country monographs on traditional system of medicine*. Kathmandu: Government of Nepal; 2007.
53. Gewali MB, Awale S. *Aspects of traditional medicine in Nepal* [Internet]. Toyama: Institute of Natural Medicine, University of Toyama, Japan [cited January 04, 2012]. Available from: http://lib.icimod.org/record/13840/files/3615.pdf; 2008.
54. Gautam M. *NPC to hold pharmacist licencing exam soon* [Internet]. Kathmandu: The Kathmandu Post [cited January 07, 2013]. Available from: http://www.ekantipur.com/the-kathmandu-post/2012/04/05/nation/npc-to-hold-pharmacist-licencing-exam-soon/233479.html; April 05, 2012.
55. Bhuvan KC, Subish P, Izham MIM. PharmD education in Nepal: the challenges ahead. *Am J Pharm Educ* 2011;**75**(2):38c.
56. *Department of pharmacy* [Internet]. Dhulikhel: Kathmandu University [cited November 12, 2012]. Available from: http://www.ku.edu.np/pharmacy/; 2012.

Pharmacy Practice in the Middle East

CHAPTER 9

Pharmacy Practice in the Kingdom of Saudi Arabia

Ahmad Almeman, Ahmed Al-jedai

Chapter Outline

1. Country background

Saudi Arabia is a wealthy country with a total population of almost 30 million. The country spans a wide area of 2.5 million km², which includes a vast desert and a highland[1]; however, the majority of people (85%) live in urban areas. The country has witnessed massive improvement with respect to socioeconomic circumstances in areas including health, education, and technology over the last few decades.

The male-to-female ratio is almost 1:1, with the younger generation overwhelmingly preponderant. The total fertility rate was reported to be almost 3% in 2012. In 2010, overall life expectancy at birth was approximately 74, with 3% of the population expected to live to be older than 65 years (Table 1).[2,3]

2. Vital health statistics

Total health expenditure has increased significantly in Saudi Arabia; there has been a significant rise from $200 per capita in 1995 to $800 per capita in 2010. One of the major problems with respect to health is a lack of reliable data and medical statistics, making it difficult to assess the real situation in the country.[4] Healthcare expenditure (9%) has grown relatively faster than that of the pharmaceutical market (8.6%). Total healthcare expenditure was reported to be USD 18 billion in 2013 and is expected to reach USD 27 billion by 2018.[5]

Immunization is obligatory in Saudi Arabia and is provided free of charge by governmental healthcare institutions (Table 2).

2.1 Morbidity and mortality statistics

The country's most common causes of death, classified according to the International Classification of Diseases (ICD-10), are as follows: diseases of the circulatory system (16.0%), conditions originating in the prenatal period (9.0%), neoplasm (4.75%), diseases of the respiratory system (4.03%), infections and parasitic diseases (3.31%), genitourinary diseases (3.09%), congenital anomalies (2.66%), endocrine, nutrition, and metabolic diseases (2.46%), and diseases of the digestive system (1.93%).[2] These statistics are consistent with those of other developing countries, with some rates recorded in Saudi Arabia exceeding those of developed countries. Despite variability, cardiovascular diseases, followed by diabetes, are the leading cause of death in most countries (Figure 1).

Hypertension and diabetes are the leading causes of cardiovascular disease, and therefore death, nationwide (Table 3). Obesity is prevalent in both men and women in the Saudi population, but it is predominantly observed in women of childbearing age.[6,7] The rate of hypertension is significantly higher in men relative to women, with prevalence rates of 29% and

Table 1: Demographics indicators, 2012

Indicator	Value	Year
Total estimated population size	29,195,895	2012
Crude birth rate per 1000 population	22.5	2012
Annual population growth rate (%)		
Total	3.19	2004–2010
Saudi	2.21	
Non-Saudi	5.61	
Age of population (%)		
<5 years	10.85	2012
<15 years	30.37	2012
15–64 years	66.89	2012
≥65 years	2.73	2012
Total fertility rate	2.87	2012
Life expectancy at birth (years)		2012
Total	73.8	
Male	72.8	
Female	75.2	
Incidence of low birth weight (%)	8.8	2011

Source: MOH, 2012.[2]

Table 2: Immunization coverage

Indicator	Percentage (%)	Year
Pentavalent vaccine[a]	97.7	2012
Oral polio vaccine (OPV)	97.7	2012
BCG vaccine	98.6	2012
MMR vaccine[b]	97.8	2012
Pneumococcal conjugate vaccine (PCV)	97.7	2012

[a]Includes diphtheria, pertussis, tetanus, *Hemophilus influenza* type B, and hepatitis B.
[b]Includes measles, mumps, and rubella.
Source: MOH, 2012.[2]

22% in urban and rural areas, respectively; both of these rates are significantly lower than those of Eastern populations (34%). Hypercholesterolemia is most common in women, particularly between the ages of 40 and 59 years. Prevalence rates for hypercholesterolemia are 9% and 11% in men and women, respectively, and could be lower than those observed in other parts of the world, such as the United States or Europe.[7]

In hospitalized patients, disease most commonly affects the cardiovascular and respiratory systems, accounting for 20% and 14% of reported cases of disease, respectively. The most common diseases are diabetes mellitus (11%), ischemic heart disease (9%), and asthma (6%).[8]

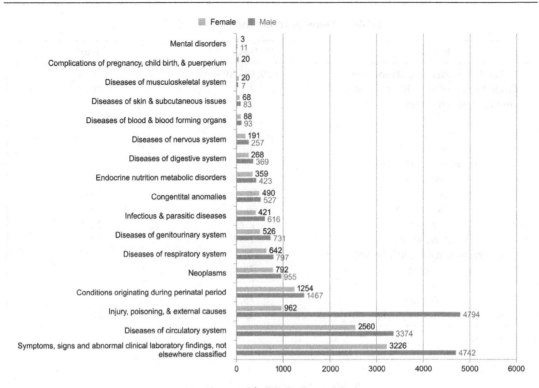

Figure 1
Causes of death among Saudis in 2012. *MOH (2012).*[2]

3. Overview of the healthcare system

The first public health department was established by King Abdul Aziz, the founder of the kingdom, in Makkah in 1925; it initially included ambulance services in order to meet the urgent need that arose at the time.[9] This department was responsible for building hospitals and centers across the country and establishing general practices with respect to medicine and medications. A Public Health Council was subsequently formed to meet the need for health services required during Hajj (pilgrimage) and Umrah seasons. The council's duty was limited to supervising medical services nationwide and providing a skilled healthcare workforce. In 1951, the need for a specialized MOH, to organize nationwide efforts and follow best practices established globally, was identified. The MOH is headed by a minister and two deputies, who are assisted by four deputy ministers. The specifics of a strategic planning process are published in detail on the official MOH Web site.[9]

The health system in Saudi Arabia has evolved substantially, from preventative services in 1950 to curative services in 1980 (Table 4). In June 2002, the Health System Law was approved for the first time, following many years of debate. The law came to fill a vacuum that had existed in healthcare regulation for more than 50 years. The importance of the Health System Law lies in the following[10]:

Table 3: Changing disease status in Saudi Arabia over 5 years

Disease Group	ICD-10	2008		2009		2010		2011		2012	
		Cases	%	Cases	%	Cases	%	Cases	%	Cases	%
Ill-defined symptoms and conditions	(R00-R99)	13,452	28.8	13,693	30.9	14,622	31.6	13,640	30.5	14,610	29.8
Diseases of circulatory system	(100-199)	8403	18	7705	17.4	7748	16.7	8607	19.2	8924	18.2
Injury, poisoning, and external causes	(S00-Y89)	8761	18.8	8130	18.3	8355	18	7702	17.2	10,402	21.2
Conditions originating during the perinatal period	(P00-P96)	4486	9.6	3773	8.5	4190	9.1	3729	8.3	3317	6.8
Neoplasms	(C00-D48)	2254	4.8	2034	4.6	2198	4.7	2028	4.5	2307	4.7
Diseases of respiratory system	(J00-J99)	1854	4	2068	4.7	1892	4.1	1824	4.1	1951	4
Congenital anomalies	(Q00-Q99)	1216	2.6	1095	2.5	1233	2.7	1214	2.7	1199	2.4
Endocrine nutrition metabolic disorders	(E00-E90)	1021	2.2	1012	2.3	1140	2.5	1193	2.7	1086	2.2
Infectious and parasitic diseases	(A00-B99)	1624	3.5	1446	3.3	1533	3.3	1427	3.2	1613	3.3
Diseases of digestive system	(K00-K93)	996	2.1	853	1.9	892	1.9	833	1.9	984	2
Diseases of genitourinary system	(N00-N99)	1468	3.1	1437	3.2	1430	3.1	1559	3.5	1626	3.3
Diseases of nervous system	(G00-G99)	614	1.3	504	1.1	525	1.1	514	1.1	565	1.2
Diseases of skin and subcutaneous tissues	(L00-L99)	269	0.6	223	0.5	231	0.5	181	0.4	179	0.4
Diseases of blood and blood-forming organs	(D50-D89)	205	0.4	244	0.6	223	0.5	268	0.6	250	0.5
Diseases of musculoskeletal system	(M00-M99)	41	0.1	32	0.1	24	0.1	24	0.1	34	0.1
Complications of pregnancy, child birth, and puerperium	(O00-O99)	49	0.1	57	0.1	52	0.1	47	0.1	40	0.1
Mental and behavioral disorders	(F06.0)	7	0	2	0	4	0	3	0	16	0
Total		46,720	100	44,308	100	46,292	100	44,793	100	44,670	100

Source: MOH, 2012.[2]

Table 4: Chronology of Saudi healthcare reforms, 1999–2009

- It defines the mandates of the MOH in relation to ensuring universal coverage and the prevention of communicable diseases.
- It defines the primary healthcare center and its responsibilities, in both public and private sectors.
- It describes alternatives to healthcare funding including government funding, insurance fund endowments, and charities.
- It mandates selecting the most appropriate alternatives in health insurance.
- The law emphasizes the importance of coordination between healthcare institutions with regard to educational and training activities, in order to meet the needs of healthcare professionals.
- It addresses the importance of research in the field of health at a national level.

Date	Authority	Law
August 11, 1999	Royal Decree No. M/10	Cooperative Medical Insurance Law
August 11, 1999	Royal Decree No. M/10	Establishment of the Council of Cooperative Health Insurance
June 3, 2002	Royal Decree No. M/11	The Health Law
2002	Cabinet Ministers Resolution	Inclusion of Saudi Working in Private Sector in Cooperative Health Insurance
January 1, 2003	Amendments	Law of Private Healthcare Institutions
March 10, 2003	Cabinet Ministers Resolution	Law of Public Authority for Food and Medicine
September 9, 2003	Royal Decree No. M/32	Cooperative Insurance Companies Control Law
2004	Amendments	The Law of Pharmaceutical Establishment and Synthetic Preparations
January 15, 2004	Royal Decree No. M/76	Law of Fertility Units, Fetuses, and Sterility Treatment
December 20, 2005	Royal Decree No. M/59	Law of Practicing Health Professions
August 28, 2007	Royal Decree No. M/71	Law of the National Unified Procurement Company for Medical Supplies
February 5, 2008	Cabinet Ministers Resolution	Establishment of the Health Endowment Fund
June 5, 2009	Ministerial Decision No. DH/1/30/6131	Cooperative Health Insurance Policy (Amended)
January 6, 2009	Ministerial Decision No. DH/1/30/6131	Implementing Regulations of the Cooperative Health Insurance Law
August 1, 2009	Cabinet Ministers Resolution	Saudi Healthcare Strategy

Source: Alfadely, 2008.

- It defines Article 31 of the Constitution, which pertains to governmental responsibility to provide free healthcare to all citizens.
- The law emphasizes the goal of achieving universal coverage to improve access to healthcare and assure equality, focusing on the importance of creating a balanced regional distribution of healthcare centers.

Currently, the concept of the healthcare system includes several modern aspects, such as patient-centered services, medical research centers, specialized tertiary and quaternary centers and hospitals, the right to choose your provider, and the right to know about other therapeutic options (Table 5). The MOH published their strategic plan and made it available to the public, allowing patients to understand their rights clearly.[9] Only 15% of hospitals, all considered large hospitals, used a complete electronic medical record (EMR) system with no paper records, whereas 81% of hospitals used partial EMR, with some components still using paper charts.[11]

The existing Saudi healthcare system has several strengths. Overall spending on healthcare is reasonable and well financed by the government; access to the system is universal and relatively equitable; the population is young with high immunization rates; there is good access to clean water and sanitation; and an extensive infrastructure exists, with many tertiary care hospitals available.[4] However, major challenges to the Saudi healthcare system remain, including, but not limited to, the following[12]:

- There is a lack of integrated and comprehensive healthcare services resulting in inefficiency, duplication, and wastage.
- As there are different healthcare sectors (e.g., MOH, Ministry Of Defense Affairs, National Guard Health Affairs, and university affiliations), the system is faced with not only governance issues but also poor coordination between these sectors.
- Access to tertiary hospitals also becomes a problem, as there is partial inequality between personnel working in these sectors and other citizens. There is poor prioritization of care, based on needs (i.e., patients with cancer compete with elective patients for care in most hospitals).
- The primary healthcare system is underdeveloped, and there is a lack of support services such as nursing homes, homecare services, and physical therapy.

Table 5: Bed rates for the Saudi population

Regions	Population	Hospital Beds	Bed Rate (per 10,000 Population)
Riyadh	7,309,966	7473	10.2
Makkah	7,471,975	6933	9.3
Medinah	1,910,998	2647	13.9
Qaseem	1,303,623	2409	18.5
Eastern	4,414,278	5111	11.6
Aseer	2,045,070	2870	14.0
Tabouk	845,857	1125	13.3
Ha'il	638,699	1095	17.1
Northern	342,498	910	26.6
Jazan	1,460,540	1800	12.3
Najran	541,344	1070	19.3
Al-Bahah	439,927	1035	23.5
Al-Jouf	471,120	471,120	28.7
Total	29,195,895	35,828	12.3

Source: MOH, 2012.[2]

Table 6: Statistics for healthcare providers

Indicator	Rate (per 10,000 Population)	Year
Physicians	244	2012
Dentists	3.41	2012
Pharmacists	5.3	2012
Nurses	47.8	2012
Allied health professionals	26.3	2012
MOH primary healthcare centers	0.77	2012
Hospital beds (all sectors), Saudi Arabia	20.9	2012
MOH hospital beds	12.3	2012
Other governmental sector hospital beds	3.8	2012
Private hospital beds	4.8	2012

Source: MOH, 2012.[2]

3.1 Human resources

The rate at which medical services are delivered to all citizens has risen rapidly, with the MOH providing approximately 60% of the country's general healthcare services. The country's total population was approximately 28 million in 2012, with an annual growth rate of 2.4% and total health expenditure of $968 per capita. Total health expenditure as a percentage of the gross domestic product (GDP) is 4.3%. There were 22 hospital beds per 10,000 population in 2009. Furthermore, there were reportedly 1529 pharmacists and 24,802 physicians in the kingdom in 2008, with 5.3 and 24.4 per 10,000 population, respectively.[4] Rates for the MOH hospital were reportedly 0.66 pharmacists and 11.6 physicians per 10,000 population (Table 6). In 2012, the number of non-Saudi pharmacists in the country was estimated at 30,000; they were distributed throughout the country and had different specialties and varied experience (Figure 2). The head of the Saudi Food and Drug Authority (SFDA) drug section stated that, bearing the population growth rate in mind, a period of approximately 17 years is required to nationalize (via "Saudization") pharmacy jobs in the kingdom. The number of Saudi pharmacy students graduating each year is estimated to reach 1000 by 2015, with an expected annual growth rate of 7–10%.[13]

4. Medicine supply systems and drug use issues

The Saudi market is perhaps the largest in the region.[14] Public expenditure on pharmaceuticals represents 40% of the country's total expenditure, including government and private expenditure combined, on pharmaceuticals (Figure 3); this translates into a per capita public expenditure on pharmaceuticals of 200 SAR ($53). The Saudi pharmaceutical market was estimated to be worth USD 2.74 billion in 2007; this accounts for 10% of the country's total health expenditure, half of which represents the expenditure of the MOH. This figure

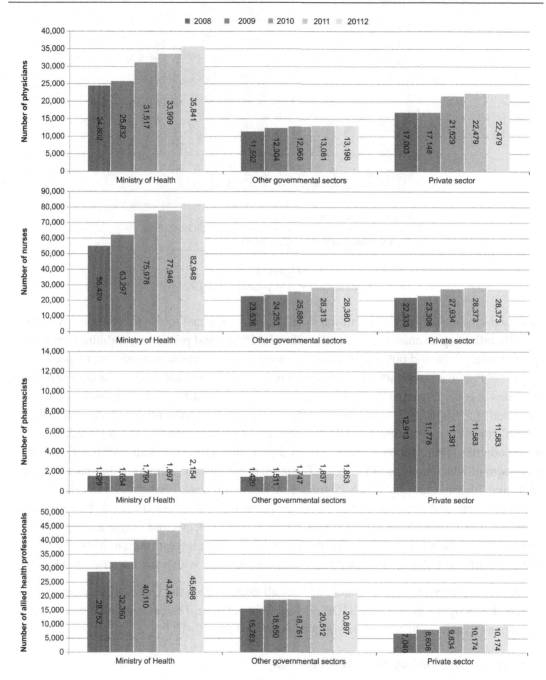

Figure 2
Distribution of total healthcare manpower in Saudi Arabia. *MOH (2012).*[2]

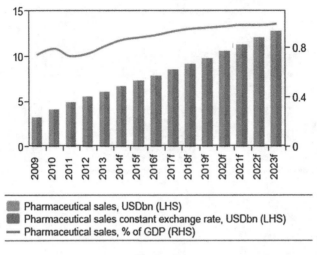

Figure 3
Pharmaceutical market growth. *BMI (2014).*[5]

increased substantially to USD 6 billion in 2013 and is expected to rise to 9 billion US dollars in 2018, reflecting an annual growth rate of 8.6%.[5] Public and private expenditure represents approximately 40% and 60% of the country's total pharmaceutical expenditure, respectively.[15,16] Public expenditure represents approximately $53 per capita. The Saudi pharmaceutical market is the largest in the Gulf Cooperation Council (GCC), and the growth rate was estimated at 5.9% in 2012. Local manufacturers account for approximately 16% of Saudi Arabia's total drug expenditure, while the majority of pharmaceuticals are imported from other countries. There are more than 27 local drug manufacturers in Saudi Arabia, the most prominent of which include SPIMACO, Tabuk Pharmaceuticals, Jamjoom Pharmaceuticals, Al-Jazirah Pharmaceuticals, SAJA Pharmaceuticals, and Riyadh Pharmaceuticals. The estimated value of the combined market for local manufacturers rose from 1.53 billion SAR in 2008 to 2.47 billion SAR in 2012. In 2008, there were 5700 registered drugs, and over-the-counter (OTC) sales reached up to 700 million SAR.[17,18] The largest foreign investor is GlaxoSmithKline (GSK), a British pharmaceutical company with a market share of 11%.[18]

Saudi Arabia purchases approximately 65% of all drugs sold in the Gulf region, with the market driven by the growth rate, GDP, and aging population. The best-selling medications according to value, volume, and groups are shown in Tables 7–10.[18]

4.1 Generic pharmaceuticals and drug pricing

Previously, prices for locally manufactured off-patent generic pharmaceutical products were 20% lower than those of the innovator's products once the patent period had expired. In contrast, prices of imported off-patent generic pharmaceutical products were 30% lower than those of the innovator's products. These pricing guidelines were regulated by the MOH to

Table 7: Top 10 therapeutic groups

Rank	Therapeutic Group	2012 Sales (USD)
1	Nonsteroidal anti-inflammatory drugs	171,566,692
2	Broad-spectrum penicillin	164,371,837
3	Cephalosporins	163,696,655
4	Proton pump inhibitors	144,940,661
5	Statins	121,560,445
6	Non-narcotic analgesics	80,117,849
7	Human insulin + analogues	79,164,989
8	Anticonvulsants	65,930,020
9	Erectile dysfunction	65,015,841
10	Antineoplastics	61,830,852

Table 8: Top 10 therapeutic groups according to volume

Rank	Therapeutic Group	2012 Sales (USD)
1	Non-narcotic analgesics	49,294,688
2	Nonsteroidal anti-inflammatory drugs	33,703,555
3	Expectorants	17,598,947
4	Broad-spectrum penicillins	17,393,249
5	Cephalosporins	15,642,423
6	Antihistamines	14,456,959
7	Topical corticosteroids	12,612,938
8	Cold preparations	10,152,407
9	Topical nasal preparations	9,294,028
10	Proton pump inhibitors	9,254,190

Table 9: Top 10 consumed brands according to value

Rank	Drug (Trade Name)	MAH**	2012 Sales (USD)
1	Lipitor	PFIZER	49,574,283
2	Augmentin	GLAXOSMITHKLINE	40,011,352
3	Klavox	SPIMACO	36,089,826
4	Nexium	ASTRAZENECA	30,158,885
5	Lyrica	PFIZER	27,357,955
6	Snafi	SPIMACO	27,320,365
7	Pantozol	ALTANA INDUSTRY	26,647,602
8	Lantus	AVENTIS	25,810,765
9	Cancidas	MERCK SHARP DOHME	24,977,351
10	Rofenac	SPIMACO	24,792,693

Table 10: Top 10 brands consumed according to volume

Rank	Drug (Trade Name)	MAH**	2012 Sales (USD)
1	Fevadol	SPIMACO	11,791,178
2	Dermovate	GLAXO SAUDI ARABIA	7,510,124
3	Panadol Extra	GLAXOSMITHKLINE	7,210,742
4	Neurobion	MERCK AG	4,875,072
5	Otrivin	NOVARTIS CONS HLTH	4,486,411
6	Mentex	Tabuk	4,348,825
7	Fevadol S.F.	SPIMACO	4,308,850
8	Rofenac	SPIMACO	4,235,587
9	Adol	Julphar	4,020,833
10	Sapofen	SPIMACO	3,868,092

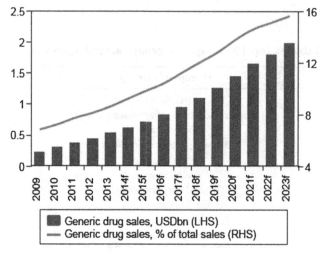

Figure 4
Generic drug market. *BMI (2014).*[5]

encourage local drug manufacturing. Generic drug manufacturing has increased significantly in 2013 and is projected to increase further by 2023 (Figure 4).[5]

Pharmaceutical prices in Saudi Arabia are currently established and regulated by the SFDA. New pricing guidelines entitled "Rules for Pricing Pharmaceutical Products" were recently implemented and are available on the SFDA Web site. The new guidelines are used by members of the Pharmaceutical Products Pricing Committee in determining drug prices. The SFDA is also able to conduct early drug pricing negotiations between companies.

November 2011 saw the implementation of new pricing guidelines that did not differentiate between national and international holders of marketing authorization with respect to pricing generic pharmaceutical products (Table 11). Based on these new guidelines, innovated product prices are reduced by 20% subsequent to registration of the first generic product. Moreover, new generic pricing schemes are applied as follows.

Table 11: New drug pricing by Saudi Food and Drug Authority

Product Order	Pricing Methodology
Innovated	The price of innovated product—20%
1st generic	The price of innovated product—35%
2nd generic	The price of 1st genetic product—10%
3rd generic	The price of 2nd genetic product—10%
4th generic	The price of 3rd genetic product—10%

Each following generic product registered will be given the same price such the price of the 4th generic product.

5. Overview of pharmacy practice and key pharmaceutical sectors

In 1997, the first residency program was established at the King Faisal Specialist Hospital and Research Center (KFSH&RC). The program subsequently evolved to become a 24-month postgraduate program with structured training in all aspects of clinical pharmacy and served as a national program under the umbrella of the Saudi Commission for Health Specialties (SCFHS).[19,20] Meanwhile, the establishment of the Scientific Board of Pharmacy, under the SCFHS, was another milestone for the pharmacy profession in the kingdom. In 2011, the postgraduate year-1 (PGY-1) residency program at KFSH&RC became the first program outside the United States to be accredited by the American Society of Health System Pharmacists (ASHPs). More programs sought the same accreditation at a later stage and became candidates.

The Saudi Pharmaceutical Society (SPS) was established in 1988 and became the only society representing pharmacists in Saudi Arabia. It now has more than 3000 members and is active in providing continuous education activities.

Pharmacy practice has evolved rapidly and now includes several special services and covers many areas throughout the kingdom. In 2012, a new vision of pharmacy practice was published by the MOH and aimed to improve clinical pharmacy and pharmaceutical care services and train personnel to reduce waste and prevent drug-related problems (DRPs). Several strategic directions have been developed to improve practices and include centralizing pharmaceutical care departments at the MOH level. This has allowed the main department to establish a number of specialized committees in several pharmaceutical domains, in order to strengthen the field. The department of pharmaceutical care at the MOH comprises four departments: the private, government, and clinical sectors, and the national drug and poison center. Each sector is further divided into several subsectors to cover the main objectives detailed in the published strategic plan for pharmaceutical care. The strategic 5-year plan has been designed with a focus on expanding pharmaceutical services and increasing personnel numbers throughout the country. Several new protocols have been established, formulated, and documented online for public and healthcare providers and involve seven domains: improving the main pharmaceutical care department, improving regional pharmaceutical care departments, improving pharmaceutical care departments in the general practitioners', improving clinical pharmacy services, improving general pharmaceutical care services, training personnel, and pharmacoeconomics. Furthermore, many newly established committees (2011–2014) include the following[21,22]:

1. Pharmaceutical technology and libraries
2. IV-admixture
3. Total quality
4. Quality assurance
5. Pharmaceutical care
6. Clinical pharmacy
7. Drug Information Center
8. Pharmacy and Hajj
9. Infectious diseases
10. Continuous pharmaceutical education
11. Pharmacy research
12. Pharmacoeconomics

Medications are provided free of charge for local residents at government and semi-government hospitals. Most private companies offer medical insurance that covers the main diseases but excludes highly priced medications such as cancer drugs and new targeted therapies. Insurance is mandatory for all expatriates but not for Saudi citizens. Some citizens prefer not to have medical insurance and therefore pay for medical treatment themselves. Accordingly, 69% of the population is covered by public health services, public health insurance, or other sickness funds and 31% is covered by private health insurance.[1]

5.1 Pharmacists' responsibilities and duties

Many hospitals provide certain pharmacy services with 24-h coverage. Some hospital pharmacies reported having an executive-level pharmacy position that meets the job profile of the Chief Pharmacy Officer or equivalent, regardless of the actual job title. The roles most closely associated with pharmacists are dispensing and on-site training, which are provided by almost all hospitals. Most military, university, and specialist hospitals have established policies and procedures for pharmacists to follow and practice. Other governmental hospitals lack such comprehensive policies, and some pharmacists work individually to establish clinical duties beyond their operational functions.

One of the main domains of practice is the identification and reporting of adverse drug events (ADEs), or pharmacovigilance duties. The vast majority of hospitals have an ADE reporting program and a medication safety committee consisting of a multidisciplinary team including physicians, pharmacists, and nurses. The duty of this committee is to review, analyze, inform, and create policies and corrective actions related to ADEs. Moreover, the number of duties involving patient counseling and review of discharge medications is increasing in Saudi hospitals. Within the past 3 years, several hospitals have implemented a variety of activities to promote medication therapy management (MTM) by pharmacists. Commonly reported activities include implementation of clinical pharmacy services, computerized prescriber order entry, recruitment of qualified clinical pharmacy staff, improvement of pharmacists' access to patient-specific data, implementation of decentralized pharmacy services, expansion of pharmacy technicians' responsibilities, and implementation of automated dispensing systems to free pharmacists from operational duties. Furthermore, the number of pharmacy-managed clinics is increasing, and they are gaining popularity. The pharmacist's role in each of these services varies significantly according to the type and size of the hospital.

6. Drug- and pharmacy-related regulations, policies, and ethics

The pharmacy profession and pharmaceuticals are regulated and controlled by various governmental agencies such as the SFDA, which regulates pharmaceuticals, medical supplies, and medical devices; the SCFHS, which regulates health-related training and licenses healthcare providers; and the MOH, which provides healthcare coverage to approximately 60% of Saudi citizens. Healthcare for the remaining 40% of Saudi citizens is provided by various healthcare sectors including the Ministry of Defense, Ministry of the Interior, National Guard, university hospitals, specialty hospitals, and the private sector. The SCFHS is also responsible for licensing, registration, and accreditation services provided to all health personnel, including pharmacists. In government schools, graduates are registered immediately subsequent to graduation without being subjected to further assessment. Conversely, private school graduates are required to complete a registration examination. However, this is subject to change in the near future, when all graduates will complete registration examinations regardless of the type of school they graduate from. Upon licensing, pharmacists can be classified into three main categories: pharmacist, pharmacist I, or consultant pharmacist. A master's or Doctor of Pharmacy (PharmD) degree with experience of at least 3 years is required for classification as a pharmacist I. Classification as a consultant pharmacist requires a PhD or PharmD, with a 1-year residency program or completion of a specialty 3-year residency program, in addition to 3 years' experience following completion of the degree program. Furthermore, pharmacists with qualifications obtained outside the kingdom must undergo a certification process at the SCFHS, and certificates must be stamped by the Saudi cultural attaché in the granting country.[23]

The national medicine policy has been in existence in Saudi Arabia for some time and was updated in 2004. The implementation plan was updated in 2005, and the SFDA was established by royal decree in 2004. Prior to this, the regulation of medication was controlled by the MOH. Drug registration and related departments were transferred to the SFDA. Currently, all medication-related national policies are implemented, monitored, and assessed by the SFDA and updated

Table 12: National medicine policies (SFAD)

Aspect of Policy	Covered
Selection of essential medicines	Yes
Medicines financing	Yes
Medicines pricing	Yes
Medicines procurement	Yes
Medicines distribution	Yes
Medicines regulation	Yes
Pharmacovigilance	Yes
Rational use of medicines	Yes
Human resource development	Yes
Research	Yes
Monitoring and evaluation	Yes
Traditional medicine	Yes

Table 13: Functions of the NMR (National Medicine Regulatory) as part of the SFDA

Functions	Covered
Marketing authorization/registration	Yes
Inspection	Yes
Import control	Yes
Market control	Yes
Medicine advertising and promotion	Yes
Pharmacovigilance	Yes
Licensing	Yes
Quality control	Yes
Clinical trials control	Yes
Other: health and herbal products, cosmetic products	Yes

regularly. The SFDA is also responsible for the governance of all pharmaceutical-related activities including product registration, manufacturing, and post-marketing issues (Tables 12 and 13).[15]

Accordingly, the SFDA is the authoritative body responsible for the medication market and manages manufacturing, registration, pricing, safety, and efficacy. In addition, the SFDA is responsible for wholesalers, private manufacturers, retail distributors, public pharmacies, medication import and export, medication testing and stores, and related activities. The only exception to this is retail pharmacies, which are still under the governance of the MOH.

7. Core pharmacy practices

7.1 Industrial pharmacy

The provision of patents for medications in Saudi Arabia is regulated by the King Abdulaziz City for Sciences and Technology.[26] Saudi Arabia is currently compliant with the

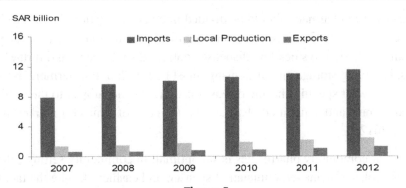

Figure 5
Estimates for medication import and export. *NCB (2012).*

trade-related aspects of the Intellectual Property Rights Agreement, which is a requirement of the World Trade Organization and further to the Gulf Consolidated Contractors. This makes the manufacturing market attractive to international investors.[14] There are currently 19 licensed and Good Manufacturing Practices (GMPs) certified pharmaceutical manufacturers in the kingdom, with no innovative research and development arms. Most of the manufacturers, work on formulating and packaging raw materials into finished products (Figure 5).

In some situations, repackaging and reproduction take place according to specific quality requirements established for original products.[16] Furthermore, there are currently four multinational manufacturers with established local manufacturing facilities in Saudi Arabia.

Domestic manufacturers hold 20% of the value share of the medication used in the kingdom.[20] Barriers to entering the markets may include the following[14]:

1. Price control by the SFDA
2. Competition with other generic manufacturers, without coordinating with legislators
3. GCC regulations
4. Registration requirements set by the SFDA

7.2 Community pharmacy practice

Community pharmacy is regulated solely by the Saudi MOH. Herbal medications and food supplements are sold in community pharmacies and subject to regulations similar to those governing medications, with some differences in the registration process. The law in Saudi Arabia has changed several times with regard to who is permitted to own a community pharmacy. Currently, only Saudi pharmacists can own and manage community pharmacies, but they cannot manage more than one. As the number of Saudi pharmacists remains low, most community pharmacists are non-Saudi. The regulations allow non-pharmacists to partner with Saudi pharmacists in establishing community pharmacies, but the manager must be a pharmacist. It also stipulates that the owner or one of the partners must be a licensed

Saudi pharmacist. The pharmacy should be divided into several sections: OTC products, cosmetics, prescription medications, and pharmaceutical preparation. The pharmacy should request special permission to stock and dispense controlled substances, and further security requirements, involving storage and dispensing, must be fulfilled. Furthermore, providing pharmaceutical care for specific chronic diseases is optional and subject to the availability of specialized equipment and a qualified pharmacists.[27] A code of ethics for marketing has been available since 2012.

The monitoring of community pharmacies is suboptimal. In community settings, the pharmacist assumes the roles of manager, clinician, dispenser, and cashier, despite the fact that he or she may not be well trained in most of these activities. Research has shown that most community pharmacists in the kingdom lack the necessary training and clinical skills. Importantly, there are substantial gaps between education and community pharmacy and community pharmacists' skills and continuous pharmaceutical education.[27,28]

Pharmacy practice in community settings has become a major issue in Saudi Arabia. The current law prohibits dispensing medications, other than those available over the counter, without a prescription. However, many pharmacies continue to dispense prescription drugs, including antibiotics, medication for chronic diseases, erectile dysfunction medication, and oral contraceptives, without prescriptions, and the only medications that are strictly regulated are controlled substances. The occurrence of this practice is primarily due to a lack of regulation enforcement by the MOH and its Directorate of Health, which attributes this issue to a lack of sufficient manpower. In large metropolitan cities, such as Riyadh, a maximum of 10 health directorate inspectors are responsible for several 1000 community pharmacies. Several practitioners and health advocates have called attention to this problem and the need for practical solutions.[29]

7.3 Hospital pharmacy

Hospital pharmacists work in hospital pharmacy services belong to the MOH as well as the private sector. Pharmacists work in this field are responsible for dispensing of medications, quality testing, formulating and re-formulating dosage forms, monitoring and reporting drug safety, and preparing budges for medications. They are also responsible for medication storage and planning for medication quantities for their hospitals. Some hospitals also have a drug reviewing committee and pharmacoeconomic unit for approval of new medications and optimizing their utilization. The specialized and university hospitals have pharmacy-managed clinics for some specialized areas, depending on the specialty of pharmacists they have. Therefore, typical day of hospital pharmacists may include the following activities:

- Managing pharmacy-related services and logistics 24/7
- Prescribing medications and ensuring their safety and efficacy
- Preparing all the medications and converting dosage forms to the applicable situation

- Reporting all the potential DRPs to the SFDA
- Contacting all healthcare provider for medication-related issues
- Participating in clinical rounds run by all healthcare providers and attending pharmacy-managed clinics
- Providing adequate statistics on medication consumptions
- Managing medication stores and planning for medication budgets
- Providing drug information services
- Conducting pharmacy-related training for under- and postgraduates
- Supervising pharmacy-related research activities

7.4 Medication promotion and marketing

The Saudi FDA represented by its pharmaceutical product advertising section/licensing department is responsible for setting the regulations for drug promotion and advertising. Under the existing regulations, no direct advertising of prescription medication is permitted. Pre-approval of advertising materials of non-prescription medications is required. The SFDA published also a national code of conduct regarding advertising and promoting medications by market authorization holders. This applied for both domestic and national manufacturers and adherence is mandatory. The code of conduct explains in details the formal process of complaints and penalties.[15]

8. Special pharmacy-related services

Several forms of specialized pharmaceutical service are provided by the kingdom's tertiary and secondary care hospitals, but access to these services is usually limited. Most tertiary hospitals provide a wide range of specialized services; however, some of these services are not available in regional or district hospitals in other regions of the kingdom. One of the well-developed specialized forms of MTM provided by pharmacists is that of anticoagulation clinics in ambulatory care settings. The role of pharmacists in these clinics varies significantly according to the type of hospital involved. Most hospitals allow pharmacists to adjust dosage, change medication, or add other anticoagulants, and some pharmacists have effective roles in monitoring anticoagulants for inpatient services. There are several other types of pharmacy-run clinic, such as cardiology, HIV, solid organ transplant, pain, oncology, and ambulatory care clinics, which are involved less frequently. The role of the pharmacist in these clinics is to ensure optimal MTM using a safe and cost-effective approach. These clinics are run by consultant clinical pharmacists who completed their education and postgraduate training in the USA, Europe, or other developed countries.

The MOH is currently advancing in many directions with respect to establishing specialized pharmacy-managed clinics. This concept is still very new to the MOH, and achieving adequacy in the required fields takes a relatively long time. The new directions of the MOH include focused training in collaboration with a number of international agencies and societies such as pain management clinics, anticoagulation clinics, infectious disease services, pharmacoeconomic units, drug information services, and pharmacy administration. Most of these services are in progress and take a long time to establish.[24,25]

The SCFHS has expanded its clinical pharmacy residency training programs to cover a number of specialized services according to the needs of the kingdom. The residency is a structured clinical training program that lasts from 2 to 3 years for each general or specialty area.[23]

8.1 Public health practice and health promotion

There are clear published guidelines concerning how marketing authorization holders advertise and promote OTC medications. Prescription medications cannot be advertised or promoted publicly, as per the National Code of Ethics.[15]

Health promotion conducted by pharmacists is not reflected in any national guidelines. However, hospital pharmacists, and to some extent, community pharmacists, continue to participate in national and international disease awareness days such as Diabetes Day, Parkinson's Day, Disability Day, Cardiac Diseases Day, Cancer Day, Rheumatoid Day, Anticoagulation Day, and many other such occasions shared by health practitioners worldwide. The participation mainly translates into health campaigns offered to the public in shopping malls or hospitals. Educational materials are distributed to patients and include brochures, booklets, and pamphlets. The majority of the participants are school students who are supervised by senior or consultant pharmacists.

There are growing numbers of pharmaceutical conferences and training courses conducted several times a year in different healthcare sectors. Some are general conferences, while others are specific workshops or training courses. Several other conferences are held by the SPS to support clinical pharmacy, pharmacotherapy, and pharmacy practice throughout the kingdom.

8.2 Pharmacy practice-related research

Practice-related pharmacy research is growing rapidly in Saudi Arabia due to increased awareness of the importance of research and the ever-increasing number of pharmacy colleges. The only peer-reviewed pharmaceutical journal in Saudi Arabia is the Saudi Pharmaceutical Journal (SPJ; impact factor 0.9 in 2013), which is published by the SPS.[30] Two other journals are currently inactive and do not include peer review. There are no official statistics on pharmacy-related papers in Saudi Arabia. Original research ranges from simple descriptive, social-pharmaceutical, or behavioral studies to advanced biopharmaceutics, pharmacogenetics, pharmacokinetics, and nanopharmaceutics. To date, there are three approved bioequivalence centers in the country and very few phase 2 or 3 multicenter trials in which clinical pharmacists are co-investigators.

Several pharmacists publish in peer-reviewed journals. In academia, faculty members are typically required to publish a certain number of papers, including original research articles and reviews, to achieve promotion. Each pharmacy school has a pharmacy practice or clinical pharmacy department. Many clinical and hospital pharmacists, particularly in tertiary care hospitals, publish their pharmacy practice work. This has supported publication and research in the domain of pharmaceutical care across the country. Furthermore, students' projects usually focus on evaluating current practices and include perception, satisfaction, and actual practices in the community or hospitals.

8.3 Clinical pharmacy services

Clinical pharmacy in hospitals started in Saudi Arabia in the mid-1970s, when clinical pharmacists from the United States introduced the concept of clinical pharmacy by establishing clinical services, such as pharmacokinetics, parenteral nutrition, and drug information services, at KFSH&RC in Riyadh. It evolved later as more Saudi clinical pharmacists completed their PharmD education and residency training in the United States. Currently, clinical pharmacy is well developed in tertiary care hospitals and to a lesser extent in MOH hospitals. Many specialized clinical services are available in Saudi Arabia including but not limited to general surgery, ambulatory care, solid organ transplantation, pediatric and adult oncology and hematology, nephrology, pediatrics, infectious disease, internal medicine, adult surgical/medical ICU, neonatology/pediatric ICU, cardiology, parenteral nutrition, pain management, therapeutic drug monitoring, drug information, anticoagulation services, and investigational drugs services. Currently, there are more than 130 clinical pharmacists in Saudi Arabia who are board certified from the Board of Pharmacy Specialties (BPS) (http://www.bpsweb.org) which is the highest number in the Arab world. With the introduction of the specialized residency training in 2013 by the SCFHS in 2013, the number of clinical pharmacists in Saudi Arabia is expected to grow rapidly. Many Saudi pharmacists are also being educated in the US who will come back and work as clinical pharmacists in the near future.

9. Pharmacy education

The college of pharmacy at King Saud University, established in 1959, was the first school of pharmacy in Saudi Arabia and the Gulf region. There were 17 students enrolled in the first year. Forty-five years passed before the second school of pharmacy was established at the King Abdulaziz University in Jeddah, where the first PharmD program began in the Gulf region.[31] Between 2004 and 2012, the total number of pharmacy colleges reached 17; the majority of these are governmental, and 11 offer a PharmD degree. By the end of 2012, the first cohort of students from only two of these colleges had completed the program.[13,32] In 2014, the number of pharmacy schools with similar academic programs and syllabi had increased to 26, indicating an urgent need for reconsideration of the contents and programs details.[32] Only eight private schools are considered to provide pharmacy education by the Saudi Ministry of Higher Education; of these, only three provide PharmD programs, and one offers a master's qualification in clinical pharmacy. There is a trend toward establishing PharmD programs rather than traditional Bachelor of Pharmacy degrees. Some colleges, such as King Saud University, offer a bachelor's degree in pharmacy with progression to a PharmD program according to specific acceptance criteria.

Most pharmacy schools have similar departmental structures, which usually include pharmaceutics, pharmacognosy and pharmaceutical chemistry, pharmacology, and pharmacy practice or clinical pharmacy departments. Most schools offer internships toward the end of the program, which are usually a year in duration. The schools share similar evaluation systems, which include short assays, multiple-choice questions, and laboratory assessment. In addition, graduation research projects in most schools include oral presentations and short reports.[31,33]

One of the major issues in education is that most school curricula are similar in structure and replicate each other, with PharmD degree courses lasting approximately 6 years. There are no significant differences between programs that offer PharmD and bachelor's degree programs with respect to clinical orientation or general content.

Some new pharmacy schools have attempted to implement newer and more innovative teaching systems. An example of this is the system adopted by the pharmacy school at Qassim University. The school uses team-based learning (TBL), which is considered one of the most advanced educational technology approaches in the health sciences. The school has been a member of the international TBL group since early 2011 and has been applying this system since then. A few publications regarding this issue have been produced by the school, demonstrating the superior impact of TBL relative to traditional systems. This technique empowers students' thinking and collaboration as key factors for success in such courses. TBL is used in core modules, including those offered during the basic sciences and pre-pharmacy years, and therapeutic modules in the professional PharmD, program. The school approach has changed and is now inclined toward the block-wise system, in which blocks are named according to function, body system, or disease state. For example, in therapeutics, such as cardiology or hematology pharmacotherapy, each student is allowed sufficient time to cover the main topics. The theme for each week involves a particular disease, such as hypertension or anemia, and all of the related pharmaceutical topics are covered.[33,34]

10. Achievements in pharmacy practice

Pharmaceutical services in Saudi Arabia have changed dramatically in recent years. The general trend has shifted from that of merely distributive pharmaceutical services to customized clinical and specialized pharmaceutical care.

Routine bedside clinical pharmacy services and specialized pharmacy-managed clinics, including military, university, and specialist hospitals and some MOH hospitals, are present in several major hospitals in the kingdom. Pharmacy-managed clinics include, but are not limited to, anticoagulation, post-transplantation, MTM, and diabetes clinics. Notably, these clinics have served as a major playground for pharmacists worldwide, and a substantial contribution to patient care is made by pharmacists on a global scale. Pharmacists identify and resolve actual and potential DRPs including those involving dosage, inappropriate medications, and safety and efficacy monitoring. Some clinical pharmacists enjoy prescribing privileges within their healthcare institutions. Practice site settings include inpatient and outpatient clinics. Many hospitals have endorsed the role played by clinical pharmacists inpatient care rounds and recognized that they should be involved in the decision-making process regarding patient care.

A growing trend in Saudi Arabia is that of the establishment of several pharmacy-related conferences and meetings including new trends in pharmacy education, pharmacoeconomic conferences, SPS meetings, and medication safety meetings. Increasing interest has been observed in recent years, and the number of attendees has also increased. Other regular workshops, meetings, and journal clubs are held in each institution on a regular basis and involve a wide variety of clinical activities and community-orientation tasks.

Clinical pharmacy research has also undergone steady growth. Many researchers have evaluated clinical pharmacy services, DRPs, national guidelines, patterns of prescribing medications, common medication problems, and evidence-based clinical services. Pharmacoeconomic and pharmacogenetics research centers have recently been established in order to contribute to the field and decision-making processes.[35] PharmD students also conduct practice-related pharmacy research that contributes to the field significantly. The number of graduates in Saudi Arabia is increasing; therefore, the number of clinical pharmacy students is also expected to increase. Moreover, some institutions have entered into contracts with well-recognized international institutes, collaborating in research and academic activities. The King Saud School of Pharmacy has established a research chair in medication safety.

11. Challenges in pharmacy practice

Each profession should endeavor to meet the challenges and difficulties that lie ahead. Nonetheless, the majority of pharmacists share the same challenges and expectations worldwide. Although the pharmacy profession has evolved significantly in Saudi Arabia, many challenges remain.[36]

Pharmacists are classified into government hospital, non-government hospital, community and retail, and university pharmacists and those employed by drug companies in different roles. Relative to the private sector, more hospital pharmacists are employed by the government; they also have greater clinical responsibility and make greater contributions to patient care. Each group of hospital pharmacists has different roles, commitments, responsibilities, and recognition.

The registration and classification processes of the SCFHS have also constituted a challenge. Since the introduction of a unified pay scale for use in all government hospitals, classification has been extremely important to practicing pharmacists, because it determines their salary levels within the pay scale. This has resulted in heavy criticism of the current classification system, as it does not take all different types of pharmacy education and training into consideration.

One of the most important challenges in Saudi Arabia is the continuous need for well-trained clinical pharmacists, who are required to run core clinical pharmacy services and provide training sites for students and residents in most major areas. Nationwide numbers of qualified faculty members and practitioners are small, and faculty members are not distributed evenly. In addition, recruitment of qualified clinical pharmacists from abroad has been a major challenge for academic health institutions and large hospitals. The worldwide scarcity of pharmacists has created a competitive market in which the package and benefits are always negotiable. The limited salaries offered by universities, relative to those provided by hospitals, have also been an issue. Finding good clinical pharmacists who would accept a relatively modest salary and competing with large health institutions, particularly those of a military nature, is very difficult.

Quality of teaching and students' perceptions were significantly affected by this particular issue. Unfortunately, due to the scarcity of clinicians, nonclinical pharmacists teach clinical therapeutics and other clinical topics in many academic institutions. There has been tendency toward recruiting physicians with higher education backgrounds in clinical pharmacology to teach therapeutics, just to meet the requirements of the education process using the best available resources. Therefore, the low number of qualified clinical pharmacists affects pharmaceutical practice as well as educational outcomes.

Although the MOH attempts to proceed with newly designed strategies that include pharmacists, limited representation of expert pharmacists in MOH committees continues to be an obstacle. Many committees have been established without the presence of practicing pharmacists, and the outcomes of these committees have been somewhat disappointing. Centralization and bureaucracy could be major contributing factors to less effective and efficient pharmacy practice in MOH hospitals.

12. Recommendations: the way forward

The pharmacy profession in Saudi Arabia is very promising and has the potential for optimization at an international level. However, there are some considerations that should be borne in mind in future:

1. Harmonization of professional standards of practice is necessary and should be performed promptly and systematically.
2. Appropriate distribution of pharmacists throughout MOH hospitals and other healthcare sectors should also be considered.

3. Pharmacy education in Saudi Arabia is currently a matter of great interest and requires standardization of curricula to meet the best available standards.
4. Collaborative work between all stakeholders to optimize pharmacy practice is of paramount importance.
5. Develop clear accreditation, registration, and classification standards and processes, with set criteria and standards nationwide.

13. Conclusions

The pharmacy profession in Saudi Arabia is evolving. There have been extensive changes and numerous challenges in the field since the late 1950s. Further development and optimization are obviously anticipated, and pharmaceutical services are expected to improve dramatically in the near future.

14. Lessons learned/points to remember

- Pharmacy profession requires a clear vision, mission and a well-designed strategy that combined all the attributes.
- Existence of multi-authority will disrupt the pharmaceutical services and create a great variability in practice.
- Education and research should be based on pharmacy practices in the kingdom and should not be separated alone.

References

1. Central Department of Statistics and Information (CDSI). *Health statistics*. Available at: http://www.cdsi.gov.sa/english/index.php?option=com_docman&task=cat_view&gid=189&Itemid=113; 2014 [accessed February 2014].
2. Ministry of Health, Saudi Arabia (MOH). *Health statistics book*. Saudi Arabia: Ministry of Health. Available at: http://www.moh.gov.sa/en/Ministry/Statistics/book/Pages/default.aspx; 2012 [accessed June 2014].
3. Yezli S, Memish ZA. Tuberculosis in Saudi Arabia: prevalence and antimicrobial resistance. *J Chemother* 2012;**24**(1):1–5.
4. World Health Organization (WHO). *Eastern midstream region, Saudi Arabia: statistics summary 2003*. Available at: http://apps.who.int/gho/data/node.country.country-SAU; [accessed January 2014].
5. Business Monitor International (BMI). *Q2 Saudi Arabia pharmaceuticals & healthcare report: includes 10-year forecasts to 2023*. Business Monitor International. ISSN:1748-2143. Available at: www.businessmonitor.com; 2014.
6. Almalki JS, Al-Jaser MH, Warsy AS. Overweight and obesity in Saudi females of childbearing age. *Int J Obes* 2003;**27**:134–9.
7. Kumosani TA, Alama MN, Lyer A. Cardiovascular diseases in Saudi Arabia. *Prime Res Med (PROM)* 2011;**1**(x):01–6. Available at: http://www.primejournal.org/PROM/abstracts/2011/May/Taha%20et%20al.htm. [accessed December 2012].
8. Alamoudi OS, Attar SM. Pattern of common diseases in hospitalized patients at a university hospital in Saudi Arabia: a study of 5594 patients. *J King Abdulaziz Univ Med Sci* 2009;**16**(4):3–12. http://dx.doi.org/10.4197/Med.16-4.1.
9. Ministry of Health Saudi Arabia (MOH). About the Ministry. Available at: http://www.moh.gov.sa/en/Ministry/About/Pages/default.aspx; 2009 [accessed June 2014].

10. Almalki M, Fitzegrald G. Health care system in Saudi Arabia: an overview. *East Mediterr Health J La Revue de Santé de la Méditerranée Orientale* 2011:784. Available at: http://applications.emro.who.int/emhj/V17/10/17_10_2011_0784_0793.pdf. [accessed November 2013].

11. Alsultan MS, Khurshid F, Mayet AY, Al-Jedai AH. Hospital pharmacy practice in Saudi Arabia: dispensing and administration in the Riyadh region. *Saudi Pharm J* 2012. http://dx.doi.org/10.1016/j.jsps.2012.05.003. Available at: http://www.sciencedirect.com/science/article/pii/S1319016412000369. [accessed February 2014].

12. Alfadley F. *Analysis of healthcare expenditure and financing in Saudi Arabia: what are the alternatives for funding healthcare in Saudi Arabia* [Master thesis]. Frankfurt (Germany): Business School of Finance and Management; 2008.

13. Bawazir S. *Number of Saudi pharmacists reaches 30,000 and 15 years is required for full Saudization.* Head of the SFDA. Alriyadh Newspaper. Available at: http://www.alriyadh.com/707880; February 7, 2012 [accessed June 2014].

14. Esquire NA, Al-Ammar MI, Esquire SM. *Healthcare and pharmaceutical industries in Saudi Arabia.* International Healthcare Affinity Group of the Business Law and Governance Practice Group. Available at: http://www.kslaw.com/Library/publication/11-09%20AHLA%20Issa,%20Al-Ammar,%20Mostafa.pdf; 2011 [accessed February 2014].

15. Saudi Food & Drug Authority (SFDA). *Pharmaceutical country profile.* Available at: http://www.who.int/medicines/areas/coordination/Saudi_ArabiaPSCP_Narrative2012-04-18_Final.pdf; 2012 [accessed February 2014].

16. Business Monitor International (MBI). *BMI Saudi Arabia pharmaceuticals & healthcare report.* Available at: http://www.businessmonitor.com; 2014 [accessed October 2014].

17. Alshaikh SA, Kotilaine J, ElZayat T, Alwazir A, Chahine P, Alrshan A, et al. The Saudi pharmaceutical sector 2011. *Infocus Rev.* Available at: http://www.qomel.com/The%20Saudi%20Pharmaceutical%20Sector%202011.pdf; 2011 [accessed February 2014].

18. Taylor L. *Saudi pharmacy market set to grow 6% annually 2011–2012.* World News. Available at: http://www.pharmatimes.com/article/11-0131/Saudi_pharma_market_set_to_grow_6_annually_in_2011-12.aspx; January 31, 2011 [accessed February 2014].

19. Qadheeb NS, Alissa DA, Al-Jedai AH, Ajlan A, Al-Jazairi AS. The first international residency program accredited by the American Society of Health-System Pharmacists. *Am J Pharm Educ* 2012;**76**(10):190.

20. Alsultan MS, Khurshid F, Mayet AY, Al-Jedai AH. *Hospital pharmacy practice in Saudi Arabia: drug monitoring and patient education in the Riyadh region.* Available at: http://www.ncbi.nlm.nih.gov/pmc/articles/PMC3824953/; 2013 [accessed February 2014].

21. Alomi. Pharmaceutical Care Department, Ministry of Health. Available at: http://www.moh.gov.sa/depts/Pharmacy/Pages/home.aspx; 2014 [accessed February 2014].

22. Saudi Commission for Health Specialties (SCFHS). *CME and accreditation portal.* Available at: http://www.scfhs.org.sa/en/CME-ADRP/Statistics/Pages/default.aspx; 2014 [accessed February 2014].

23. King Abdulaziz City for Science and Technology (KACST). *Kingdom of Saudi Arabia.* Available at: http://www.kacst.edu.sa; [accessed February 2014].

24. Saudi Food & Drug Authority (SFDA). SFDA Regulation (2007) Institutions and Pharmaceutical Products Guidelines. Available at: http://www.sfda.gov.sa/ar/drug/drug_reg/DocLib/ExecutiverolesforInstitutionsandPharmaceuticalProductslaw.pdf; 2007 [accessed February 2014].

25. Al-Hassan M. Community pharmacy practice in Saudi Arabia: an overview. *Internet J Pharmacol* 2009;**9**(1). Available at: http://ispub.com/IJPHARM/9/1/5301.

26. Al-Arifi MN. The managerial role of pharmacist at community pharmacy setting in Saudi Arabia. *Pharmacol Pharm* 2013;**4**:63–70. Published Online January 2013. Available at: http://dx.doi.org/10.4236/pp.2013.41009. [accessed February 2014].

27. Haifa. *The Saudi top ten medications include antibiotics, antidepressants, and sexual medications.* Mekkah Newspaper. Available at: http://www.makkahnewspaper.com/makkahNews/societyhuman/26373/26373#.U8v4 tJR_sS4; 2014 [accessed February 2014].

28. Al-Wazaify M, Matowe L, Albsoul-Younes A, Al-Omran OA. Pharmacy education in Jordan, Saudi Arabia, and Kuwait. *Am J Pharm Educ* 2006;**70**(1):18. PMC1636892. Available at: http://www.ncbi.nlm.nih.gov/pmc /articles/PMC1636892/. [accessed February 2014].
29. Alhujairi Y. *Pharmacy sector faces a huge lack of well-trained Saudi pharmacists*. Alyaum Newspaper. Available at: http://www.alyaum.com/article/3056990; 2012. [accessed November 2012].
30. Saudi Pharmaceutical Journal. Production and hosting by Elsevier B.V. on behalf of King Saud University. Peer review under the responsibility of King Saud University. Available at: http://www.journals.elsevier.com/ saudi-pharmaceutical-journal/; 2004 [accessed February 2014].
31. Albukairi A. *Twenty-six unrecognized pharmacy schools in the kingdom*. Alshareq Newspaper. Available at: http://www.alsharq.net.sa/2013/02/28/744000; 2013 [accessed January 2014].
32. Asiri YA. Emerging frontiers of pharmacy education in Saudi Arabia: the metamorphosis in the last fifty years. 2011 http://dx.doi.org/10.1016/j.jsps.2010.10.006. Available at: http://www.sciencedirect.com/science/ article/pii/S1319016410000964; [accessed February 2014].
33. Almeman AA, Al-Worafi Y, Saleh M, Alorainy M. Perception of Pharm D students towards team-based learning methods in College of Pharmacy, Qassim University. In: *Team-based learning Collaborative 12th annual TBLC conference February 28–March 2, 2013*. California (USA): San Diego Marriott Mission Valley San Diego.
34. Almeman AA, Al-Worafi Y, Saleh M. Team-based learning (TBL) as a new learning strategy in pharmacy college, Saudi Arabia: student's perception. *Univers J Pharm* 2004;**3**(3):57–65. Available at: http://ujponline.com/wp-content/uploads/2013/03/10-UJP-14375-Rs.pdf. [accessed June 2014].
35. Alsaggabi A. Pros and cons of pricing and reimbursement: Saudi Arabia health care system. President of ISPOR Chapter, KSA. In: *Power point presentation, ISPOR 1st conference Saudi Arabia, Riyadh*. 2013.
36. Albejaidi FM. Health care system in Saudi Arabia: an analysis of structure, total quality management and future challenges. *J Altern Perspect Soc Sci* 2010;**2**(2):794–818. Available at: http://www.japss.org/upload/16. Fahd[1].pdf. [accessed June 2013].

CHAPTER 10

Pharmacy Practice in Iraq

Inas Rifaat Ibrahim, Abdul Rasoul Wayyes

Chapter Outline

1. Introduction

1.1 Country background

Iraq is the eastern gate of the Arab world, with a population of 34 million.[1] Ancient Iraq was known as Mesopotamia (Babylonian and Sumerian empires) and featured early records of medical texts and drug therapy on cuneiform clay tablets in the 6th millennium BC.[2] Some of these remedies are still in use in today's pharmacopeia.[3] The country is rich in petroleum and natural resources. Two famous rivers, the Tigris and the Euphrates, flow from the north of its area to the south embracing a fertile land that is suitable for agriculture and settlement. Iraq is divided into 18 governorates, and more than 26% of the population lives in the capital city Baghdad. The official language is Arabic, and in addition, the Kurdish language is spoken by the Kurdish community in the northern governorates. The majority of Iraqis are Muslims. Further demographic characteristics are presented in Table 1.

An astounding development was seen in the economic and health status of Iraq during the early 1950s. Then it suffered three periods of decline, the Iraq–Iran War (1981–1988), the Gulf War (1991–1998), and the U.S.-led invasion (2003–2011).[4,5] The whole country has been subjected to an immense shortage of human resources; people were banned from traveling outside the country as well as from using advanced technology in communications.[6,7] With the U.S. invasion in 2003, the infrastructures of Iraq were destroyed. Collapse in security, deadly sectarian violence, and killing and kidnapping of scientific personnel resulted in the escape of more than 3 million Iraqis to other countries.[8] The country today is facing many challenges left by the wars and U.S. invasion.

1.2 Health sector and system

The first health unit in Iraq was established in 1905 and managed by a physician and health inspector. In 1914, a public health management office was founded, which was renamed later the Public Health Directorate. This was changed to the Ministry of Health (MOH) during the establishment of the Kingdom of Iraq in September 1921. Between the 1950s and the early 1980s a sophisticated health system was seen in Iraq.[9,10] Health care and treatment services were and still are offered free of charge to the population through the facilities of the MOH, the major provider and regulator of health service. These facilities include public hospitals, primary health care

Table 1: Sociodemographic characteristics of Iraq

Indicator	Category	Value
Urban area	–	67.5%
Literacy	–	74.1%
Ethnic groups[a]	Arab	75–80%
	Kurdish	15–20%
	Turkoman, Assyrian, and others	5%
Age structure[b]	0–14 years	38%
	15–64 years	58.9%
	65+ years	3.1%
Median age	–	21.1 years
Sex ratio (males/100 females)	–	104
Crude birth rate/1000 of the population	–	38.1
Annual population growth rate	–	3.4
Dependency ratio	–	75
Health expenditure	–	9.7% of GDP
Average temperature	July–August	>48°
	January	<0°

[a]The Kurdish community has formed recently an autonomous region of its own.
[b]About 68.8% of the population today is under the age of 30 years.

centers, and preventive and curative activities (MOH facilities are presented in Table 2). All these facilities are supervised by directorates of health, which are distributed throughout the 18 governorates (each governorate has one directorate, except Baghdad, which has three directorates of health).[11] Yet, the country does not possess social or private insurance organizations.

Until 2003, health services reached about 97% of the urban and 79% of the rural society. Owing to the imposed embargo by the United Nations in 1991–2003, the Iraqi health system was influenced greatly by the limited budget allocation. Per capita spending on health was reduced by 90%.[12] This resulted in poor medical supplies, spread of infectious and communicable diseases, an increase in the infant and mother mortality, and a decrease in the average life expectancy. Births with congenital malformations as a result of weapons of war is the greatest burden facing Iraq today (the top 10 causes of stillbirths in Iraq are presented in Table 3). MOH-recorded statistics of 2012 concerning the congenital malformations and stillbirths were 3593 and 7676 of all live births (1,131,632) across the country.[13]

The generalized violence and conflicts that followed the 2003 war led to the fleeing of physicians, pharmacists, and other health workforces because they or their families were the preferred targets of the terror that settled in the country.[14,15] After 2011, the MOH adopted new strategies to improve the access and quality of health services and rebuild war-ravaged hospitals and health centers. Good efforts were made to stem the deficiency of the medical staff and encourage the

Table 2: Iraqi public health facilities

MOH Facilities	Number
Directorates of health	21
General and specialized public hospitals	173
Teaching hospitals	66
Primary health centers headed by medical doctors	1266
Primary health centers headed by health workers	1272
Number of ambulances	2309

Obtained from the Iraqi MOH annual report.[13]

Table 3: The top 10 causes of stillbirths in Iraq for the year 2012

Causes	Percentage
Maternal care related to the fetus and amniotic cavity and delivery problems	27.0
Disorders originating in the perinatal period	21.4
Maternal factors and complications of pregnancy, labor, and delivery	18.0
Respiratory and cardiovascular disorders specific to the perinatal period	6.5
Congenital malformations	5.2
Disorders related to the length of gestation and fetal growth	4.7
Edema, proteinuria, and hypertensive disorders in pregnancy	3.2
Hypertensive diseases	1.8
Congenital malformations of the nervous system	1.5

Obtained from the Iraqi MOH annual report.[13]

return of those who had migrated. Per capita health expenditure has increased from US$39.21 in 2004 to US$164.00 in 2012 owing to increased oil revenue and increased MOH-allocated budget.

1.3 Morbidity and mortality in Iraq

Statistics on births and death are available only from the MOH. In all Iraqi governorates there are registration offices affiliated with the MOH for birth and death information. These events are recorded in unified certificates for public and private health facilities and then transferred to the registration offices of the MOH. Physicians write death certificates exclusively. The total deaths in Iraq for the year 2012 were 134,096 for the whole population. The percentage of male deaths is higher (55.2%) than that of females (44.8%) (mortality indicators for Iraq are presented in Table 4). The top 10 diseases causing death are heart failure, cerebrovascular diseases, external forces causing death, ischemic heart diseases, renal failure, septicemia, respiratory distress syndrome, senility, diabetes mellitus, and malignant tumor of the gastrointestinal tract. Records on health and diseases are collected on a monthly basis via the health information system and from surveys of the MOH in collaboration with the World Health Organization (morbidity causes in Iraq are presented in Table 5).[16]

Table 4: Mortality indicators for Iraq for the year 2012

Indicators	Rate
Crude death rate/1000 of the population	3.9
Death due to violence/10,000 of the population	6.3
Death due to immunodeficiency/10,000 of the population	0.0002
Infant mortality (under 1 year)/1000 live births	19.9
Child mortality (under 5 years)/1000 live births	24.2
Maternal mortality/100,000 live births	25.8
Hospital death/1000 inpatients	17.4

Obtained from the Iraqi MOH annual report.[13]

Table 5: Top 10 causes of morbidity in Iraq for the year 2012

Name of Disease	Percentage
Intestinal infectious diseases	5.7
Respiratory and cardiovascular disorders specific to the prenatal period	2.7
Pregnancy with abortive outcome	2.6
Ischemic heart disease	2.3
Acute lower respiratory infections	2.2
Influenza and pneumonia	2.2
Diseases of the urinary system	2.1
Heart diseases	1.5
Chronic lower respiratory diseases	1.5
Hemorrhagic and hematological disorders of fetus and newborn	1.4

Obtained from the Iraqi MOH annual report.[13]

2. Pharmacy practice

2.1 Pharmaceutical sector

Public and private sectors are the major components of the health system and pharmaceutical sector in Iraq. In both sectors, the provision of health is mainly through the clinical services; public health service is poorly addressed. It is worth mentioning here that pharmacists in Iraq are allowed to work in both sectors on the same day. According to data from the Syndicate of Iraqi Pharmacists (SIP) there are 11,857 pharmacists in Iraq; slightly more than half of them (53.06%) are females. However, it is expected that the female ratio will increase to 66% in 2015. Only 3.14% of pharmacists have a master's degree and 1.30% have a doctorate's qualifications. Pharmacists' ages vary between the 50s and younger generations; the majority of pharmacists (75%) are 22–48 years of age. Thus, the ability to offer pharmacy services extends to more than 2 decades for the older pharmacists and to more than 4 decades for the lower age group.

2.2 Private versus public sectors

The model of the public sector is hospital-oriented, capital-controlled, and inadequately suited to meet the requirements of the current demographic changes in the population.[9] The MOH is the main body responsible for the regulation of the public sector and the distribution of medical staff and other health workers. This sector still suffers a shortage in the supply of medicines, inadequate medical supplies, and poor utilization of informational technology. Yet, the distribution of pharmacists in the public health facilities does not meet the local need. On the other hand, the private sector is strong, offers around 50% of the health services, and was able to compensate for the shortfall in the public sector after the conflict of 2003.[12] Health settings of the private sector include private hospitals (96), physicians' clinics (10,000–12,000), scientific drug bureaus (396), drugstores (344), and community pharmacies (6140), all providing services for profit. The cost of visiting a private physician's clinic ranges between US$15 and US$25; in limited cases it could exceed US$50 for highly qualified doctors. Private clinics and community pharmacies are almost widespread throughout the entire country. However, the drugstores and scientific drug bureaus are often clustered together in the centers of Iraqi cities. All these settings of the private sector should be owned and managed by licensed pharmacists and open on a full-time basis throughout the week except on Friday. They are routinely subject to inspection by a selected committee of the MOH and other committees of the SIP; both work jointly to regulate the private sector. A household national survey from 2010 indicated that most members of the society were satisfied with the primary care services offered by the public and private sectors. The first and most popular source of primary care was the private clinics, while the public health setting was the preferred choice for the poorer people. Public clinics were indeed free; there was little evidence of informal payments to ensure the provided services.[17]

2.3 Medicine supply and distribution

Before 2003, the supply of medicines occurred mainly through Kimadia, the operational arm of the MOH, which was founded in 1964 in Iraq. It is the state company and was the only body responsible for the procurement and distribution of drugs and medical appliances (imported or locally produced) from the center to the end-user facilities.[12] However, this function was reduced to the supply of medicines to the health facilities of the MOH after the conflict of 2003. As of this writing, the scientific drug bureaus occupy the major role in the supply of medicines for both sectors because of the openness of the Iraqi pharmaceutical market to the international pharmaceutical environment. They import medicines and medical supplies from international pharmaceutical industries on a wholesale basis. The supply of medicines in Iraq is best described in Figure 1. It was estimated that around 70% of the available medicines are imported by the private sectors.[12] According to regulation, the imported pharmaceutical product and the manufacturer should be registered at the MOH. Postmarketing surveillance is the responsibility of the MOH in coordination with the SIP.

2.4 Industrial pharmacy and pharmaceutical technology

The public production factories in Iraq are Samara Drugs Industries (SDI), Nineveh Drug Industry, Arab Company for Antibiotics Industries, Abu Ghurayb Veterinary Production, Amiriyah Serum and Vaccine Institute, Baghdad Factory for IV Solutions and Medical Gases Production, Baghdad South Saline Production, and Dawrah Foot and Mouth Disease Vaccine Production Facility.[12] Less than 25% of the consumed medicines in the country are manufactured locally. SDI was the main drug factory originally, established by the Iraq–Soviet economic and technical cooperation treaty in 1959 to produce about 160 products of various dosage forms. In the 1980s, it was split from the MOH and became an independent construct

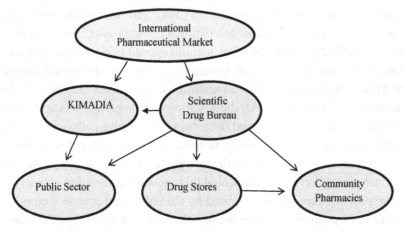

Figure 1
The supply of medicines in Iraq.

affiliated with the Ministry of Industry. It has three production sites: Samara Drug Factory, Baghdad Factory for Medical Gases, and Babylon Factory for Disposable Syringes and Medical Gases. The production of SDI before 2003 was sold to the MOH and then distributed by Kimadia drug channels to various health settings. As of this writing, SDI works as a separate factory and sells medicines for both the MOH and the private sector. There are several[24] small private factories for various dosage forms. Pharmaceutical promotion and production under license are still not active and poorly controlled and regulated in Iraq.

2.5 Community pharmacy practice

The appearance of the first apothecary in history was in Baghdad in 754 AD; it was managed by the scientist Jaber Ibn Hayyan, the founder of chemistry science (721–815 AD).[18] Today, there are thousands of community pharmacies distributed widely throughout the country. All are privately owned and managed by licensed pharmacists. International chain pharmacies are lacking in Iraq. The SIP regulates the practice of community pharmacies. Like other Middle Eastern countries, a baccalaureate degree is the first professional degree.[19] According to regulation, the distance between adjacent pharmacies should be more than 25 m; pharmacist attendance is required during working hours. However, some pharmacists have adhered less to the regulations, which has led to the intrusion of unauthorized individuals in the private sector. It is no small fact that these venders have weakened the crucial role of community pharmacists. This phenomenon is highly recognized in developing countries.[20]

In general, community pharmacies in Iraq are relatively small (the minimal required area is $20\,m^2$) and highly accessible to the public either for purchasing medicines or for seeking for medical advice. The daily working hours depend on the type of pharmacist's license. The part-time license is given to the pharmacists who are engaged in the public sector in the morning. That is, their pharmacies start daily work at 4:00 PM. In contrast, the full-time license is offered to pharmacists who are retired or resigned from the public sector. Public–pharmacy interaction is best described by the frequent visits to the community pharmacies (once or more per month); however, the professional performance of pharmacists is poorly addressed by the society.[21] More studies reflecting the real image of community practice as well as public attitudes about the profession of pharmacy in Iraq are warranted.

The daily practice of community pharmacists includes dispensing medicines on a prescription–nonprescription basis, preparation of some admixtures (such as syrups, ointments, and capsules) in response to medical prescription, substitution of unavailable medicine with an alternative one, counseling on minor illness, monitoring adverse drug effects, providing products for children, and providing medical supplies. Additionally, some pharmacies nowadays have free services for body weight, blood pressure, and blood glucose measurements using advanced electronic devices. Dispensing of medicines still follows the traditional method in which the practicing doctor prescribes a specific treatment, then the patient goes to a pharmacy to get it dispensed. Pharmacists in Iraq frequently seize the available opportunity in dispensing medicines to provide the necessary medical advice. However, information available from the province of Basra showed that dispensing generic medicines instead of the prescribed brand was an unacceptable practice to physicians. Fear of therapeutic failure, inadequate training of the pharmacist, and interfering with the physician's choice were the main reasons mentioned by the physicians in Iraq.[22]

2.6 Pharmacy education

Several public and private colleges of pharmacy are distributed throughout the various governorates of Iraq. The first pharmacy college, the Royal College of Pharmacy and Chemistry, was established in 1936 in Baghdad and affiliated with the University of Baghdad, the largest university in the country. At the time of this work, there are 17 colleges of pharmacy; all offer pharmacy teaching in the English language. Twelve colleges are public, affiliated with the Ministry of Higher Education and Scientific Research (MOHEASR). The five private colleges run under the patronage of a private investor. International accreditation is not fully applicable in Iraq. All pharmacy colleges offer a baccalaureate degree of pharmacy after 5 years (10 semesters) of study and follow the same pharmacy curriculum (the curriculum of Iraqi colleges of pharmacy is explained in Table 6). In addition, the public colleges offer high

Table 6: Curriculum of pharmacy colleges in Iraq

Year	Course No.	Modules
1st	1	Human Biology, Principles of Pharmacy Practice, Analytical Chemistry, Computer Sciences, Mathematics and Biostatistics, Medical Terminology.
	2	Human Anatomy, Pharmaceutical Calculations, Medical Physics, Organic Chemistry, Histology, Human Rights.
2nd	1	Organic Chemistry II, Medical Microbiology, Physical Pharmacy I, Physiology I, Democracy, Arabic Language.
	2	Communication Skills, Organic Chemistry III, Medical Virology and Parasitology, Physical Pharmacy II, Physiology II, Pharmacognosy I.
3rd	1	Inorganic Pharmaceutical Chemistry, Pharmacognosy II, Pharmaceutical Technology I, Biochemistry I, Pathophysiology.
	2	Organic Pharmaceutical Chemistry I, Pharmacology I, Pharmaceutical Technology II, Biochemistry II, Pharmacognosy III, Pharmacy Ethics.
4th	1	Pharmacology II, Organic Pharmaceutical Chemistry II, Clinical Pharmacy I, Biopharmaceutics, Public Health.
	2	Pharmacology III, Organic Pharmaceutical Chemistry III, Clinical Pharmacy II, General Toxicology, Industrial Pharmacy I.
5th	1	Organic Pharmaceutical Chemistry IV, Industrial Pharmacy II, Applied Therapeutics I, Clinical Chemistry, Clinical Laboratory Training, Clinical Toxicology, Graduation Project.
	2	Pharmacoeconomics, Applied Therapeutics II, Therapeutic Drug Monitoring, Advanced Pharmaceutical Analysis, Hospital Training, Dosage Form Design, Pharmaceutical Biotechnology.

diploma, M.Sc., and Ph.D. programs in different disciplines of pharmacy. The Doctor of Pharmacy degree program is currently not pursued in Iraq. All pharmacy colleges in Iraq accept both males and females (with no gender discrimination). The criteria for accepting students depend on their high school grade average, which should be more than 95 for the public pharmacy college and not less than 90 for the private. In past years, the number of pharmacy students has increased remarkably (more than 800 students in each college). This is due to the ongoing establishment of private pharmacy colleges. Student fees in private colleges range from US$5000 to US$7000 each year. However, pharmacy education at the public colleges is free of charge.

The colleges' applied strategy of teaching pharmacy plays a crucial role in the professional performance after graduation.[23] The pharmacy teaching method in Iraq is still characterized by a traditional way of teaching, an information-oriented format, and overcrowding of students in the classrooms.[24] Pharmacy students get an enormous amount of knowledge mainly through lectures, reading, and, to a lesser extent, practice. However, the pharmacy practice in Iraq has witnessed an increased number of qualified pharmacists and improvement in pharmaceutical care services. Owing to the critical and volatile status of Iraq, much of the qualified teaching staff have fled Iraq, searching for safe living in other countries. In an attempt to improve the quality standards of education and increase the number of pharmacists wishing to pursue a good career in the future, the MOHEASR has adopted a promising strategy of providing scholarships for postgraduate studies in the United States, the United Kingdom, Australia, European countries, and East Asia.

2.7 Hospital practice

All pharmacy graduates are obliged to enroll in a medical gradation program of the MOH for a period of 3 years. In the first, the rotation period, pharmacists have to work in the public teaching hospitals as "intern-pharmacists." Then, they are distributed by the MOH to work for 2 years in the public health centers that are scattered throughout the country's rural areas. Upon completion, they get the title "practitioner-pharmacist," which allows them to own their private work license (part-time license). During these 3 years, most pharmacists acquire good pharmaceutical knowledge that enhances their skills during their practice. Another opportunity for around 100 intern-pharmacists every year is an engagement in the clinical pharmacy program after passing a special exam at the MOH. Clinical pharmacists are excluded from the allocation to the far rural areas and are eligible to get a private work license upon completing the first year of the rotation period. The good income from the private sector along with the limited role in the public hospitals have encouraged most pharmacists to discontinue the public work at the MOH, seeking their own professional work. A pharmacist shift toward private practice in developing countries had been reported frequently.[25]

3. Achievements

- Despite the dramatic changes that weakened the country for 3 decades, pharmacy in Iraq continues to provide the required pharmaceutical care in both the public and the private sectors. The private pharmaceutical sector in Iraq can be considered as the strongest in the Arab region and the most promising in terms of investment.
- The number of graduate pharmacists has increased during the past 10 years to reach more than 1000 graduates owing to the expansion and increased number of pharmacy colleges. Many Middle East pharmacists have graduated from the College of Pharmacy of the University of Baghdad since its establishment in 1936.
- The joint collaboration between the MOH and the SIP contributes for better regulations and policies that suit the reality of pharmacy practice in the country. The SIP is one of the important influential institutions in Iraq concerning pharmacy-related issues.
- The adopted clinical pharmacy program of the past 2 decades offers a good opportunity for pharmacists in providing the current trend toward patient care.

4. Challenges

- The volatile political status of Iraq is the major challenge facing the MOH today, interfering with its adopted plans and strategies for improvement.
- The effective medical graduation program, which requires that all pharmacy graduates be employed in the public services, is indeed a burden that should be addressed.
- Research and information in particular to the practice of pharmacy is lacking in Iraq. Challenges facing this field and requirements for its development are weakly comprehended.
- Intercountry variation in pharmacy colleges, absence of international collaboration, and a shortage of well-trained faculty staff are other challenges facing Iraqi pharmacy education.

5. Recommendations

- Decision-makers at all levels in the MOH and MOHEASR should articulate new strategies to engage pharmacists of both sectors in providing public health services such as smoking cessation programs, TB control programs, and obesity control. Efforts should be made to improve the current role of pharmacists in public settings.
- The increased number of pharmacy students must be controlled and accommodated to compensate the excessive increase in the number of community pharmacies throughout the country. Collaboration with international pharmacy schools may improve the qualification standards of pharmacists and help in the development of ideas for a better pharmacist's role in Iraq.
- Research on pharmacy practice should be encouraged and funded by both the MOH and colleges of pharmacy to provide the needed evidence before any future policy or plan is adopted.

6. Conclusions

Pharmacy in Iraq is characterized by the presence of public and private sector settings and personnel. It had been affected by a variety of reasons including 32 years of an atmosphere of conflicts, an uncontrolled private sector, profit orientation, a lack of learning skills, a limited role of hospital pharmacists, and the present gap between pharmacy colleges and the real practice of pharmacy. Despite recent plans to improve the practice of pharmacy, there is a need for future pharmacists who have sufficient skills to meet the escalating social demand. There is a paucity of research pertaining to the profession of pharmacy in both the public and the private sectors. Additionally, little value is given to pharmacy research that has taken place outside the public hospitals. Addressing this will enhance the effective role of the pharmacist in providing efficient patient care and monitoring the rational use of medicines by the society.

7. Lessons learned

- The political instability of Iraq interferes with the MOH plans and strategies for providing the optimum goal of the health care.
- The decline in the health system needs an articulation of new policies that address to some extent the rapid change in the Iraqi population demography rather than the total reliance on the MOH government-allocated budget.
- Despite the witnessed success of the private sector, it is still struggling with the uncoordinated policies of the MOH that still embrace the old concepts and do not value the benefit of this field in supporting the public sector.

Acknowledgments

A special thank you goes to Dr Manal Younus (Specialized Clinical Pharmacist at MOH) and Dr Imad A. Al-Naimi (Consultant and Clinical Microbiologist, Department of Pharmacy/Alyarmouk University College) for their valuable efforts in providing the required country documents of the health system. The authors also thank Dr Kawkab Saour (Professor at College of Pharmacy/University of Baghdad), the library staff in the Iraqi Council of Deputies, and the pharmacist Haider Al-Amiry (Director of Jawharat Alrafidin Scientific Bureau) for help in providing the required information.

References

1. Iraq. Central Statistical Organization. *Annual abstract statistics*. Baghdad: Ministry of Planning; 2012.
2. Roux G. *Ancient Iraq*. NY (USA): Penguin Group; 1993.
3. Stol Marten. *Epilepsy in Babylonia*. Groningen (the Netherlands): Styx Publication; 1993.
4. Burnham G, Malik S, Al-Shibli A, Mahjoub A, Bager A, Baqer Z, et al. Understanding the impact of conflict on health services in Iraq: information from 401 Iraqi refugee doctors in Jordan. *Int J Health Plann Manage* 2012;**27**:e51–64.
5. Wilson F. The health care revival in Iraq. *Ann Intern Med* 2004;**141**:825–8.
6. Godichet O, Ghanem V. Iraqi system of primary health care: a communitarian system of family medicine under a dictatorship framework. *Contemp Nurse* 2004;**17**:113–24.

7. Sansom C. The ghost of Saddam and UN sanctions. *Lancet Oncol* 2004;**5**:134–45.
8. UNICEF. UNICEF humanitarian action for children. New York (USA) [cited September 7, 2012]. Available from: http://www.unicef.org/hac.
9. World Health Organization-Regional Health System Observatory (WHO-EMRO). *Health system profile-Iraq.* Cairo (Egypt). 2006.
10. International Pharmaceutical Federation. FIP Global Pharmacy Report. Work Force Report 2009. Netherlands [cited August 3, 2012] Available from: www.fip.org/hr.
11. World Health Organization. Iraq health information system review and assessment. [Cited December 20, 2013]. Available from: http://applications.emro.who.int/dsaf/libcat/EMROPD_110.pdf.
12. USAID (IZDIHAR-USAID). *Pharmaceutical and medical products in Iraq.* 2007. Contract No. 267-C-00-04-00435-00.
13. Iraq M.O.H.. *Annual report for the year 2012.* Baghdad: Ministry of Health; 2012.
14. Bristol N. Iraq's health system requires continued funding commitment. *Lancet* 2006;**368**:905–6.
15. Zarocostas J. Exodus of medical staff strains Iraq's health infrastructure. *BMJ* 2007;**334**:865.
16. Iraq MOH. *Health information system review and assessment.* Baghdad: Ministry of Health; 2011.
17. Burnham G, Hoe C, Hung Y, Ferati A, Dyer A, Al Hifi T, et al. Perceptions and utilization of primary health care services in Iraq: finding from a national household survey. *BMC Int Health Hum Rights* 2011;**11**:15.
18. Meri J. *Medieval Islamic civilization.* London: Routledge; 2006.
19. Kheir N, Zaidan M, Younes H, El Hajj M, Wilbur K, Jewesson P. International pharmacy education and practice in 13 middle eastern countries. *Am J Pharm Educ* 2008;**72**:133.
20. Rabbani F, Cheema FH, Talati N, Siddiqui S, Syed S, Bashir S, et al. Behind the counter: pharmacies and dispensing patterns of pharmacy attendants in Karachi. *J Pak Med Assoc* 2001;**51**:149–53.
21. Ibrahim Inas R, Al Tukmagi Haydar F, Wayyes Abdulrasoul. Attitudes of Iraqi society towards the role of community pharmacist. *Innovations Pharm* 2013;**4**:1–10.
22. Sharrad A, Hassali M, Shafie A. Generic medicines: perceptions of physician in Basrah, Iraq. *Australas Med J* 2009;**1**:58–64.
23. Devlin M, Samarawickrema G. The criteria of effective teaching in a changing higher education context. *Higher Educ Res Dev* 2010;**29**:111–24.
24. Saleh A, Al-Tawil N, Al-Hadithi T. Teaching methods in Hawler college of medicines in Iraq: a qualitative assessment from teachers' perspectives. *BMC Med Educ* 2012;**12**:59.
25. International Pharmaceutical federation (FIP). *FIP Global Pharmacy Report. Work Force Report.* 2009. Netherlands.

CHAPTER 11

Pharmacy Practice in Jordan

Qais Alefan, Abdulsalam Halboup

Chapter Outline

Pharmacy Practice in Developing Countries. http://dx.doi.org/10.1016/B978-0-12-801714-2.00011-3

1. Introduction

1.1 Country background

Jordan is located in the Middle East. It shares borders with Saudi Arabia to the east and south, Iraq to the northeast, Syria to the north, and Israel and the Palestinian territories to the west. Jordan has an area of 89,213 km^2 and is divided into three provinces (north, middle, and south). Jordan has a population of 6.714 million people,[1] of whom more than 70% are under 30 years of age. People between the ages of 15 and 24 years comprise 22% of the total population.[2] Jordan is an upper middle-income country with a per capita gross national income of US$4950. It is ranked the world's fourth poorest country in water resources.[3] Jordan's economy depends highly on tourism. Tourism is the largest export sector, with a contribution of more than $800 million to the national economy, and accounts for about 10% of gross domestic product (GDP). Services account for more than 70% of GDP and more than 75% of jobs.[2] In terms of human development relative to middle-income countries, Jordan is above average. Jordan spends more than 25% of its GDP on human development, education, health care, retirement funds, and social safety nets. School enrollment rates at all levels of education are close to those rates in countries at Jordan's income level. The demand on health care services and education is increasing because of the growing population in Jordan.[3]

2. Vital health statistics

2.1 Statistics on morbidity and mortality

The first leading cause of death in Jordan is cardiovascular disease, which contributes to 38% of all death cases. Cancer comes in second and contributes to 14% of all death cases, and trauma comes in third and contributes to 11%.[4,5] The mortality rate for those under 5 years of age (per 1000 live births) in Jordan declined from 28 in 2000 to 19 in 2013.[6] The neonatal mortality rate (per 1000 live births) was 19 in 1990 for both genders and declined to 11 in 2013. The infant mortality rate (per 1000 live births) for both genders was 24 in 2000 and declined to 16 in 2013. The adult mortality for those between 15 and 60 years of age per 1000 population for both genders was 310 deaths in 1990 and the number declined to 229 in 2012.[7] Infectious disease, diarrhea, respiratory infection, and hepatitis are the leading causes of morbidity as reported from health care facilities in Jordan, especially among children; however, polio has been eradicated since 1991.[5] The incidence rate of tuberculosis per 100,000 population in 2000 was 8.1 and the number declined to 5.8 in 2012, and the prevalence of this disease in the same population was 10 in 2000 and declined to 8.5 in 2012.[7]

3. Overview of the health care system

3.1 Human resources for health

Jordan is considered the training center for health professions in the region. It provides many countries in the region with a health workforce. However, Jordan lacks a comprehensive plan and strategy to fulfill the local and regional needs.[5] As of 2009, the Jordan health sector employs 57,000 health care providers, of which 56% are in the private sector and the rest are in the public sector.[70] The public sector in Jordan employs 40% of practicing physicians, 7% of pharmacists, and 64% of nurses (i.e., all nursing categories).[5] The total number of practicing physicians in Jordan in 2012 was 17,284, which is higher than that in most other countries in the region. The number of dentists was 6357; the number of nurses in all categories (i.e., registered, associated degree, assistant, and midwife) was 29,812 in 2012.[8] At the end of December 2013, the total number of pharmacists was 15,583; 59% were female.[9]

3.1.1 Public sector

The Ministry of Health (MOH), which was established in late 1950, offers preventative treatment and health control services and public health insurance. In addition, it manages the health education and training institutions and oversees health care services offered by the public and private sectors. It is considered the largest provider of health care in Jordan. In addition to its governmental annual budget, the MOH receives additional funds from the Civil Insurance program in the form of insurance premiums. In 1997, Jordan established a health sector reform project in cooperation with the World Health Organization (WHO) and the World Bank.[10] Training and certifying general and specialist doctors is the responsibility of the Jordan Medical Council. The Higher Health Council formulates and supervises the implementation of national health policies in their hospitals, their health centers, and the Jordan Food & Drug Administration (JFDA).

The Royal Medical Services (RMS) provides health care services to the members of the Jordanian Armed Forces, security personnel, and their families. Most of its budget comes from the Ministry of Finance. There are eight hospitals under the umbrella of the RMS. In addition, the Jordan University Hospital (JUH), the King Hussein Medical Center, and the King Abdullah University Hospital (KAUH) provide health care services to the employees of the Jordan Universities and their families, private patients, and patients who are referred from the MOH and RMS hospitals and medical centers.

3.1.2 Private sector

The private sector provides high technological capacity and quality of services and holds a large number of the country's medical expertise. The Private Hospitals Association (PHA) is a private voluntary nonprofit organization. It was established in 1984. It represents the private hospitals' interests in Jordan and includes independent private hospitals and medical centers. The PHA has gained notable reliability locally and internationally. This was achieved by providing an advanced level of health care services and always seeking to implement the highest international standards to develop medical services offered in Jordan. In 2013, there were 45 PHA members.[11]

3.1.3 Nongovernmental and international organizations

The National Center for Diabetes Endocrinology and Genetics (NCDEG) is an independent nonprofit organization, which provides health care services, education, and training on issues related to diabetes, endocrinology, and genetics.[12] In addition, the United Nations Relief and Works Agency (UNRWA) runs 24 primary health care centers, 8 women's program centers, and 172 schools serving more than 1.9 million Palestinian refugees in Jordan.[13] The Jordanian Red Crescent Society provides health care services during emergencies and for refugees in Jordan, especially Syrian refugees.[14]

3.2 Primary, secondary, and tertiary health services

The MOH in Jordan provides primary, secondary, and tertiary health services throughout its health centers as well as public and private hospitals. In 2013, there were 103 hospitals in Jordan and 12,081 beds and the population/bed ratio was 541. Additionally, there were 1510 health centers and clinics including comprehensive and primary health centers distributed throughout the country.[14]

3.3 Financing of health care

The general government expenditure on health included 65.5% of total health expenditures and 25% as out-of-pocket expenditures in 2011[7]. The MOH budget accounted for 6.3% of the government budget, and total expenditure on health was 8.4% of the GDP. Total expenditure on health per capita was US$505 for the same year.[15] Public sources were considered the primary health care financing sources (i.e., Ministry of Finance), which accounted for about

61.95% of health care financing. The second largest source was the private sector, accounting for 34.42%, whereas 3.63% was from donors.[16] Public health care expenditures accounted for 66.85% of total health care expenditures, followed by private health care expenditures (31.34%), nongovernmental organizations (1.14%), and the UNRWA (0.67%).[16]

3.4 Health insurance

Around 82.3% of the Jordanian population has insurance (some data show that more than this percentage are insured, because some people have multiple insurance coverage). Health care insurance in Jordan is covered by four schemes. The MOH is the largest insurer, covering 35% of the population, followed by the RMS, covering 27%; the UNRWA, covering 8%; private insurance, covering 10%; and University Hospitals (UHs), covering 2.3%. However, about 17.7% of the Jordanian population is still without formal insurance.[17]

3.5 Medicine expenditure

According to a National Health Accounts report in 2011, total health expenditure as GDP was 8.4% compared to 9.4% of the GDP in 2003, with 3.1% of health expenditure on medicines. On the other hand, more than 3.08% of the GDP was pharmaceutical expenditures.[18] Almost one-third of total health care expenditures went for pharmaceuticals and accounted 13.81 and 22.12% of public and private health care expenditures, respectively. That put Jordan among the highest countries all over the world based on pharmaceutical expenditures.[5]

4. Medicine supply systems and drug use issues

4.1 Important local manufacturers and importers

Jordan has a well-developed high-quality local manufacturing sector. Currently there are 16 pharmaceutical companies that manufacture mostly generics or branded generics. All 16 companies are Good Manufacturing Practice (GMP)-certified based on WHO GMP standards. Seven are European Medicines Agency certified, and two are FDA certified.[19] The Jordanian Association of Pharmaceuticals Manufacturers (JAPM) is a nonprofit organization established in 1996 to be the representative body of manufacturers and medical appliances. The JAPM is a voluntary association that has members from almost all the pharmaceutical companies in Jordan. Jordanian pharmaceutical companies that are member of the JAPM are presented in Table 1. Other companies that are associated members of the JAPM are presented in Table 2. Jordan pharmaceutical industries are export driven. Jordan pharmaceuticals are now exported worldwide to more than 60 countries. Almost 90% of the exports are exported to the Arab countries.[20]

Drug importers in Jordan represent 84 medicine agents and around 160 subagents. All companies registered with the JFDA as wholesalers and drug importers for pharmaceutical products must have a storage facility in which the product can be stored before distribution.[19]

Table 1: JAPM members

No.	Company Name	Year Established	Registered Capital, Million JD	Number of Employers	Location
1	The Arab Pharm. Mfg. Co. Ltd.	1962	20.0	856	Amman
2	Dar Al-Dawa Develop & Invst. Co.	1957	20.0	786	Amman
3	Hikma Pharmaceuticals	1977	29.8	1.004	Amman
4	The Jordanian Pharm. Mfg. Co.	1978	20.0	478	Amman
5	Arab Center for Pharm. & Chem.	1983	5.0	260	Amman
6	United Pharmaceuticals	1989	3.0	382	Amman
7	Hayat Pharm. Ind. Co. Ltd.	1993	9.5	166	Amman
8	RAM Pharma	1992	5	189	Sahab
9	MID Pharma	1993	15.0	312	Amman
10	Pharma International	1994	28.8	460	Amman
11	Jordan Sweden Medical & Strz.	1996	7.0	175	Amman
12	TQ PHARMA	2007	10.0	86	Amman
13	Jordan River Pharm. Ind.	1999	7.5	80	Amman
14	Amman Pharmaceutical Industries	1989	6.0	250	Amman

Source: Jordan Association of Pharmaceutical Manufacturers.

Table 2: JAPM-associated members

No.	Company Name	Location
1	Arab Pharmaceutical Industry Consulting Company	Amman
2	International Pharmaceutical Research Center (IPRC)	Amman
3	ACDIMA BioCenter	Amman
4	Jordan Center for Pharmaceutical Research (JPRC)	Amman
5	Triumpharma, Inc., Product Development & Clinical Evaluation Center	Amman
6	Pharmaceutical Research Center (PRC)/Jordan University of Science and Technology	Irbed
7	PharmaquestJo Drug Evaluation & Research	Amman
8	RUM Calibration	Amman
9	NutriDar	Amman
10	EFADA Medical Industries Co. Ltd. (SUCTON)	Amman

Sources: Jordan Association of Pharmaceutical Manufacturers.

The importers make deliveries to retail pharmacies and private hospitals all over the country. The Amman area accounts for about 65% of all transactions.[21]

4.2 Prescribing and dispensing

Medication prescribing in Jordan is the physician's responsibility. However, dispensing is the pharmacist's responsibility. Several factors play a major role in influencing the physician prescribing behavior, such as the quality image of the pharmaceutical company and trust. Physicians' prescribing behavior is also influenced by a variety of incentives such as cash payment, free samples and small gifts, and financing for international conference participation. Clinical effectiveness is the most important factor that influences physician prescribing behavior in Jordan. The second factor is the dosage form and daily recommended dose; and the third factor is the cost of the prescribed medication. A 2014 study showed that community pharmacists were the main source of information about medicines for physicians (77%), the second source was medical representatives (65.4%), and 20.2% of physicians reported that the JFDA was a source of information about costs.[22]

4.3 Self-treatment

Self-medication can be defined as the self-consuming of medication without getting advice from a physician for either diagnosis or treatment. Self-treatment may lead to several health problems: misuse of over-the-counter (OTC) medication, concurrent use of several medications, and use of home remedies to treat potentially serious diseases, which may lead to misdiagnosis or masking of potential health problems.[23,76] In Jordan, like in many other developing countries, patients can purchase a large number of medicines, including antibiotics, without prescription, except for narcotics and major tranquilizers. According to a study conducted in Amman to evaluate self-medication patterns, self-medication behavior was a common health care practice among Jordanians (42.5%). Several reasons were behind this finding according to the study: minor diseases do not need a physician visit, long waiting times in the physician's clinic, and the desire to save money. Unfortunately, a small percentage of patients were engaged with a pharmacist for therapeutic consultations.[23]

4.4 Medicine prices

The JFDA is the authority responsible for fixing prices for prescribing and OTC medications. The price-setting criteria use various methods to calculate the price of the drug in the domestic market in Jordan. For the originator, the mechanism of pricing uses various methods (mathematic formula based on CIF/FOB prices; the median price based on the country basket; the price in the country of origin, with local margin adjustment; the export price to the Saudi Arabia market; and the reference price at the country of origin). The method that provides the lowest price is adopted and the price is given. In practice, the most commonly used method is based on the price in Saudi Arabia and it is adjusted every year to decrease prices only.[24] For the branded originator, the price is set around 80% of the originator company's prices, whereas subsequent branded takes the lowest price in the Jordanian market. For imported generics, the price is fixed according to the price of the country of origin, the price of neighboring countries, and the price in the Middle East and North Africa region.[26]

4.5 Traditional and complementary medicines

Medicinal plants are considered sources of variety of certain medicinal substances that are widely used to treat either infectious or chronic disease.[26] The majority of developing country populations who are seeking health rely on medicinal products regardless of their being licensed or not.[27] Complementary alternative medicine is commonly used in Jordanian cancer patients.[28] A lot of medicinal plants are available on the market without license or regulations to control their proper use. In addition, many herbalists are not educated and not trained and they gain expertise from their predecessor.[61] According to a study conducted in Jordan to investigate the prevalence of the use of complementary and alternative medicine (CAM) among infertile couples, the result showed that 44.7% of the study sample were CAM users. The majority of CAM users were females. In addition, the most commonly used CAMs were herbs and spiritual healing. The need for health care providers to increase awareness is necessary to encounter this excessive herb use and more research is needed in this field.[29] A 2013 study was conducted to explore the prevalence of the use of medicinal plants among patients with chronic kidney disease, hypertension, and dyslipidemia in Jordan. About 7.6% of participants reported using herbs and most of them were elderly and predominantly females. The most common herbal product used was *Hibiscus sabdariffa*.[30] A similar study was conducted on Jordanian diabetic patients who attended the NCDEG, in Amman. The study found that 16.6% of the participants reported using herbs, 44% of CAM users were in the age group 51–60 years, and 59.6% of them were females. The most commonly used herbal product was green tea.[31]

5. Overview of pharmacy practice and key pharmaceutical sectors

5.1 Breakdown of pharmacy-related human resources

According to the Jordan Pharmaceutical Association (JPA), the total number of registered pharmacists in 2014 was 15,583; 59% of them were female.[9] The percentage of pharmacists in the private sector comprises about 90%, whereas 10% are in the public sector and UHs.[32,34] Pharmacists in Jordan represent 16.3 per 10,000 of the population.[8]

5.2 Statistics on human and capital workforce

According to an MOH report, Jordan has 16.3 pharmacists per 10,000 of population.[8] About 62% of the Jordanian total population lives in the middle region governorates (Amman, Zerka, Madaba, and Balqa), which accommodate 72% of the health workforce. On the other hand, the north region governorates (Irbed, Ajlon, Jarash, and Mafraq) represent 29% of the total Jordanian population and accommodate 19% of the health workforce. In the south region governorates (Aqaba, Ma'an, Karak, and Tafelah), the percentage of the total population matched with the percentage of health care workforce was 9%.[33]

6. Drug- and pharmacy-related regulations, policies, and ethics

6.1 Inspection of pharmaceutical premises

The JFDA is the official authority that approves, registers, and prices of the pharmaceutical products. Imported pharmaceutical products should be declared to the JFDA and have pro forma invoice approval.[19] JFDA inspector activities cover manufacturing and pharmacies. The JFDA inspector team has grown from 8 to 12 personnel in the past few years. Their efforts have achieved a reduction in the number of counterfeit items from being available at 61 pharmacies in 2007 to 12 in 2008.[19]

According to Article 35 of the drug and pharmacy law, it is not allowed to advertise, for promotion purposes, drugs or any substances that have medicinal characteristics or infant milk formula or any supplemented food in any media, whether readable, visual, or audible, unless approved by both the Minister of Health and the JPA, with the exception of medicinal product publications and information directed at health authorities in which such information is authenticated.[35]

6.2 Drug registration

For registration of generic pharmaceutical products, the manufacturer's technical dossier must comply with the International Conference on Harmonization guidelines along with bioequivalence data. For an originator pharmaceutical product to be registered in Jordan, it must be registered in the origin country in addition to being registered at least for 1 year in a country with a highly developed regulatory system. For the cost of drug registration in Jordan, the fee for registering an originator pharmaceutical product is US$2000, whereas the fee is US$1000 for generic registration.[33] According to the JFDA, registration of a new drug must be completed within 180 days. The average registration time is around 90 days.[32]

6.3 Quality control

The JFDA has a well-equipped quality control lab with 56 staff members. The JFDA states that if the drug that has been on the market for more than 2 years and achieves seven consecutive successful batches, it does not need to go through quality control inspection for all batches, and only random batches should be quality control inspected. However, for drugs procured by public sector agencies, the joint procurement department states that quality testing for each single batch should be carried out.[32]

6.4 Professional associations

The JPA is the representative body of pharmacists. It was established in 1957 in adherence to Pharmaceutical Law No. 10 in the same year. Pharmacists in Jordan cannot practice their profession until they have a membership in the JPA, which is mandatory in Jordan.[36] For registration in the JPA, pharmacists should pass 1440 credit hours of training in pharmacy and be supervised by a licensed pharmacist and then sit for a pharmacy board exam.[37]

7. Pharmacy practices

7.1 Country perspective

Many studies reveal that pharmaceutical care services save patients' lives, influence expenses, and improve patient quality of life.[38–40] According to a study on the expectations of physicians regarding expanding pharmaceutical care services in Jordan, generally, Jordanian physicians agree on the concept of pharmaceutical care services. Rather, they accept the traditional role of the pharmacist in educating the patient about his or her medications. However, they have had bad experiences with pharmacists providing pharmaceutical care services. They do not think that pharmacists are ready to practice pharmaceutical care services.[41] Pharmacists have very good attitudes toward the implementation of pharmaceutical care practice but a number of barriers that limit the pharmaceutical care practice implementation in Jordan have been identified. These barriers include the level of understanding of pharmaceutical care practice, lack of a private counseling area, difficulties in communicating with physicians, and lack of access to patient medical records.[42] Establishing Master of Clinical Pharmacy and PharmD programs, increasing the publications about the role and benefit of pharmaceutical care services in decreasing drug therapy problems, improving communication with physicians, and modifying the undergraduate curriculum to become more focused on pharmaceutical care and therapeutics may help to solve implementation barriers.[42]

The Jordanian government has a strong commitment regarding health and education programs. Pharmacy education and practice in Jordan are thriving; this is demonstrated by the increase in the number of pharmacy schools and pharmacy students. Before 2009, there were eight pharmacy schools (two public and six private); all of them use English as the instruction language.[43] Now, there are 14 pharmacy schools.

7.2 Hospital pharmacy practice

Hospital pharmacy departments are expected to optimize the preparation, dispensing, and distribution of medications. So, it is necessary to have policies and regulations for handling medication safely.[44] The total number of hospitals in Jordan according to a statistical report in 2012 was 103 and the total number of beds was 12,081.[8] Hospital pharmacy practice provides services to all patients. These services include dispensing and distribution of medication, processing medication orders, providing drug information services, participating in quality improvement programs, participating in hospital activities, and ensuring the availability of medications with affordable prices.[45] However, in a study conducted to evaluate job satisfaction and job-related stress between community pharmacists and hospital pharmacists in Amman

City, pharmacists in the hospital setting were more satisfied than pharmacists in the community setting. Therefore, pharmacists' job satisfaction should be enhanced to improve pharmacists' job motivation and competence. Consequently, this will improve pharmaceutical care practice and increase productivity.[46] Another study was conducted to assess the factors that contribute to medication errors in Jordanian hospitals. The study found that the highest level of medication errors was committed by nurses (48.4%), compared to 31.7 and 11.1% committed by physicians and pharmacists, respectively. Additionally, the leading causes of medication errors were heavy workload (41.4%) and new staff (20.6%).[47]

7.3 Industrial pharmacy practice

The JAPM is a voluntary, nonprofit association, was established in 1996 as a devoted specific sector association, and is considered the representative body of pharmaceutical manufacturers and medical appliances, which is a key sector of the Jordanian economy. There are 14 pharmaceutical companies that are members of the JAPM; they are pioneer the exporting sector owing to their high quality and excellent reputation. Eighty-one percent of the pharmaceutical production is exported to foreign markets.[20] The Arab Pharmaceutical Manufacturing Company (APMC) was the first pharmaceutical company to be established in Jordan; it was established in 1962 and launched its product to the Jordanian market in 1966. In the late 1980s, the APMC started exporting to North African countries.[25] Jordan joined the World Trade Organization in 2000. This membership conveyed a variety of benefits, including reduced trade barriers to exports and lower tariffs, more access to foreign products, and enhanced international relations.[48] In addition, Jordan signed the bilateral Free Trade Agreement (FTA) with the United States, which was fully implemented in 2010. The Jordan–United States FTA expanded trade relationships by reducing export barriers, increasing intellectual property protection, and playing an important role in boosting the Jordan–United State economies.[49] The pharmaceutical industry in Jordan was established in 1962, when a company was begun with capital amounting to JD150,000. In mid-1970, three companies were established, and in 1980, three new pharmaceutical companies joined the pharmaceutical market. In the 1990s, remarkable development was witnessed in the pharmaceutical sector. This development resulted from capital inflow during the Gulf War as well as from laws and regulations that facilitated investments in Jordan.[50] The pharmaceutical industry in Jordan comprises 25 pharmaceutical companies marketing in over 60 countries worldwide, including the Middle East, South Africa, Europe, and North America.[8] Jordanian pharmaceutical companies import raw, processed, and developed pharmaceutical material from the international market such as the United States, China, and India.[51] The Jordanian pharmaceutical market is made up of 75% imported products and 25% locally manufactured products.[52] The total value of the pharmaceutical market in Jordan in 2008 was US$350 million; approximately 80% corresponds to imported products. The public pharmaceutical sector comprises 40%, whereas the private sector comprises 60%. The pharmaceuticals spent per capita represent US$80.[19]

7.4 Community pharmacy practice

Community pharmacy practice in Jordan is still developing, like other community pharmacy in the Middle East. In 2005, the number of registered community pharmacies was 1500.[53] In 2014, according to the JPA, there were 2220 community pharmacies in Jordan. About 77% of them are located in the middle region, 18% are located in the north region, and 5% in the south region of Jordan. All are inspected at least two times a year.[9] Community pharmacists contribute to decreased morbidity and mortality in the community setting. Approximately 60–70% of the Jordanian population has insurance and the community pharmacies are still the primary health care facility before physician clinics. In addition to dispensing, patient counseling is still the integral service all over the community pharmacy, especially counseling on OTC medications.[54] Nowadays, the role of the community pharmacist has expanded to be more patient-oriented in ideal pharmacies, especially after the establishment of the clinical pharmacy and PharmD programs in Jordan.

Chain pharmacies in the private pharmaceutical sector provide a high quality of health care services with qualified, well-trained pharmacists. Also, drug information centers (DICs) provide online services 24 h a day, helping people know more about the appropriate use of medications. The first chain pharmacy in Jordan was established in 2001, with home drug delivery services being offered.[53] There are 11 chain pharmacies distributed in Jordan, the largest of which has 76 branches.[55] A public opinion survey was administered to explore the societal perspective on the role of community pharmacists and OTC medication. The study revealed that 62% of participants sought advice from the community pharmacist when a condition was not serious enough to visit the physician; more than 60% of participants reported that they bought antibiotics without prescriptions. In addition, more than half of participants (58.8%) reported that they follow the directions on the packet of the OTC products.[56] Another study was conducted to show the problems and causes of irrational use of drugs in Jordan and Syria. Although the main problems of irrational drug use in Jordan and Syria were almost the same, they varied in the percentage of occurrence. These problems included excessive use of antibiotics and antidiarrheals, overprescribing of nonsteroidal anti-inflammatory drugs, self-prescribing medications, common use of antibiotics to treat minor upper respiratory infections, and prescribing by trade names. According to the study, the consequences of irrational use of drugs were poor patient medical record, lack of patient education about medication and disease, no family physician system, lack of standard treatment guidelines, and lack of progressive education for doctors and pharmacists.[57] Also, the average clinician–patient consultation time and pharmacist–patient dispensing time was short, which led to drug-related problems taking place.[10] Another study conducted in Jordan to evaluate patient perception regarding generic medicine showed that the high cost of medicines in Jordan is the main driving reason to choose generic medicines. Moreover, involvement of the patient in treatment options results in more medication adherence and health improvement.[58] Faculties of pharmacy in Jordan have conducted many pharmaceutical and health campaigns to increase awareness and improve health promotion among the public. In addition, pharmaceutical care free days were conducted by pharmacy students to help people take responsibility for their health, educate and counsel patients about medications, and educate them on how to manage their chronic diseases.

7.5 Medicine marketing and promotion

Pharmacists as medical representatives play a core role in many companies and make a bridge between selling companies and customers. Medical sales representatives promote pharmaceutical products to physician with various specialties, leading to improving the sales force by increasing pharmaceutical product prescriptions. Pharmaceutical companies in Jordan can be categorized into two types: generic (Jordanian) companies and nongeneric (multinational, foreign) companies. Nongeneric companies are the originators of the pharmaceutical product. However, generic companies mimic the originator after the pharmaceutical products patency has expired. A study was conducted in Jordan to compare the factors affecting medical representative performance between nongeneric and generic pharmaceutical companies. The results showed significant differences between generic and nongeneric pharmaceutical companies regarding many factors together: differences in wage system, sales target, evaluation, training schedule, promotional system, and personal traits and skills, as well as significant differences in medical representative performance, were found between generic and multinational pharmaceutical companies.[59]

8. Special pharmacy-related services and activities
8.1 Clinical pharmacy

The primary role of the clinical pharmacist is to provide a safe, efficacious, and accurate dose, which finally considers cost-effectiveness and leads to improvement in quality of life.[60] Many studies have revealed the positive role of clinical pharmacy services in improving patients' clinical and economic outcomes.[61,62] In Jordan, the physicians' acceptance rate of clinical pharmacy and their acceptance of clinical pharmacists as health care members was 69.4%,[63] which indicates the crucial role of the clinical pharmacist in increasing health care awareness and improving quality of life and reducing drug-related problems.[64] Clinical pharmacists in Jordan function as resources for drug information to other health care professions and patients, they participate in medical rounds, and give recommendations regarding medication dosing and adjustment, drug interactions, dilutions, and rate of infusion. They educate patients about their disease and counsel them regarding their medication during hospitalization and before discharge. In 2009, the Department of Clinical Pharmacy was implemented in teaching at the hospital of the Jordan University of Science and Technology (JUST) in an effort to provide health care services. Also, in the same year the King Hussein Cancer Center (KHCC) in Amman fully implemented a clinical pharmacy department and established a collaborative agreement with St. Jude Children's Research Hospital in Tennessee for advanced training of Jordanian clinical pharmacists.[63,65] The Department of Clinical Pharmacy at KAUH comprises 12 clinical pharmacists who provide services to all hospital wards and units. Clinical pharmacy services in Jordan are provided freely to most MOH hospitals, RMS hospitals, and UHs in collaboration with the Faculty of Pharmacy at JUST and JU. At this time, there is no clinical pharmacist job title in the Jordanian Ministry of Health. The benefit of the implementation of clinical pharmacy appears obviously in a study conducted in the Health Center of the JUST. The study involved hyperlipidemic patients who attended an outpatient clinic and were closely followed by clinical pharmacists for 6 months. After the 6-month study period 94.5% of the intervention group reached the treatment goal compared to 71.2% of the control group.[66] Another study was conducted in an outpatient clinic in RMS in Jordan. The study enrolled patients with diabetes type 2 who attended an outpatient clinic and were followed for 6 months. The results showed a 0.8% reduction in Hb1c in the intervention group compared with 0.1% reduction in the group followed by a traditional team. A study was conducted to reflect the importance of clinical pharmacists' contribution to the care of patients with chronic obstructive pulmonary diseases (COPD) by making an intervention focusing on patient education about COPD, counseling patients about their medications and the proper use of inhalation technique. In addition, an assessment of patients' willingness to adhere to their medication was made and the patients were referred to smoking cessation programs if necessary. The results showed significant improvement in COPD knowledge and medication beliefs and significant decrease in patient admission rates compared with controls.[64] Another study was conducted to assess the impact of clinical pharmacists' services on the cost of drug therapy for patients admitted to the intensive care units at Al-Hussein Hospital at the RMS in Amman. The study compared the consumption quantities of drugs over two periods of time. Each period was 10 months long. Clinical pharmacist services were implemented in the second period. The results showed that the total reduction in drug cost in the 10-month duration after implementation of clinical pharmacy practice was JD149,946.80 (US$211,574.90), which represents a 35.8% average drug saving compared to the first period.[67] The difficulties that limit the implementation of clinical pharmacy services may be summarized in the following: Clinical pharmacy services are relatively new in Jordan. There is a lack of institutional policies that describe the role, responsibilities, and clinical pharmacist position as a health care member. Also, the clinical pharmacist concept in Jordan is not fully developed and has weak communication with other professions.

8.2 Drug and poison information

Provision of drug information is an integral part of the extended role of the pharmacist. This role includes educating, monitoring, and caring for patients in collaboration with other health care professionals. In Jordan, DICs in public and private sectors provide accurate and up-to-date drug information to health care providers and patients.

The Jordan Drug Information and Toxicology Center belongs to the RMS and serves by providing timely, accurate, up-to-date, and evidence-based information for pharmacists, health care professionals, and the public. The DIC at KAUH provides free, precise, up-to-date, and evidence-based drug information for health care and the community. The National

Drug and Poison Information Center at JUH was established in 2004. The center covers three major areas: information services, clinical services, and analytical toxicology services. The Jordan National Drug Formulary is considered an easy reference for health care providers on rational drug use. The JFDA Web site serves the community by providing drug information and alerts and warnings on medications. In a study conducted in Jordan on hospital-based pediatricians about sources of information used when prescribing for children, 75% reported that Lexicomp's drug information handbook was the most frequently used when prescribing for children; 22% claimed that they discussed with a hospital pharmacist when they faced difficulties in prescribing for children.[68] Another study conducted on community pharmacies in Amman about drug information resources found that all community pharmacies had at least one reference book. However, most of these resources were out of date. The *Monthly Index of Medical Specialties* was the most commonly used reference in community pharmacy (64.7%). On the other hand, 40.4% had Internet access, whereas 19.2% depended on medical representatives for medical information.[69]

8.3 Health promotion and public health services

8.3.1 Smoking cessation clinic

Jordan is a country with high reported smoking rates. Around 48% of men are smokers, and among woman, the reported figure is 5%. However, this percentage is probably underestimated, because woman in Jordan underreport smoking owing to cultural and social reasons.[70] Jordan has signed the Framework of Conventional Tobacco Control agreement and antismoking policies exist in Jordan. Unfortunately, they are not fully implemented in public and private sectors.

On the other hand, Jordan is considered one of the few countries in the region that has initiated smoking cessation services. The MOH has three smoking cessation clinics, distributed in each of the north, middle, and south regions. They provide counseling and pharmacotherapy free of charge for smokers who want to quit. Another smoking cessation clinic is found in the KHCC. The clinic provides counseling and pharmacotherapy for cancer patients mainly, as well as smokers from the general population. Tobacco dependence training has increased over recent years. Since 2011, around 200 health care professionals (i.e., physicians, dentists, pharmacists, and nurses) have been trained in tobacco dependence treatment (TDT). In addition, 327 teachers and counselors have been trained in tobacco control and TDT. Pharmacological treatments that are available and approved in the smoking cessation clinics include nicotine replacement therapy (e.g., patches, gums, and lozenges) and varenicline. Bupropion is not registered in the JFDA and is available only in the KHCC.[71]

8.4 Research in pharmacy practice

Pharmacy practice in Jordan is still developing, but it took a good position compared with pharmacy practice in developing countries. This improvement in pharmacy practice mostly resulted from the initiation of Master in Clinical Pharmacy and PharmD programs in two public universities, JUST and JU. Likewise, research in pharmacy practice is still developing in Jordan. However, the literature contains a satisfactory number of published articles on pharmacy practice. In Jordan, most research has been conducted to evaluate the impact of clinical pharmacy services to justify the importance of implementing such services. The following few studies are examples of the research in pharmacy practice in Jordan.

A study was conducted to evaluate the impact of clinical pharmacy management in type 2 diabetic patients in outpatient diabetes clinics in Jordan. The patients were grouped into an intervention group, in which clinical pharmacist services (patient education and treatment recommendations) were given, and a control group (e.g., patients received the usual treatment from the clinic). The results showed a reduction in the mean HbA1c by 0.8% in the intervention group. However, the control group showed an increase of 0.1% in the HbA1c. Systolic and diastolic blood pressure, fasting blood glucose, total cholesterol, LDL, and triglycerides levels were evaluated and showed significant improvement in the intervention group compared to control group.[72]

Another study was conducted to evaluate the ability of health care professionals (e.g., specialists in airway disease, general practitioners, pharmacists, assistant pharmacists, nurses, and respiratory therapists) to demonstrate the correct use of some inhalers using a standardized checklist. Specialists scored the highest in inhaler technique demonstration skills. However, all health care professionals scored poorly on demonstrating the correct use of a powder inhaler compared with a pressurized metered-dose inhaler. The results also showed that participants who attended training workshops showed improvement in inhaler skills and scored significantly higher in all devices compared with nonattendees. The study concluded that health care professionals in Jordan should be up to date with inhaler skills, especially with dry powder inhalers, and educational workshops on inhaler technique significantly improved health care professionals' ability to demonstrate these skills.[73]

Another study was conducted to evaluate sources, patterns, and appropriateness of antibacterial drug consumption and showed that 45% of all antibacterial drugs were consumed without prescription, 23.2% through self-medication, and 23.1% through pharmacist recommendation. Moreover, inappropriate use of antibacterial drugs was seen in 29.9% of prescribed drugs and 34% of nonprescribed drugs. The results also showed that antibiotic misuse and abuse were common among Jordanians. The study concluded that regulations are needed to control inappropriate use of medications and increase awareness about the consequences of inappropriate use.[74]

9. Pharmacy education

9.1 History

The first school of pharmacy in Jordan was established as a department of the Faculty of Medical Sciences at Yarmouk University by a royal decree in 1979. The department then was transferred into an independent faculty on 19 September 1983. Three years later (i.e., September

1986) the Faculty of Pharmacy became affiliated with JUST. The second school was established in the University of Jordan in 1980.

9.2 Curriculum

Faculties of pharmacy in Jordan offer academic programs that require completion of 165 credit hours to obtain a bachelor degree in pharmacy. Pharmacy practice in Jordan is still developing and the focus on pharmaceutical care is still weak. According to a study conducted in eight Jordanian universities (two public and six private) about pharmaceutical care-oriented courses in pharmacy curricula, one public university (JUST) and two private universities (Al-Isra'a University and Philadelphia University) allocated a high percentage of pharmaceutical care courses in their curricula, which comprised 20% of total pharmacy courses, compared with other universities. None of the six universities have patient-oriented program training. The problem facing this program comes from the slow change in the education programs and lack of pharmaceutical care jobs.[75]

9.3 Degrees

All pharmacy schools (i.e., public and private) in Jordan offer Bachelor of Pharmacy programs. However, students in Hashemite University have the advantage of choosing between two tracks (i.e., Industrial Pharmacy and Pharmacy Management) in their final year. A PharmD program is offered by two public schools (i.e., JUST and University of Jordan).

A Ph.D. program is offered by the University of Jordan only,[76] while an M.Sc. program is offered by seven pharmacy schools in Jordan, of which, two are public schools (i.e., JUST and University of Jordan)[77] and five are private (i.e., Al-Ahliyya Amman University, Isra University, Al-Zaytoonah University of Jordan,[78] Petra University,[79] and Applied Science Private University[80]).

9.4 A lists on important colleges of pharmacy with locations

In Jordan, there are 14 pharmacy schools. Of which, 5 are public while 9 are private. The following table presents these schools (Table 3).

9.5 Achievements in pharmacy practice

Achievements in pharmacy practice in Jordan can be presented as follows:

- Establishment of Master of Clinical Pharmacy and PharmD programs in two public universities: JUST and the University of Jordan.
- The implementation of clinical pharmacy services in tertiary hospitals in Jordan such as KAUH, JUH, KHCC, and King Hussein Medical City.
- Establishment of the job description of clinical pharmacist by the MOH.

Table 3: Pharmacy colleges in Jordan

No.	University	Establishment Year	Public/Private	Programs Offered
1	Jordan University of Science and Technology (JUST)	1979	Public	Bachelor of Pharmacy, PharmD, M.Sc. program
2	The University of Jordan	1980	Public	Bachelor of Pharmacy, PharmD, M.Sc. program, Ph.D.
3	Yarmouk University	2013	Public	Bachelor of Pharmacy
4	Mutah University	2013	Public	Bachelor of Pharmacy
5	Hashemite University	2013	Public	Bachelor of Pharmacy
6	Al-Ahliyya Amman University	1990	Private	Bachelor of Pharmacy, M.Sc. program
7	Isra University	1991	Private	Bachelor of Pharmacy, M.Sc. program
8	Applied Science Private University	1991	Private	Bachelor of Pharmacy, M.Sc. program
9	Petra University	1991	Private	Bachelor of Pharmacy, M.Sc. program
10	Philadelphia University	1991	Private	Bachelor of Pharmacy
11	Al-Zaytoonah University of Jordan	1993	Private	Bachelor of Pharmacy, M.Sc. program
12	American University of Jordan	2011	Private	Bachelor of Pharmacy
13	Zarqa University	2011	Private	Bachelor of Pharmacy
14	Middle East University	2014	Private	Bachelor of Pharmacy

9.6 Challenges in pharmacy practice

The following points summarize the main challenges in pharmacy practice in Jordan:

- Jordan is a country with limited natural resources. The lower salary scale for qualified health care providers compared with Gulf Cooperation Council countries, Europe, and United States forces qualified health care providers to look for job opportunities outside the kingdom.[81]
- The workload of hospital pharmacists and the absence of technology utilization (e.g., automatic dispensing robots).
- Pharmacy curricula in universities are not being updated accordingly and many pharmacy programs still lack focus on pharmacy practice courses and training.
- Many pharmacies in Jordan are owned by nonpharmacists. This makes the pharmacy business-oriented rather than patient- and customer-oriented.
- Lack of specific pharmacist–patient training and pharmacy infrastructure and flow are considered barriers to getting involved in the pharmaceutical practice in many pharmacies.[54]
- Lack of institutional and governmental policies that describe the responsibilities of the clinical pharmacist.

9.7 Recommendations: way forward

Pharmacy leaders believe that the pharmacy profession should be redirected in education and practice toward pharmaceutical care services by changing the undergraduate pharmacy curriculum to be more related to pharmaceutical care services.[75] In addition, using innovative methods to improve students' ability to learn new skills concerning pharmaceutical care practice, such as adding practical courses that discuss identification, analysis, and prevention of drug therapy problems, must be a priority for all pharmacy schools in Jordan.[82] Using automated dispensing cabinets in hospital pharmacies significantly reduces medication errors during dispensing, distribution, and administration. It also frees pharmacists to focus more on direct patient care.[83] Pharmacy schools should update their curricula according to changes in the pharmacy profession that have taken place in more developed countries. Curricula should also be expanded to encourage critical thinking, improve problem-solving skills, learn how to collaborate with other health care professionals, and decision-making during pharmaceutical intervention.[84] Implementation of clinical pharmacy services in hospitals will improve patients' quality of life, decrease medication-related problems, and enhance patients' adherence to medication by improving patients' knowledge about diseases.

10. Conclusions

Pharmacy practice in Jordan is mainly seen as community and hospital pharmacy. Although Jordan is self-sufficient with regard to number of pharmacists, clinical pharmacy services are still developing in Jordan. On the other hand, the Jordanian industrial pharmaceutical sector is very important to Jordan's economy. Pharmaceutical industry in Jordan occupies a good position in the local market and abroad because of its high quality and affordable prices. Although some achievements in pharmacy practice have happened in Jordan, challenges continue to exist from different aspects.

References

1. Department of Statistics — Jordan [Internet]. Department of Statistics. [cited April 08, 2015]. Available from: http://www.dos.gov.jo; 2015.
2. About Jordan | United Nations — Jordan [Internet]. About Jordan | United Nations. [cited April 08, 2015]. Available from: http://www.un.org.jo; 2015.
3. Jordan | Data [Internet]. World Bank. [cited April 08, 2015]. Available from: http://data.worldbank.org/country/jordan; 2015.
4. Fa'ouri M, Najdawi F. *Patterns of childhood injuries*; 2002.
5. WHO. *Country cooperation strategy for WHO and Jordan 2008–2013*. 2010.
6. Mortality rate, under-5 (per 1000 live births) | Data | Table [Internet]. World Bank. [cited April 09, 2015]. Available from: http://data.worldbank.org; 2015.
7. World Health Organization. *World health statistics*; 2014.
8. MOH. *Statistical book*; 2012.
9. JPA. Total Number of Pharmacist [Internet]. Available from: http://www.jpa.org.jo/; 2014.

10. Otoom S, Batieha A, Hadidi H, Hasan M, Al-Saudi K. Evaluation of drug use in Jordan using WHO prescribing indicators. *East Mediterr Health J Rev Sante Mediterr Orient Al-Majallah Al-Sihhiyah Li-Sharq Al-Mutawassit* 2001;**8**(4–5):537–43.

11. History & Overview [Internet]. Private Hospitals Association. [cited April 09, 2015]. Available from: http://www.phajordan.org/; 2015.

12. Welcome to NCDEG | The National Center for Diabetes Endocrinology and Genetics [Internet]. National Center for Diabetes, Endocrinology and Genetics. [cited April 09, 2015]. Available from: http://www.ncd.org.jo/; 2015.

13. UNRWA [Internet]. UNRWA. [cited April 09, 2015]. Available from: http://www.unrwa.org/; 2015.

14. Jordan Red Crescent [Internet]. Jordan: Jordan Red Crescent. [cited November 17, 2013]. Available from: http://jnrcs.org/; 2015.

15. WHO | Jordan [Internet]. WHO. [cited November 17, 2013]. Available from: http://www.who.int/countries/jor/en/; 2011.

16. HHC. *Jordan National Health Accounts 2010–2011*; 2013.

17. Ajlouni Musa T. *Division of Health System and Services Development (DHS)*. August 2011.

18. NHA. *Jordanian National Health Accounts*. March 2011.

19. Conesa S, Yadav P, Bader R. *Analysis of the pharmaceutical supply chain in Jordan*. July 2009. p. 30.

20. JAPM [Internet]. Jordanian Association of Pharmaceutical Manufacturers. [cited April 09, 2015]. Available from: http://www.japm.com/; 2015.

21. Mohammad T.S. Sabbagh. Private communication of Dr. Mohammad T.S. Sabbagh, CEO of Sabdrugsz.

22. El-Dahiyat F, Kayyali R, Bidgood P. Physicians' perception of generic and electronic prescribing: a descriptive study from Jordan. *J Pharm Policy Pract* 2014;**7**(1):7.

23. Yousef A-MM, Al-Bakri AG, Bustanji Y, Wazaify M. Self-medication patterns in Amman, Jordan. *Pharm World Sci PWS* January 2008;**30**(1):24–30.

24. JFDA [Internet]. *Laws and Regulations*. Available from: http://www.jfda.jo/IF_Laws.aspx; 2015.

25. GIH. *Jordan pharmaceutical sector*; June 2007.

26. Mahasneh AM, El-Oqlah AA. Antimicrobial activity of extracts of herbal plants used in the traditional medicine of Jordan. *J Ethnopharmacol* 1999;**64**(3):271–6.

27. Afifi FU, Abu-Irmaileh B. Herbal medicine in Jordan with special emphasis on less commonly used medicinal herbs. *J Ethnopharmacol* September 1, 2000;**72**(1–2):101–10.

28. Afifi FU, Wazaify M, Jabr M, Treish E. The use of herbal preparations as complementary and alternative medicine (CAM) in a sample of patients with cancer in Jordan. *Complement Ther Clin Pract* November 2010;**16**(4):208–12.

29. Bardaweel SK, Shehadeh M, Suaifan GA, Kilani M-VZ. Complementary and alternative medicine utilization by a sample of infertile couples in Jordan for infertility treatment: clinics-based survey. *BMC Complement Altern Med* 2013;**13**(1):35.

30. Wazaify M, Alawwa I, Yasein N, Al-Saleh A, Afifi FU. Complementary and alternative medicine (CAM) use among Jordanian patients with chronic diseases. *Complement Ther Clin Pract* August 2013;**19**(3):153–7.

31. Wazaify M, Afifi FU, El-Khateeb M, Ajlouni K. Complementary and alternative medicine use among Jordanian patients with diabetes. *Complement Ther Clin Pract* May 2011;**17**(2):71–5.

32. MOH [Internet]. *Annual statistical book*. p. 292. Available from: http://www.jordan.gov.jo/; 2011.

33. Ajloni M. *Human resources for health country profile*; January 2010. p. 116.

34. MOH. *Annual statistical book*; 2013. p. 320.

35. JFDA. *Drug & Pharmacy Law* [Internet]. [cited February 04, 2015]. Available from: http://www.jfda.jo/.

36. Amwal invest. *Pharmaceutical Sector* [Internet]. p. 39. Available from: http://www.amwalinvest.com/archive; August 2010.

37. Jordan Pharmacists Association | [Internet]. Jordan Pharmacists Association | [cited April 09, 2015]. Available from: http://jpa.org.jo/; 2015.

38. Al-Lawati JA, Muula AS, Hilmi SA, Rudatsikira E. Prevalence and determinants of waterpipe tobacco use among adolescents in Oman. *Sultan Qaboos Univ Med J* 2008;**8**(1):37.

39. Lazarou J, Pomeranz BH, Corey PN. Incidence of adverse drug reactions in hospitalized patients. *JAMA J Am Med Assoc* 1998;**279**(15):1200–5.

40. Winterstein AG, Sauer BC, Hepler CD, Poole C. Preventable drug-related hospital admissions. *Ann Pharmacother* 2002;**36**(7/8):1238–48.

41. AbuRuz S, Al-Ghazawi MA, Bulatova N, Jarab AS, Alawwa IA, Al-Saleh A. Expectations and experiences of physicians regarding pharmaceutical care and the expanding role of pharmacists in Jordan. *Jordan J Pharm Sci* 2012;**5**(1).

42. AbuRuz S, Al-Ghazawi M, Snyder A. Pharmaceutical care in a community-based practice setting in Jordan: where are we now with our attitudes and perceived barriers? *Int J Pharm Pract* April 2012;**20**(2):71–9.

43. Kheir N, Zaidan M, Younes H, El Hajj M, Wilbur K, Jewesson PJ. Pharmacy education and practice in 13 Middle Eastern countries. *Am J Pharm Educ [Internet]* 2008;**72**(6). [cited July 30, 2013]. Available from: http://www.ncbi.nlm.nih.gov/.

44. Franckef DE. American Society of Hospital Pharmacists. *J Am Pharm Assoc* 2006;**34**(12):365–7.

45. Pharmacy Services, Jordan Hospital [Internet]. Pharmacy Services, Jordan Hospital. [cited April 09, 2015]. Available from: http://jordan-hospital.com/; 2015.

46. Khalidi DA, Wazaify M. Assessment of pharmacists' job satisfaction and job related stress in Amman. *Int J Clin Pharm* 2013;**35**(5):821–8.

47. Al-Shara M. Factors contributing to medication errors in Jordan: a nursing perspective. *Iran J Nurs Midwifery Res* 2011;**16**(2):158.

48. WTO I Jordan - Member information [Internet]. WTO I Jordan — member information. [cited February 22, 2014]. Available from: http://www.wto.org/.

49. OUSTR. Jordan Free Trade Agreement I Office of the United States Trade Representative [Internet]. [cited February 22, 2014]. Available from: http://www.ustr.gov/.

50. Al-Shaikh M, Torres I, Zuniga M, Ghunaim A. Jordanian pharmaceutical companies: are their marketing efforts paying off? *Health Mark Q* April 2011;**28**(2):174–89.

51. Tashtoush W. *Jordan medicine marketing in the Hashemite Kingdom of Jordan* [unpublished master's thesis]. [Mafraq.]: Al-Albeit University; 2000.

52. Mawajdeh S, Bader R, Otoum S, Jarrar L. *Medicine prices, availability and affordability in Jordan*. August 2007.

53. Al-Wazaify M, Albsoul-Younes A. Pharmacy in Jordan. *Am J Health Syst Pharm* 2005;**62**(23):2548–51.

54. Shilbayeh SA. Exploring knowledge and attitudes towards counselling about vitamin supplements in Jordanian community pharmacies. *Pharm Pract Internet* 2011;**9**(4):242–51.

55. Al-Abbadi I, Qawwas A, Jaafreh M, Abosamen T, Saket M. One-year assessment of joint procurement of pharmaceuticals in the public health sector in Jordan. *Clin Ther* 2009;**31**(6):1335–44.

56. Wazaify M, Shields E, Hughes CM, McElnay JC. Societal perspectives on over-the-counter (OTC) medicines. *Fam Pract* April 2005;**22**(2):170–6.

57. Otoom SA, Sequeira RP. Health care providers' perceptions of the problems and causes of irrational use of drugs in two Middle East countries. *Int J Clin Pract* May 2006;**60**(5):565–70.

58. El-Dahiyat F, Kayyali R. Evaluating patients' perceptions regarding generic medicines in Jordan. *J Pharm Policy Pract* June 13, 2013;**6**(1):3.

59. Musleh YA, Al-Dmour HH. Factors affecting medical representatives' performance in generic and non-generic pharmaceutical companies in Jordan: a comparative study. *Dirasat Adm Sci [Internet]* 2010;**36**(2). [cited February 03, 2015]. Available from: http://journals.ju.edu.jo/DirasatAdm/article/view/227.

60. Schott W, Stillman K, Bennett S. *Effects of the global fund on reproductive health in Ethiopia and Malawi: baseline findings*; 2005.

61. Von Muenster SJ, Carter BL, Weber CA, Ernst ME, Milchak JL, Steffensmeier JJ, et al. Description of pharmacist interventions during physician–pharmacist co-management of hypertension. *Pharm World Sci* 2008;**30**(1):128–35.

62. Westerlund T, Marklund B. Assessment of the clinical and economic outcomes of pharmacy interventions in drug-related problems. *J Clin Pharm Ther* 2009;**34**(3):319–27.

63. Al-Azzam SI, Shara M, Alzoubi KH, Almahasneh FA, Iflaifel MH. Implementation of clinical pharmacy services at a university hospital in Jordan. *Int J Pharm Pract* November 26, 2012.

64. Jarab AS, AlQudah SG, Khdour M, Shamssain M, Mukattash TL. Impact of pharmaceutical care on health outcomes in patients with COPD. *Int J Clin Pharm* February 1, 2012;**34**(1):53–62.

65. Tuffaha HW, Abdelhadi O, Omar SA. Clinical pharmacy services in the outpatient pediatric oncology clinics at a comprehensive cancer center. *Int J Clin Pharm* February 2012;**34**(1):27–31.

66. Tahaineh L, Albsoul-Younes A, Al-Ashqar E, Habeb A. The role of clinical pharmacist on lipid control in dyslipidemic patients in North of Jordan. *Int J Clin Pharm* April 2011;**33**(2):229–36.

67. Aljbouri TM, Alkhawaldeh MS, Abu-Rumman AE, Hasan TA, Khattar HM, Abu-Oliem AS. Impact of clinical pharmacist on cost of drug therapy in the ICU. *Saudi Pharm J [Internet]* December 2012. [cited September 24, 2013]. Available from: http://linkinghub.elsevier.com/retrieve/pii/S1319016412001296.

68. Mukattash TL, Nuseir KQ, Jarab AS, Alzoubi KH, Al-Azzam SI, Shara M. Sources of information used when prescribing for children, a survey of hospital based pediatricians. *Curr Clin Pharmacol* November 11, 2013.

69. Maani M, Ball D, Wazaify M. Drug information resources at community pharmacies in Amman, Jordan. *Int J Pharm Pract* June 1, 2009;**17**(3):151–5.

70. Belbeisi A, Al Nsour M, Batieha A, Brown DW, Walke HT, et al. A surveillance summary of smoking and review of tobacco control in Jordan. *Glob Health* 2009;**5**(18):18.

71. Feras Hawari, Hiba Ayub, Nour Obeidat, Malek Habashneh. Jordan guidelines for tobacco dependence treatment.

72. Jarab AS, Alqudah SG, Mukattash TL, Shattat G, Al-Qirim T. Randomized controlled trial of clinical pharmacy management of patients with type 2 diabetes in an outpatient diabetes clinic in Jordan. *J Manag Care Pharm* 2012;**18**(7):516–26.

73. Basheti IA, Qunaibi EA, Hamadi SA, Reddel HK. Inhaler technique training and health-care professionals: effective long-term solution for a current problem. *Respir Care* 2014;**59**(11):1716–25.

74. Al-Bakri AG, Bustanji Y, Yousef A-M. Community consumption of antibacterial drugs within the Jordanian population: sources, patterns and appropriateness. *Int J Antimicrob Agents* November 2005;**26**(5):389–95.

75. Albsoul Younes A, Wazaify M, Alkofahi A. Pharmaceutical care education and practice in Jordan in the new millenium. *Jordan J Pharm Sci* 2008;**1**(1):83–90.

76. The University of Jordan [Internet]. Amman: The University of Jordan. [cited February 26, 2014]. Available from: http://www.ju.edu.jo/home.aspx; 2014.

77. Jordan University of Science and Technology [Internet]. [cited April 09, 2015]. Available from: http://www.just.edu.jo/; 2015.

78. Al-Zaytoonah University of Jordan [Internet]. Al-Zaytoonah University of Jordan. Available from: http://www.zuj.edu.jo; 2015.

79. Pharmacy & Medical Sciences [Internet]. [cited February 03, 2015]. Available from: https://www.uop.edu.jo/faculties/.

80. Faculty of Pharmacy [Internet]. [cited February 03, 2015]. Available from: http://www.asu.edu.jo/Faculties/.

81. Khammash T. *The Jordanian health sector*; 2012.

82. Bulatova NR, Aburuz S, Yousef AM. An innovative pharmaceutical care practical course. *Adv Health Sci Educ* May 1, 2007;**12**(2):211–22.

83. Grissinger M. Safeguards for using and designing automated dispensing cabinets. *Pharm Ther* September 2012;**37**(9):490–530.

84. Toklu HZ, Hussain A. The changing face of pharmacy practice and the need for a new model of pharmacy education. *J Young Pharm* June 2013;**5**(2):38–40.

CHAPTER 12

Pharmacy Practice in Qatar

Nadir Kheir

Chapter Outline

Pharmacy Practice in Developing Countries. http://dx.doi.org/10.1016/B978-0-12-801714-2.00012-5

Table 1: Qatar's demographic indicators

Indicators	Year								
	2011	2010	2009	2008	2007	2006	2005	2004	2003
Population (in thousands)	1733	1715	1639	1448	1226	838	796	755	724
Natural increase rate/1000 population	10.9	10.2	10.0	10.5	11.3	14.8	14.9	15.6	16.0
Crude birth rate/1000 population	11.9	11.4	11.2	11.9	12.8	16.8	16.8	17.4	17.8
Total fertility rate (15–49) years	2.1	2.1	2.3	2.3	2.4	2.7	2.7	2.8	3.0
Life expectancy at birth									
• Male	NA	NA	NA	NA	77.8	75.9	75.3	76.8	74.4
• Female	NA	NA	NA	NA	77.9	75.7	75.8	76.5	74.7
Total	78.6	78.4	78.2	NA	77.8	75.8	75.5	76.7	74.6

Adapted from the HMC annual health report 2012.

1. Country background

The State of Qatar, an Arab Emirate that lies on the northeastern coast of the Arabian Peninsula, has a population of approximately 1.7 million people, of which approximately 80% are expatriates.[1] Gas and oil produced and exported from this small country make it one of the countries with the highest gross domestic product (GDP) per capita in the world. Qatar is also known as one of the two least-taxed sovereign states in the world.[2] Table 1 shows the demographic indicators as per the 2012 report.[3] Qatar is also a member of the Gulf Cooperation Council (GCC), which is composed of Bahrain, Kuwait, Oman, Saudi Arabia, Qatar, and United Arab Emirates (UAE), all sharing similar economic and cultural characteristics. Qatar is now considered the region's wealthiest state due to its enormous oil and natural gas revenues. As a result, the country is undergoing rapid development, which has significant implications for demographic and health indicators.[4]

Qatar is, politically, a stable middle eastern country and has not been affected by the political turbulence seen in recent years in the region. This, in part, is due to less youth unemployment, lower food price inflation, and a stable political system.[5]

2. Vital statistics

The increased population of Qatar following the oil and gas boom and the parallel developments and modernization projects reflected in a greater demand for health care services explain the rise in the number of health care providers during 2005–2015 from 4707 (1.48 health care providers per 1000 population) to 11,949 (2.24 health care providers per 1000 population).[6] In addition to the growing number of health care professionals, numerous

Table 2: Environmental burden by disease category (DALYs/1000 capita) per year

Disease	World's Lowest Country Rate	Country Rate	World's Highest Country Rate
Diarrhea	0.2	0.9	107
Respiratory infection	0.1	0.2	71
Malaria	0.0	–	34
Other vector-borne disease	0.0	–	4.9
Lung cancer	0.0	0.1	2.6
Other cancers	0.3	0.3	4.1
Neuropsychiatric disorders	1.4	1.7	3.0
Cardiovascular disease	1.4	1.7	14
COPD	0.0	0.3	4.6
Asthma	0.3	0.7	2.8
Musculoskeletal disease	0.5	0.7	1.5
Road traffic injuries	0.3	2.8	15
Other unintentional injuries	0.6	1.8	30
Intentional injuries	0.0	0.3	7.5

Source: http://www.who.int/quantifying_ehimpacts/national/countryprofile/qatar.pdf.

new internationally recognized institutions have launched their initiatives in Qatar, thus considerably improving the quality of the health care system in the country.

The crude death rate in Qatar declined from 1.88 in 2001 to around 1.15 per 1000 in 2012.[7] This reduction was accompanied by an upward shift in life expectancy at birth. The decline in the crude death rate and the increase in the life expectancy at birth reflect that Qatar is entering the age of noncommunicable disease. According to reports, there has been a massive increase in public spending on health care in Qatar, placing the country at the top of the per capita health expenditure list among the Gulf Cooperation Council.[8] This is reflected in significant low environmental burden of disease, as can be seen in Table 2.

3. Overview of the health care system

As per statistics published by the Hamad Medical Corporation (HMC),[3] the population in Qatar per physician was 444, population per general practitioner (GP) was 949, and population per hospital bed was 716. Road traffic accidents and poisoning were ranked as the leading causes of death (22.4%). The infectious disease with the highest incidence rate per 10,000 was chicken pox (39.07%). Other statistical data are shown in Table 3. Manpower in the health care sector is found in Table 4.

Compared to the 2008 numbers of manpower, in 2012 the number of medical staff working in the HMC and Supreme Council of Health (SCH) increased by 19%.[3] The number of doctors increased by 35%, dentists by 6%, and nurses by 17%.

The State of Qatar started to establish a primary health care system as early as 1954 to cope with the increase in population. In 1978, the Ministry of Health launched primary health care

Table 3: Health care statistics

Indicator	Data (2010 Statistics)
Total population	1,759,000
Life expectancy at birth M/F (years)	78/79
Probability of dying under 5 years of age (per 1000 live births)	8
Probability of dying between 15 and 60 years M/F (per 1000 population)	69/48
Total expenditure on health as % of GDP (2010)	1.8
Per capita total expenditure on health at average exchange rate (US$)	1489
Density of pharmaceutical personnel (per 10,000 population)	12.59 (2006 statistics)

Source: HMC Report, 2012.

Table 4: Health manpower indicators in the period from 2003 to 2010

Indicator	Year							
	2010	2009	2008	2007	2006	2005	2004	2003
No. of doctors per 10,000 population	31.4	20.1	22.5	20.8	27.6	26.3	25.2	22.4
No. of dentists per 10,000 population	5.7	3.7	5.6	4.0	5.2	4.9	4.2	3.9
No. of nurses per 10,000 population	59.5	48	58	56.8	73.8	72.7	62	55.8
No. of pharmacists per 10,000 population	10.9	7.0	9.1	9.6	12.6	12.4	11.2	10.1
No. of other health care providers per 10,000 population	26.0	18.9	22.4	21.7	27.1	25.8	22.1	19.8

Source: HMC Report, 2012.

services through health centers that covered various parts of the country with comprehensive health and medical services (preventive and curative). The aim was to raise the health standard of the community as a whole. These services were planned with the objective of being the first health defense line, as well as being a broad base that would provide support to the hospitals. However, primary health care services encountered many challenges during their development, ranging from overuse of hospital services for minor ailments by patients to an overall concept among health professionals that their role was only curative. Recently, Qatar launched its National Health Strategy (NHS), which is a comprehensive program of reforms aligned with the Qatar National Vision 2030 that is expected to advance Qatar's health care vision of creating a world-class, patient-centered health care system.[9] The NHS provides a guiding work plan, under seven goals, with 35 specific projects and associated implementation plans to achieve the goals of Qatar National Vision 2030. It is a strategy for reform with far-reaching and fundamental changes across Qatar's entire health care system. The NHS is very ambitious and describes the introduction of disease management, health insurance, and greater integration between the government and the private sector, all of which are expected to provide huge opportunities for the pharmacy profession but would require a highly skilled, patient-focused workforce. The strategy advocates a community pharmacy network supported by appropriate policy and process, decreasing the reliance on hospitals for filling drug prescriptions, leading to increased efficiency and enhanced access. These plans demonstrate the national leadership that will be necessary to provide the impetus for a transformation of pharmacy practice to being an effective patient-centered service provided by competent pharmacists and supported by technicians and automation.

The SCH is the executive arm of the central government authority responsible for health laws, policies, and standards, in addition to practitioner registration, certification, accreditation, and services.[10] The main (but not only) provider of health care services in Qatar is the HMC, which encompasses a national public sector hospital group that manages numerous public sector hospitals, warehouses, pharmacies, and facilities and provides shared services to these organizations.[11] Hamad General Hospital is the largest hospital under the HMC, and it provides free (for Qataris) and subsidized (for non-Qataris) health care and pharmaceutical services and products. There are around 24 primary health care centers distributed in Qatar, all of which provide primary care services, pharmacy services, and medical assistance to Qataris and the expat population in a community setting across Qatar. The number of total visits to health centers reached 3,817,356 in the year 2012, with an increase of 40.9% compared to the year 2008.[3]

Various other government or semigovernment hospitals and clinics benefit from pharmaceutical distribution services from the HMC Warehouse (e.g., Qatar Petroleum Medical Services, Sidra Medical and Research Center, Aspetar Orthopedic and Sports Medicine Hospital, and armed forces and police hospitals). Aside from pharmacies in hospitals and health clinics, pharmaceutical services are also provided from the private market, which has over 196 private community pharmacies.

The health services' private sector is witnessing rapid growth in Qatar. In 2000, the first private hospital was opened, and as of this writing, there are five private hospitals, 128 medical clinics, and over 130 dental clinics (based on 2006 statistics).[3]

Several internationally accredited recognized institutions have contributed to the improvement of Qatar's health care system since 2005. For instance, the Pasteur Institute, Imperial College, University of Pittsburgh, Weill Cornell Medical College, Heidelberg University Hospital, and Mayo Clinic have all contributed to advancing the clinical, laboratory, diagnostic, and research facilities in Qatar. Moreover, the Joint Commission International accreditation, which began in 2005, has greatly improved the quality of health care management in this country.[12] However, the expected increases in population, and the additional nine hospitals and 18 primary health care centers being developed to meet that increase, mean that significantly more health care workers, including pharmacists, will be needed. As a result, the National Health Workforce Development Advisory Committee was established in April 2012 to bring together all the health care and education and training providers in Qatar and develop and deliver the National Workforce Plan, which will identify how to manage the huge demand for skilled health workers.

A major development in health care in Qatar was the creation of the Qatar Council for Healthcare Practitioners (QCHP; http://www.nhsq.info/strategy-goals-and-projects/national-health-policy/qatar-council-for-healthcare-practitioners/qatar-healthcare-practitioners) under the SCH to ensure that the workforce in Qatar is appropriately qualified and supported to deliver a consistently high quality of patient care. This was one of the stated deliverables of the NHS, and it was established in 2013 as a nonprofit government body that regulates the health care practice and medical education in the country. One of the QCHP's departments is the accreditation department (QCHP-AD), which was formed and tasked with improving health care quality in collaboration with other stakeholders and national and international partners. The QCHP-AD started a process of accrediting medical and other health care-related educational institutes and programs to help health care practitioners to stay competent at all times. One of the three divisions of the QCHP is the Division of Medical Education and Continuing Professional Development. This division is concerned with developing mechanisms to regulate and accredit activities of medical education (or continuing professional development) and to monitor such activities to ensure their adequacy, quality, and compliance with national and international accreditation standards. The Continuing Professional Pharmacy Development Program of the College of Pharmacy at Qatar University was the first to be nationally accredited by the QCHP.

4. Medicine supply systems and drug use issues

4.1 Drug purchases

The GCC, which includes Qatar, the Kingdom of Saudi Arabia (KSA), Oman, Bahrain, Kuwait, and the UAE, coordinates medicinal purchases through a joint agreement. This arrangement has been in place since the first Ministers' Council for GCC States in 1976, with the objective of procuring some of the medicinal products that were hard to obtain because of either the small quantity needed or their high price.[12] Drug purchases are made through a joint tender undertaken by the GCC Permanent Drug Committee. This policy has ensured the use of the same drugs by all member states in terms of the manufacturing companies and led to the improvement and application of quality assurance and quality control procedures as well as drug bioequivalence across the board. In 2008, a GCC Common Market was established and is expected to increase the intra-GCC generic market imports. Two GCC countries (KSA and UAE) have predominantly generic-drug pharmaceutical industries.

4.2 Drug pricing and insurance

The number of medications (pharmacological products) registered in Qatar is around 8000 products.[3] Drug pricing in the past did not segregate between public and wholesale or between brand name medications and generics, and the earning ratios were equal. The year

2011 witnessed a strong pharmaceutical market growth due to several factors, including consumer price inflation and liberalization of pharmaceutical pricing.[5] However, since the adoption of an open market policy, prices of all medicines in Qatar have been regulated, and the SCH imposed a cap on the prices of at least 5000 registered medicines in an effort to contain inflation of prices.

The government health insurance system has been liberalized since the year 2000; and this had supported prescription drug expenditures. A national health model based on purchasing insurance covering all Qatar residents (national and expatriate populations) is due to be implemented in 2016. This new insurance system will have implications on pricing, drug policy, availability, and access in this country.[5] The plan is that Qatar's health system will make a phased transition toward a national health insurance-based model in line with Qatar's 2011–2016 health care development strategy.

4.3 Pharmaceuticals

There is still no mature drug manufacturing plant in Qatar; hence the drug market predominantly relies on drug exports. Unlike patented (branded) drugs, which have the main share of the market, generic drugs contribute a small part of the country's drug purchases. Most generics are imported from Middle Eastern manufacturers. Forecast reports estimate that by 2017, generic-drug spending will account for around 14% of all pharmaceutical spending.[5] However, Qatar has started plans for a local drug manufacturing industry, and in 2010 the first phase of a three-phase plant was opened. This could be the early beginnings of an expanded drug manufacturing market in the country, which could curb the total reliance on imported drugs and reduce drug prices.

Currently, and because of a small market and the regulation that a local agent for participating in public tenders is required, international drug manufacturers operate through a local distributor. The leading agent of international drug companies in Qatar has a market share of more than 50% and has its own chain of community pharmacies.[5]

Qatar prohibits direct-to-consumer advertising of drugs. The majority of the international pharmaceutical companies market their products in the country through a local agent (who must also be of Qatari nationality).

5. Drug- and pharmacy-related regulations, policies, and ethics
5.1 Drug-related regulations

In Qatar, as well as in the majority of the GCC countries, drugs are classified into two major classes: prescription and over the counter. Examples of prescription medicines are antibacterials (excluding metronidazole), corticosteroids (excluding inhalers, nasal sprays, 1% topical hydrocortisone ointment), dextromethorphan-containing cough preparations, PDE-5 inhibitors, androgens and growth hormones, antidepressants, and immune modulators (tacrolimus, pimecrolimus). However, and until the time of writing this chapter, most other drugs can be purchased from community pharmacies with no need for a prescription. Qatar does not allow direct-to-consumer advertising of medicines. In this, Qatar joins all the GCC countries in banning this activity. The Department of Pharmacy and Drug Control is the governmental agency responsible for drug registration in the country, herbal drugs and supplements (including natural health products), and regulations related to controlled drugs in the private market.

5.2 Pharmacy-related issues

The practice of pharmacy in Qatar has witnessed rapid change and development since around 2007 as a result of a number of national initiatives that included accreditation programs of health care services, opening (and ultimately international accreditation) of the first and only national college of pharmacy, and a trend toward recruitment of holders of advanced degrees in pharmacy practice (PharmD, masters in clinical pharmacy). From a policy point of view, Qatar's National Health Strategy of 2011–2016 articulated its goal of developing a comprehensive world-class health care system and advocated the introduction of disease management, health insurance, and greater integration between the government and the private sector.[9] The Executive Committee for the strategy described a community pharmacy network supported by appropriate policy and process, decreasing the reliance on hospitals for filling drug prescriptions, leading to increased efficiency and enhanced access.[13] A new role for community pharmacies in delivering health services in Qatar in the future is being crafted, and this shall encompass a range of areas, including developing a pharmacy network, reviewing existing laws and regulations, setting requirements for continuous professional education, and assessing the need for efficient information-technology systems. At the time of writing this chapter, the Department of Pharmacy and Drug Control is taking steps toward preparing to pilot a community pharmacy model as proposed in its Community Pharmacy Strategy (Project 1.6 in the NHS).

Because there is no autonomous professional pharmacy association or society that regulates the practice of pharmacy and represents or promotes the profession of pharmacy in Qatar,[14] these roles fall under the jurisdiction of the SCH, and a pharmacy law provides the legal framework that governs the practice. However, as part of the NHS and its associated projects, a new pharmacy law regulating pharmaceutical services will be prepared, taking into consideration the many new developments that have taken place with respect to pharmacy practice in Qatar. Project 1.6 of the NHS also recommends the development of a modern national pharmacy regulatory framework that incorporates global best practices and establishes a unified national drug information (DI) unit within the SCH made up of staff from individual hospital units. It also proposes the creation of a central database to capture all reported adverse drug events and the launch of a 24-hour hotline accessible to patients, caregivers, and all health care workers.

While the potential for witnessing a world-class pharmacy practice in Qatar within the coming years exists, however, and has a strong basis, the current pharmacy practice (especially in the community pharmacy sector) still emulates the practice elsewhere in the GCC region (both its strengths and its weaknesses).[15] Continuation of this limited role in the community and ambulatory practice can only deepen the already existing gap between pharmacists and other health care providers. For example, it had been reported that physician acceptance of specific clinical pharmacy services (e.g., advising physicians and monitoring drug regimens) was related to the exposure they already had to these contemporary pharmacy services.[16] Nevertheless, in hospitals, clinical pharmacy programs are expanding, with many pharmacists holding advanced clinical pharmacy specializations or PharmD degrees. Some pharmacists have even started asthma and diabetes management programs in some primary health care facilities. At these sites, interprofessional interactions are being realized.

In terms of the public's perception of pharmacists in Qatar, El-Hajj and colleagues reported the findings of a pilot study in which they identified a poor understanding of the role of the community pharmacist's by the public.[17] The researchers identified barriers in the patient–pharmacist interaction including insufficient contact time and unsatisfactory pharmacist knowledge.

The fifth edition of the Qatar Pharmacy Law, published first in 1983, regulates the profession of pharmacy, including issues around pharmacy personnel qualifications, pharmacy practice, ethics, and drug companies. The pharmacy law restricts the sale and preparation of any drug products to qualified pharmacists. Only Qatari nationals (over the age of 21 years) can own a pharmacy in Qatar. However, a licensed pharmacist must manage the pharmacy. The law emphasizes ethical issues in practicing pharmacy; for example, Article 8 states that "…The pharmacist should observe accuracy and trustworthy in all his dealings. He should keep the dignity of his profession. The relation between him and his colleagues should be on the basis of mutual respect and strong cooperation in the service of the patients…." However, Subarticle 8.c instructs that "a pharmacist is banned from discussing the treatment prescribed in the medical prescription with the patient or bearer of the prescription." In an environment in which pharmacists are expected to promote patient autonomy and empowerment, this clause is a demonstration of the need to update the law to reflect these contemporary pharmacy services, which Qatar has embarked on at full speed in recent years.

6. Core pharmacy practice

So far, most pharmacists practicing in Qatar are expatriates and the majority of pharmacists received their degrees in Egypt, India, or Jordan.[15] Practice opportunities resemble those in other regional countries and are primarily in private community pharmacies, publicly funded hospitals, and public health and private clinics.

6.1 Pharmacy practice research

Pharmacy practice has been rapidly advancing in all health care settings in the State of Qatar.[16,18] Nevertheless, it has been observed that pharmacists' advancement in terms of research involvement is slow compared to the pace of the current practice changes. Two Qatar-based studies (2013 and 2014) have documented the needs for research capacity building among hospital-practicing pharmacists in Qatar.[19,20]

Research efforts should align with national priorities in which pharmacists can contribute to better patient care outcomes.[21] The Hamad Medical Corporation, in alliance with the National Health Strategy, aims to be a leading health organization in the region. In addition, the NHS has clearly indicated the need to prioritize cancer and cardiovascular care research due to the high prevalence of related diseases in Qatar and the Middle East region. Awaisu and colleagues (2014) reported that the majority of pharmacists in Qatar have indicated that they did not have previous research experience, and a substantial proportion (60% of the surveyed sample) perceived a lack of adequate training as a major barrier to conducting research.[19] However, a number of structured pharmacy practice research capacity building programs for hospital pharmacists as well as other health care professionals have since been conducted or advertised.

6.2 Hospital pharmacy

Eight hospitals under the HMC provide health care services for the entire population of Qatar. Three general hospitals (Al Wakra, Al Khor, and Dukhan) care for people in densely populated areas outside Doha. The Rumailah, Women's, National Center for Cancer Care and Research (NCCCR), Hamad General, and Heart hospitals provide emergency services and specialist care, as well as treat people with specific rehabilitation needs and patients with cancer or heart conditions and provide maternity and pediatric care for women and newborns (Table 5).

The pharmacy services in the hospital sector are rapidly developing in Qatar. With the inauguration of new large hospitals (Al Wakra, Al Khor, the Heart Hospital), more pharmacists with either PharmD qualification or clinical or hospital pharmacy experience have been recruited. In 2006, a cohort of pharmacists including several Qatari nationals completed an in-house foundation program in clinical pharmacy, and over half of these are now working

Table 5: Hospitals in Qatar

Hospital	Care Category	Bed Capacity
NCCCR	Tertiary	60
Al-Wakra Hospital	General	190–260
Hamad General Hospital	Tertiary	600
Heart Hospital	Tertiary	116
Rumailah Hospital	Continuing care	520
Women's Hospital	Tertiary	330
Al Khor Hospital	General	110
Cuban Hospital	General	75

NCCCR, National Center for Cancer Care & Research.
Source: Information provided from the Office of the Executive Director of Pharmacy at Hamad Medical Corporation.

as clinical pharmacists. Several government hospitals have also motivated pharmacists to obtain advanced pharmacy degrees and attend clinical ward rounds to make real contributions to inpatient care.

Hospital pharmacy departments enjoy a degree of autonomy in running their own services within the hospital borders; but all public hospitals fall under the administrative control of the HMC, and all pharmacy directors report to an executive director of pharmacy at the HMC, who sits at the top of pharmacy services in HMC. Several specialized hospital pharmacy services have been introduced in the HMC's hospitals as mentioned in more detail elsewhere in this section.

Pharmacy personnel in all HMC pharmacy services include a skilled mix of staff pharmacists, clinical pharmacists, informatics pharmacists, pharmacy technicians, trainee pharmacists, and administrative staff. Pharmaceutical services are provided to inpatients and outpatients. Service quality standards are ensured through the use of protocols and procedures. Table 6 depicts the current numbers of pharmacists and pharmacy technicians in all HMC hospital pharmacies.

Hamad General Hospital (HGH) is the largest of all HMC hospitals and has well-established clinical pharmacy services that cover intensive care, internal medicine, surgical, and pediatric wards in addition to an emergency department. In 2013, the continuing education (CE) program at HGH was accredited by the US Accreditation Council of Pharmacy Education (ACPE). This tertiary hospital also hosts the oldest and only drug information (DI) service in the country. The DI service is run by an experienced pharmacist and a small team of pharmacists and it provides its services to HGH as well as to all HMC hospitals and clinics. The head of the DI service represents the pharmacy department at HGH on its Pharmacy and Therapeutics Committee. Drug information services were also established in other tertiary hospitals (like in Al Wakra and Al Khor hospitals).

Al Wakra Hospital, the Heart Hospital, and the NCCCR are good examples of the emerging tertiary care hospitals in the country. These Joint Commission International (JCI)-accredited

Table 6: Public hospitals and their pharmacy services

Name of Hospital	No. of Pharmacists	No. of Technicians	Total
Hamad General Hospital	163	80	243
Al Wakra Hospital	70	13	83
NCCCR[a] Hospital	31	11	42
Women's Hospital	54	6	60
Al Khor Hospital	40	17	57
Cuban Hospital	17	5	22
Rumailah Hospital	49	20	69
Heart Hospital	37	19	56

[a]NCCCR, National Center for Cancer Care & Research.
Source: Information provided from the Office of the Executive Director of Pharmacy at Hamad Medical Corporation.

multispecialty hospitals operate under the HMC umbrella. Services offered in Al Wakra include cardiology, dental care, ear, nose, and throat (ENT); general medicine; general surgery; intensive care; renal medicine (including dialysis); obstetrics and gynecology; ophthalmology; orthopedics; pediatric medicine (including intensive care); and urology. The pharmacy departments at these hospitals oversee medication procurement, storage, dispensing, and utilization throughout the hospital. Clinical pharmacy services are well established and pharmacists deliver a variety of patient-centered care. Clinical pharmacists are involved in outpatient clinics and, in the case of the Heart Hospital, they serve at the heart failure clinic and the anticoagulation clinic. There is now more focus on ambulatory and outpatient care in the Heart Hospital; clinical pharmacists also expanded their services to the cardiac rehabilitation program.

Al Wakra's pharmacy offers the first pharmacy-managed anticoagulation clinic in Qatar. It also has robotic solutions for intravenous admixture preparations, robotic dispensing, and an automated unit dose-packaging system. New services provided are patient postdischarge phone follow-up services and pictogram-aided counseling. New services planned are medication management clinics and pharmacy-centered diabetes clinics. In the NCCCR and the Heart Hospital, pharmacists routinely provide clinical pharmacy to most of the inpatients, and counseling services are well developed.

The outpatient dispensary outlets in all hospitals still constitute one of the major activities of all pharmacy staff, and through this service, medicines are procured, stored, and supplied to outpatients and discharged patients. All hospitals harbor inpatient pharmacy services, sterile compounding services, emergency pharmacy, extemporaneous preparation units, narcotics, and medical stores.

Clinical pharmacy involvement at the ward level is increasing, and the aim is to ensure the safe, effective, and economical use of drugs to all patients. Clinical pharmacists routinely provide information on drugs to the medical, nursing, and paramedical staff and patients. They also provide patient-centered services on admission, during the patient's stay, and upon discharge. Most clinical pharmacists provide discharge counseling, albeit their numbers do not cover all wards in most of the cases. The progress in clinical pharmacy is made by a regular flow of graduates from Qatar's national university and a new set of prerequisites for recruitment at the hospital pharmacy level. Clinical pharmacy experience and, in some cases, an advanced pharmacy degree (e.g., PharmD) feature in advertisement for new pharmacy posts much more than they had in the past.

All hospitals are involved in providing supervision of Qatar University's pharmacy students during their experiential training. Preceptors are recruited and provided with a structured program of supervision by the Structured Pharmacy Experiential Program Coordinator, and the program is compulsory for all students from the second to the fourth academic pharmacy years.

CE has been provided in some of the HMC hospital pharmacies since 2004.

As of this writing, the pharmacy corporation at HMC is developing a competency framework and evaluation system for pharmacists. Other pharmacy services at the HMC level include a pharmacist orientation program, accredited residency program, investigational drug services, bar coding, and smart pump projects.

It is anticipated that Qatar will open, very shortly, one of the most anticipated medical education, research, and health care centers in the country. Sidra Medical and Research Center will provide the latest in medical education and biomedical research and is planning to provide specialized care in obstetrics, gynecology, and pediatrics. Among its planned 4500 employees, Sidra will present an excellent opportunity for employment of Qatari-based clinical pharmacists and graduates from its College of Pharmacy at Qatar University.

6.3 Community pharmacy

There are more than 170 privately owned community pharmacies in Qatar. All community pharmacies recruit a mix of licensed pharmacists and pharmacy technicians and are either single or chain pharmacies. Services provided by the community pharmacies are the traditional services, which are dispensing prescribed and over-the-counter drug products and selling a range of health-related products (natural health products, supplements, nutritional products, minor/small medical devices for personal use, etc.). As of this writing, no advanced or specialized services are provided (for example, medical management or drug utilization reviews), albeit these services are being planned following the approval of Project 1.6 of the NHS. There is an expectation that the community pharmacy practice shall play a pivotal role in the future when Qatar's health strategy is fully implemented. This will be accompanied, and helped, by a new insurance policy, and patients seen at primary care facilities for minor health conditions shall utilize community pharmacies more often and be provided with high-level clinical services from the community pharmacy outlets. Table 7 provides data related to the current volume of prescription dispensed at the community pharmacies and other pharmacies.

Qatar's prescription drug market is estimated to increase from QR1.32 billion (US$363 million) in 2012 to QR2.34 billion (US$643 million) by 2017.[5]

Table 7: Prescriptions dispensed and pharmacy personnel at various pharmacies

Type of Pharmacy	Items Dispensed in 2012	Number of Pharmacies	Number of Pharmacists	Pharmacists/ Pharmacy	Items/Pharmacy/ Annum
Private	4,849,104	173	538	3.11	28,030
PHCC	6,077,742	21	171	8.14	289,416
HMC	6,495,301	25	255	10.20	259,812
Other	830,634	8	34	4.25	103,829
Total	18,252,780	227	998	4.40	1840

PHCC, Primary Health Care Corporation; HMC, Hamad Medical Corporation.
Source: Ref. 5.

7. Special pharmacy-related services

7.1 Primary health care

Primary health care (PHC) is the first level of contact for individuals, the family, and the community with the national health system and "addresses the main health problems in the community, providing health promotion, preventive, curative and rehabilitative services accordingly."[22] Pharmacists have always played a key role in primary care with respect to their traditional role in medicine supply. In so many countries, pharmacists remain the only health professional affordable and readily accessible to patients.[23] In 2001, the Board of Pharmacy Specialties in the United States of America began certification of pharmacists practicing in the area of ambulatory care. This is a more advanced role than the traditional role in which pharmacists are simply expected to react to health care decisions taken by other members of the health care team. The expectation of a contemporary ambulatory care pharmacy is one in which pharmacists become an integral part of the provision of integrated and accessible health care services. This includes roles such as addressing patient-centered medication needs, developing sustained partnerships with patients, and practicing in the context of family and community medicine. The new understanding of an ambulatory care pharmacist is one in which the pharmacist focuses on direct patient care and medication management for ambulatory patients, long-term patient–provider relationships, wellness and health promotion, triage and referral, and patient education and self-management.[24]

The place of community pharmacy in the "ambulatory" care service chain in Qatar is still ill-defined and immature. As stated elsewhere, community pharmacy still lacks any cognitive service provision such as smoking cessation, asthma (or chronic disease) clinics, and medication management. The onus is on the implementation of the NHS plans related to community pharmacies and on the efforts of individuals who might establish enhanced services in some community outlets.

On the secondary level, however, primary health care in Qatar is provided through 21 centers operating across the State of Qatar. Clinical services delivered by these centers include general practice, family medicine, cardiology, well woman care, antenatal care clinics, well baby care and vaccinations, noncommunicable disease care, dental clinics, dietary clinics, premarital examination, and ophthalmology, ENT, and audiology clinics. The pharmacy workforce comprises around 173 pharmacists distributed as shown in Table 7. A total of 47 pharmacists working at the PHC pharmacies possess some sort of postgraduate qualification (masters in clinical pharmacy, postgraduate diploma, etc.). Pharmacists provide patient counseling and drug reconciliation services. Future services include clinical pharmacy, medication use review, and medication optimization service.

7.2 Chronic disease management

To date, no specialized pharmacy cognitive services have been established in the ambulatory or community practice. In primary care, an asthma clinic has been functioning in the Qatar

Petroleum Medical Services. This asthma clinic provides asthma-specific education and management to patients presenting with asthma in the medical services of this state-owned oil and gas company. The clinic's team is composed of a clinician, a pharmacist, and a nurse. Patients are provided with tailored education, asthma medication, and asthma action plans. In PHC, plans are under way to provide medication utilization reviews. However, in the hospital sector, at least two anticoagulation clinics are functioning with a major contribution from pharmacy (http://marhaba.com.qa/anti-coagulation-clinic-opens-at-al-wakra-hospital/).

8. Pharmacy education in Qatar

8.1 Background

Qatar's only national pharmacy program was opened in 2007 at Qatar University, making it the newest public college of pharmacy in the Gulf region at the time this chapter was being written. Admission to the program requires completion of a US-based pharmacy college admission test as a component of the application process.[15] Admission also requires attending a structured interview, in addition to providing a personal statement and references. The college had secured international accreditation from the Canadian Council on Accreditation of Pharmacy Programs (CCAPP) in 2008, making it the first and only pharmacy program accredited by the CCAPP outside Canada. The college had its plans for a PharmD degree approved in early 2007 and was CCAPP-accredited in 2013. The PharmD degree program was designed to meet Western accreditation standards and to provide advanced professional training opportunities for students wishing to pursue specialized clinical careers.

The College of Pharmacy at Qatar University adopts a strategy of involvement with health care policy and practice in the country by linking with multiple practice sites and multiple local stakeholders such as hospital, community, and other pharmacy practitioners, as well as supporting organizations.[18] The deliberate strategy of adopting an intimate involvement of stakeholders in the college's plans, experiential training, and invited lectureships presents a model that is rarely seen in the region. This partnership model demonstrates concerted efforts by the college to play an effective role toward developing a practice of pharmacy of high standards in line with its vision, which is "advancing healthcare in Qatar and the world through excellence and innovation in pharmacy education, research and service."

The first baccalaureate and PharmD graduates from Qatar's College of Pharmacy entered the workforce in 2011 and 2012, respectively. As per the strategic planning of the pharmacy services at the main government provider (HMC), pharmacy technicians will start to provide most of the preparative and dispensing services and most pharmacists will be deployed to provide clinical pharmacy services using the pharmaceutical care approach outside of the pharmacy units.[18]

A pharmacy technician program has also been opened in Qatar. This program is in the Qatar branch of the College of the North Atlantic (CNA-Q), and its graduates are trained to support local pharmacists in the delivery of competent health care.[15] In 2013, the CNA-Q received accreditation by the CCAPP (in addition to the national accreditation received from the SCH), making it also the first pharmacy technician program outside Canada to be accredited by the CCAPP. As of this writing, the pharmacy technician program has 57 students enrolled, showing a 19% growth rate overall, with 25% of the students being sponsored in the current semester.

8.2 Continuing professional development

Until the development of the Continuing Professional Pharmacy Development Program (CPPD) at the College of Pharmacy (CPH) in Qatar University in 2008, there had been no national platform for professional development of pharmacists in Qatar. This made it necessary that the CPH take the lead to establish this mandate. In its strategic plan, the mandate of the CPPD emphasized the commitment of the program to the continuing professional development of pharmacists in Qatar and is aimed at supporting lifelong learning to ensure optimal patient care. Five stakeholder meetings were held to establish links and get pharmacy practitioners involved in the program. The CPPD initiated communications to plan collaborations with important health care providers in the country, especially the SCH, the Medical Education unit at HMC, and several community pharmacy groups. A nationwide survey was disseminated in October 2010 to explore the educational needs and self-perceived competency levels of pharmacists in Qatar. On June 13, 2013, the Qatar Council for Health Practitioners at the SCH officially declared the CPPD of the College of Pharmacy accredited as a provider of continuous medical education and professional development for health practitioners. This makes Qatar University College of Pharmacy's CPPD the first accredited continuous professional pharmacy development provider in Qatar. Additionally, in March 2014 the ACPE awarded the CPPD accreditation as a Continuing Professional Development (CPD) provider. Recently, the name of the CPPD program of the College of Pharmacy was changed into the Continuing Professional Development to emphasizes its interprpfessional nature.

8.3 Interprofessional education

Accreditation standards for the various professions now list interprofessional education experiences as an integral component of any education program in health care. To contribute to the maturation of the skill and attitude of effective interprofessional collaboration, CNA-Q conducts an annual health sciences skills competition, the only event of its kind in the region. This initiative has helped increase interaction and sharing of knowledge and expertise among students of different disciplines, including Qatar University's College of Pharmacy, the College of Arts and Sciences' Human Nutrition and Public Health, the University of Calgary–Qatar's School of Nursing, and CNA-Q's pharmacy technician program.

8.4 Simulation in education

There is an increasing recognition in Qatar of the importance of simulation in health sciences education. Simulation techniques are now widely perceived as a valid, viable, and frequently preferred means of teaching and evaluating competence in health care professions. This is especially true in instances in which interdisciplinary learning experiences continue to grow. As a result, the Qatar Simulation Consortium was established, with representation from the Sidra Medical and Research Center, the University of Calgary's (Qatar) School of Nursing, Weill Cornell's (Qatar) School of Medicine, and Qatar University's School of Pharmacy. The consortium continues to flourish, and before long, it is hoped that students from these disciplines shall experience shared learning in an environment supported by simulation technology in addition to other proven teaching and learning strategies.

9. Achievements

- So far, the most significant achievement in pharmacy practice in this country could be considered the sharp rise in the number of pharmacists who have either completed postgraduate courses in pharmacy practice or subscribed to higher degrees while practicing pharmacy in Qatar. A qualified workforce forms a strong foundation that is needed to elevate the standard and status of pharmacy. There are several factors that could be attributed to the phenomenon we are witnessing in this respect. One factor is the competitive environment created by a stream of young graduates from a local, but internationally accredited, pharmacy program. The mere presence of graduates who have received pharmacy syllabi that are contemporary and advanced presents a motive for existing pharmacists to seek higher qualifications that would help them provide services comparable to those provided by their younger but highly capable peers. Another factor that could explain this phenomenon is the new emerging health care environment created by the launching of the NHS and the impending plans for a new set of licensing requirements that demand a high level of skills and expertise from pharmacists applying for license renewal or registration to practice.
- The speed of the introduction of clinical pharmacy services in the hospital sector is another achievement. Clinical pharmacy practice has been embraced in several hospitals, and new recruitment requirements that include clinical pharmacy experience are emerging as a result.
- Finally, more pharmacy services are being accredited as CPD providers, and more pharmacists attend CE activities. This is a sign of quality and commitment to lifelong learning. It is another important element that ensures the creation of a strong and committed pharmacy workforce in Qatar.

10. Challenges

- It could be argued that the most important challenge facing pharmacy practice in Qatar is to maintain and build on the advances achieved so far. There is undoubtedly a rapid development in clinical pharmacy expansion, continuing professional development, and best pharmacy practices brought about by active accreditation processes and the establishment of Qatar's National College of Pharmacy.

- The NHS was also a powerful driver for the change, backed by a clear political will. But these achievements and developments require a good deal of focused effort to take them forward and to be able to identify their key performance indicators to keep track of their progress.
- Another likely challenge is the complete integration of pharmacy (and pharmacists) into a health care formula that had traditionally perceived pharmacy as a profession that circles around drug inventories and availability. While this perception is rapidly being replaced by one that recognizes pharmacists as health care workers with unique skills and expertise with regard to medications and their utilization, this change of heart is still limited to the large and emerging hospitals. Much work needs to be done to provide evidence supporting a new image. New generations of graduates from medical, nursing, and pharmacy programs that share classrooms and projects in interprofessional undergraduate education environments, a practice that has already started in Qatar, will help remove the barriers and misconceptions.
- Most importantly, the immediate challenge facing any future plans for contemporary pharmacy practice that falls in line with the ambitions of Qatar's NHS is harmonizing visions and efforts of the various directorates within the SCH so they could work synergistically to make the required changes. While a degree of autonomy and independence is always a health sign, this independence should not be a hindrance, but rather a strength.

11. Recommendations: way forward

- Qatar's health care is moving in the right direction. Pharmacy in Qatar is rapidly changing and pharmacists are embracing a new culture of lifelong learning and commitment for self-development.
- However, these exciting developments require a great deal of committed effort to follow them through. Fortunately, Qatar does not lack the financial resources to sustain the successes achieved so far and to build on them.
- The community pharmacy practice is poised to play a pivotal role in the near future when Qatar moves toward a primary health care model. For community pharmacy services to play the role articulated in the approved strategic plans, radical changes have to be made. An advanced information technology that supports seamless patient care must be built and piloted. Advanced and enhanced pharmacy practice services have to be planned and pharmacists trained to apply the skills required for these services to take place.
- The current pharmacy law has to be revised and updated, and a set of pharmacy regulations should be written and enforced. Competency standards should be developed or adapted, and pharmacists should receive the necessary information and training on how to apply the required standards in their practice.
- As these activities take place, pharmacy in primary health care and the hospitals must continue its efforts toward excellence in practice while acknowledging the new role of the community pharmacy practice in an integrated health care environment. A new culture of continuity of care should be targeted.

- The way forward, in a nutshell, requires total awareness of the requirements and promises for a world-class health care system and deliberate and harmonized effort to achieve it.

12. Conclusions

Qatar is positioning itself to be specialized in education and health care and to act as a bridge between the GCC and the rest of the world. The country is actively working through a strategic plan to turn an oil-dependent economy into an economy that is found on high-quality education, health services, and knowledge-based specialties, including research in biomedical sciences. The health care system of Qatar is focused on its mandates, and a national health strategy guides its development. For the first time, pharmaceutical services are placed at the heart of the strategic plans for a strong primary care system, and the evidence shows that steps are being taken to meet this mandate. It would not be surprising if, in few years, we see Qatar's health care, and specifically pharmacy practice, presenting itself as a model in the region. However, there are challenges facing the ambitious plans, and these must be tackled.

13. Lessons learned/points to remember

- Qatar's health care, and pharmacy practice as an integral part of it, is advancing rapidly.
- Pharmacy practice is changing and this change is supported by many enabling factors, mainly, focused leadership, a vibrant profession, and a continuous flow of fresh graduates from an accredited national pharmacy college.
- The rapid change is faced by a set of challenges, and these must be confronted and addressed.

Acknowledgments

The author acknowledges and thanks Dr Moza Sulaiman H. Al Hail (Executive Director of Pharmacy, HMC, Doha, Qatar) for facilitating the provision of information and data related to hospital pharmacies in Qatar.

References

1. Qatar Information Exchange [Internet]. *Population.* [cited October 13, 2013]. Available from: http://www.qix. gov.qa/portal/page/portal/qix/subject_area?subject_area=176; 2011.
2. Maps of the world.com. *Qatar GDP.* [cited November 14, 2013]. Available from: http://www.mapsofworld. com/qatar/economy/gdp.html; 2011.
3. Qatar. *Hamad Medical Corporation annual health report 2012.* Department of Epidemiology and Medical statistics. Doha: HMC; 2013.
4. Alrouh H, Ismail A, Cheema S. Demographic and health indicators in Gulf Cooperation Council nations with an emphasis on Qatar. *J Local Glob Health Perspect* 2013;**2013**:3.
5. *Qatar pharmaceuticals and health care report.* Business Monitor International; 2013.
6. Bener A, Ma Al. Health services management in Qatar. *Croat Med J* February 2010;**51**(1):85–8.
7. Qatar Statistical Authority (QSA) [Internet]. Doha [cited September 14, 2014]. Available in: http://www.qsa. gov.qa/QatarCensus/GeneralInfo.aspx on the 2 September 2012; 2012.

8.   Hamad Medical Corporation [Internet]. [cited October 13, 2014]. Available from: http://www.hamad.qa/en/press/healthcare_in_qatar/healthcare_in_qatar.aspx.

9.   National Health Strategy [Internet]. Doha: Supreme Council of Health [cited June 19, 2012]. Available from: http://www.nhsq.info/; 2011.

10.   Qatar. Supreme Council of Health. Available from: http://www.sch.gov.qa/sch/En/scontent.jsp?smenuId=46; 2012.

11.   AMEInfo.com. Hamad Medical Corporation globally recognized. http://www.ameinfo.com/108288.html; 2012.

12.   The Executive Board of the Health Ministers' Council of the GCC States [Internet]. [cited September 21, 2014]. Available from: http://sgh.org.sa/enus/grouppurchasing/whatisgrouppurchasing.aspx.

13.   Executive Committee, S. H. C. *Qatar national health strategy 2011–2016*; 2011.

14.   Wilbur K. Continuing professional pharmacy development needs assessment of Qatar pharmacists. *Int J Pharm Pract* 2010;**18**(4):236–41.

15.   Kheir N, Zaidan M, Younes H, El Hajj M, Wilbur K, Jewesson P. Pharmacy education and practice in 13 Middle Eastern countries. *Am J Pharm Educ* 2009;**72**(6):1–13.

16.   Zaidan M, Singh R, Wazaify M, Tahaineh L. Physicians' perceptions, expectations, and experience with pharmacists at Hamad Medical Corporation in Qatar. *J Multidiscip Healthc* 2011;**4**:85–90.

17.   El Hajj MS, Salem S, Mansoor H. Public's attitudes towards community pharmacy in Qatar: a pilot study. *Patient Prefer Adherence* 2011;(5):405–22. http://dx.doi.org/10.2147/PPA.S22117. Available from: http://www.dovepress.com/publicrsquos-attitudes-towards-community-pharmacy-in-qatar-a-pilot-stu-peer-reviewed-article-PPA.

18.   Kheir N, Fahey M. Pharmacy practice in Qatar: challenges and opportunities. *South Med Rev* 2011;**4**:45–9.

19.   Awaisu A, Bakdach D, Elajez RH, Zaidan M. Hospital pharmacists' self-evaluation of their competence and confidence in conducting pharmacy practice research. *SPJ* 2014. http://dx.doi.org/10.1016/j.jsps.2014.10.002.

20.   Elkassem W, Pallivalapila A, Al Hail M, McHattie L, Diack L, Stewart D. Advancing the pharmacy practice research agenda: views and experiences of pharmacists in Qatar. *Int J Clin Pharm* 2013;**35**(5):692–6.

21.   Allen SJ, Christensen D, Clark TR, Eckel VF, Gouveia WA, Hay JW, et al. Advancing pharmacy practice through research: a 2004 perspective. *J Am Pharm Assoc* 2004;**44**(5):621–8.

22.   WHO. *Declaration of Alma-Ata (International Conference on Primary Health Care, Alma-Ata, USSR, September 6–12, 1978)*. [cited September 27, 2014]. Available from: URL: http://www.who.int/publications/almaata_declaration_en.pdf?ua=1.

23.   Smith F. Private local pharmacies in low-and-middle income countries: a review of interventions to enhance their role in public health. *Trop Med Int Health* 2009;**14**(3):362–72.

24.   Board of Pharmacy Specialists. Available from: http://www.bpsweb.org/specialties/AmbulatoryCarePharmacy.cfm [accessed 10.05.14, (Archived by WebCite® at http://www.webcitation.org/6PSla13FY)].

CHAPTER 13

Pharmacy Practice in Palestine

Waleed M. Sweileh, Sa'ed H. Zyoud, Mahmoud S. Al-Haddad

Chapter Outline

1. Country background

The occupied Palestinian territories (OPT) are a small area in the Middle East, west of the Jordan River.[1,2] The two geographical areas that make up the OPT are the West Bank (including East Jerusalem) and the Gaza Strip. The Israeli occupation of these territories started after the Six-Day War in 1967.[1] The international community has denied the Israeli occupation of the Palestinian territories and uses the phrase OPT to describe them.[3] Parts of the OPT came under the legal and political control of the Palestinian National Authority (PNA) after the Oslo Accords in 1993.[2] Israeli occupation and its full military control are still present in 61% of the West Bank (Area C). As of this writing, parts of the West Bank area are under the control of the PNA, while the Gaza Strip split from the Palestinian Authority in 2007 after the internal conflict between different Palestinian parties. From 1948 until 1967,

Pharmacy Practice in Developing Countries. http://dx.doi.org/10.1016/B978-0-12-801714-2.00013-7

the West Bank was under the control of Jordan, and the Gaza Strip was under the control of Egypt, although limited authority had been exercised in Gaza by the All-Palestine Government from September 1948 until 1959. Before 1948, the West Bank and Gaza Strip were part of Mandatory Palestine under British governance, formed in 1922. According to the Palestinian Central Bureau of Statistics, the total number of Palestinian people in 2011 was 4,168,858. Gender distribution is as follows: 50.8% are males and 49.2% are females. Age distribution shows that 2.9% of the Palestinian population is above 65 years of age.[1] In 2011, the reported natural increase in population, crude birth rate, and fertility rate were 2.9%, 29.1/1000, and 4.3, respectively.[4] Almost all Palestinians belong to one ethnic group, which is Arabic ethnicity. According to World Bank data, the gross domestic product (GDP) for the West Bank and Gaza Strip was US$11.26 billion in 2012, while the GDP growth rate was −4.4% and the rate of inflation was 2.8% in 2009.[5]

2. Vital health statistics

The health status and health services in Palestine were discussed in detail in a series of publications in the journal *Lancet* by a public health research team at Birzeit University[2] as well as by the annual health report published by the Palestinian Ministry of Health (MOH).[6] Many fatal and disfiguring infectious diseases such as schistosomiasis, leprosy, diphtheria, plague, poliomyelitis, and rabies have been eliminated from Palestine. Few cases of other infectious diseases, such as meningococcal meningitis, brucellosis, HIV/AIDS, hepatitis, tuberculosis, diarrhea, and pneumonia, are still present in Palestine. Immunization coverage is close to 100% in Palestine.[7]

The major health burden in Palestine is the noncommunicable diseases, such as cardiovascular diseases, hypertension, diabetes, and cancer. In 2006, the rate of reported hypertension and diabetes was higher than 10%.[4,8] Cross-sectional studies done in Ramallah governorate showed a rate of diabetes mellitus between 9.8 and 12% at ages 30–65 years.[9–11] In 2011, the cancer incidence rate was 64.2 per 100,000 of population, with breast cancer ranking first, followed by colon and stomach cancer. Reports from the MOH showed that the rate of cancer incidence and mortality is on the rise.[6]

According to the Palestinian MOH, there has been a progressive decline in the crude death rate over the years. The crude death rate in 2011 was 2.6 and 2.7 per 1000 of population in the Gaza Strip and West Bank, respectively. In 2011, the infant mortality rate was reported to be 18.8 per 1000 live births. The top leading causes of death in the West Bank as reported in 2011 were cardiovascular diseases followed by cancer and cerebrovascular diseases.[6]

3. Overview of the health care system

The key player in health services in Palestine is the Palestinian government through the MOH. Many pharmaceutical departments are available within the MOH to ensure the enforcement of MOH laws and legislation and to enhance the quality of pharmaceutical services provided to patients. These departments are the Dangerous Drugs Department, Drug Control Department,

Table 1: Numbers of health personnel in Palestine[1]

Specialty	Palestine	Ministry of Health
Physicians	8093	3124
Dentists	2117	285
Pharmacists	4084	412
Nurses	7010	3572
Midwives	577	284

Drug Import and Export Department, Pharmaceutical Policy Department, Quality Control Department, and Drug Registration Department.[6] All these departments work hand in hand to control the drugs available on the Palestinian market and to monitor all practices by pharmaceutical institutions. Therefore, this would protect patients and enhance the quality of all the services provided to them. Other major providers of health in Palestine include the United Nations Relief and Works Agency for Palestine Refugees in the Near East (UNRWA), Palestinian nongovernmental organizations (NGOs), Palestinian Military Medical Services (PMMS), and private for-profit organizations. The bulk of health services and health expenditures are provided by the Palestinian MOH through 458 primary health care centers distributed throughout Gaza and the West Bank. The international refugee agency UNRWA operates 102 primary health care centers that provide free medical services to Palestinians in refugee camps in Gaza and in the West Bank.[12] The NGO sector operates 206 primary health care centers and general clinics, while the PMMS operates 23 primary health care centers and clinics distributed through different districts in the West Bank and Gaza Strip.[6] There are 81 governmental hospitals in Palestine. The total number of beds in governmental and nongovernmental hospitals is 5414, with an average of 13 beds per 10,000 inhabitants.[1] The majority of these beds are general, while less than 25% of beds are specialized.[6] Overall, there are 4048 licensed pharmacists, 8093 physicians, and 7587 nurses and midwifery personnel in Palestine. This means that there are 10 pharmacists, 20 physicians, and 18.7 nurses per 10,000 population in Palestine.[13] Table 1 shows the number of health personnel in Palestine as reported in 2011.[1] According to the National Health Accounts 2000–2008 report published in 2011, Palestinian health expenditures increased from 400 million New Israeli Shekels (NIS) in 2000 to NIS900 million in 2008 (US$1.00=NIS3.58 in 2008). In addition, according to the same report, the health expenditure percentage of the GDP increased from 9.5% in 2000 to 15.6% in 2008.[14]

4. Medicine supply systems and drug use issues

In Palestine there are five manufacturers of drugs for human use, which cover approximately 50% of the local pharmaceutical market. All five are in the West Bank; one was in the Gaza Strip, but it is no longer functioning owing to Israeli restrictions on goods allowed to enter Gaza. The major Palestinian pharmaceutical companies are Quds Pharmaceuticals (Jepharm), Birzeit Pharmaceuticals, Beit Jala Pharmaceuticals, and Pharmacare Pharmaceuticals.[15] The Paris Protocol and joint Customs Envelope, which outlined the economic relations between Israel and Palestine, have many implications for the Palestinian pharmaceutical market. The joint Customs Envelope has maintained free one-way flow for Israeli manufacturers as well as foreign companies licensed in Israel into the Palestinian market.[16] These agreements have resulted in a deterioration of the Palestinian pharmaceutical industry. Furthermore, the joint Customs Envelope has contributed to the developing Israeli pharmaceutical market and deteriorating Palestinian pharmaceutical industry by applying Israeli standards on importing and exporting pharmaceutical products and raw materials to and from Palestine. Palestinian manufacturers have to obtain a license and approval from Israeli authorities prior to importing or exporting drugs to or from Palestine.[17] Therefore, to import drugs from any country, a Palestinian agent has first to register the products in Israel. This has resulted in the absence of cheap generics from China, India, or Eastern Europe from the Palestinian market, since Israel registers products mainly from Western countries. In addition, this has resulted in the loss of the neighboring markets in Israel and in the Arab countries. Israeli delegates have to visit the manufacturing institutions as a requirement of the registration process. However, Israeli inspectors refuse to inspect Palestinian pharmaceutical companies owing to security reasons. In addition, Arab countries refuse to send delegates to an occupied country.[16] Long procedures and restrictions for importing and exporting drugs and raw materials have presented real challenges for local manufacturers. The joint Customs Envelope also raised the prices of drugs in Palestine since Palestine was considered to be in the same socioeconomic zone as Israel, whereas in reality, there is a big difference in terms of socioeconomic level between Israel and Palestine. This has resulted in equal pricing of imported drugs from multinational companies in Palestine and Israel. Owing to the trade barriers mentioned earlier and the absence of real competition, the MOH procurement prices are 4.4 times higher than UNRWA prices and 7 times higher than the international procurement prices, with a total of US$105 million spent in 2005 on pharmaceutical products, which amounts to 20% of the MOH budget on health expenditures. It must be mentioned that medicines available in the public sector are bought through government tenders. Drug prices are normally higher in Palestine compared to the neighboring Arab countries.[18] The lowest generic product in the West Bank public sector was 4.5 times higher than that in countries with the same level of GDP, such as Syria. This has resulted in a high percentage of the Palestinian population being unable to afford medicines in the private sector, as around 47% of the population is below the poverty line. Drug prices are fixed throughout the country, by which a sticker obtained from the Palestinian Pharmacist Union is fixed on the medicine package indicating its price. Retail markups of medicines are regulated by the MOH in agreement with the Palestine Pharmacists' Association (PPA). An average of 25% markup is given to locally manufactured products and 10–15% is given to imported products.[18] Approximately 50% of the pharmaceutical market in Palestine is held by Israeli and foreign pharmaceutical companies. The major foreign pharmaceutical contributors are Teva and Novartis.

5. Overview of pharmacy practice and key pharmaceutical sectors

Modern pharmacies in Palestine began in the 1920s. Before then, pharmacy practice focused mainly on folk and traditional medicines through special shops, which continued to exist in the form of herbalists. Among the first Palestinian pharmacists was Dr Fakhri Jdai, who started the pharmacy profession in Yafa in 1923.[19] In 1957, the Jordanian Pharmaceutical Association (JPA) was established with two operating centers, one in Amman and one in Jerusalem. Since both Jordan and the West Bank of Palestine were under Jordanian rule, Palestinian and Jordanian pharmacists had to register at the JPA to become licensed for work in the pharmacy profession. In 1973, and as a consequence of the physical separation of Jordan and Palestine by the Israeli occupation, a branch of the JPA located in East Jerusalem started functioning to serve Palestinian pharmacists and to organize the pharmacy profession in the West Bank. From the 1940s until the 1980s, most Palestinian pharmacists obtained their pharmacy professional degree from the American University of Beirut or Damascus University, or the University of Cairo. As of this writing, there is no published code of ethics for pharmacists in Palestine. Furthermore, there is no set of competency standards to evaluate pharmacists who graduate from different countries. The current Palestinian pharmacy legislation focuses on pharmacy and the pharmacist registration process, structure and area of the pharmacy premises, and controlled drug regulations.[20] However, the Palestinian legislation barely focuses on standard pharmacy practice. According to a 2011 health report, there were 4048 licensed pharmacists, at a ratio of pharmacists to population of 100:100,000. Of these, 412 were working in the governmental sector. There were approximately 1000 pharmacy technicians and assistants in Palestine. Most of them work in the private sector.[13]

6. Drug- and pharmacy-related regulations, policies, and ethics

The PPA is the organizational body of pharmacists in Palestine. This body was established in 1957 as a joint body with the pharmaceutical association in Amman, Jordan. The PPA has recently adopted new regulations regarding pharmacy practice, particularly those pertaining to establishing a private community pharmacy service. The regulations were set so that one community pharmacy per approximately 3000 inhabitants is permitted to be established. The regulations also include the physical specifications of the premises, whether it is a private community pharmacy or a drugstore. Such specifications include area, distance from nearest community pharmacy, and qualifications of pharmacist in charge. The PPA has a set of ethics upon which pharmacists' conduct should be judged. The General Directorate of Pharmacy in the MOH functions nationally to perform the following functions that address pharmaceutical regulations: marketing authorization/registration, inspection, import control, licensing, market control, quality control, medicine advertisement and promotion, clinical trial control, and pharmacovigilance. Registration of medicines in Palestine does not follow the mutual recognition mechanisms. Therefore, pharmaceutical products need to be registered before marketing. The number of registered pharmaceutical products in Palestine is approximately 7000 (http://pharmacy.moh.ps/index/RegisteredProducts/Language/ar). Regulations regarding governmental inspections of the pharmaceutical market and activities are also available. Inspection includes local manufacturers, public pharmacies and stores, private wholesalers, retail distributors, and pharmacies and dispensing points in health facilities.[13,21] There are also regulations pertaining to import of medicines. However, there are no regulations regarding inspection of imported pharmaceutical products at authorized ports of entry. Pharmaceutical activities in Palestine require licensing from the Palestinian MOH. Licensing is granted for importers, wholesalers, and distributors. Domestic and international manufacturers have to comply with good manufacturing practices (GMP) per governmental regulations. However, no regulations regarding good distribution or good pharmacy practice exist. Limited quality control testing for pharmaceutical products present in the Palestine market is available. Such limited testing is performed through collection of samples from the market by governmental inspectors.[22] It has been reported that 4% of the collected samples fail to meet the quality standards. Pharmaceutical promotion in Palestine is not regulated. Furthermore, there is no national code of conduct concerning advertising and pharmaceutical promotion. Regarding controlled medicines, morphine, fentanyl, and pethidine are the most commonly reported controlled medicines in Palestine.[23] Although Palestine is a signatory of several international conventions regarding narcotic drugs, there are no laws regarding the control of narcotics and psychotropic drugs.[23]

7. Core pharmacy practices

7.1 Hospital pharmacy

There is no documented history of hospital services in Palestine. However, based on personal communications with senior physicians, it is believed that hospital services in Palestine started as early as 1900 in some major cities in Palestine, such as Yafa. The current status of hospital services in Palestine is shown in Table 2.[1]

As of this writing, all hospitals have a pharmacy department; however, very few offer clinical pharmacy services inside the hospital. Actually, hospital pharmacy in Palestine is not a well-defined subsection of pharmacy practice. Hospital pharmacy is seen mainly in governmental hospitals. Such hospital pharmacies have a small window for dispensing medications for in- and outpatients. No or limited patient counseling or pharmaceutical care services or pharmacy research activities are performed by hospital pharmacies in Palestine. Furthermore, compounding activities are very limited and pharmacists try to avoid compounding, especially in chemotherapy preparations. Nurses are more involved in chemotherapy preparation than pharmacists in the Palestinian governmental hospitals. Several projects have been carried out to upgrade such activities, including the rational drug use project funded by the French Agency. The rational use of medicines project funded by the French government focused on training governmental pharmacists, including hospital pharmacists, on rational drug use and chemotherapy preparation.[24]

7.2 Industrial pharmacy

Industrial pharmacy in Palestine has witnessed a great advancement in the past 20 years. Table 3 shows the list of current pharmaceutical manufacturers in Palestine with their year of establishment.[1] Palestinian pharmaceutical companies have obtained local certificates of ISOs and GMP.[13] Pharmacare, Birzeit-Palestine, and Jerusalem Pharmaceutical companies have

Table 2: Number of hospitals in Palestine and indicator of hospital quality as reported in 2011[1]

Indicator/Palestine, 2010	Palestine	Ministry of Health
No. of hospitals	76	25
Population/hospital ratio	53,268	161,936
No. of beds	51,105	3.002
Population bed ratio	807	1349
Beds per 10,000 population	12.6	7.4

Table 3: List of pharmaceutical companies in Palestine

Company	Location	Year Established
Jordan Chemical Laboratory	Beit Jala/Bethlehem	1968
Jerusalem Pharmaceutical Company	Al-Bireh/Ramallah	1969
Birzeit-Palestine Pharmaceutical Company	Birzeit/Ramallah	1973
Pharmacare	Beitunia/Ramallah	1986
Medical Arab Supply Company	Gaza	1981

succeeded in exporting medicines to Africa, Europe, and Russia. Most pharmaceutical manufacturers in Palestine lack research and development as well as discovery of new drug entities. Furthermore, Palestine lacks manufacturing capabilities of pharmaceutical raw materials. However, all Palestinian pharmaceutical companies have the capability to produce formulations and repackage finished dosage forms.

7.3 Community pharmacy

Community pharmacy in Palestine is still traditional. There are approximately 1000 community pharmacies in West Bank and East Jerusalem. There are no chain pharmacies in Palestine. However, several trials were made to initiate such activity in the past. Most pharmacists working in community pharmacies in Palestine are graduates of Palestinian national universities. No professional development or continuing pharmacy education exists for community pharmacists in Palestine. Community pharmacies in Palestine are engaged mainly in dispensing medications, and most drugs, including antibiotics, are dispensed as nonprescription. Self-medication is common practice in Palestine, and in most cases, community pharmacists are the first-line health care providers for most people with minor aliments or for medical consultation.[25–27] According to regulations, all community pharmacies must have a laboratory area for compounding. However, compounding practices are very limited in Palestine.[28] Female pharmacists are dominating the scene in community pharmacies in Palestine. According to regulations, only pharmacists can own a community pharmacy and only those with no other full-time job are allowed and granted permission to own a community pharmacy.

7.4 Medicine marketing and promotion

Medicine marketing and promotion have witnessed great advancement since 2005. In the past, most medical representatives were chemists and biologists. Currently, there are hundreds of pharmacists working as medical representatives for local and international manufacturers. Medical representatives for foreign companies receive good training in pharmaceutical promotion and marketing compared to those working in local pharmaceutical companies. Promotion is mainly through free medical samples for physicians and scientific conferences and workshops held by a pharmaceutical association or physician association. For community pharmacists, promotion is made through the bonus policy, which creates a good profit margin. Prices of medicines in Palestine are fixed through an official label on the product. The most commonly dispensed drugs in Palestine are antibiotics and analgesics.[29] Most expensive drugs, such as chemotherapy drugs, are available through medical insurance from governmental pharmacy services.

8. Special pharmacy-related services and activities

In 2006, An-Najah National University established the first poison control and drug information center (PCDIC) in Palestine. The PCDIC was established by Dr Ansam Sawalha, who is a pioneer in toxicology and poisoning.[30] The center is run by clinical toxicologists, pharmacists, and researchers.[31] The PCDIC offers free telephone services both to the public and to the medical community. The PCDIC is the first and only specialized center in Palestine that offers such services. During its first years of establishment, the PCDIC received thousands of calls regarding medical poisoning and emergency treatment of such cases. The center is also engaged in clinical toxicology research and pharmacoepidemiology activities. The PCDIC is also working on improving awareness regarding toxic and hazardous materials through its annual poison prevention week held each April. The PCDIC is run by a clinical toxicologist and a group of consultants in the fields of pharmacology and pharmacy, herbal specialists, clinical pharmacists, pediatric specialists, and others.[30] In Palestine, there is no specialized pharmacovigilance center or adverse drug reaction (ADR) advisory committee. However, the Palestinian MOH has developed an official standardized form for reporting ADRs. No database is available nationally or at the MOH level pertaining to ADR data.

Research in pharmacy practice in Palestine was initiated by a group of researchers at An-Najah University. The group has published many articles in the field of pharmacy practice, pharmacy education, clinical pharmacology/toxicology, and public health. However, research in pharmacy practice in Palestine still needs more efforts to reshape the profession in the future.

9. Pharmacy education

Pharmacy education in Palestine started in the mid-1990s (Table 4). The initiative to start pharmacy education in Palestine was begun in early 1990 at An-Najah National University in Nablus and Al-Azhar University in the Gaza Strip. As of this writing, there are four

Table 4: Pharmacy programs offered in universities in Palestine[32-36]

University Name	Faculty Name	Year Established	University Type	Pharmacy Degrees Offered	Curriculum–Credit Hours
Al-Azhar University–Gaza	Faculty of Pharmacy	1992	Public, nonprofit	• Bachelor in Pharmacy. • M.Sc. in Pharmacy in all the above majors. • M.Sc. in Clinical Nutrition	B.Sc. 170
An-Najah National University–Nablus	College of Medicine and Health Sciences/ Department of Pharmacy	1994	Public, nonprofit	• Bachelor in Pharmacy. • Doctor of Pharmacy • M.Sc. in Pharmacy in Pharmaceutical Sciences • M.Sc. in Clinical Nutrition	B.Sc. 170 PharmD 240
Birzeit University–Birzeit	Faculty of Nursing, Pharmacy, and Health Professions	2009	Public, nonprofit	• Doctor of Pharmacy	210
Al-Quds University–Jerusalem	Faculty of Pharmacy	2002	Public, nonprofit	• Bachelor in Pharmacy.	172
Hebron University–Hebron	College of Pharmacy & Medical Science	2010	Public, nonprofit	• Bachelor in Pharmacy.	172

universities in the West Bank that offer pharmacy education and one in the Gaza Strip. An-Najah National University (established in 1994), Al-Quds University (established in 2002), Birzeit University (established in 2010), and Hebron University (in the process of starting a pharmacy program) all have pharmacy programs. The program in the Gaza Strip is at Al-Azhar University.[32-36] Table 4 shows a list of universities in the West Bank, year of establishment, types of pharmacy degrees offered, and number of credit hours in their pharmacy curriculum.[32-36] Prior to 1994, most pharmacists working in the West Bank studied and were trained outside Palestine, mainly in Jordan, Syria, and Egypt. The four pharmacy schools in the West Bank have a 5-year bachelor of science (B.Sc.) program, which requires the completion of at least 10 full semesters with a total of 163–176 credit hours and 1440 h of training at community pharmacies, hospitals, or industry. Birzeit University has a pharmacy doctor program and does not have a B.Sc. degree in pharmaceutical sciences. An-Najah University has B.Sc. in pharmacy and PharmD programs. Most students in colleges of pharmacy in Palestine are females. In general, students who enroll in the B.Sc. 5-year program study basic sciences such as mathematics, chemistry, and physics in the first year of study. During the following 4 years of study, pharmacy students take biomedical and pharmaceutical courses. All pharmacy students in Palestinian universities are required to finish a total of 1444 practical hours in any pharmacy settings before graduation. The language used in teaching in all pharmacy programs is English. The College of Pharmacy at An-Najah University is being restructured to be a division of the College of Medicine and Health Sciences. The PharmD program at Birzeit University is structured to be part of the College of Nursing, Pharmacy, and Health Sciences. The other colleges of pharmacy in Palestine exist as independent colleges. The concept of department is being remodeled at the pharmacy program at An-Najah University with three general departments: pharmaceutical technology, clinical pharmacy, and pharmaceutical chemistry. At Al-Azhar University, they have departments similar to those at An-Najah University in addition to a pharmacology/toxicology department. The other programs of pharmacy in Palestine have no well-defined departments.[20]

The PharmD program at An-Najah National University awards the doctor of pharmacy degree after the completion of 48 weeks of clinical training consisting of 8 consecutive 6-week rotations in various medical specialties such as pediatrics, internal medicine, and surgery at governmental and private hospitals as well as at Najah teaching hospital. This program started in 2006 with the objective of introducing a new clinical component to pharmacy education and practice in Palestine. The program was designed to meet the increased need for high-quality hospital-based pharmacy services in Palestine. An-Najah University also has a graduate clinical pharmacy program that offers a master's of science (M.Sc.) degree in clinical pharmacy after the successful completion of theoretical and practical courses consisting of 36 credit hours and 36 weeks of clinical rotations. The M.Sc. clinical pharmacy program started in 2003 as a joint program with the Palestinian MOH with the objective of improving clinical pharmacy services at the MOH. An-Najah National University has started a graduate program in pharmaceutical sciences with emphasis on various pharmacy disciplines.[20]

All pharmacy graduates from the national universities can register with the PPA and get their practice license without sitting for any exam. On the other hand, all pharmacy graduates from universities outside Palestine have to sit for written and oral exams in the PPA prior to getting a license to practice pharmacy services in Palestine. According to current regulations and laws implemented by the PPA and MOH, continuing pharmacy education is not mandatory and there are no relicensure procedures.

10. Achievements

Definitely, the presence of several colleges of pharmacy in Palestine has provided the Palestinian community with a qualified number of pharmacists who initiated several pharmaceutical services that were lacking in the past. In the field of education, the introduction of PharmD programs and graduate programs in clinical pharmacy and pharmaceutical sciences has advanced pharmacy practice in Palestine. Research in Palestine was led by a group of pharmacists who helped in starting clinical and basic research in Palestine.

Palestinian pharmaceutical manufacturers have increased their share of the market with time, while the share of imported medicines has started to decrease. This was achieved through continuous development of pharmaceutical manufacturing in Palestine.

The pharmaceutical services in the Palestinian government have also advanced in the past 10 years. The development of an updated essential drug list, Palestinian National Formulary, and therapeutic protocols were all published and nationally discussed. Advancements in poison control and management have been seen since 2005 and were led by a group of pharmacists particularly.[30,31]

11. Challenges

Owing to the political instability of the country and the low level of available resources, both public health institutions and pharmacists face many challenges.

For public health institutions it is difficult to maintain a good level of pharmaceutical services provided to patients, difficult to have long-term plans for pharmaceutical services, and difficult to expand the pharmaceutical services to certain Palestinian areas that are under full Israeli control. In addition, pharmacy graduates have great challenges in terms of choosing their career. Owing to the presence of many Israeli colonies surrounding the Palestinian cities in the West Bank, it is very difficult to expand the areas of residence in these cities. Thus pharmacy graduates who mainly prefer to work in the community setting, which provides them more freedom and is more profitable in that they can sell over-the-counter and prescription drugs, medical supplies, and cosmetics, have to work within limited areas in their cities. This has caused the presence of a saturated market for pharmacy graduates. Graduates have the options of working in the industrial field mainly as medical representatives or continuing their M.Sc. or Ph.D. studies or leaving the country and working overseas. As of this writing, new graduates in the West Bank cannot open their own community pharmacies immediately. First they have to register their applications in the PPA and wait until their turn comes. The queue might take several years. Therefore, practice options are limited for pharmacy graduates in the West Bank. Creation of jobs in hospitals and clinical settings might decrease the pressure on new graduates.

On the other hand, owing to the presence of the Gaza Siege, the recurrent Israeli attacks on Gaza, the split between the PNA in the West Bank and the Hamas Party in the Gaza Strip, as well as the difficulty for residents in the West Bank to visit the Gaza Strip and vice versa, it is very difficult to define and evaluate the actual practices for pharmacists and pharmaceutical institutions in the Gaza Strip. In the Gaza Strip, Hamas has its own government, which sets the regulations and has control over all practices in the Gaza Strip. Trade barriers forced by Israel on Palestinian manufacturers present a real challenge to them in that they are forced to get permissions and licenses for every shipment in and out of Palestine. In addition, limited markets and high operating costs are main barriers for their development.

At the educational level, the pharmacy curriculum, particularly the PharmD curriculum, needs to be upgraded to international standards to pursue international accreditation. All pharmacy programs in Palestine have local accreditation only and in most cases the curriculum is based on an individual vision rather than global or international vision for pharmacy education and practice. Relicensure and continuing professional development of Palestinian pharmacists remain the most debatable future issues and the real future challenge in the pharmacy profession in Palestine.

Finally, research in pharmacy needs to be focused on social and professional issues related to pharmacy practice. Although several articles have been published from Palestine in the fields of social pharmacy and pharmacy practice, the current vision and research in pharmacy in Palestine are centered on traditional chemistry research and herbal-based chemistry research.

12. Recommendations

All parties involved in the pharmacy profession must combine their efforts to promote pharmacy practice and pharmacy education in Palestine. The presence of five colleges of pharmacy in Palestine has led to a higher number of pharmacy graduates who are currently facing serious employment problems given the limited opportunities for pharmacists both in government and in the private sector. The Palestinian pharmaceutical association needs to upgrade and reshape the pharmacy profession by adopting modern patient-oriented pharmacy practices instead of the business-oriented practices. Both An-Najah and Birzeit universities need to pursue international accreditation for their PharmD programs. Laws and regulations regarding the pharmacy profession need to be revisited and upgraded. For example, laws and regulations regarding chain pharmacies need to be discussed at all levels and approved by the pharmaceutical association and MOH. This is an important step owing to the financial restraints and the limited opportunities for most pharmacists to start a new independent pharmacy business. Research in clinical pharmacology, pharmacoepidemiology, and drug utilization is highly required to obtain baseline data on the drug situation in Palestine. Continuing pharmacy education and professional development must be part of the relicensure requirements. Finally, universities and the MOH should work together to establish clinical pharmacy residency programs to create needed clinical pharmacy specializations.

13. Conclusion

Pharmacy practice in Palestine is still progressing. Continuing pharmacy education is needed to upgrade pharmacists and pharmacy services in Palestine. Pharmacy education needs better organization to meet international standards. Clinical pharmacy services are still primitive and collaboration with the pharmaceutical association and MOH is required to implement such services.

14. Lessons learned

1. Regulation regarding many aspects of pharmacy practice are required.
2. Pharmacy education and research need to be coordinated and upgraded.
3. Clinical pharmacy services need to be implemented.
4. Professional pharmacy development is highly needed.
5. Collaboration between industry, community, government, and universities regarding pharmaceutical services is needed.

References

1. Palestinian Central Bureau of Statistics. *Palestine in figures 2011*. [cited January 30, 2013]. Available from: http://www.pcbs.gov.ps/portals/_pcbs/downloads/book1855.pdf; 2012.
2. Giacaman R, Khatib R, Shabaneh L, Ramlawi A, Sabri B, Sabatinelli G, et al. Health status and health services in the occupied Palestinian territory. *Lancet* 2009;**373**(9666):837–49.
3. The Security Council. *Resolution 446 (1979)*. (doc.nr. S/RES/446(1979)). [cited January 31, 2013]. Available from: http://unispal.un.org/UNISPAL.NSF/0/BA123CDED3EA84A5852560E50077C2DC; March 22, 1979.
4. Palestinian Central Bureau of Statistics. *Palestinian family health survey*. [cited January 30, 2013]. Available from: http://82.213.38.42/PCBS_NADA3.1/index.php/ddibrowser/116/download/276; 2006.
5. World Bank Group. *Countries and economies 2013*. [cited September 23, 2014]. Available from: http://data.worldbank.org/country; 2014.
6. Ministry of Health. *Health status in Palestine 2011*. [cited January 30, 2013]. Available from: http://www.moh.ps/attach/441.pdf; 2012.
7. Ministry of Health, Palestinian Health Information Center. *Health status in Palestine 2013*. [cited December 22, 2014]. Available from: http://www.moh.ps/attach/704.pdf; 2014.
8. Abu-Irmaileh BE, Afifi FU. Herbal medicine in Jordan with special emphasis on commonly used herbs. *J Ethnopharmacol* December 2003;**89**(2–3):193–7.
9. Abdul-Rahim HF, Husseini A, Giacaman R, Jervell J, Bjertness E. Diabetes mellitus in an urban Palestinian population: prevalence and associated factors. *East Mediterr Health J* January–March 2001;**7**(1–2):67–78.
10. Husseini A, Abdul-Rahim H, Awartani F, Giacaman R, Jervell J, Bjertness E. Type 2 diabetes mellitus, impaired glucose tolerance and associated factors in a rural Palestinian village. *Diabet Med* October 2000;**17**(10):746–8.
11. Husseini A, Abdul-Rahim H, Awartani F, Jervell J, Bjertness E. Prevalence of diabetes mellitus and impaired glucose tolerance in a rural Palestinian population. *East Mediterr Health J* September–November 2000;**6**(5–6):1039–45.
12. Aker MB, Taha AS, Zyoud SH, Sawalha AF, Al-Jabi SW, Sweileh WM. Estimation of 10-year probability bone fracture in a selected sample of Palestinian people using fracture risk assessment tool. *BMC Musculoskeletal Disord* 2013;**14**:284.
13. Palestinian Ministry of Health, World Health Organization. *Pharmaceutical country profile—Palestinian National Authority 2011*. [cited December 22, 2014]. Available from: http://www.who.int/medicines/areas/coordination/PalestinePSCP_NARRATIVE-PAL_2011-08-10Final.pdf.
14. Palestinian Central Bureau of Statistics. *National health accounts 2000–2008, main findings*. [cited January 30, 2013]. Available from: http://www.moh.ps/attach/278.pdf; 2011.
15. Abu Alia A. *The Palestinian pharmaceutical industry*. [cited December 22, 2014]. Available from: http://archive.thisweekinpalestine.com/i110/pdfs/June%20-%20110%20-%202007.pdf; 2007.
16. Naqib F. *Economic relations between Palestine and Israel during the occupation era and the period of limited self rule*. [cited December 22, 2014]. Available from: http://www.erf.org.eg/CMS/uploads/pdf/2015%20Naquib%20website.pdf; 2000.

17. Almi O. *Captive economy—the pharmaceutical industy and the Israeli occupation.* [cited December 22, 2014]. Available from: http://whoprofits.org/sites/default/files/captive_economy_0.pdf; 2012.
18. The World Bank. *Reforming prudently under pressure: West Bank and Gaza health policy report, health financing reform and the rationalization of public sector health expenditures.* [cited January 30, 2013]. Available from: http://web.worldbank.org/WBSITE/EXTERNAL/COUNTRIES/MENAEXT/WESTBANKG AZAEXTN/0,contentMDK:22264372~pagePK:141137~piPK:141127~theSitePK:294365,00.html; 2009.
19. Zochrot. *Remembering Yafàs al-Ajami neighborhood.* [cited December 22, 2014]. Available from: http://zochrot. org/uploads/uploads/cd7c6d613af3226ebb1b0c6a285ace01.pdf; 2007.
20. Sweileh WM, Al-Jabi SW, Sawalha AF, Zyoud SH. Pharmacy education and practice in West Bank, Palestine. *Am J Pharm Educ* April 07, 2009;**73**(2):38.
21. Sweileh WM, Arafat RT, Al-Khyat LS, Al-Masri DM, Jaradat NA. A pilot study to investigate over-the-counter drug abuse and misuse in Palestine. *Saudi Med J* December 2004;**25**(12):2029–32.
22. Palestinian National Authority-Ministry of Health. *Good manufacturing practices inspection Aide-Memoir.* [cited December 22, 2014]. Available from: http://pharmacy.moh.ps/Content/Laws/9CvORqjBt6jOsghsCptw8 FBg_ocX4rGJYY3Zobq38t6hBDtFa.pdf; 2007.
23. General Directorate of Pharmacy-Palestinian Ministry of Health. *Conditions & rules.* [cited December 22, 2014]. Available from: http://pharmacy.moh.ps/index/condition/Language/en; 2014.
24. Palestinian Economic Council for Development & Reconstruction. *Central medical stores in Nablus.* [cited December 22, 2014]. Available from: http://www.pecdar.ps/etemplate.php?id=841; 2010.
25. Sweileh W. Self-medication and over-the-counter practices: a study in Palestine. *J Al-Aqsa Unv* 2004;**8**:1–9.
26. Al-Ramahi R. Patterns and attitudes of self-medication practices and possible role of community pharmacists in Palestine. *Int J Clin Pharmacol Ther* July 2013;**51**(7):562–7.
27. Sawalha AF. A descriptive study of self-medication practices among Palestinian medical and nonmedical university students. *Res Soc Adm Pharm* June 2008;**4**(2):164–72.
28. Zaid AN, Al-Ramahi R, Shahed Q, Saleh B, Elaraj J. Determinants and frequency of pharmaceutical compounding in pharmacy practice in Palestine. *Int J Pharm Pract* February 2012;**20**(1):9–14.
29. Sawalha AF, Sweileh WM, Zyoud SH, Al-Jabi SW, Shamseh FF, Odah A. Analysis of prescriptions dispensed at community pharmacies in Nablus, Palestine. *East Mediterr Health J* July 2010;**16**(7):788–92.
30. Sawalha AF. Poison control and the drug information center: the palestinian experience. *Isr Med Assoc J* November 2008;**10**(11):757–60.
31. Zyoud SH, Al-Jabi SW, Bali YI, Al-Sayed AM, Sweileh WM, Awang R. Availability of treatment resources for the management of acute toxic exposures and poisonings in emergency departments among various types of hospitals in Palestine: a cross-sectional study. *Scand J Trauma Resusc Emerg Med* 2014;**22**:13.
32. Al-Azhar University. Faculty of Pharmacy. [cited February 22, 2015]. Available from: http://www.alazhar.edu .ps/Eng/Pharmacy.htm; 2015.
33. An-Najah National University. Department of Pharmacy. [cited February 22, 2015]. Available from: http://fmhs.najah.edu/node/21; 2015.
34. Birzeit University. Faculty of nursing, pharmacy and health professions. [cited February 22, 2015]. Available from: http://www.birzeit.edu/faculties/nursing-pharmacy-health-professions; 2015.
35. Al-Quds University. Faculty of Pharmacy. [cited February 22, 2015]. Available from: http://www.alquds.edu/en/faculty-of-pharmacy.html; 2015.
36. Hebron University. College of Pharmacy & Medical Science. [cited February 22, 2015]. Available from: http://www.hebron.edu/index.php/en/academic-programs/faculties/pharmacy-medical-science; 2015.

CHAPTER 14

Pharmacy Practice in Yemen

Yaser Mohammed Ali Al-Worafi

Chapter Outline

Pharmacy Practice in Developing Countries. http://dx.doi.org/10.1016/B978-0-12-801714-2.00014-9
267

1. Country profile

Yemen is situated in the southwest corner of the Arabian Peninsula with a population of approximately 24 million.[1] It is among the least developed countries in the world. Yemen's health situation is considered the worst in the region. The total expenditure on health per capita (US$) is 122 and the total expenditure on health as a percentage of GDP is 5.2.[2]

2. Vital health statistics

Yemen's health situation is considered the worst in the region, Yemen has a high rate of mortality and malnutrition, high infant mortality (75 per 1000 lives births), and under-5 mortality (96 per 1000 lives births).[3] Tables 1 and 2 show the health expenditures and top 10 diseases in Yemen.

3. Overview of the health care system

The Yemeni health system consists of a public sector and private sector. The public health sector is organized into three levels: primary health care (PHC), secondary health facilities,

Table 1: Health indicators and expenditures in Yemen

1	Gross national income per capita (PPP international $)	2500
2	Life expectancy at birth m/f (years)	63/67
3	Probability of dying under five (per 1000 live births)	77
4	Probability of dying between 15 and 60 years (per 1000 population, males/females)	237/180
5	Total expenditure on health per capita (US$, 2010)	122
6	Total expenditure on health as % of GDP (US$, 2010)	5.2

Source: World Health Organization country profiles.[3]

Table 2: Top 10 causes of morbidity and mortality in Yemen

Rank	Morbidity	Mortality
1	Diarrheal diseases	Infectious and parasitic diseases, including diarrhea
2	Malnutrition	Diseases of the respiratory disease
3	Complication of pregnancy and delivery	Diseases of the digestive system
4	Acute respiratory disease	Complications of pregnancy, child birth, and puerperium
5	Malaria	Injuries and poisoning
6	Bilharziasis	Diseases of the circulatory system
7	Tuberculosis	Others
8	Accidents	
9	Hepatitis B virus	
10	AIDS, leprosy	

Source: Regional Health Systems Observatory, EMRO, World Health Organization.[4]

and tertiary health facilities. Primary health care starts at the rural community level and is mainly focused on primary health programs, providing first-level curative care. The PHC units are supported by PHC centers, run by one doctor, and they have laboratory and X-ray facilities. The secondary health facilities consist of the regional hospitals. These facilities are more specialized in curative services and receive cases from the PHCs. The tertiary health facilities are the national hospitals providing specialized care.[5]

The Ministry of Public Health and Population is responsible for the health sector and is one of the largest public employers in the country. However, there are other public organizations involved in financing, planning, and provision of health services. These consist of the Ministry of Finance, Ministry of Planning and International Cooperation, Ministry of Civil Service, the two autonomous hospitals, the Health Manpower Institutes and the military and police health services. The health system in Yemen suffers from shortcomings in construction and organization, inadequate staffing, low quality of health care, shortage of essential medicine, and lack of government budget. Table 3 shows the health indicators in Yemen.

There are no official statistics about the total number of pharmacists in Yemen. The only officially available statistics according to the Ministry of Public Health and Population is the number of pharmacists registered in the Ministry. However, according to the Yemen Pharmacists Syndicate (2010), the estimated number of registered pharmacists in Yemen is greater than 4000.[9–12]

4. Medicine supply systems and drug use issues

The Supreme Board of Drugs and Medical Appliances (SBDMA) and Ministry of Public Health and Population (MoPH) are responsible for the regulation of pharmacy practice,

Table 3: Health indicators in Yemen

Health Indicator	2008	2009	2010	2011
Number of population	21,843,554	22,492,035	23,153,982	23,832,569
Number of physicians	6226	6468	6599	6469
Number of dentists	535	587	573	572
Number of inhabitants per physician	3508	3477	3509	3684
Number of nurses	11,845	12,211	12,785	12,685
Number of nurses per physician	2	2	2	2
Number of beds	15,184	16,095	16,534	16,695
Number of inhabitants per bed	1439	1397	1400	1428
Number of licensed community pharmacies			3092	3315
Number of licensed drug stores			2703	4133
Number of pharmacists (public hospitals)			1010	994
Number of pharmacists (community pharmacies)			3092	3315
Number of technicians (public hospitals)			1372	1420
Number of technicians (drug stores)			2703	4133

Source: Ministry of Public Health and Population.[2,6–8]

**Table 4: Top 10 local medicines in Yemen based
on sales in Yemeni Riyals**

Rank	Medicine
1	Amoxicillin plus others
2	Paracetamol
3	Sildenafil citrate
4	Amoxicillin
5	Tadalafil
6	Cetirizine
7	Metronidazole plus others
8	Ciprofloxacin
9	Pantoprazole plus others
10	Diclofenac sodium

Source: The Supreme Board of Drugs and Medical Appliances, 2011.

registration, and drug procurement. The Yemen Pharmacists Syndicate is responsible for offering the license for pharmacists to work in pharmacies; the license for operating a pharmacy should be obtained from the Ministry of Public Health. Only a pharmacist who has at least a bachelor's degree in pharmacy or pharmaceutical science can legally open a pharmacy in Yemen. The Supreme Board of Drugs and Medical Appliances is under the supervision of the MoPH.

Currently, there are about 500 foreign pharmaceutical companies and more than 13,000 brand medicines registered in Yemen. In 2012, the Ministry of Public Health and Population and the SBDMA started a new policy to ensure the quality of medicines in Yemen. The policy stipulates that to renew the registration of medicines currently marketed or to register new medicines in Yemen, companies must first register with the executive boards of the Health Ministers Council for Gulf Cooperation Council (GCC) states or the Gulf Central Committee for Drug Registration, or register the drugs in the United States; otherwise registration would be canceled. This policy will lead to decreasing the number of registered companies and number of registered medicines.[10,13–17] Table 4 shows the top 10 local medicines. Tables 5–7 show the top 10 imported medicines, exporting countries, and imported materials.

4.1 Medicine availability, affordability, and price components

Despite the presence of drug companies in Yemen, the availability and affordability of medicines are major concerns. Most Yemenis make huge sacrifices to buy the necessary medicines for their health. Public sector access is poor compared to the availability of medicines in the private sector. Lower-priced generics are relatively affordable compared to original brands. Compared with international reference prices, the lowest-priced generic medicines available in the private sector vary from very cheap to expensive. Most branded Drugs are priced much higher than the reference prices (75% had a median price ratio of

Table 5: Top 10 imported medicines in Yemen based on sales in Yemeni Riyals

Rank	Medicine
1	Sera and vaccines
2	Ceftriaxone
3	Diclofenac sodium
4	Amoxicillin plus others
5	Codeine phosphate plus others
6	Cetirizine
7	Multivitamin plus others
8	Amoxicillin
9	Paracetamol
10	Tri-B vitamin

Source: The Supreme Board of Drugs and Medical Appliances, 2011.

Table 6: Top 10 exporting countries

Rank	Medicine
1	Egypt
2	India
3	Syria
4	Denmark
5	Germany
6	United Kingdom
7	Switzerland
8	Jordan
9	France
10	United Arab Emirates

Source: The Supreme Board of Drugs and Medical Appliances, 2011.

Table 7: Top 10 imported raw materials in Yemen

Rank	Medicine
1	Amoxicillin
2	Clavulanate potassium
3	Paracetamol
4	Clarithromycin
5	Cefaddroxil
6	Metronidazole
7	Clavulanate potassium plus others
8	Pseudoephederine
9	Ketoprofen
10	Ethanol

Source: The Supreme Board of Drugs and Medical Appliances, 2011.

(MPR)>7). The price components of medicine in Yemen consist of wholesale mark-up, retail mark-up, taxes, storage and transportation, custom duty, drug support fund, bank charges, and cost/insurance/freight (CIF).[5,10,18]

5. Overview of pharmacy practice and key pharmaceutical sectors

The first pharmacy in Yemen was opened in 1875 in Aden, and the second pharmacy was opened in1876. In 2010, the first chain pharmacies were established in the capital Sana'a. Since then, many chain pharmacies have been established in Sana'a and other cities.[10]

The estimated number of registered pharmacists in Yemen is greater than 4000, according to the Yemen Pharmacists Syndicate (2010). However, this may not be the actual total number of pharmacists because there are about 1000 pharmacists graduating each year from the Yemeni universities and other countries and that are not registered in the Syndicate. They are working outside Yemen in the Kingdom of Saudi Arabia, Emirates, and other countries for many reasons, such as a lack of jobs and low salaries in Yemen and more attractive work environments outside Yemen.[10-12] The Ministry of Health and Medical Council classify the pharmacy professionals as the following (Table 8):

Table 8: Classifications of pharmacy professionals in Yemen

No	Level	Certificate
1	Technician	Diploma degree in Pharmacy
2	Pharmacist	Bachelor of Pharmacy or Pharmaceutical Sciences
3	Specialist	Master degree of Pharmacy or Pharmaceutical Sciences
4	Consultant	PhD degree of Pharmacy or Pharmaceutical Sciences

Source: Pharmacy regulation and Law Yemen.[19]

6. Drug- and pharmacy-related regulations, polices, and ethics

The SBDMA and MoPH are responsible for the regulation of pharmacy practice, registration, and drug procurement. Local and foreign pharmaceutical industries distribute medicines in two ways: directly to the pharmacies and drug stores through their supply offices in each city in Yemen and through subagents who distribute the medicines to the pharmacies and drug stores. Pharmaceutical marketing plays an important role in the pharmaceutical industry. Each company hires a medical representative to visit hospitals, clinics, pharmacies, drug stores, and physicians to market their products. Physicians receive brochures, free medical samples, commissions, televisions, mobile phones, free tickets, foods, money to cover conference fees, percentages of total sales, and other gifts to prescribe their products. There is a strongly a need to implement a code of ethics in pharmaceutical marketing in Yemen as the pharmaceutical companies are focusing only on maximizing their profits.[10,13-17]

7. Core pharmacy practices

7.1 Hospital pharmacy

The total number of public health facilities in Yemen is 4059, including referral hospitals, general hospitals, district hospitals, and PHC units. The total number of private health care facilities in Yemen is 3641, including hospitals and polyclinics.[2] There are no differences between public and private hospitals in terms of focusing on dispensing of medications and workforce issues as the majority of dispensers are nonpharmacists, either pharmacy technicians or others. Public hospitals either do not have pharmacies inside the hospitals or the medications are not available.[10] Usually, there is a community pharmacy attached to or in front of each hospital; however, such pharmacies are not actually under the control of the hospitals. The daily working hours are about 8 h for five or six days weekly. Generally, the main duty of pharmacists working in hospitals is merely dispensing medications, either prescribed or over-the-counter drugs.

7.2 Industrial pharmacy

There are nine local pharmaceutical manufacturers in Yemen.[10] The Yemen Drug Company (YEDCO) was set up in 1964 by the Yemeni government in cooperation with private investors. It was established as a company specialized in the marketing of medicinal drugs. YEDCO initiated its work by importing drugs from foreign companies and then marketing and distributing them locally. In 1982, YEDCO established the first medicinal factory for drugs in Sana'a. Today, YEDCO produces more than 60 medicinal products. In 1993, Shiba Pharma, the second pharmaceutical company, was established in Sana'a. More than 134 products produced by Shiba Pharma have been approved and sold in Yemen and are exported to countries in the Middle East and Africa. The local pharmaceutical industry covers approximately 10–20% of the total market. Yemen is a member of the Arab Union of the Manufacturers of Pharmaceuticals and Medical Appliances, and it ranks 11th among Arabic countries in medicine production. Yemen spends about US$263 million a year on pharmaceutical drugs, according to the national Supreme Drugs Authority. Most of this expenditure is spent on importing medicines from 50 countries through 400 importers.[10] Few pharmacists are working in the pharmaceutical industry. The daily working hours are about 8 h for five days weekly.

7.3 Community pharmacy

Pharmacists working in community pharmacies in Yemen work 8–12 h daily, six days per week. Most community pharmacies are not open on Fridays. Many community pharmacy dispensers in Yemeni community pharmacies are nonpharmacists.[10] Community pharmacy dispensers in Yemen dispense prescribed medications without prescriptions, including analgesics, antibiotics, antipsychotics, cardiovascular medications, and others. The dispensing of medications without prescriptions in Yemen is a big problem affecting people's health and health resources. Most community pharmacy dispensers are not registered pharmacists and they do not know the harmful impacts of dispensing prescribed medications on people's health. Community pharmacy dispensers in Yemeni community pharmacies make diagnoses, prescribe, and dispense medicines to treat many diseases, even though they lack knowledge and authority.

Several factors cause the problem of dispensing prescribed medications without a valid prescription as well as making diagnoses in Yemeni community pharmacies: "Most Yemenis do not go to physicians because that they cannot afford the treatment in private hospitals or clinics, and generally there is no medical insurance. Unfortunately, the government hospitals and medical centers are the worst in the country. Also, care in these facilities is mostly reserved for patients who have relatives working in the hospital or having relationships with influential people. Furthermore, patients are required to buy everything starting from the papers used to write prescriptions to the medicines. People are also unaware of the dangers of buying prescription medicines without a valid prescription. The Ministry of Public Health and Population and the Supreme Board of Drugs and Medical Appliances fail to regulate, control, and monitor prescribing. No policy exists requiring dispensers to be qualified and registered as pharmacists. Anyone with money in Yemen can open a pharmacy by renting a license from a pharmacist and hiring non-qualified persons to work in the pharmacy."[10]

7.4 Medicine marketing and promotion

There are about 500 foreign pharmaceutical companies and more than 13,000 brand medicines registered in Yemen. Pharmaceutical marketing plays an important role in the pharmaceutical market. Each company hires a medical representative to visit hospitals, clinics, pharmacies, drug stores, and physicians to market their products. Physicians may receive brochures, free medical samples, commissions, televisions, mobile phones, free tickets, foods, money to cover conference fees, percentages of total sales, and other gifts to prescribe their products.[10]

8. Special pharmacy-related services and activities

Clinical pharmacy services were implemented at the end of 2010 in few community pharmacies and private hospitals. Clinical pharmacy services include medication therapy management, pharmaceutical care services for selected diseases, and health screening. There are few researchers in Yemen investigating pharmacy practice issues.

A Yemeni Pharmacovigilance Center (YPVC) was established in early 2011 in the capital Sana'a with the following objectives: "early detection of adverse drug reactions (ADRs); detection of increase in frequency of (known) adverse reaction; identification of risk factors and possible mechanisms underlying adverse reactions; estimation of quantitative aspects of benefit/risk analysis and dissemination of information needed to improve drug prescribing and regulation; prevention of adverse drug reactions; drug quality surveillance; encouraging rational and safe use of drugs and communication with international institutions working in pharmacovigilance." To achieve its objectives, YPVC has visited many hospitals (government and private) and pharmacies (government and private) to increase their awareness toward ADR detection, ADR assessment, ADR reporting, and quality of medicines. YPVC published ADRs reporting and pharmaceutical product quality for health care professional in English and for public in Arabic.[24]

9. Pharmacy education

9.1 Introduction

In Yemen, there are 4 public and 12 private colleges of pharmacy. In 2008, all of the 4 public colleges and 3 of the private colleges are recognized by the Ministry of Higher Education and Scientific Research (MOHESR). The establishment of pharmacy colleges in Yemen has been relatively new. The first public pharmacy faculty (college) was established in 1987 in Sana'a. It was first a department in the Faculty of Medicine and Health Sciences, University of Sana'a. The first group of students graduated in 1993. It became a separate faculty in 2002. The second public pharmacy college was established in 1995 in Aden. It was first a department in the Faculty of Medicine and Health Sciences, University of Aden. It became a separate college in June 2009. The third public pharmacy faculty (college) was established in 2005 in Thamar as a department in the Faculty of Medicine and Health Sciences, University of Thamar. The fourth public pharmacy faculty (college) was established in 2011 in Hodeidah University. It is as a department of Clinical Pharmacy in the Faculty of Medical Sciences. It offers two programs: bachelor of pharmacy and the doctor of pharmacy (PharmD).

The three private colleges of pharmacy offer a diploma of pharmacy as well as a bachelor's degree in pharmacy. The University of Science and Technology established the first private college of pharmacy as a department within the College of Medical Sciences. It offers a diploma of pharmacy and bachelor of pharmacy. In 2010–2011, the College of Pharmacy, University of Science and Technology started a PharmD program. The duration of a bachelor's degree program in all public and private colleges is 5 years. The program is taught in English, with Arabic language used in a few courses, such as Arabic and Islamic subjects.[10–12]

9.2 Pharmacy college admission requirements

Educational and other specifications or minimum competencies required for admission to pharmacy colleges that a student must satisfactorily complete to be accepted are often stated in terms of admission requirements. These criteria are highly variable between the governmental or public and the private sector schools. Currently, there is intense competition for admission to pharmacy colleges due to the limited places in the public colleges. In an attempt to select the best candidates, colleges generally follow the center selection criteria set by Acceptance Committee under supervision of MOHESR, which include screening students on the basis of their academic achievement and assessing their performance on a test set by the college as an acceptance examination. The private sector sets their own acceptance criteria, which include the minimum pass of a high school examination and the ability to pay the tuition fees yearly. Although most public colleges utilize essentially the same type of admission criteria, the validity and the outcome evidence indicating the relationship between admission criteria and pharmacy graduate performance in pharmacy practice are not strong and consistent.[10–12]

9.3 Pharmacy programs and degrees offered

The system of Yemeni pharmacy degrees in the public and private colleges is summarized in Table 9 and Figure 1.

Table 9: Comparison between public and private colleges

	Public Colleges		Private Colleges	
Degree offered	Faculty of Pharmacy, Sana'a University (established in 1987)	Bachelor's and master's in pharmacology, pharmaceutics, and pharmacognosy; Master's and PhD in pharmacology and public health (under supervision of Faculty of Medicine and Health Sciences)	College of Pharmacy, University of Science and Technology (established in 1997)	Diploma of pharmacy, Bachelors of pharmacy, and doctor of pharmacy
	Faculty of Pharmacy, Aden University (established in 1995)	Bachelor degree of pharmaceutical sciences	College of Pharmacy Queen Arwa University	Diploma of pharmacy and Bachelors of pharmacy
	Faculty of Pharmacy, Thamar University (established in 2005)	Bachelor degree of pharmaceutical sciences	College of Pharmacy, Dar Alsalam International University for Science and Technology (established in 1987)	Diploma of pharmacy and Bachelors of pharmacy
	Faculty of Pharmacy, Hodeidah University (established in 2011)	Bachelor of pharmacy and doctor of pharmacy (PharmD)		

	Public Colleges	Private Colleges
Language	English, with Arabic language used in a few courses such as Arabic and Islamic subjects	English, with Arabic language used in a few courses such as Arabic and Islamic subjects.
Duration of study (years)	Diploma (2–3), Bachelor (5), Master (3) and PhD (3–5)	Diploma (2–3), Bachelor (5), and PharmD (6)
Admission criteria	Grades of higher secondary school (≈>90%) plus university examination	Minimum pass of high school examination
Tuition Fees	Free	Range from 2500 to 5000 US dollars
Student gender status	Integrated (male > female)	Integrated and segregated (male > female)
Students admitted/ year	Range from 100 to 250 in each school	Range from 10 to 30 in each school
Accreditation	National (from the Ministry of Higher Education and Scientific Research (MOHESR))	Only three schools accredited from national (from MOHESR)
Credit hours	174–190	174–190
Teaching methods	Traditional (lecture based)	Traditional (lecture based)

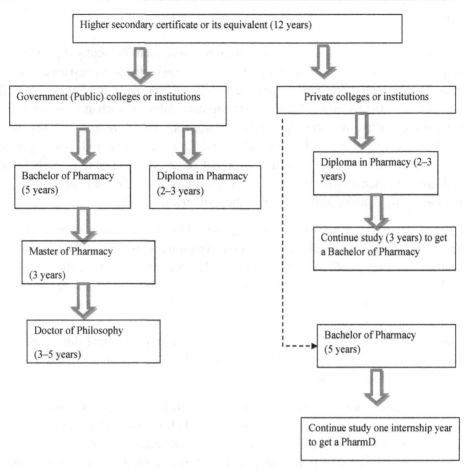

Figure 1
System of Yemeni pharmacy degrees.

9.4 Students

According to the Central Statistics Organization in Yemen, the percentage of male students is about 70% in both public and private pharmacy colleges. The number of pharmacy students admitted yearly in the recognized public and private pharmacy colleges and schools in Yemen is more than 500.

Female students across all colleges face different challenges, as the pre-university sex-segregated school system has a huge impact on their education at the college level. The cultural assumption that women should marry rather than to exercise their civic responsibilities dominates in Yemeni community. There is also a perception that college-educated women are less likely to marry. Female students are also less likely than male students to receive financial assistance or to participate in some clinical training outside the university campus during their study at pharmacy colleges.[10–12]

9.5 Staff

The Faculty of Pharmacy, Sana'a University, employs more than 30 faculty members as professors, associate professors, assistant professors, lecturers, teaching assistants, and technicians. There is collaboration between the Faculty of Pharmacy and Faculty of Medicine and Health Sciences and Faculty of Science to teach many subjects, such as anatomy, histology, physiology, biochemistry, microbiology, and other subjects. There are many faculty working as visiting lecturers (including professors and others). Graduates with high grades get the opportunity to work as a teaching assistant, after that getting a scholarship to study for a master's degree and then a PhD outside of Yemen, such as in the United States, United Kingdom, Germany, Canada, Malaysia, and other countries.

The Faculty of Pharmacy in Aden currently employs 23 faculty members as professors, associate professors, assistant professors, lecturers, teaching assistants, and technicians. There is a lack of staff in other public faculties in Yemen. The private pharmacy colleges also suffer from a lack of staff. Even the University of Science and Technology, which was the first private college of pharmacy in Yemen, is suffering from a lack of staff. Many of the staff members are not satisfied with their work in Yemen. The migration of academic staff from Yemeni universities as well as pharmacy colleges was reported from the Ministry of Immigrates affairs. Most of the pharmacy staff migrated to Saudi Arabia, United Arab of Emirates, Malaysia, and other countries.

In a personal interview with five staff members (two professors and three assistant professors) working in Saudi universities and two PhD holders working in Malaysia about their reasons for migrating from Yemen, they mentioned the following reasons: low salaries in Yemen, high cost of living, lack of facilities in colleges of pharmacy, and lack of jobs. Although there is a shortage of academic staff in pharmacy colleges, it is difficult to get a position because the hiring procedures are very difficult, especially in the public universities. in addition, the interviewees mentioned the lack of funds to attend conferences or workshops, lack of the research facilities and funds, inadequate teaching facilities, an absence of databases and good references (either electronic or textbooks), the general work environment in Yemen, and the attractive work environments outside Yemen.[10–12]

9.6 Pharmacy curriculum

Public and private pharmacy colleges in Yemen adapted their curricula from the curriculum of Faculty of Pharmacy, Sana'a University. Table 10 and Figure 2 show the pharmacy curricula in Yemen.

The credit hours range from 174 to 190 h. The sixth year in the PharmD program is 30 credit hours; each credit hour consists of 1 week of training at the hospital.

Table 10: Pharmacy curriculum in Yemen

Year	Curriculum
First year	General Chemistry, General Physics, Physical Chemistry, Biology, English Language, Arabic and Islamic Culture
Second year	Pharmaceutics, Analytical Chemistry I, Physiology, Biostatistics, Psychology, Organic Chemistry I, Anatomy and Histology, Business Administration and Botany
Third year	Organic Chemistry II, Analytical Chemistry II, Biochemistry, Microbiology, Pharmaceutics II and Pharmacognosy
Fourth year	Phytochemistry, Toxicology, Public Health, Pathology, Pharmaceutics III, Medical Chemistry I, and Pharmacology
Fifth year	Medical Chemistry II, Industrial Pharmacy, Clinical Pharmacy, Quality Control of Drugs, Applied Pharmacognosy, Therapeutics, Hospital and Community Pharmacy Practice, First Aid, and Graduation Research Project

Source: Sana'a University, 2012 and Aden University, 2012.[12]

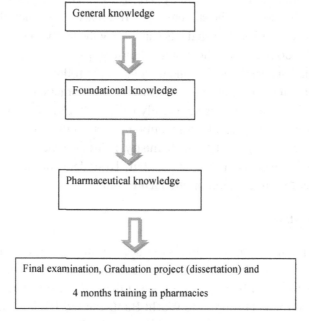

Figure 2
General structure of BSc pharmacy curriculum.[19]

The pharmacy curriculum has been designed to provide pharmacy students with all the necessary information and knowledge on both basic and pharmaceutical sciences to help them in the practice of pharmacy. Knowledge of the basic sciences, such as chemistry, biology, physics, and mathematics, is necessary not only for studying but also for conducting pharmaceutical research. Patient-focused education is an essential component of pharmacy education in developed countries, such as the United Kingdom and the United States.

However, undergraduate pharmacy programs in Yemen remain influenced by traditional pharmaceutical sciences with limited application of knowledge to patient care. Generally, the basic subjects are being taught as a core knowledge approach to applied pharmaceutical sciences. Basic science content must be maintained in pharmacy curricula, according to the American Council on Pharmacy Education accreditation standards and guidelines.[20] There is no balance between the science and practice subjects. There are few clinical and pharmacy practice subjects and an absence of clinical training in pharmacy curricula in Yemen.[10–12]

9.7 Teaching methods

There are different teaching methods used by different pharmacy colleges in Yemen: traditional lecture approach, tutorials, seminars, practicals, and research. In Yemen, e-learning is not officially being used in the public higher education sector. Students do not have access to the Internet at their place of study as well as they do not have computers. Generally, the lecturers still use the old traditional system by writing on the board and asking the students to write or distribute the handouts to the students. The references are generally not available in the college or university libraries. The students cannot buy the textbooks due to their economic status and they usually do not have scholarships, fellowships, or other external funds. The assessment of students' academic achievement includes the following: quizzes, midterm examination, oral examination, small research, assignments, practical examination, and final examination. The examination language generally is English. Each student is required to finish all the courses and do a research (graduation project) in the final year. The research is in pharmacognosy, pharmacology, medicinal chemistry, pharmaceutics, and public health. Due to the large number of students and shortage of staff, 10 students do their graduation research project together under the supervision of one faculty staff.[12]

9.8 Quality of education

There is no proper quality system for higher education in Yemen; colleges of pharmacy get their accreditation from MOHESR, which was established in 1990. However, there is an increasing interest in establishing quality assurance and accreditation systems in higher education in Yemen. Through the World Bank-funded Higher Education Learning and Innovation Project (a US$ 5 million credit), MOHESR developed the National Strategy for the Development of Higher Education, which was approved by the Yemeni Government in 2006 following extensive stakeholder consultation. A major step was taken, namely the development of a proposal to establish a Higher Education Quality Assurance Council (QAC). The QAC, which was approved by the Republican Decree No. 21 0/2009 in August 26, 2009, opened the way for the development of an institutional quality assurance function at the national level. The project's development objective is to create conditions that allow for the enhancement of the quality of university programs and graduate employability.[12]

9.9 Pharmacist training

There are huge challenges facing standards of initial education and internship training for newly graduated pharmacists. These challenges are based on the different regulations set by different colleges in the private sector and the public. There is no universal regulation setting up the criteria for education and training of pharmacists and pre-registration trainee pharmacists for continuous professional pharmacy programs in any pharmacy college in Yemen.[12]

9.10 Licensure of pharmacy professionals

There is no regulation that requires pharmacists in Yemen to pursue additional training after graduation, nor is continuing education openly encouraged. Moreover, there is no continuous professional pharmacy program in any of Yemen's pharmacy colleges.[11,12]

9.11 Education satisfaction

Most Yemeni pharmacists are not satisfied with the pharmacy curriculum in Yemen, especially those who graduated from the private colleges. The author of this chapter surveyed10 graduated pharmacists from public colleges and 10 from private colleges: 90% of them were not satisfied. They highlighted many reasons, such as the lack of facilities during study, the curriculum was not updated, lack of the clinical pharmacy and pharmacy practice courses, no clinical practice during the study, and nonqualified lecturers in the private colleges.[10–12]

9.12 Recommendations for improving pharmacy education

This section presents some practical recommendations that may strengthen pharmacy education and lead to better outcomes in both patient-centered care and more qualified practicing pharmacists:

- Pharmacy curriculum in Yemeni universities should be updated to meet the requirements of those working in public health services, pharmaceutical care services, and clinical pharmacy services.
- Pharmacy curricula should be designed to provide outcomes that meet the actual needs of the current and developing practices of pharmacy.
- Special interest should be given to the integration of objectives, learning activities, and the assessment of the pharmacist-physician relationship into professional training programs. Pharmacy colleges should be encouraged to promote such standards. An American national survey showed that pharmacist-physician interaction is one of the topics covered in communication courses in colleges of pharmacy.[21]
- Colleges of pharmacy should provide significantly more time and effort toward developing and updating the curriculum to improving pharmacy practice and healthcare in Yemen.

Collaboration with Ministry of Public Health and Population, Pharmaceutical Industries, Public and private hospitals, pharmacies, companies and Ministry of Higher Education and Scientific Research should occur to address all of the needs and then develop a plan to improve the pharmacy education and practice in Yemen. There could be a collaboration with pharmacy schools in the United States to benefit from their experience.

- Teaching strategies can be improved by introducing new teaching methods, such as problem-based learning, team-based learning, case discussion, and simulation-based education.
- Sites for practice and application of the taught knowledge should be established via collaboration with university teaching hospitals, government hospitals, private hospitals, community and hospital pharmacies and pharmaceutical industries, and the establishment of training facilities within the colleges such as drug information centers, Theraapeutic Drug Monitoring (TDM) and Total Parenteral Nutrition (TPN) laboratories, and simulation pharmacies (for teaching purposes).
- Collaboration between pharmacy colleges and MOHESR is needed to address the reasons for the shortage of the academic staff and provide solutions. Providing pharmacy colleges with more scholarships for their teaching assistants can help in solving the problem.
- Collaboration with international universities for hiring faculty staffs as visiting lecturers is required.
- Establishing a PhD study program covering different areas in pharmacy is needed.
- Increasing the number of the private colleges and institutions of pharmacy is needed.
- Any established quality assurance system should take into consideration the following points:
    - Reflecting the vision for pharmacy practice and education that has been developed through profession-wide consensus
    - Allowing appropriate input from all stakeholders, including students and the public
    - Ensuring that educational programs are evidence-based and competency-based and of high quality
    - Meeting the needs of the people, the pharmacists, and their country
    - Evaluating programmatic outcomes as well as institutional structures and processes
    - Being transparent and free of inappropriate influences and appearances of conflicts of interest in its development and implementation
    - Promoting and fostering self-assessment and continuous quality improvement of educational institutions
    - Being accountable to the appropriate governmental authorities[22]
- The licensure examination is not required for pharmacy practice in Yemen. To solve this issue, Yemen needs an obligatory licensing examination, which all graduates must pass to practice the pharmacy to ensure the quality of the working pharmacists in Yemen. The examination should include theory and practice.
- There is no continuing professional development in Yemen. Overall professional development and educational training for pharmacists is an important component of improved pharmacy practices. Participation in continuous education (CE) activities provides

assurance that practitioners are maintaining and updating their professional knowledge, and serves as a proxy for assuring ongoing competence to practice. Pharmacy colleges may assist in this by establishing CE centers. Policymakers should encourage the establishment of a pharmacists' professional re-registration system, which can be accompanied by an obligatory and hours' credited type of continuous professional development in pharmacy practice topics.

- Pharmacy colleges should revise their mission to serve the pharmaceutical care needs of the society through education, patient care, research and public service, and the colleges should interact with the community through numerous patient-oriented service commitments. Faculty members can be advised to conduct community outreach initiatives and increase the awareness of the peoples about their health. Pharmacy students can participate in a variety of public and charitable outreach projects, including helping to administer immunizations in the community and consulting patients regarding their medicines. Establishing drug and poison information centers is necessary to the public as well as health care professionals to provide them with a comprehensive information about drug use, side effects, drug–drug interaction, and treatment. Conducting lectures, seminars, and workshops through CE programs is required for pharmacists as well as the public to improve the awareness of the community pharmacists, hospital pharmacists, physicians, nurses, and other health professionals as well as the public about the new role of the pharmacist in the pharmaceutical, public, and clinical services rather than dispensing. Increased faculty participation in community services such as lectures, brochures, media, and symposium is required. Establishment of a good relationship with the pharmaceutical industry in Yemen is necessary, as well as active participation in improving the quality of their products.

- Pharmacy education research is vital for the continuing development and improvement of the educational experience of both the learners and the faculty staff. Such research should include various aspects of the educational phases including curriculum design and structure, curriculum implementation, and student evaluation. Other research areas may include the factors that may influence the education success as well as other issues related to pharmacy practice in Yemen. Authorities need to place these research themes as a priority with appropriate financial support.

- Finally, the development of optimal pharmacy education in Yemen should be progressed through an action plan that first seeks to "identify local needs, the pharmaceutical services needed to meet these needs, the competences needed to provide these pharmaceutical services and the education required to achieve/ensure these competences."[23] The Pharmacy Education Action Plan of the World Health Organization (WHO) United National Educational, Scientific and Cultural Organization International Pharmaceutical Federation is oriented toward identifying locally determined needs and pharmaceutical services and using those to facilitate comprehensive education development and achievement of competencies, which in turn are required to meet the local services.

10. *Achievements in pharmacy practice*

Currently, there are nine local pharmaceutical industries in Yemen. The local pharmaceutical industry covers approximately 10–20% of the total market. There are about 500 foreign pharmaceutical companies and more than 13,000 brand medicines registered in Yemen. But in 2012, the Ministry of Public Health and Population and the SBDMA started a new policy to ensure the quality of medicines in Yemen. The policy stipulates that to renew the registration of medicines currently marketed or to register new medicines in Yemen, companies must first register with the executive boards of the Health Ministers Council for GCC states or the Gulf Central Committee for Drug Registration, or register the drugs in the United States; otherwise, registration would be canceled. This policy should decrease the number of registered companies and number of registered medicines.

There is a slow shift from traditional drug dispensing to a patient-centered approach in pharmacy practice. Clinical pharmacy services were implemented at the end of 2010 in few community pharmacies and private hospitals. Clinical pharmacy services implemented were medication therapy management, pharmaceutical care services for selected diseases, and health screenings. There are few researchers in Yemen investigating pharmacy practice issues.

The establishment of the Yemeni Pharmacovigilance Center in early 2011 in the capital Sana'a is one of the important achievements in pharmacy practice.

11. *Challenges of pharmacy practice in Yemen and recommendations*

The following list summarizes the major challenges to pharmacy practice in Yemen and what can be done to address them:

- Community pharmacies and drug stores in Yemen are still focused on dispensing and selling medicines and nonpharmacological products. Community pharmacists need to be educated about their new roles in the pharmaceutical, public, and clinical services, rather than simply dispensing.
- Physicians, nurses, other healthcare professionals, and the public need to be educated about the new roles of the pharmacists in providing pharmaceutical care, public, and clinical services.
- There is a lack of clinical pharmacists in hospitals because the Ministry of Public Health and Population hires few pharmacists in their hospitals and clinical centers when compared to job vacancies for physicians and others. The pharmacies in most hospitals are either not available or have few medicines available. Therefore, there is a need to establish a pharmacy in each hospital in Yemen, which will create job vacancies for pharmacists. Moreover, a law should be enacted and regulations made that lead to the acceptance of the new role of the pharmacists in the hospitals to provide pharmaceutical care and clinical pharmacy services.

- Increasing public awareness is required about the importance of treatment and diagnosis by authorized physicians, rather than relying on unqualified staff at pharmacies and drug stores to diagnose and prescribe treatment. Taking medicines without identifying the real problems can lead to serious adverse effects on people's health.
- Counterfeit medicines in Yemen are a major problem. Steps need to be taken to increase awareness on the part of pharmacists, healthcare professionals, and the public about the dangers and potentially bad outcomes from using these counterfeit medicines.
- The lack of staff in pharmacovigilance centers in Yemen is a challenge. Sufficient staffing is needed to activate the pharmacovigilance roles and activities in Yemen. Hiring better trained staff is necessary to improve the services of pharmacovigilance center in Yemen.
- Marketing the pharmacovigilance center role and activities through media, workshops, general lectures, brochures, and educational materials is needed to increase the awareness of health care professionals.
- There is a need to conduct further research about the various issues facing pharmacy practice in Yemen. This requires support from the policymakers and universities so that researchers can conduct studies.
- The increase in pharmacies and drug stores operated by unqualified persons in the last 5 years has created a major challenge for the development of legitimate pharmacy practice in Yemen. Steps must be taken to address this problem.
- More private colleges and institutions of pharmacy are offering a bachelor degree of pharmacy without being officially recognized by the Ministry of Higher Education and Scientific Research. The large number of pharmacists graduating from those colleges undermines pharmacy practice in Yemen. Greater regulation of pharmacy colleges is needed to curtail the number of unaccredited pharmacy colleges and graduates.
- There is an urgent need for laws and regulations that require pharmacy and drugstore owners to hire qualified and registered pharmacists, as these professionals are the only ones that have the right to legally dispense medications. Also, there is a need to implement and enforce penalties to punish those who are not following these laws and regulations.
- There is a need for a registration examination to ensure the quality of the working pharmacists in Yemen; the examination should be theoretical and practical.
- Poor counseling among community pharmacy dispensers was reported in Yemen.[25] There is a need for collaboration between the official pharmacy colleges and the Ministry of Public Health and Population to develop a policy requiring pharmacists to attend yearly continuous medical education courses, as it is very important that pharmacists update their knowledge of pharmacy practice and other issues.

12. Conclusions

Pharmacy practice in Yemen is still in its infancy and it faces major hurdles. Many developments are needed, including updating the pharmacy curriculum; updating, implementing, and enforcing the pharmacist law; developing a standard for patient pharmaceutical care services and the quality of the pharmacy workforce; and increasing the awareness among the public, physicians, other healthcare professionals, and policy makers about the value of pharmacists. The first pharmacy in Yemen was opened in 1875 in Aden, and the second pharmacy opened in1876. In 2010, the first chain pharmacies were established in the capital Sana'a. There are nine local pharmaceutical industries in Yemen, which cover approximately 10–20% of the total market. The Yemeni Pharmacovigilance Center was established in early 2011 in the capital Sana'a. Clinical pharmacy services were implemented at the end of 2010 in a few community pharmacies and private hospitals.

The author hopes that pharmacy practice in Yemen will improve in the near future and pharmacists take seriously their new role in providing pharmaceutical care and clinical pharmacy services.

13. Lessons learned

- Establishing the appropriate systems and setting up suitable regulations are essential requirements and are the first step to establish and develop better pharmacy practice.
- Without enforcement, regulations become just documents that have nothing to do with practice.
- Collaboration is needed between stakeholders to improve pharmacy practice, and collaboration with international organizations is an additional benefit.
- Development takes time, however, as long as there is some progress, great expectations are never lost.

Acknowledgments

I would like to thank my wife for her support during each step in this work. I would also like to thank the pharmacists Ibrahim Mahmoud Alsaman and Tammam Noman Saeed for their help for the information collection.

This chapter reflects the opinion of the author and does not necessarily reflect any organization in the Republic of Yemen.

References

1. Central Statistics Organization. *Annual report*. [cited September 29, 2013]. Available from: http://www.cso-yemen.org/content.php?lng=arabic&id=623; 2012.
2. Ministry of Public Health and Population. *Annual statistical health report*. [cited March 1, 2013]. Available from: http://www.mophp-ye.org/arabic/docs/Report2011.pdf; 2011.
3. WHO. *Country profiles: Yemen*. Available at: http://www.emro.who.int/emrininfo/index.asp?Ctry=yem; 2005. [accessed on 03.09.12].
4. Health System Profile Yemen, Regional Health Systems Observatory- EMRO, World Health Organization. [cited March 1, 2013]. Available from: http://gis.emro.who.int/HealthSystemObservatory/PDF/Yemen/Full%20Profile.pdf; 2006.

5. USAID/Public expenditure review, health sector republic of Yemen, 1999–2003. [cited March 1, 2013]. Available from: http://www.phrplus.org/Pubs/Tech096_fin.pdf; 2003.

6. Ministry of Public Health and Population. *Annual statistical health report.* [cited March 1, 2013]; Available from: http://www.mophp-ye.org/arabic/docs/Report2010.pdf; 2010.

7. Ministry of Public Health and Population. *Annual statistical health report.* [cited March 1, 2013]. Available from: http://www.mophp-ye.org/arabic/docs/Report2009.pdf; 2009.

8. Ministry of Public Health and Population. *Annual statistical health report.* [cited March 1, 2013]. Available from: http://www.mophp-ye.org/arabic/docs/Report2008.pdf; 2008.

9. Yemen Pharmacists Syndicate. First preparatory meeting Sana'a, http://www.14october.com/news.aspx?newsno5108803; 2010 [accessed 01.03.13].

10. Al-Worafi YM. Pharmacy practice and its challenges in Yemen. *Australas Med J* 2014;**7**(1):17–23.

11. Al-Worafi YM. Pharmacy education in Yemen. *Am J Pharm Educ* 2013;**77**(3):65.

12. Al-Worafi YM. The challenges of pharmacy education in Yemen. *Am J Pharm Educ* 2014;**78**(8):146.

13. Yemen Drug Company (YEDCO). [cited September 3, 2012]. Available from: http://www.yeco.biz/yecoeng/modules.php?name=yedco&pa=showpageyedco&pid=1; 2012.

14. Shiba Pharma for Pharmaceutical Industries. [cited September 3, 2012]. Available from: http://www.shibapharma.com/; 2012.

15. Supreme Board of Drugs and Medical Appliances (SBDMA) annual report. [cited September 3, 2012]. Available from: http://sbd-ye.org/; 2011.

16. Ministry of Public Health and Population. [cited March 1, 2013]; Available from: http://www.mophp-ye.org/arabic; 2012.

17. Supreme Board of Drugs and Medical Appliances (SBDMA). [cited March 1, 2013]. Available from: http://www.sbdye.org/; 2012.

18. WHO/HAI. Medicine prices, availability, affordability and price components. A synthesis report of medicine price surveys undertaken in selected countries of the World Health Organization Eastern Mediterranean Region. Cairo, World Health Organization Regional Office for the Eastern Mediterranean. [cited March 1, 2013]. Available from: http://applications.emro.who.int/dsaf/dsa904.pdf; 2008.

19. Pharmacy regulation and Law Yemen. http://www.yemen-nic.info/db/laws_ye/detail.php?ID=11755 [accessed 01.03.13] http://www1.umn.edu/humanrts/arabic/Yemeni_Laws/Yemeni_Laws69.pdf; 2002 [accessed 01.03.13].

20. Accreditation standards and guidelines for the professional program leading in pharmacy leading to the Doctor of Pharmacy degree. Accreditation Council for Pharmacy Education (ACPE). Available at: https://www.acpe-accredit.org/pdf/ACPE_Revised_PharmD_Standards_Adopted_Jan152006.pdf [accessed 01.08.13].

21. Beardsley RS. Communication skills development in colleges of pharmacy. *Am J Pharm Educ* 2001;**65**:307–14.

22. International Pharmaceutical Federation. FIP Statement of Policy on Good Pharmacy Education Practice. http://www.fip.org/www/uploads/database_file.php?id=302&table_id= [accessed 01.08.13].

23. Anderson C, Bates I, Beck D, Brock TP, Futter B, Mercer H, et al. The WHO UNESCO FIP pharmacy education taskforce. *Hum Resour Health* 2009;**7**:45.

24. Al-Worafi YM. Comment on:"Pharmacovigilance in the middle east". *Drug Safet J* 2014;**37**(8):651–2.

25. Al-Worafi YMA. Appropriateness of metered-dose inhaler use in Yemeni community pharmacies. *J Taibah Univ Med Sci* 2015.

Pharmacy Practice in Africa

CHAPTER 15

Pharmacy Practice in Egypt

Tarek Mohamed Elsayed, Gihan H. Elsisi, Mahmoud Elmahdawy

Chapter Outline

1. Country background

Egypt is located in Northern Africa, bordering the Mediterranean Sea, between Libya in the west and occupied Palestine and the Red Sea in the east and north of Sudan. It includes the Asian Sinai Peninsula. With its location in the northeast corner of Africa, Egypt has been the cultural bridge between the African continent and the Middle East for millennia.

While 97% of the 1 million km^2 that constitutes Egyptian land is desert, the world's longest river, the Nile, runs through it, and for 6000 years civilization has flourished on its banks. Egyptian culture has consistently changed across various periods of time from Pharaonic to Coptic Christian to Arabic Islamic culture. Currently, the great majority of its population are

Pharmacy Practice in Developing Countries. http://dx.doi.org/10.1016/B978-0-12-801714-2.00015-0

Table 1: Trends of demographic indicators for Egypt

Demographic Indicator	2013
Total population (millions)	82.06
Population, female (% of total)	49.78
Population ages 0–14 (% of total)	31.14
Population ages 15-64 (% of total)	63.11
Population ages 65 and above (% of total)	5.76
Population growth (annual %)	1.6
Population density (people per km^2)	82.43
Fertility rate, total (births per woman)	2.77
Birth rate, crude (per 1000 people)	23.18
Death rate, crude (per 1000 people)	6.49
Rural population	46,751,621

Source: World Bank.[1]

Muslims, with a Christian minority below 10% of the population. The official language is standard Arabic, with several Arabic dialects used in everyday matters.

Egypt has a rapidly growing population. In July 2013, the population in Egypt reached 82.06 million.[1] The aging population is expected to continue increasing each year (Table 1). The national median age estimated in 2014 was 25.1 years. Egypt is considered a lower middle-income country, with a gross national income per capita of $3160 in 2013, a population below the international poverty line of US$1.25 per day of 1.7% in 2012, and a poverty head-count ratio at the national poverty line (% of population) of 25.2% in 2011. Ranked 112 in the human development index, of 177 countries, it had an adult (15+ years) literacy rate of 73.9% in the period from 2008 to 2012.[2]

Politically, Egypt is a constitution-based republic. This consists of a mixed legal system based on Napoleonic civil law and Islamic religious law and judicial review by a Supreme Court and a Council of State.[3] After independence from British colonialism and the ousting of the last Egyptian king, Farouk, in 1952 by the military movement led by General Mohamad Nageeb, General Gamal Abdel Naser, the second president of Egypt, led a transition to socialist rule in the 1950s and 1960s. The Egyptian economy showed gradual transformation from a socialist one toward a market-based economy starting in the 1970s.[4]

The opening of the country to the world economy allowed continued economic growth through the years as well as implementation of various economic reforms to balance economic inequalities as well as to reduce foreign debt (Table 2).[5] Despite some social improvements and a growing economy, widespread public dissatisfaction with basic living conditions and high levels of poverty remained and spurred the Arab Spring revolution in 2011. The uprising caused economic growth to slow down in the following years owing to the political uncertainty along with a significant reduction in tourism.[3]

Table 2: Macroeconomic indicators for Egypt

Indicator	2012
GDP per capita (US$)	3187
GDP per capita, PPP (US$)	6700
GDP real growth rate (%)	2.2
Labor force (millions)	26.42
Population below poverty line	20% (2005 est.)
Unemployment rate	13.5%
Public debt (% of GDP)	88%
Tax burden (% of GDP)	19.5%
Budget deficit (−)	−10.8%
Official exchange rate against US$ (as in July 2014)	£E7.15

Source: Egypt overview.[1]

2. Vital health statistics

Egypt has shown a consistent overall improvement in health indicators that surpassed the regional averages. There is a marked reduction in the crude death rate, infant mortality rate, under 5 years death rate, and maternal mortality rate.

Egypt showed a decline in population growth rate from 2.75% in 1966 to 1.6% in 2013. The prevalence of adult risk factors such as raised blood pressure and glucose is lower than the regional average in both males and females, while obesity and tobacco use are higher. Polio eradication is sustained, with ongoing elimination of filariasis, schistosomiasis, and measles. However, hepatitis B and C continue to be a public health problem in Egypt, which has the highest prevalence of hepatitis C (HCV) in the world.[6] The strong homogeneity of HCV subtypes found in Egypt (mostly 4a) suggests an epidemic spread of HCV through the past practice of parenteral therapy for schistosomiasis.[7] Tables 3 and 4 show the top 10 diseases causing mortality and morbidity in Egypt, respectively.[5]

Like many other developing countries, the achievement of diminished communicable disease burden is challenged by a large and rapidly growing noncommunicable disease burden including mental health-related diseases (Table 5). Also, lifestyle factors and risk-taking behaviors such as smoking, substance abuse, lack of exercise, overconsumption of fatty and salty foods, nonuse of seat belts, and nonobservance of traffic rules contribute to a significant proportion of the overall mortality and morbidity.[8]

The World Health Organization (WHO) (2013) reported a 26% and 9% prevalence of hypertension and diabetes mellitus in the Egyptian adult population, respectively. Around 1% of the population is blind, mainly due to cataracts; a high prevalence of trachoma is reported in some governorates. The incidence of cancers is approximately 110–120 cases per 100,000 of the population.

Table 3: The top 10 diseases causing mortality in Egypt

Disease	Rank
Essential primary hypertension	1
Intracerebral hemorrhage	2
Fibrosis and cirrhosis of the liver	3
Hepatic failure	4
Atherosclerosis	5
Elevated blood glucose level	6
Arterial embolism and thrombosis	7
Acute myocardial infarction	8
Cerebral infarction	9
Other	10

Source: National Health Accounts.[5]

Table 4: The top 10 diseases causing morbidity in Egypt

Disease	Rank
Infectious gastroenteritis	1
Spontaneous labor	2
Cesarean section	3
Acute appendicitis	4
Iron deficiency anemia	5
Respiratory distress syndrome	6
Broncho pneumonia	7
Acute tonsillitis	8
Forearm fracture	9
Nonspecific renal colic	10

Source: National Health Accounts.[5]

The four most common cancers in the country are breast, liver, bladder, and lymph node. With regard to the Tobacco-Free Initiative, there have been three increases in tobacco tax in the year since the revolution and the current Minister of Finance has passed a decree for the tobacco industry to apply the band roll system on all tobacco product packs in Egypt. Egypt has become the leading country in the world with an estimated road traffic death rate per 100,000 of 41.6.

There was a consistent improvement in drinking water sources and sanitation facilities from the year 1990 to 2012 and an increased total expenditure on health in the same period that is above the regional average.

While public expenditure on health in terms of budget share seems to be low in Egypt, the overall spending at 3.7% of GDP is also low, compared to other comparable income countries. The Ministry of Health and Population (MOHP) budget, as part of the entire government budget, increased from 2.2% in 1995/1996 to 3.3% in 2000/2001and the MOHP expenditure per capita increased from £E26.8 in 1996 to £E56.7 in 2001.

Table 5: Health care indicators in Egypt

Health Indicator	Egypt	Regional Average	Global Average
Life expectancy at birth (years)	71	68	70
Crude death rate in (%) 1970/2012	15.8/6.5	n.a.	n.a.
Under 5 years mortality rate (per 1000 live births)	21	57	48
Probability of dying between 15 and 60 years M/F (per 1000 population)	196/120	194/139	187/124
Maternal mortality ratio (per 100,000 live births, 2013)	45	170	210
Prevalence of HIV (per 100,000 population)	8.1	68	511
Prevalence of tuberculosis (per 100,000 population)	29	180	169
Prevalence of hepatitis C (%)	14.7	n.a.	3%
Use of improved drinking water sources (%) 2011, total	99.3	n.a.	n.a.
Use of improved sanitation facilities (%) 2011, total	95.0	n.a.	n.a.
Routine Expanded Program on Immunization (EPI) vaccines financed by government (%) 2012	100.0	n.a.	n.a.
Malaria (%) 2008–2012, antimalarial treatment among febrile children	0.0	n.a.	n.a.
Total expenditure on health per capita (Intl $)	323	n.a.	n.a.
Total expenditure on health as % of GDP	5.0	n.a.	n.a.

Source: Egypt: health profile.[9]

3. Overview of the health care system

Egypt is the second most populous country recognized by the WHO's Eastern Mediterranean region.[8] Egypt's health care system is pluralistic and complex (Figure 1), combining both public and private providers and financiers. Public investment in the health system has been declining since 2005.[10] This has forced financing from private households (out-of-pocket) to continue rising, distinguishing it further as the single largest source of health financing (Figure 2).
To date, pharmaceutical expenditures have been the largest; they account for 34% of overall health spending, which is a relatively high percentage in comparison to other health systems.[10] The expenditure on pharmaceuticals mostly comes from out-of-pocket spending owing to the limited budget and the lack of information and education about proper use of pharmaceuticals.

Health care services are provided through public sector entities, mainly the MOHP and the state-owned Health Insurance Organization (HIO), as well as other ministries and other public sector entities such as the Curative Care Organization, Teaching Hospitals and Institutes, and nongovernmental organizations involved in health, which are nonprofit organizations in addition to private insurance plans (Egycare). The MOHP owns and operates a large network of hospitals and outpatient facilities. Each public entity runs its own facilities following the MOHP regulations, while the private sectors have their own set of regulations and standards.

The largest source of health insurance for Egyptians remains the HIO, essentially a social health insurance system that is supposed to complement the tax-financed services provided by

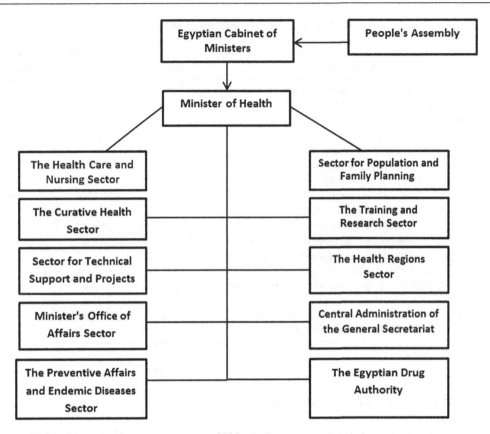

Figure 1
Organization of the health system in Egypt. *Source: Organizational chart of the MOHP in Eygpt.*[11]

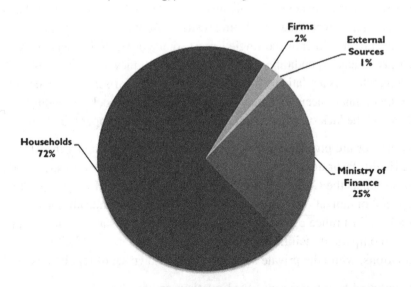

Figure 2
Egyptian health investments 2008–2009. *Source: National Health Accounts, 2010.*[5]

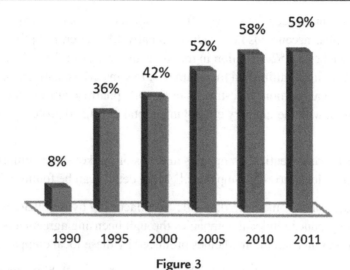

Figure 3

Development in health insurance coverage. *Source: Health Insurance Organization Report.*[13]

the MOHP. The aim of this organization is to provide universal health care coverage for all Egyptians. While this organization has not achieved this goal, its coverage has continued to rise significantly since 1990 (Figure 3). As such, the HIO represents the second largest health financing organization in Egypt.[12]

The number of health facilities has been growing rapidly since 1995. These consist of both public and private facilities with varying services and amenities. The number of physicians, dentists, pharmacists, and nursing and midwifery personnel are above the regional average. In 2009, there were 28.3 physicians, 4.2 dentists, 16.7 pharmacists, and 35.2 nurses and midwifery personnel per 10,000 people registered in Egypt.[12]

4. Medicine supply systems and drug use issues

The pharmaceutical sector in Egypt is one of the oldest strategic sectors in the country, founded in 1939 with the establishment of Misr Company for Pharmaceutical Industries. The Egyptian pharmaceuticals market, estimated at around US$4.1 billion at retail prices or US$48 per capita in 2010, is considered the largest in the Middle East and North Africa (MENA) region, accounting for around 30% of the regional market. Pharmaceutical companies in Egypt fall into three categories: public sector companies, subsidiaries to the Holding Company for Pharmaceuticals (Holdipharma); private sector companies; and multinational companies. Before 1990, the sector was heavily dominated by public companies. Since then, the private sector has constituted the highest share after starting a privatization program. Currently, there are 119 licensed pharmaceutical plants in Egypt, eight of which are public companies. Their major activity is the production of formulations from pharmaceutical starting material, with some production of pharmaceutical starting materials (APIs) and repackaging of finished dosage forms.[14]

Local production of pharmaceuticals covers 93% of local consumption, with 7% made up of highly specialized pharmaceuticals not produced locally. Moreover, Egypt's exports of pharmaceuticals reached US$270 million in the financial year 2011/2012. They are mainly retail medicaments, with semifinished medicaments, raw materials, antisera, and vaccines constituting only a small portion. Investments in Egypt's pharmaceutical industry currently stand at £E26 billion, with the industry employing a total of 39,500 professional staff and production workers.

In 2012, the top 10 pharmaceutical companies in terms of market share comprised 5 multinational and 5 local private companies.[15] More details can be found in Table 6.

Around 30% of local sales come from domestic manufacturing by multinational corporations, and about 35% are produced in local companies through licensing agreements, while the remaining ratio represents generic medicines produced by these local companies.

Egypt is in the preliminary stages of establishing a successful health biotechnology sector. This sector emerged from existing pharmaceutical and generics companies that have an interest in recombinant technology products for their business. The production includes diagnostic kits, vaccine production, and antibiotics manufacturing.[16]

Egypt is one of the four countries in the region that are major producer of vaccines. The goal of the region is to become self-sufficient in its need for quality-assured vaccines.

Production of vaccines started in Egypt with a small laboratory established in 1881 by the Health Department. The smallpox vaccine was produced for the first time in Egypt in 1893, followed by the rabies vaccine in Kasr El-Ainy–Pasteur Institute in 1907. In 1939, the state-owned General Organization for Vaccines & Sera was established. Since its success at producing cholera vaccine for the first time in Egypt in 1939, progress has continued. It was converted to the Holding Company for Biological Products & Vaccines (VACSERA) by a

Table 6: The top 10 pharmaceutical companies in Egypt

	Corporation	YTD 2012 in Millions	Growth (%)
1	GlaxoSmithKline	335	19.1
2	Novartis	317	15.0
3	Pharco	219	14.6
4	Sanofi Aventis	204	13.3
5	EIPICO	183	14.8
6	Amoun Pharmaceutical Company	152	7.8
7	Pfizer	134	20.3
8	EVA Pharma	102	10.4
9	SIGMA	93	18.1
10	M.S.D	81	30.1

Source: Egypt; country brief.[15]

presidential decree in 2003.[17] Currently, VACSERA is the only producer of vaccines and sera in Egypt and is one of the main blood banks. It produces a wide range of products including vaccines, immunoglobulins, biopharmaceuticals, veterinary products, blood products and derivatives, therapeutic fluids, and diagnostic media.[18] The technical capacity of the national regulatory authority for vaccines in Egypt is still weak and needs to be strengthened to meet functional requirements. Cooperation was established with the WHO to assist in establishing Egypt as a prequalified producer of vaccines and biologicals and a regional reference laboratory for vaccine quality control.[8] Currently, VACSERA has a large number of laboratories that operate according to international standards. Among these laboratories are the WHO Regional Reference Lab for Polio and the WHO Influenza National Reference Center.

Although Egypt's pharmaceutical expenditure per capita is still one of the lowest in the MENA region, Egypt is the largest consumer of pharmaceuticals in this region, with an annual increasing pharmaceutical spending reaching about US$2.48 billion by the end of 2009. Consumption is expected to continue increasing at a compound annual growth rate of 11.4%.[19]

Legal provisions exist to govern the licensing and prescribing practices of prescribers. Furthermore, legal provisions restricting dispensing by prescribers do exist. Prescribers in the private sector do dispense medicines. There are regulations requiring hospitals to organize and develop drug and therapeutics committees (DTCs).

In public health care facilities, prescribing by International Nonproprietary Name (INN) is compulsory; however, only 37.5% of prescribed medicines are in INN. The average number of medicines prescribed per patient contact in these facilities is 2.3, and 88.47% of prescribed medicines are on the national Essential Medicines List. Of prescribed drugs, 91.2% are dispensed to patients and only 45.2% of dispensed medicines are adequately labeled.

Also, legal provisions in Egypt exist to govern dispensing practices of pharmaceutical personnel. Substitution of generic equivalents at the point of dispensing is allowed in public and private sector facilities.

National health insurance and the Ministry of Health have an approved formulary that is updated every 2 years; government hospitals are required to adhere to such list, and when generics do exist, they might be preferred owing to the price advantage.[14] The pharmacovigilance (PV) department at the ministry has accomplished a great national input in establishing a national adverse drug reaction (ADR) monitoring network and linking pharmacists to it.

The drug market, as everywhere, is regulated by prescribers (physicians), patients, and pharmacists who are currently playing a crucial role in drug price control, especially after establishment of a pharmacoeconomic unit that evaluates the cost and effectiveness of drugs and performs cost–benefit analyses and budget impact analyses to affect decisions on a policy level. Pharmacists are active members of established pharmacy and therapeutics committees. Also, formularies and an essential drug list are discussed in committees in which pharmacists have a heavy presence and their clinical and scientific opinion counts; however, there is more opportunity in this area and room for improvement. Decisions based on evidence-based medicine practices and adhering to latest clinical practice guidelines (standard treatment guidelines) for selected diseases are an uphill battle for pharmacists in terms of implementation, but it is a great opportunity to curb a huge irrational use of medicine and consequent expenditures.[10]

Medicine prices in Egypt are considered the lowest in the region. Publicly produced medicines are heavily subsidized. In Egypt, there are legal or regulatory provisions affecting pricing of medicines, which are aimed at the level of manufacturers/wholesalers/retailers and are applied to all types of medicines in the market.

The government runs an active national medicine price monitoring system for retail prices. Regulations exist mandating that retail medicine price information should be publicly accessible. The data available regarding drug prices in Egypt are from the WHO/Health Action International pricing survey conducted in Egypt in 2004. Compared to international reference prices, the median price ratio for generics was 0.95 in the public sector, while no originators were found there. The private sector had higher prices (1.69 for generics, 2.73 for originators).[14]

5. Overview of pharmacy practice and key pharmaceutical sectors

The practice of pharmacy and pharmaceutical preparations in ancient Egypt may date back to thousands of years before Christ. The physician-priests of Egypt were divided into two classes: those who visited the sick and those who remained in the temple and prepared remedies for the patients.[20] Egyptians are thought to be the first to write medical texts describing illnesses and drug therapies.[21] The first known documentation for this practice is the Kahun Papyrus.[22] The so-called Kahun Gynaecological Papyrus is one of the largest manuscripts dating from the late Middle Kingdom (1850–1700 BC), a 34-paragraph document divided into sections. Each section has detailed information about a specific medical problem or complaint. The details include symptoms and advice on how to address the patient in offering his or her diagnosis and, finally, a recommended treatment is suggested. No mention is made, however, of the likely prognosis. This process of described symptoms, diagnosis, report, and treatment makes up 17 sections.[23]

The Edwin Smith Papyrus, which dates back to 1550 BC, is another important document, which includes descriptions of several remedies and diagnoses of various traumas. Egyptians were the first to perform surgery and use splints and bandages. The Ebers Papyrus, which has been dated back to 1500 BC, contains the most information on drug remedies and names of over 900 specific drugs. Remedies contained ingredients of plant, animal, and mineral origin in addition to the use of magic in some cases.[24] Many dosage forms are prescribed in these scripts, including infusions, decoctions, macerations, inhalations, gargles, poultices, and the same types of preparations the older pharmacists of today would still recognize. Tools for compounding, such as mortars of wood or stone, and containers for storage made of pottery and glass were also used.[22]

Currently, Egypt has the fourth highest number of pharmacists per 10,000 of population in the world, after Malta, Japan, and Jordan, with around 16.8 pharmacists per 10,000 of population.[25] The number of pharmacies per 10,000 of population is the highest in the world (around 6.5 pharmacies for each 10,000 of population). Moreover, the average number of graduates per school is the highest in the world (480 students). With such a large number of graduates, the number of pharmacists relative to population is expected to increase further. Pharmacists in Egypt are employed in various sectors, including enforcement, drug information, pharmaceutical product sales and promotion, manufacturing, research, academia, and hospital and community pharmacy. The number of licensed pharmacists in all sectors in Egypt reached 139,479 in the year 2011; 15,457 of them are working in the public sector. This is a large increase compared to the number of registered pharmacists in 1997, which was only 36,500 pharmacists. The majority of pharmacists in Egypt work in community pharmacies, followed by hospitals as well as industrial, academic, and research institutions. Pharmacists are also involved in other professional practices, including forensic services, biomedical laboratories, the cosmetic industry, veterinary medicine, and military pharmacy services. Furthermore, a large number of Egyptian pharmacists work abroad, mainly in Arab countries. However, information about human resources in the pharmaceutical sector in Egypt remains fragmented and there is no adequate information or statistics about the distribution of pharmacists in various sectors.

6. Drug- and pharmacy-related regulations, policies, and ethics

Access to essential medicines/technologies as part of the fulfillment of the right to health is recognized in the Egyptian constitution and national legislation. Encouraging the Egyptian and Arab pharmaceutical industry and ensuring availability at affordable prices are features of the Health Sector Reform Program in 2010. To accomplish these goals, an Egyptian national medicine policy does exist and was updated in 2005. It covers selection of essential medicines, medicine financing, procurement, distribution, regulation, rational use, PV, monitoring, and evaluation, in addition to human resources development. Its implementation is regularly monitored/assessed by the Egyptian Drug Authority (EDA).[14]

The EDA is responsible for protecting people's health through regulation of the safety and quality of pharmaceutical products; regulation and legislation of pharmacy practice; availability of high-quality medicines at affordable prices; strategic planning; policy-making for the sector; the setting of standards of pharmaceutical services for both hospital and community; orchestration and integration of all reviewing and analysis processes for product registration, lot releases, and market monitoring; enhancement of public awareness of possible adverse actions of medicines, dangers of drug misuse, and warnings against counterfeited medicines; the support of programs for improving pharmacy education and continuous training of pharmacists; and cooperation with relevant international organizations, for example, the WHO, to improve standards of pharmaceutical products and practices. Funding for the EDA is provided through the regular government budget as well as through fees imposed for services provided. A computerized information management system is in place to store and retrieve information on processes that include registrations, inspection, etc.

The EDA has three suborganizations that work cooperatively and synergistically to ensure the achievement of the EDA mission. These are the Central Administration of Pharmaceutical Affairs (CAPA), National Organization for Drug Control and Research (NODCAR), and National Organization for Research and Control of Biologicals (NORCB).

The CAPA has four departments. The Registration Department is responsible for registration of medicines for human and veterinary use, food supplements, medical devices, cosmetics, and insecticides. Pricing of medicines for human and veterinary use and food supplements and collection of samples of these products from manufacturing and distribution facilities are within the discretion of this department.

The Licensing and Pharmacists' Services Department issues licenses for facilities that are involved in manufacturing, distributing, selling, or promoting pharmaceutical products. The Inspection and Control Department oversees activities of pharmaceutical manufacturing facilities, distributors, public and private pharmacies, and scientific offices. The Importation and Exportation Department issues permits for importation and custom release of narcotics, raw materials, finished products, and medical devices.

In Egypt, manufacturers, importers, wholesalers, and distributors of pharmaceutical products must be licensed. NODCAR is a component of the Ministry of Health established in the year 1976 under Presidential Decree 382/1976. The aim of NODCAR is to ensure the good quality, safety, and effectiveness of marketed local and imported pharmaceutical products. To ensure this, marketing authorization is not allocated to any product unless it obtains the necessary certificate of compliance from NODCAR. These products are subjected to various chemical, physical, microbiological, biological, and pharmacological quality control tests to ensure that they conform to appropriate standards of identity, strength, quality, and purity. The products tested by NODCAR include pharmaceutical products, raw materials, cosmetics, medical devices, veterinary products, household insecticides, medicinal plants, natural products, and materials (packaging and filling materials). Testing of biological products is under the authority of NORCB. Testing is done to ensure the safety, quality, and efficacy of all imported and domestic biologicals. Testing is done for product registration, for public procurement prequalification, and routinely for quality monitoring in public and private sectors and when there are complaints or problem reports in compliance with requirements of the WHO and the International Organization for Standardization.[26] In January 2012, the Egyptian Ministry of Health and

EDA announced the launch of new PV guidelines for marketing authorization holders. These laws make the reporting of adverse drug effects compulsory for firms and are part of a wider increase in focus on regulatory activity in the field of PV in Africa, which helps in combating soaring rates of drug counterfeiting.[27]

As Egypt is a member of the World Trade Organization (WTO), a new intellectual property rights law came into force on 4 June 2002 aiming at the implementation of the WTO Agreement on Trade-Related Aspects of Intellectual Property Rights (the TRIPS Agreement). Pharmaceuticals are included in this law; however, it contains TRIPS-specific flexibilities and safeguards, including compulsory licensing provisions, that can be applied for reasons of public health, such as the Bolar exception and parallel importing provisions. The Bolar provision, sometimes called the "regulatory exception," allows manufacturers of generic drugs to use the patented invention to obtain marketing approval without the patent owner's permission and before the patent protection expires. The generic producers can then market their versions as soon as the patent expires.[28]

All pharmaceutical products marketed in Egypt require an MOH registration number before they can be traded or given to people, which is the authority of CAPA. The CAPA registration process starts by receiving a registration submission request with the required data, which include assay methods, in vitro dissolution, and bioequivalence and stability studies in addition to pharmacology information.

In Egypt, legal provisions exist to control the promotion and/or advertising of prescription medicines. CAPA is responsible for regulating the promotion and/or advertising of medicines. Direct advertising of prescription medicines to the public is prohibited and preapproval for medicine advertisements and promotional materials by the Technical Committee for Drug Control in CAPA is required prior to submission through the media. Guidelines and regulations exist for advertising and promotion of nonprescription medicines. However, there is no national code of conduct concerning advertising and promotion of medicines by marketing authorization holders.

Pharmacist registration is compulsory in Egypt in order to practice. No evaluation exam is required for pharmacists graduating from Egyptian pharmacy schools. For pharmacists graduating from foreign schools, an evaluating exam is required.

In addition to CAPA, the Egyptian pharmacists syndicate (EPS) has a role in regulating the profession. Pharmacists' membership in the EPS is compulsory. There is a code of conduct that governs the professional behavior of pharmacists.[14]

6.1 Drug price control

Because of the socioeconomic implications of pharmaceutical drug prices, Egypt has a binding price control system for drugs. The prices are controlled by the government (MOHP). Pricing of the products is decided by the pricing committee at CAPA. In the event of a violation, both the producer and the retailer would be subject to severe punishment. The drug price control system is consistent with the TRIPS Agreement (Article 8 (1)), which allows TRIPS members to adopt measures necessary to protect public health and nutrition.[28]

The MOHP is also the final decision-maker for pharmaceutical and health technology reimbursement in the public sector through its approved drug tender lists. CAPA, part of the MOHP, is the final decision-maker for market authorization and pricing and is responsible for postmarket surveillance and price regulation. The marketing authorization is granted by CAPA within 12 months of the day of application submission. Pricing decisions are based on international pricing considerations in compliance with the pharmaceutical Egyptian price regulations. CAPA is the final pricing decision-maker of the first price. Currently, there are two prices for each drug. The first price is the mandated public government price and the second price is the tender price for every market-authorized drug included in the Tender Drug List. Drug manufacturers just recommend prices for new medicines and then the pricing committee evaluates this price to be approved or not, according to its external reference pricing, and sets the approved price. According to the latest pricing decree issued as of this writing, No. 499/2012, CAPA reevaluates pricing of drugs (first price, i.e., public price) every 5 years. It also reevaluates pricing of drugs upon request of the drug manufacturer in the case of changed costs. In addition, reevaluation also takes place in the case of new indications or a foreign currency exchange rate change of 15%. A pharmacoeconomic study for high technology products may be provided upon request. The price of the product can be changed upon appearance of other lower prices for the same product in any country.[29]

The Egyptian government uses a variety of strategies to keep many medicines at an affordable price, including subsidization through the public sector and drug pricing. The main strategy is the investment in the public sector firms, which play an important role in making affordable drugs accessible. While these firms are commonly criticized for "poor profitability, the relative inefficiency, and the low labour productivity," they constitute 30% of the local drug consumption needs at affordable prices.[30] Another strategy is pricing. Reasonably priced medicines have long been widely available in Egypt, in part because of a strong local pharmaceutical industry, although private sector retail pharmacy prices for the lowest priced generics were, on average, 68% higher than public sector procurement prices for the same medicines. Nevertheless, patients in Egypt rely heavily on private pharmacies as many products are not subsidized and not manufactured by the public sector firms.[31] Such prices put a heavy burden on families with modest incomes. Consequently, Egyptian citizens in the low-income bracket are not guaranteed access to medicines.

Before September 2009, the pricing committee in the Ministry of Health determined the profit margin ceiling for various types of medicine through the "cost-plus system." The profit margin ceiling was 15% for essential drugs, 25% for nonessential drugs, and 40% for over-the-counter drugs. In the year 2009, two pricing systems for the registration of new medicines in the market, one for branded pharmaceuticals and the other for generic drugs, were adopted. Under this system, the price of branded drugs is set 10% lower than their cheapest retail price in 36 countries in which the drug is available; however, this does not mean that the drug should be registered in all 36 countries. For generic drugs, the price is decreased by a fixed percentage below the similar branded drug price, which is 30% for companies licensed by the Ministry of Health and certified by international agencies, 40% for companies licensed by only the Ministry of Health, and 60% for companies that do not possess manufacturing facilities. This new system is expected to increase medicine prices compared to the previous prices that were cheaper by 80 and 90% compared to branded drugs.[19]

As for the pricing of orphan drugs, although it is an issue of high priority for decision-makers to provide access to orphan drugs, manufacturers attempt to maximize their prices within the constraints of domestic pricing policies to recoup the substantial research and development costs from a small number of patients. This translates to higher prices of orphan drugs that render them inaccessible.

7. Core pharmacy practices

The pharmacy profession is responsible for ensuring equity, accessibility, and affordability of essential drugs and vaccines to the entire Egyptian population. The significant role of the pharmaceutical industry in Egypt, which covers more than 90% of local drug consumption, demonstrates the importance of the pharmacy profession in promoting the health of Egyptians and overall national economic development.

7.1 Hospital pharmacy

There are 1969 hospitals in Egypt,[14] 539 of them are public ones.[32] Regulations require hospitals to organize and develop DTCs. Many challenges face hospital pharmacy practice in Egypt. For many years, the role of the hospital pharmacist was limited to procurement, dispensing, and counseling. Until the late 1990s, shortages in hospital pharmacists contributed to this limitation. Moreover, many problems, including lack of training, education, and administrative framework, delayed the initiation of clinical pharmacy practice in Egyptian hospitals.

Clinical pharmacy services and clinical pharmacy awareness are rapidly increasing nowadays in many governmental and private hospitals. The Hospital Pharmacy Department within the Ministry of Health has devoted a sincere effort to putting forth standardized clinical pharmacy implementation guidelines that include a clinical pharmacist job description, a hospital pharmacist job description, criteria for establishment of clinical pharmacy units and drug information services, clinical pharmacy staff development, facilities and infrastructure, and a drug information pharmacist job description.

Field hospital pharmacists are contributing to patient care in many ways; specialized medical centers are witnessing clinical pharmacists attending bed rounds with physicians and regularly making pharmacotherapeutic recommendations, identifying and resolving drug therapy problems, preparing intravenous admixtures, compounding total parenteral nutrition preparations, and performing aminoglycoside dosing. They also actively participate in patient counseling and nurse education. Many hospital pharmacists are now active members of pharmacy and therapeutics committees within their respective hospitals, making an effort to align with physicians to follow standard treatment guidelines.[33]

Hospital pharmacists' duties include administrative duties, clinical service patient care, drug distribution, drug control, ensuring medication safety, and activities for quality and performance improvement (Table 7).

7.2 Industrial pharmacy

Currently, there are 119 licensed pharmaceutical manufacturers in Egypt. They are mainly involved in the production of formulations from pharmaceutical starting materials with limited involvement in the production of APIs and some involvement in the repackaging of finished dosage forms.[14] Being one of the biggest pharmaceutical industries in the region, the Egyptian pharmaceutical industry recruits a large number of pharmacists. They perform many duties, including manufacturing, quality assurance and control, drug registration, research and development, marketing, and clinical trials. Many of them are holders of postgraduate qualifications in pharmaceutical technology, chemistry, and other industry-related disciplines. There are no statistics for the workforce in the pharmaceutical industry in Egypt. Current regulations require the executive director of a pharmaceutical plant to be a pharmacist with pharmaceutical industry experience.

Table 7: Hospital pharmacist duties

Pharmacy and Therapeutic Committees
• Overseeing policies and procedures related to all aspects of medication use within an institution
• Managing the formulary system
• Medication use evaluation
• Adverse drug event monitoring and reporting, medication error prevention
• Development of clinical care plans and guidelines
Continuous education and staff development
Clinical Services and Patient Care
• Pharmaceutical care
• Drug information center services
• Patient counseling
Clinical pharmacokinetics consults
Drug Distribution and Control
• Procurement: Drug selection, purchasing authority, making decisions regarding products, quantities, product specifications
• Drug storage and inventory control, proper environmental control (i.e., proper temperature, light, humidity, and conditions of sanitation, ventilation, and segregation)
• Bulk compounding, packaging, and labeling
• Dispensing of medications including unit dose dispensing

7.3 Community pharmacy

The largest number of pharmacists in Egypt work as community pharmacists. There are around 59,79810 community pharmacies in Egypt.[14] The number of pharmacies per 10,000 of population is the highest in the world (around 6.5 pharmacies for each 10,000 of population).[25] As of this writing, there is no regulation in Egypt for chain pharmacies. Moreover, community pharmacy ownership is restricted to holders of a bachelor degree of pharmacy and a pharmacist is allowed to own a maximum of only two pharmacies.[34] A community pharmacy must be managed by a registered pharmacist after 1 year in practice as a provisionally registered pharmacist. They are present in all areas of Egypt from big cities to small villages and provide pharmaceutical care to their customers. However, a few chain pharmacies do exist in Egypt by managing pharmacies owned by several pharmacists. A dispute has been ongoing for several years between these chain pharmacies, which seek legalization, and the Egyptian Pharmacist Syndicate, which refuses their presence. Payment to community pharmacies is largely out of pocket and may be covered by the National Health Insurance Program in listed community pharmacies.[13] The role of the community pharmacist is essential in the provision of pharmaceutical care. In addition to dispensing of prescription drugs and extemporaneous preparation, community pharmacists recommend nonprescription drugs for treatment of simple ailments, monitor drug therapy, and perform tests to monitor disease control, such as blood pressure, blood sugar, and cholesterol monitoring. They also perform public health activities to promote healthy lifestyles, including healthy nutrition, combating drug abuse, smoking cessation, and physical activities. Many consumers refer to pharmacists in seeking advice about their symptoms and get information about local physicians they should visit for treatment. Many problems face the community pharmacy business in Egypt. The large increase in their number in previous years and the expected increase owing to large numbers of pharmacy graduates have affected their revenues negatively. Moreover, the new requirements for opening a community pharmacy, especially the minimum area, which has been increased from 25 to 40 m^2,[34] will reduce the ability of many pharmacists to have their own business. This problem is further complicated by the rise in property prices in the past few years.

Owing to the less competitive salary structure of community pharmacists and absence of a motivating career pathway, it is difficult to staff thousands of pharmacies across Egypt with a licensed pharmacist at all times, although this is required by law. In minor cases, a pharmacist is not present behind the counter and a technician or pharmacy assistant is rather present. This is of great relevance, because in April 2014 Egypt approved its list of prescription-only medicines (POMs) and over-the-counter (OTC) products. To augment patient safety practices and for better enforcement of current laws, such a referenced list would assist community pharmacists in making selections of OTC products. OTC products will not be offered an advantage in terms of registration period required, pricing decisions, etc.

7.4 Medicine marketing and promotion

The Hospital Pharmacy Department has collaborated in the establishment of ethical promotion guidelines. Canadian and Australian guidelines were taken as references. In addition, the
Ministry of Health has recently approved a POM/OTC classification list to help itemize
molecules that can be dispensed OTC without a prescription and items requiring a valid
physician's prescription prior to dispensing. There are no available statistics regarding the
workforce in the medicine marketing sector.

8. Special pharmacy-related services and activities

In Egypt, there are legal provisions in the Medicines Act that provide for PV activities
as part of the EDA mandate. This is being carried out by the National Office for Handling
and Reduction of Medication Errors (MEs). This is a national office established within the
hospital pharmacy administration in CAPA for the purpose of detecting, learning, and reducing MEs. PV is regulated by the Egyptian Pharmacovigilance Center of the
Egyptian Ministry of Health. Medication error reports can be submitted online through the
EDA Web site.[35] Legal provisions also exist requiring the marketing authorization holder to
continuously monitor the safety of its products and report to the EDA. The reporting of ADRs
by health care professionals is optional. The PV center has seven full-time staff members (six
pharmacists and one administrative assistant). An official standardized form for reporting
ADRs is used and information pertaining to ADRs is stored in a national ADR database,
reviewed, and analyzed. Also, an ADR bulletin is published. Although Egypt became a
member of the WHO Global Drug Monitoring Program in 2001,[36] ADR reports are not sent
to the WHO collaborating center in Uppsala. There is a national ADR or PV advisory committee able to provide technical assistance or causality assessment, risk assessment, risk
management, case investigation, and, where necessary, crisis management including crisis
communication in Egypt.[37]

Radiopharmacy in Egypt has gone through some developments. Since the early 1960s until
the late 1990s, production of radiopharmaceuticals in Egypt took place in the radioisotope
production laboratory at the Egyptian Authority for Atomic Energy. With the commissioning of a second research reactor in 1998, radioisotope production capability was enlarged.[38]
The end of the 1990s witnessed the entry of private companies into the production of
radiopharmaceuticals.[39] By July 2009, Egypt's first new-generation cyclotron production
facility was completed by GE Healthcare in partnership with the Children's Cancer Hospital Egypt (CCHE), the largest pediatric oncology center of its kind in the Middle East and
Africa. A PETtrace 6 cyclotron with a complete radiopharmacy suite was installed at the
CCHE.[40] Nonetheless, there are no similar radiopharmaceutical units in public or private
hospitals in Egypt.

9. Pharmacy education

Pharmacy education has an important role in the development of science and technology research and continued professional development to meet the global challenges and new technological developments in pharmaceutical sciences. Egypt has one of the oldest pharmacy schools in the region. The first modern pharmacy program offered in Egypt dates back to 1824, when the ruler of Egypt, Mohamed Ali Pasha, founded the Medicine and Pharmacy School as part of a hospital established in Abu Zaabal, in the province of Cairo. It was then transferred to the Citadel area in 1829 and then to Kasr El-Aini street, its current situation, in 1837. The appointed dean of the school was the eminent French doctor, Klute Bey.[41] The first pharmacists graduated from this school were 25 students, in the year 1832, and they studied for 5 educational years. Postgraduate programs were introduced in 1941, when the school was affiliated with Fuad I University. At this time, only master and diploma programs were introduced, to be followed in 1951 by the introduction of the Ph.D. in pharmaceutical sciences. It was only in 1955 when a governmental decree was issued to establish a faculty of pharmacy as an independent entity.[42]

As of this writing, the bachelor degree of pharmaceutical sciences (B. Pharm. Sci.) is a 5-year pharmacy education program; however, radical changes have been applied to update the curriculum. This program includes basic, pharmaceutical, medical, social, behavioral, management, health, and environmental sciences as well as pharmacy practice.

Since 1995, Egypt has seen a dramatic change in the funding landscape of its universities. Starting in the late 1990s, many privately funded schools of pharmacy have been established. All private universities in Egypt are mandated to follow the same process of legal recognition and approval by the Ministry of Higher Education and the Supreme Council of Universities, on the basis of the presidential decrees issued for the establishment of those institutions.[43] Students must receive science training in high school, and final examination results are the primary criteria for selection into a public program. However, private universities have their own admission procedures that comply with the Egyptian Ministry of Higher Education's rules and regulations.

Approximately, 6750 students were admitted to public schools in the 2003 academic year. A private pharmacy school is permitted to enroll a maximum of 400 students per year. Accordingly, total public/private admissions are estimated to range from 11,000 to 13,000 students per year.[44] Egyptian universities produce a higher number of pharmacists than required by the country (Table 8).

Egypt has the largest number of pharmacy schools among the Middle East countries (currently 24) (Table 9), making Egypt the major exporter of pharmacy graduates in the Middle East.[44] Over 75% of all students admitted to pharmacy programs in 13 Middle Eastern countries obtain their pharmacy education in Egypt.

Table 8: The ratio of pharmacists to population with comparison to the Middle East countries

Country	No. Pharmacists (Density/1000)	Students Admitted/Year
Egypt	138,000 (1.7)	11,000–13,000
Iraq	13,775 (0.5)	250–500
Jordan	8414 (1.4)	500–1000
Kuwait	722 (0.3)	25–50
Lebanon	4732 (1.2)	250–350
Oman	1551 (0.5)	100–150
Palestine	~1400 (0.9)	400–500
Qatar	530 (0.9)	20
Saudi Arabia	5485 (0.2)	>650
Syria	8862 (0.5)	250–500
UAE	1656 (0.4)	450–550
Yemen	2638 (0.1)	200–250
All	~188,000	14,000–17,500

Source: Pharmacy education and practice in 13 Middle Eastern countries.[44]

Most of the public Egyptian universities provide master, doctor of philosophy, and diploma in many disciplines of pharmaceutical sciences, including clinical and social pharmacy. In addition, a postgraduate program in four Egyptian universities called a clinical pharmacy program, which offers the PharmD degree, has been started. These universities are Alexandria University, Helwan University, Cairo University, and Tanta University.

Teaching of clinical pharmacy began in the pharmacy school at Tanta University in 1980 by a group of visiting professors from the United States, who gave lectures and trained some of the school academic staff on this new discipline in pharmaceutical education. Clinical pharmacy departments were established at many pharmacy schools in public universities (e.g., Cairo University, Helwan University, and Alexandria University) and private universities (e.g., German University) all over Egypt by 2005.[45]

Departments of pharmacy practice and clinical pharmacy within each university offer several courses to introduce the student to clinical pharmacy practice and to develop skills integrated with knowledge, which enables the student to improve his or her practice of pharmacy. The student would be equipped to promote, develop, and assess clinical pharmacy services within his or her profession, which will ensure the best outcomes for the patients. The course content in many universities for undergraduate students is a construct of clinical pharmacy, clinical pharmacy practice, first aid, pharmacokinetics, clinical pharmacokinetics, pathophysiology, and pharmacy administration. Courses offered for postgraduate students are hospital pharmacy, community pharmacy, clinical pharmacokinetics, drug information, drug promotion, marketing, applied therapeutics, and clinical data interpretation.

Another clinical pharmacy program is being run in MOHP hospitals to provide intensive training in clinical pharmacy services and pharmaceutical care practice to the pharmacists.

Table 9: Characteristics of pharmacy schools in Egypt[43]

School of Pharmacy	Average Class Size[a]	Funding Source[a]	Location (City)	Year Established[a]
Ahram Canadian University	210	Private	Giza	2004
Ain Shams University	600	Public	Cairo	1995
Al-Azhar University-Cairo/Assiut	700/383	Public	Cairo/Assiut	1965/1993
Alexandria University	1500	Public	Alexandria	1955
Assiut University	900	Public	Assiut	1957
Beni Swef University	360	Public	Beni Swef	1994
Cairo University	1500	Public	Cairo	1925
Egyptian Russian University	280	Private	Cairo	2006
Future University in Egypt	300	Private	Cairo	2006
German University in Cairo	450	Private	Cairo	2003
Helwan University	400	Public	Helwan	1994
Mansoura University	1200	Public	Mansoura	1972
Minia University	330	Public	Minia	1995
Misr International University	450	Private	Cairo	1997
Misr University for Science & Technology	500	Private	Giza	1997
Modern Sciences & Arts University	300	Private	Giza	2003
Modern University for Technology & Information	200	Private	Cairo	2010
Nahda University	300	Private	Beni Swef	2007
October 6th University	850	Private	Cairo	1997
Pharos University	350	Private	Alexandria	2006
Sinai University	300	Private	Arish	2006
Suez Canal University	250	Public	Ismailia	1993
Tanta University	1200	Public	Tanta	1973
Zagazig University	1200	Public	Zagazig	1976

[a]Data on funding source and year of establishment were obtained from the Web sites of each of the listed schools. Data on average class size were obtained from the responses of schools to the survey and, for nonrespondents, from the respective school's Office of Student Affairs through a personal communication with a school's academic/administrative official.

The so-called Clinical Pharmacy Fellowship Training Program has been developed with the cooperation of CAPA within the MOHP, the leader of the control of pharmaceuticals in Egypt. This entity has been able to positively influence pharmaceutical development through a decree establishing a clinical pharmacy unit and drug information center in every public and private hospital to empower and educate patients on their medications. The fellowship program is managed by the Hospital Pharmacy Administration in collaboration with the High Commission for Medical Specialties and directed at pharmacists with previous experience in hospital pharmacy. It is a 2-year full-time program composed of a practical part and a theoretical part comprising 80 and 20%, respectively. Training is performed by both physicians and clinical pharmacists within teaching hospitals according to a syllabus provided by University College Cork in Ireland, as are the exams.[46] Furthermore, the use of pharmaceuticals will continue to develop as the MOHP Health Technology

Assessment and Pharmacoeconomic Unit works to better utilize pharmaceutical resources and expenditure.

10. Achievements in pharmacy practice

Many achievements have been reached on many fronts with respect to the pharmacy profession in Egypt. Egypt being the largest producer and even exporter of trained pharmacists in the Middle East is an undeniable achievement. Most pharmacy schools in Egypt, especially the public ones, have postgraduate programs in various disciplines of pharmaceutical sciences. A great expansion of the pharmaceutical industry in Egypt has been made. The number of licensed pharmaceutical manufacturers in Egypt has reached 119. Their production covers more than 90% of the local consumption and many products are being exported to the Middle East, Africa, and Eastern Europe. Strict policies are in place to ensure affordability and quality of medicines in Egypt. Drug price control and involvement of the public sector in pharmaceutical production has made medicine prices in Egypt the lowest in the region. Expansion is now going on in biotechnology products and radiopharmaceuticals. Clinical pharmacy services and clinical pharmacy awareness are rapidly increasing in many governmental and private hospitals. Hospital pharmacy administration at the Central Administration for Pharmaceutical Affairs has introduced guidelines and procedures toward assisting in proper application and practice of clinical pharmacy in Egyptian hospitals. These guidelines for clinical pharmacy practice will serve as a tool for all to work consistently for good pharmacy practice and the benefit of patients. The guidelines focus on standards of clinical pharmacy practice that describe the work flow of clinical pharmacy service and explain the necessary documentation involved. It is believed that such guidelines are able to steer good management practice in conductive environments toward fulfillment of the customer's needs.[5]

Postgraduate programs especially in the field of clinical pharmacy have shown a dramatic increase since 2005. Furthermore, the Hospital Pharmacy Administration has established a clinical pharmacy fellowship training program for the first time in Egypt and the Middle East, to inject the field force with fresh graduates who are dedicated and experienced. The Clinical Pharmacy Fellowship Program is a full-time 3-year program.[46]

Also, a proposal has been submitted to the Supreme Council of Higher Education to extend pharmacy education to 6 years, rather than 5 years, to give the opportunity for practical rotation and experiential training to students.

11. Challenges in pharmacy practice

Producing graduates with a high competency level and keeping them updated through their career pathway is a big challenge. Unfortunately some Egyptian pharmacy graduates are of moderate quality, as most public governmental pharmacy schools lack the necessary tools and funds to graduate a competitive pharmacist. Egypt has traditionally had the largest number of graduating pharmacists across the Middle East and they are recruited across the region, particularly in the Gulf region. Private colleges of pharmacy have better resources in terms of lab equipment, but across the board the majority of schools lack experiential pharmacy training in their pharmacy curricula. Nevertheless, some public schools are seeking international accreditation and affiliations with esteemed universities and academic institutions worldwide for the betterment of the educational system.

Unfortunately no recertification for pharmacy licensure is mandated for Egyptian pharmacists, and pharmacy graduates are not required to take a board exam prior to licensure. The Ministry of Health, in collaboration with the pharmacy syndicate, is seeking to mandate a recertification program for all licensed pharmacists, to enforce staying up to date with the medical literature. On the positive side, many pharmacists are opting to self-pursue postgraduate programs, including, but not limited to, American board certification in selected therapeutic areas, clinical pharmacy fellowships, pharmacy doctorate programs, and clinical pharmacy diplomas offered at many universities.

A gap exists between the career pathway for community pharmacists, for example, and pharmacists in the industry or in hospital settings. Community pharmacists have been reported to attend fewer continuing education events compared to hospital pharmacists in Egypt.[47] Owing to the less competitive salary structure of community pharmacists and absence of a motivating career pathway, it is difficult to staff thousands of pharmacies across Egypt with a licensed pharmacist at all times, although required by law. As a developing nation, an emphasis on better allocation of health care resources and improving income and salary structure of medical professionals in general, and pharmacists in particular, will help reduce rates of expert immigration to the Gulf region in particular. Public hospital services can be improved by letting pharmacists get involved in new projects and activities in hospitals, and when they are successfully accomplished, bonuses as motivational incentives should be given, particularly when such projects do have a budget impact analysis, essentially offering a fee for service structure and better motivating pharmacists for innovative outside the box thinking.

As with the rest of the world, unauthorized dispensing of narcotics is illegal. The law requires all narcotic prescriptions to be stamped, and a monthly inventory of pharmacies with license to sell narcotics takes place to ensure adherence to national law regarding dispensing controlled substances, while not preventing such medicines from reaching patients who actually need them.

Although Egypt has made some achievements in some areas of API manufacturing, such as antibiotic API production using biotechnology, it is still behind in API manufacturing in general. Most APIs and excipients needed for pharmaceutical manufacturing are imported. A lot of investment, research, and cooperation between universities and industry are needed for this sector to progress. In addition, counterfeiting does remain a challenge for the Egyptian market, owing to uneven enforcement and a highly fragmented market. This is compounded by a sprawling drug distribution segment, with more than 45,000 smaller pharmacies selling over 8000 different forms of product. In total, fake, expired, or illegal drugs are estimated to comprise anywhere between 10 and 15% of the local market. The issue received renewed prominence in early February following a multibillion dollar shipment of counterfeit Avastin cancer drugs to the United States that was initially thought to have originated from Egypt. While further investigations revealed that the drugs had actually originated in Turkey, with the shipment's paperwork having been routed through a front company in Egypt, the scandal prompted the Egyptian Ministry of Health to reassert its commitment to policing the sector. Although medication shortage is a global trend, it seems to be magnified in Egypt at the time of writing. It is a challenge that we are facing nowadays, particularly in the post-January 25th revolution era, in that Egypt's credit rating has dropped and hence local manufacturers have had difficulty paying for 100% of bulk material cost up front, which has added to the problem of worldwide drug shortages due to logistic reasons.

To alleviate the problem of medication shortage and its consequences, Egypt has launched a department specifically dealing with medication shortage issues. The functions of this department are:

- Assisting prescribers and pharmacists with therapeutic alternatives
- Forecasting potential pharmaceuticals expected to be on the drug shortage list
- Facilitating communication between stakeholders (industry, regulatory authority, prescribers) to minimize negative consequences of the problem
- Publishing a monthly newsletter outlining drugs on the shortage list (nationally/internationally) to spread awareness to prescribers and pharmacists alike.

There are a number of problems facing the pharmaceutical services. The laws and regulations covering various aspects of the work of the Secretariat for Pharmaceutical Affairs in the Ministry of Health, such as licensing of pharmaceutical firms to produce medicines, registration of medicines, and inspections, are outdated and need revision. There are problems connected with storage and transportation of medicines and with maintenance of up-to-date inventories at the various levels of the health care system. The management skills of staff need to be upgraded and an appropriate information system developed to facilitate performance monitoring and evaluation.

Concerns have been expressed regarding the expected impact of the WTO agreement on TRIPS on the national pharmaceutical industry and on access to medicines. National laws and bylaws have been updated to prepare for expected developments.

There is a great need to promote the rational use of medicines and to train health professionals in this regard. There is also a need to improve communication between pharmacists and doctors to facilitate the prescribing of generic medicines.

12. Recommendations: way forward

As a developing nation, an emphasis on better allocation of health care resources and improving income and salary structure of medical professionals in general, and pharmacists in particular, will help reduce rates of expert immigration to the Gulf region in particular. Public hospital services can be improved by allowing greater involvement in new projects and activities in hospitals, and when they are successfully accomplished, bonuses as motivational incentives should be given, particularly when such projects do have a budget impact analysis, essentially offering a fee for service structure and better motivating pharmacists for innovative outside the box thinking.

13. Conclusions

Better enforcement tools are needed to follow up on project progress, new ministerial decrees, adaptation of new guidelines, etc. Periodic follow up is essential to ensure that work done is up to current adopted standards. To structure a cohesive medical team, the pharmacist's role is essential and vital for better patient care and better allocation of health care resources, utilizing pharmacists' knowledge and expertise to efficiently assist health care professionals.

14. Lessons learned/points to remember

- Egypt is the largest producer of pharmacists in the MENA region.
- The Egyptian pharmaceutical industry is the biggest in the MENA region.
- Egypt is one of the four main producers of vaccines in the MENA region.
- Pharmaceutical policies in Egypt succeeded making medicines more affordable despite several economical challenges.
- Collaboration between multiple stakeholders (academia, government, etc.) is crucial to improve the quality of health care in Egypt.
- Continuous updating of guidelines, protocols, and procedures is imperative to ensure desired quality standards in our health care system.
- Clinical pharmacy is a main pillar for improving patient care in the Egyptian health care system; better support toward implementation will result in the highest degree of success.
- A lot of effort should be made to improve the pharmacy profession and increase the efficiency of graduates.
- The pharmaceutical industry in Egypt is still behind many developing countries in API production.

References

1. *Egypt overview* [internet]. Washington, DC: World Bank [cited November 27, 2014]. Available from: http://www.worldbank.org/en/country/egypt/overview; 2013.
2. *Egypt: country statistics* [internet]. Geneva: UNICEF [cited November 27, 2014]. Available from: http://www.unicef.org/infobycountry/egypt_statistics.html; 2013.

3. *CIA Factbook* [internet]. Washington, DC: Central Intelligence Agency [cited November 27, 2014]. Available from: https://www.cia.gov/library/publications/the-world-factbook/geos/eg.html; 2013.

4. Shukrallah A, Khalil M. Egypt in crisis: politics, health care reform, and social mobilization for health rights. In: Jabbour S, editor. *Public health in the Arab world.* Cambridge (New York): Cambridge University Press; 2012. p. 477–88.

5. National Health Accounts 2007–2008: Egypt report. In: *Health systems 20/20 project.* Bethesda (MD): Abt Associate Inc.; 2010.

6. Mohamoud YA, Mumtaz GR, Riome S, Miller D, Abu-Raddad LJ. The epidemiology of hepatitis C virus in Egypt: a systematic review and data synthesis. *BMC Infect Dis* June 24, 2013;**13**:288.

7. *Global Alert and Response: Hepatitis C* [internet]. Geneva: World Health Organization (WHO) [cited November 27, 2014]. Available from: http://www.who.int/csr/disease/hepatitis/whocdscsrlyo2003/en/index4.html; 2014.

8. *Country Cooperation Strategy for WHO and Egypt 2010–2014* [internet]. Geneva: World Health Organization [cited November 27, 2014]. Available from: http://www.who.int/countryfocus/cooperation_strategy/ccs_egy_en.pdf; 2010.

9. *Egypt: health profile* [internet]. Geneva: World Health Organization (WHO) [cited November 27, 2014]. Available from: http://www.who.int/gho/countries/egy.pdf?ua=1; 2014.

10. *Summary key findings: National Health Accounts 2008/2009* [internet]. Washington, DC: United States Agency for International Development (USAID) [cited November 27, 2014]. Available from: http://egypt.usaid.gov/en/procurement/Documents/keyfindings_nha2008_09EN.pdf; 2009.

11. *Organizational chart* [internet]. Cairo: Ministry of Health and Population [cited November 27, 2014]. Available from: http://www.mohp.gov.eg/about/OrgChart/default.aspx; 2014.

12. *Health System Profile Egypt.* Cairo: Regional Health Systems Observatory, EMRO, World Health Organization; 2006.

13. *Health Insurance Organization Report 2011* [internet]. Cairo: Health Insurance Organization [cited November 27, 2014]. Available from: http://www.hio.gov.eg/Ar/Pages/default.aspx; 2011.

14. *Egypt: pharmaceutical country profile* [internet]. Cairo: Ministry of Health and Population/World Health Organization (WHO) [cited November 27, 2014]. Available from: http://www.who.int/medicines/areas/coordination/Egypt_PSCPNarrativeQuestionnaire_27112011.pdf; 2011.

15. *Egypt: country brief* [internet]. Cairo: MSD Egypt. Available from: http://www.msd-egypt.com/assets/pdf/EGYPT%20COUNTRY%20BRIEF.pdf; 2013.

16. Abdelgafar B, Thorsteinsdóttir H, Quach U, Singer P, Daar A. The emergence of Egyptian biotechnology from generics. *Nat Biotechnol* 2004;**22**(S):DC25–30. [cited November 27, 2014]. Available from: http://joint centreforbioethics.ca/rss/news/documents/nature_egypt.pdf.

17. *VACSERA history* [internet]. Cairo: VASCERA [cited November 27, 2014]. Available from: http://www.vacsera.com/index.php/about-us/vacsera-history; 2014.

18. *The Holding Company for Biological Products and Vaccines (VACSERA)* [internet]. Cairo: VASCERA [cited November 27, 2014]. Available from: http://www.b2match.eu/fp7health2011/participants/19; 2014.

19. *Sectoral survey: pharmaceutical industry in Egypt* [internet]. Cairo: Economic Research Division, Alexandria Bank [cited November 27, 2014]. Available from: http://www.alexbank.com/Uploads/documents/research/pharmaceutical%20industry%20in%20Egypt.pdf; 2010.

20. *Pharmacy* [internet]. Encyclopaedia Britannica Online, Academic ed., London: Encyclopædia Britannica Inc. [cited November 27, 2014]. Available from: http://www.britannica.com/EBchecked/topic/455192/pharmacy; 2014.

21. Shapiro AK, Shapiro E. *The powerful placebo: from ancient priest to modern physician.* Maryland: JHU Press; 2010.

22. *The ancient Egyptians, the Greeks and the Romans, pharmacy history* [internet]. Canberra: Pharmaceutical Society of Australia [cited November 27, 2014]. Available from: http://www.psa.org.au/history-2/chapter-2-the-ancient-egyptians-the-greeks-and-the-romans; 2014.

23. Smith L. The Kahun Gynaecological Papyrus: ancient Egyptian medicine. *J Fam Plann Reprod Health Care* 2011;**37**:54–5.

24. Whitelaw WA. *The Proceedings of the 10th Annual history of medicine days.* Faculty of medicine the University of Calgary. Health Sciences Centre, Calgary, AB; March 23–24, 2001.

25. *Global pharmacy workforce report* [internet]. Geneva: International Pharmaceutical Federation (FIP) [cited November 27, 2014]. Available from: http://www.fip.org/files/members/library/FIP_workforce_Report_2012. pdf; 2012.

26. *Egyptian Drug Authority* [internet]. Cairo: Ministry of Health and Population [cited November 27, 2014]. Available from: http://eda.mohp.gov.eg/; 2014.

27. *Egyptian Pharmaceutical Vigilance Center* [internet]. Cairo: Egyptian Drug Authority [cited November 27, 2014]. Available from: http://epvc.gov.eg.allium.arvixe.com/viewpage.aspx?Pid=3; 2014.

28. Balat M, Loutfi M. The TRIPs agreement and developing countries: a legal analysis of the impact of the new intellectual property rights law on the pharmaceutical industry in Egypt. *Web J Curr Leg Issues* 2004. [cited November 27, 2014]. Issue 2. Available from: http://webjcli.ncl.ac.uk/2004/issue2/balat2.html.

29. *Egyptian Pricing Decree no 499/2012.* Cairo: Egyptian Drug Authority (EDA) [cited November 27, 2014]. Available from: http://eda.mohp.gov.eg/; 2012.

30. Abdelgafar B. *The illusive trade-off.* Toronto: University of Toronto Press; 2006.

31. *Medicine prices in Egypt.* Cairo: Unpublished Report submitted by World Health Organization (WHO) and Health Action International (HAI) at the WHO/HAI Post-Medicine Price Survey Workshop; 2007.

32. *Ministry of Health Hospitals* [internet]. Cairo: Ministry of Health and Population [cited November 27, 2014]. Available from: http://www.mohp.gov.eg/Guidelines/DocLib/moh.ppt; 2014.

33. Egypt. Egyptian Drug Authority. *Egyptian clinical pharmacy standards of practice.* 1st ed. Cairo: Ministry of Health and Population; 2014.

34. *Egypt. Specifications of pharmacies and stores. Minister of Health Decree No. 380/2009.* Cairo: Ministry of Health and Population; 2009.

35. *National medication error reporting form* [internet]. Cairo: Ministry of Health and Population [cited November 27, 2014]. Available from: https://docs.google.com/forms/d/12CGMvEMO1sDN1yqeT8O5QIndZ SwkTrEimm6ep1f9ulg/viewform?fbzx=7743618757993279564; 2014.

36. Edwards R, Biriell C. *Pharmacovigilance.* 2nd ed. West Sussex: John Wiley & Sons Ltd; 2007.

37. Egypt. *Concerning the regulations of Pharmacovigilance and Pharmaceutical Products safety for Marketing Authorization Holders. Minister of Health Decree No. 2/2010.* Cairo: Ministry of Health and Population; 2010.

38. Rajeh M. *Radiopharmaceuticals production activities in Egypt* [internet]. Vienna: International Atomic Energy Agency [cited November 27, 2014]. Available from: http://www.iaea.org/inis/collection/NCLCollection Store/_Public/29/061/29061177.pdf; 1998.

39. *Femto trade for scientific services* [internet]. Cairo: Femto Trade Co. [cited November 27, 2014]. Available from: http://www.femtoegypt.com/about.html; 2014.

40. *GE healthcare in Egypt* [internet]. Cairo: General Electric Egypt [cited November 27, 2014]. Available from: http://www.ge.com/eg/b2b/healthcare; 2014.

41. Gad MZ. *Making pharmacy education in Egypt fit for the future. Final wrap up meeting for the Tempus project JEP 31028-2003.* Witten-Herdecke, Germany: Witten-Herdecke University; September 24, 2007.

42. *Faculty of Pharmacy, Cairo University: history and facts* [internet]. Cairo: Cairo University [cited November 27, 2014]. Available from: http://www.pharma.cu.edu.eg/English/AboutFaculty/Overview.aspx; 2014.

43. Soliman AM, Hussien M, Abdulhalim AM. Pharmacoeconomic education in Egyptian schools of pharmacy. *Am J Pharm Educ* 2013;**77**(3):57.

44. Kheir N, Zaidan M, Younes H, Hajj ME, Wilbur K, Jewesson PJ. Pharmacy education and practice in 13 Middle Eastern countries. *Am J Pharm Educ* 2008;**72**(6):133.

45. Wafaa ME. Clinical pharmacy in Egypt. *IJPTP* 2010;**1**(2):18–9.

46. *Egyptian clinical pharmacy fellowship* [internet] Cairo: Ministry of Health and Population [cited November 27, 2014]. Available from: http://eda.mohp.gov.eg/Pharma/Clinical.aspx?Main=Services&Serviceid=5&Sub main=serv16; 2014.

47. Mohamed Ibrahim OH. Assessment of Egyptian pharmacists' attitude, behaviors, and preferences related to continuing education. *Int J Clin Pharm* 2012;**34**(2):358–63.

CHAPTER 16

Pharmacy Practice in Sudan

Abubakr Abdelraouf Alfadl, Gamal Khalafalla Mohamed Ali, Mirghani A. Yousif, Mohammed Fadlalla Ahmed Babekir

Chapter Outline

1. Country background

Sudan is a large country, with an area of 1,861,484 km^2. The vast country hosts climatic, ethnic, tribal, cultural, and religious diversities. It is bordered by seven countries: Egypt, Eritrea, Ethiopia, South Sudan, the Central African Republic, Chad, and Libya. The population of Sudan was estimated at 33.5 million following the secession of the Republic of South Sudan in July 2011, with an annual growth rate of about 2.24%.[1] About 52% of the inhabitants live in rural areas, roughly about 40% are settled in urban areas, and the rest (8%) live as nomads.[2] Most of the population is concentrated in the middle of the country, mainly in the states of Gadaref and Khartoum. This concentration has been caused, on the one hand, by propulsive factors like war and drought in other part of the country, and on the other hand, by the pull factors such as aggregation of economic activities and the labor market in the center

Pharmacy Practice in Developing Countries. http://dx.doi.org/10.1016/B978-0-12-801714-2.00016-2

of the country. The last census in 1993 indicated that 44% of the population was under 15 years. The literacy rate is estimated at 61.1%, and it is even worse for women.[2]

In 1994, the government adopted the federal system. Currently, the powers of governance are distributed between the federal government, 15 states, and 144 localities.[1] The system is founded upon a multi-tier government: federal, state, and local governments. The federal government exercises its power over the whole country. However, significant responsibilities for social services have been decentralized to the states and localities. In the health sector, the administration and delivery of public health services has been decentralized. The Federal Ministry of Health (FMoH) retains responsibilities for overall policy, and legislation, as well as the posting and continuing professional development of health personnel, and the adminis- tration of 15 tertiary hospitals in Khartoum State. The states have responsibility for health centers and hospitals, while the localities are responsible for other primary health care (PHC) facilities that comprise the first level of the health care pyramid, such as dispensaries. A number of problems appeared during the implementation of the federal system, the most prominent being uneven distribution of financial and human resources between states and between rural and urban areas.

Sudan is rich in terms of natural and human resources, but economic and social developments have been below expectations. The gross domestic product (GDP) per capita was US$395 in 2001, with subsequent annual increases to US$570 in 2004, US$589 in 2005, and US$2700 in 2011.[3] Agriculture is the backbone of economic and social development, with 62% of the population employed in agriculture. Agriculture contributes 33% of the gross national prod- ucts, and 95% of all earnings.[4] Despite the domination of agriculture in Sudan's economy, the role of the industrial sector is becoming increasingly important for growth in urban areas. As a consequence of the implementation of economic reform packages in 1992, encouraging results in curbing macroeconomic imbalances and inflation were obtained. However, wide- spread poverty, highly skewed income distribution, and inadequate delivery of social services remain serious problems.

2. Vital health statistics

The nutrition situation in Sudan is poor, characterized by high levels of underweight and chronic malnutrition, as well as persistently elevated levels of acute malnutrition. Nationally, one third (32.2%) of children under the age of 5 years in Sudan are moderately or severely underweight. Pneumonia, malaria, diarrhea, and malnutrition usually still represent the major causes of under-5 illness and deaths. The result of Sudan Household Health Survey (SHHS) showed clear decline in infant mortality rate from nearly 80/1000 live births (LBs) in the mid-1990s to 57/1000 LBs in 2010.[4] The under-5 mortality rate in Sudan, which was esti- mated at 130/1000 LBs in the mid-1990s, declined to 102/1000 LBs in 2006,[5] and finally stood at 78/1000 LBs in 2010 (SHHS 2010). The most recent survey (SHHS 2010) estimated maternal mortality rate to be 216/100,000 LBs at the national level (225/100,000 LBs rural and 194/100,000 LBs urban).[4] Malaria is a leading cause of morbidity and mortality in Sudan. Symptomatic malaria accounts for 17.5 of outpatient clinic visits and approximately 11% of hospital admissions.[6]

3. Overview of the health care system

The modern health care system in Sudan is one of the oldest in Africa. Initially, it was established to provide medical services to the colonial army and its civil administration. The health system was western oriented, urban based, and emphasized curative service.[7]

On achieving independence, Sudan inherited a disciplined health care system. The quality of services was given priority and the service was free for all. Since then, the health care infrastructure has undergone considerable expansion. However, the distribution of health facilities remained concentrated in the urban areas, namely Khartoum and the Central region. Therefore, distance is considered as the bigger barrier for access to health services for rural residents, which may be why about 25% take modern treatments without consultation and 19% take traditional treatments.[1] Despite this, traditional, complementary, and alternative medicine still remains unregulated. However, a directorate has been set up recently in the Sudan Medical Council (SMC) to help the regulation of the traditional, complementary, and alternative medicine.[1] On the other hand, the ratio of medical doctors, nurses, and midwives is 1.23 per 1000 population.[1] This means Sudan is still within the critical shortage zone according to the World Health Organization (WHO) benchmark of 2.3 health care professionals per 1000 population.

The Sudanese health care system is divided into primary, secondary, and tertiary levels of care, which are under the three tiers of government, though with some overlapping of responsibilities. The lowest is the PHC level and service delivery is through PHC units, dressing stations, dispensaries, and health centers. These facilities are under the responsibility of the locality. The health center is the referral point for the lower-level facilities and, in principle, is staffed by a medical doctor, medical assistants, and nurses. In addition, vertical programs, in particular those for tuberculosis and the expanded program on immunization, work through the primary level facilities but also sometimes establish independent posts in peripheral areas. The state governments provide the secondary level of health care and the service delivery is through general referral hospitals (which also provide some primary care). Finally, the federal government is responsible for tertiary care through highly specialized services in teaching hospitals and national specialized centers in Khartoum State, such as the renal transplantation center and the national center for radiotherapy. However, some states, such as Khartoum and Gazera, also provide tertiary care through state-owned hospitals.

Health services are provided through different partners (in addition to federal and state Ministries of Health, Ministry of Social Care, Ministry of National Defence, and Ministry of

Interior), such as universities and the private sector (both for profit and not-for-profit organizations). However, there is no coordination between these different levels. Health care services provided by the government are comprehensive; where physical facilities are not established, particularly in very remote areas in Khartoum State, mobile health services are provided. As a result of the much-enhanced construction efforts to achieve equitable access to public health facilities, some improvement in the health infrastructure has been achieved in recent years.

The economic liberalization policy has led to a tremendous growth of private health care. Under this policy, private facilities may be established anywhere in the country. Public sector doctors are allowed to run their own private clinics outside office hours or to work in private hospitals, provided their public services are not compromised. Being profit driven, private facilities are concentrated in places where there is a demand, leading to an accumulation in urban and better-off rural areas, particularly in Khartoum State and, to some extent, Gazera State. They are also perceived to be of better quality than government services. The growth in private hospitals is driven mainly by the customers' need. It is not surprising, then, that the focus of these hospitals is mainly on curative selective services and mainly accessed by the better off.[8] The bulk of the private health care facilities are single-doctor clinics. An expansion of private secondary and tertiary care facilities is limited to few states, such as Khartoum and Gezira States. It is necessary to note that growth in the private sector should relieve some of the pressure of demand for health services, allowing the government to concentrate more on the provision of services for the poor.

The private not-for-profit health care system is operated by international and national nongovernmental organizations (NGOs). A set of specialized health care systems also exist for specific subsets of the Khartoum State population. These systems include health care services operated by large firms for their employees and their relatives. Often, such facilities are in urban areas. However, they also exist on large plantations in rural areas, such as Khartoum Refinery Hospital in Al-Giely area (Table 1).

Total government health expenditure was estimated at 6.2% of the GDP in 2010 and per capita health expenditures at US$ 122 in the same year. Government health expenditure was 27.8% of the total health expenditure of the country, with a total per capita public expenditure on health of US$ 33.9. The government annual expenditure on health represents 9% of the total government budget.[9]

The National Health Account for 2008 estimated national health expenditure originating from households' funds at about 64%, with 29% from public funds, 4% from international donors, and the remaining 3% originating from employers.[1] However, the breakdown of health expenditure by health function shows that health spending is more related to tertiary care (curative care 60%, pharmaceuticals 23%, health administration 6%, and 5% on other health-related functions) than pro-poor services such as primary and preventive care (only 4%).[1]

Table 1: Health facilities in Sudan

Number	Health Facility	Number
1	Public hospitals	416
2	Public health centers	1900
3	Functioning public health units	3299
	Total number of public health facilities	**5615**
4	Private hospitals	170
5	Specialists' clinics	1146
6	General practitioners' clinics	961
7	Private laboratories	1224
8	Dentists' clinics	100
9	Community pharmacies	2972
10	Veterinary clinics	68

Source: *General Directorate of Pharmacy, Annual Statistical Report.*[10]

The value of the Sudanese pharmaceutical market in the year 2012 was estimated to 300 million dollars and includes both domestically produced and imported medicines and medical supplies with no significant growth. It is such a small market when compared to the overall pharmaceutical market in the Arab region, which is estimated to be 15 billion dollars. The share of import seems overwhelming at 72%, while national production represents only 28%.[10]

4. Overview of pharmacy practice and key pharmaceutical sectors

Clearly, an adequate pharmaceutical service, ideally provided by pharmacists, is a vital component of PHC. This is recognized by the WHO, and several subsequent publications of the WHO emphasize the role of the pharmacist in the health care system. In the following subsections, the authors tried to highlight issues such as medicine supply as a vital role in pharmaceutical services and human resources and their distribution between urban/rural areas; public/private, etc.; it is recognized and accepted that conditions of pharmacy practice vary widely between different areas/sectors due to the fact that the number of pharmacists is less than desirable. Also, the benefits that are attained from the direct supervision of the pharmacist in ensuring the quality of pharmaceutical products and services throughout the distribution chain cannot be realized in areas where there are insufficient numbers of pharmacists, or at least persons with formal pharmaceutical training (Table 2).

In Sudan, three bodies are working collaboratively to regulate pharmacy practice: the SMC, Directorate General of Pharmacy (DGoP), and the National Medicines and Poisons Board (NMPB). The SMC is responsible for issuing the license for a pharmacist to practice, ensuring ethical practice, and also designing professional curricula development criteria for pharmacy education.

Table 2: Assessment of dispensing practices in Khartoum State tertiary hospitals

Domain	Theme	Percentage[a]
Dispensing personnel		51.0
	Qualification	68.5
	Quality of services	66.7
	Administrative issues	51.4
	Training	40.7
	Therapeutic committee	27.8
Dispensing environment		**60.6**
	Design	56.6
	Hygiene	69.5
	Administrative	55.6
Dispensing process		**50.3**
	Administrative	56.2
	Pharmaceutical care	44.4

[a]For dispensing personnel and dispensing process, percentages were calculated based on number of personnel (out of N = 30) who satisfied certain requirements based on study conducted by Elhassan, G.O. et al. (2015, unpublished). For the dispensing environment, percentages are based on number of facilities (N = 8) that satisfied certain requirements.

4.1 Industrial pharmacy and pharmaceutical technology

In Sudan, the pharmaceutical industry was started in the 1950s by the Sudanese Chemical Industries; until the end of the 1980s, the number did not exceed seven plants. A breakthrough occurred after the Revolution of Salvation, when the number of licensed factories increased to 24.[11]

These 24 pharmaceutical manufacturing factories are producing medicines, cosmetics, paramedicals, and medical gases. From these 24 manufacturers, five produce cosmetics, paramedicals, and medical gases, whereas the other 19 produce medicines in various forms. Some manufacturers export to neighboring countries.

To support the domestic pharmaceutical industry, the government has adopted a number of policies. These policies include exemption of imported raw materials (i.e., active pharmaceuticals and excipients), packaging materials, and all equipment and devices needed to meet requirements of the good manufacturing practice from any governmental charges. The FMoH has approved policy to encourage the flourishing of the national pharmaceutical industry. This policy gives priority in registration to the locally manufactured medicines. It also allows foreign investors who are interested in establishing a pharmaceutical plant in Sudan to apply for registration of their medicines manufactured abroad, as if they are locally manufactured, on the condition that they complete the construction of the local factory within 2 years. To protect the local producers against overwhelming the Sudanese pharmaceutical market with cheap medicines imported from abroad, mainly India and China, local producers can potentially benefit from regulatory support of the import bans on selected essential medicines

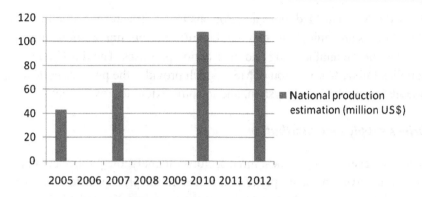

Figure 1

National pharmaceutical production estimation. *Source: General Directorate of Pharmacy, Annual Statistical Report.*[10]

(e.g., NMPB does not register a medicine that has been locally produced by at least two manufacturers; the originator product is exempted) (Figure 1).

Being a market-driven industry, it is the policy of the government medicine procurement agency to give preference margins by conducting a separate tender restricted to local manufacturers. This is because the purchase of locally produced medicines from domestic manufacturing plants can be economically attractive, especially if they compete with overseas suppliers. In addition, the advantages of local manufacturers comprise the payment in local currency, cheaper communication and transport costs, and frequent inspection by the NMPB, the medicine regulatory authority of Sudan; there is no need for a quality test because items are only tested before release. Finally, the Procurement Act (2010)[12] has required that public firms purchase their needs from local manufacturers, unless public firms could show that overall costs (including the landed cost) of imported goods are at least 10% less than those produced by the local firms. However, although support to local pharmaceutical manufacturers is a reasonable policy priority, this should not be at the cost of less access to essential medicines due to higher prices. Additionally, this policy may distort the market, as local small companies may not even attempt to be competitive.[13] It is therefore recommended that the government seeks other ways to support the national pharmaceutical industry without affecting accessibility to essential medicines.

4.2 Governmental pharmaceutical sector

The governmental pharmaceutical sector is divided into three bodies. The first is the Planning and Policy body, which is represented by the Directorate General of Pharmacy, FMoH. It is responsible for setting plans for the pharmaceutical sector, formulation of the National Medicine Policy and the monitoring of its implementation, development of the Essential Medicines List (EML), and the setting of training policies and national training programs for pharmacists working in the public sector. The second body is the regulatory one, which is represented by the National Medicines and Poisons Board. It is responsible for setting and enforcing legislations and guidelines that regulate registration, importation, and quality control of medicines and their manufacturing and distribution premises. The third body is the Central Medical Supplies Public Corporation (CMS), which provides the pharmaceutical supply for the governmental or public health system, and to some extent to private sector.

4.3 Medicines supply and distribution

In order to ensure access to medicines, three sectors—namely, the public sector, private sector, and NGOs—are involved in the supply of medicines. In the private sector, there are 24 manufacturers of pharmaceuticals. In addition, there are about 296 and 1477 private wholesalers and retail pharmacies respectively throughout the country. Approximately 57% of the retail pharmacies are in three towns of Khartoum State (Figures 2 and 3).

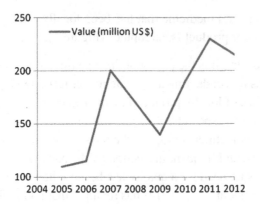

Figure 2

Value of imported medicines (2005–2012). *Source: General Directorate of Pharmacy, Annual Statistical Report.*[10]

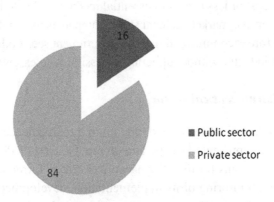

Figure 3

Public sector to private sector in Sudanese pharmaceutical market (2012).

In as far as public supply system is concerned, there is a Central Medical Supplies Public Cooperation, which was established in 1991 as a semi-autonomous body to facilitate the selection, procurement, storage, and distribution of medical supplies for the public sector. Central Medical Stores is the national center for procurement, storage, and distribution of medical supplies in Sudan. It was established in 1935 as a department in the Sudan Medical Services, and then transferred to the current building in 1954 as a department in the Ministry of Health, under the new name of the Central Medical Supplies. In February 1991, the Central Medical Supplies became a parastatal organization under the Organization Act 1991, which allowed the new organization to exercise the maximum possible autonomy within the framework of the Government of Sudan. It was subsequently renamed the Central Medical Supplies Public Corporation (widely known as CMS).

Before CMS was given autonomy, all medicines and medical supplies that it procured and warehoused were given free of charge to public health facilities. However, from 1992, and since becoming a semi-autonomous organization, CMS has worked on a cost-recovery system, to be in line with the cost-recovery policy that is implemented by government at all health facilities in the public health sector of Sudan.

In its efforts to contain the problems of those who cannot pay for their medicines, in 1996, the government announced a project for free treatment at hospital emergency units. The emergency free medicines project was intended to increase access for those who need emergency treatment in hospital casualty departments, regardless of their ability to pay. According to this project, all patients are entitled to receive free services including medicines, during the first 24 hours of admission. The CMS receives a special budget from the Ministry of Finance and National Economy (MOF) for the free distribution of emergency medicines at hospital emergency departments. The medicines are distributed on monthly basis after their value has been deposited in the CMS account. The budget allocated for this was SDG 60 million (around US$20 million) in the current fiscal year, which accounted for more than 35% of CMS sales. The CMS serves 73% of sales to the public, 26% to private pharmacies, and 1% to others. There is also public procurement through the Revolving Drug Fund, health insurance, police, and military medical facilities. Public procurement is governed by a number of laws and regulations, such as the Medicine Act, Procurement Act, and Accounting Procedures Act (Figure 4).

The United Nations Development Programme is a key partner to the Global Fund to Fight HIV/AIDS, Tuberculosis and Malaria (GFATM) and is the UN agency assuming the role of Principal Recipient of GFATM grants in Sudan. The FMoH has undertaken efforts to achieve this through the establishment of a separate Procurement and Supply Management (PSM) Unit, which was under the General Directorate of Pharmacy (GDP). However, recently, a ministerial decree designated the CMS as the preferred PSM implementation partner in Sudan, in line with the recent decision by the Ministry of Health regarding the integration of PSM interventions within the CMS. In addition to the increase in access to these services, there are several activities aimed at increasing demand for HIV, TB, and malaria services in Sudan (Figure 5).

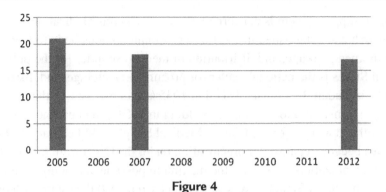

Figure 4

Share of CMS in Sudanese pharmaceutical market. *Source: General Directorate of Pharmacy, Annual Statistical Report.*[10]

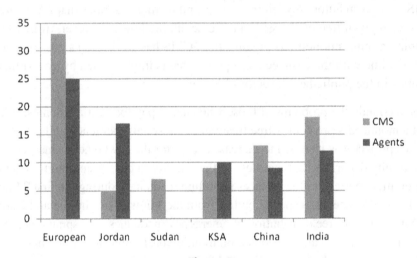

Figure 5

Contribution of some countries in the Sudanese pharmaceutical market (2012). *Source: General Directorate of Pharmacy, Annual Statistical Report.*[10]

4.4 Drug regulations and policies

The history of medicines regulation in Sudan dates back to 1939 when the Pharmacy and Poisons Ordinance (PPO) was first enacted.[14] The Central Board of Public Health (CBH) was vested with the responsibility of administering the provisions of Act, which included registration of graduate pharmacists, licensing of drug establishments (wholesale and retail) and control of poisons used for industrial, agriculture, and horticultural purposes. In order to execute its functions, the CBH delegated its functions to authorized standing committees. Regulation of the drug law was further complemented by Prohibited Goods Ordinance administered by customs, while sanctions were provided by the Penal Code and the code of Criminal Procedure Ordinance. The PPO was repealed with subsequent enactment of the

Pharmacy and Poisons Act, 1963. The main areas of departure included provisions related to marketing authorization of pharmaceutical products based on the need, quality, efficacy, and safety parameters. In addition, the Act provided for licensing of pharmaceutical manufacturing activities. The 1963 Act was superseded by the Pharmacy and Poisons Act 2001, and finally the Medicines and Poisons Act was enacted in 2009.

The Act regulates the compounding, sale, distribution, supply, dispensing of medicines and provides different levels of control for different categories (e.g., medicines, poisons, cosmetics, chemicals for medical use, medical devices).[13] The sector is guided by the 25-Year National Pharmaceutical Strategy (2005–2029), from which the National Drug Policy (NMP) (2005–2009) has been developed.

The NMPB is the Supreme Federal Authority vested with powers to organize, control, and monitor the operations of import, manufacture, storage, pricing, transport, and use of drugs, cosmetic preparations, medical requisites, and pharmaceutical preparations. Any person aggrieved by any decision issued by any of the technical committees may appeal to the Board within 15 days of the date of the decision and the decision of the Board shall be final in that respect. If any person is aggrieved by the decision of the Board, he or she may appeal to the court within 15 days of the date of his being notified with the decision.

A National Drug Policy was defined for 2005–2009, assessed in 2007, and to be updated in the context of the new Health Strategic Plan. The public sector ensures drug sales in hospitals, health centers, and basic community health units. The private sector operates through 19 licensed manufacturers (two of which are co-owned by the military), about 80 wholesalers and 2306 retailers (community pharmacies and drugstores). The National Health Insurance Fund (NIHF) also operates its own pharmacies provides medicines to patients consulting in its health centers.

The term "wholesale pharmacy" is not applicable in Sudan. So, pharmacies are either public pharmacies (pharmacies at public hospitals or those that belong to the governmental supply system) or private retail pharmacies. Therefore, there are approximately 3519 pharmacies in total. About 1456 of these are public pharmacies, which represent about 41% of the total number of pharmacies. There are 57 registered NGO in Sudan; none of them have a pharmacy[11] (Figure 6).

The pharmaceutical premises that are responsible for wholesaling of medicines for both public and private sector are called "pharmaceutical companies." There are local agencies for either multinational and/or generic medicines companies. In Sudan, the total number of companies that import medicines is around 283.[15] These agents are mostly stationed in Khartoum (98%), the capital, and are used to supply medicines either through direct sales to different health settings in other states or through appointing subagents at states' levels. For the pharmaceutical premises, operating licenses are issued for public sector pharmacies, private retail pharmacies, local agencies, drug stores, and pharmaceutical manufacturers. For the first four, the license is issued by the regional pharmacy authority (State Directorate of

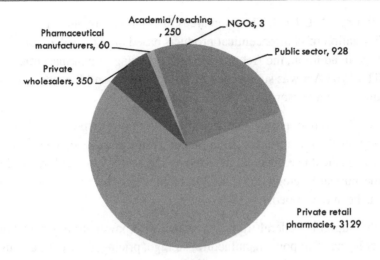

Figure 6

Distribution of pharmacist workforce by employment sector (2009). *Source: Assessment of human resources at the pharmaceutical sector.[11]*

Pharmacy). For the pharmaceutical manufacturers, the license is issued by the National Medicines and Poisons Board.[14]

4.5 Medicine pricing and financing

Prices of medicines are extremely high compared to neighboring countries and household income, especially in private sector outlets. These high prices, combined with irrational drug prescription practices and rampant self-medication, probably contribute to the very high out-of-pocket (OOP) expenditures on drugs reported in the National Health Accounts. More than 40% of OOP on health are related to medicines.[16] The Pharmacy and Poisons Act regulates pharmaceutical prices in Sudan. The NMPB uses medicine cost and freight total (i.e., wholesalers add a fixed percentage to the price they pay for the manufacturers from abroad) to fix the different maximum percentage markups for all medicines. This is done through two stages of the distribution. The wholesaler's profit is 15% of the total costs to their central warehouses in Khartoum, the capital city of Sudan; the retailer's profit is 20% of the wholesaler's price.[17] No active national medicines price monitoring is available, but several studies consider that the current pricing system is of limited benefit in controlling escalating medicines prices in Sudan. In one study,[15] the cost and freight prices of 23% was found to be more than 10 times higher than the International Reference Price published by Management Sciences for Health. Furthermore, lower prices at the public central medical store did not help much in controlling the prices in private sector, as retail pharmacies sell the low cost tender items from CMS at the retail price set by their wholesalers.

The current National Essential Drug List (NEDL) was last edited in 2007. Although it is supposed to have been printed and distributed, it is not available in a lot of health facilities. Activities are underway to develop and approve standard treatment guidelines for 10 diseases. However, studies conducted by the Rational Drug Use Department of the GDP/FMoH and the Drug Fund (RDF) have documented overprescription practices for both antibiotics (ranging from 31% to 65% in reviewed prescriptions) and injections (ranging from 11% to 36% in reviewed prescriptions).[14] To respond to this pressing issue, the Quality Directorate of the FMoH has set up a Consultative Council for Respiratory Medicines and issued an Antibiotic Policy for Respiratory Infections.[14]

Private expenditure in pharmaceuticals largely surpasses public expenditure. The 2008 National Health Accounts (NHA) reported that more than 40% of OOP expenditures in health are related to medicines.[16] The total annual expenditure in health (THE) in 2010 was US$ 3755.5. The total pharmaceutical expenditure (TPE) during the same year was US$ 1349, which accounts for 2.2% of GDP and makes up 36% of THE.[16] This very high level of OOP drug expenditures may be due to high drug prices, irrational prescription or dispensation practices, high level of self-medication, or all of the above. A public program provides free medicines and vaccines to under-5 children and pregnant women, as well as patients suffering from malaria, tuberculosis, sexually transmitted disease, and HIV/AIDS.

In 1996, the government made social health insurance (HIS) compulsory for all employees of public and private sectors. This coverage includes 75% of the cost of medicines on its approved list of essential medicines. The beneficiaries pay the remaining 25% of their prescription and pay the full cost of medicines prescribed out of the list.[18]

However, a study conducted in 2005 revealed that 10 years after its initiation, the HIS still provides limited insurance coverage for only 13% of the population.[8] Most (85%) of the insured individuals are public sector employees, 6% are members of the informal sector, 4% are poor families, 3% are families of martyrs, and 2% are students.[19]

4.6 Practice-related regulations and policies

The SMC is the national body that regulates the practice of doctors, dentists, and pharmacists in Sudan. This council is responsible for the temporary registration of pharmacists after graduation and before finishing their internship period. To become permanently registered with the SMC, pharmacists must work for 1 year in the public sector after graduation and pass the registration examination. In 2009, this period of public sector service was reduced to 3 months. After passing the examination, the pharmacists are given a permanent license that allows them to practice in different pharmaceutical sectors. At the present time, no license renewal is required. Upon completion of training, pharmacists are permanently licensed by the SMC. Also, the SMC is by law responsible for establishing ethics for all medical practice. Thus, the SMC receives, handles, and judges complaints against pharmacists.

Sudan has lacked effective systems for the collection and analysis of the data on human resources for health that are needed for evidence-based policy-making and the planning of health services.[20] According to SMC, there was a total of 7685 registered pharmacists.[12] The actual number of actively practicing pharmacists is not known. This figure includes pharmacists who have died, migrated abroad, changed jobs, or retired. There is no system for registration renewal or updating information in the register. Also, the percentage of females from this number could not be calculated because the existing data need to be updated and validated. The number of foreign-registered pharmacists is about 40.[11] Data on the newly registered pharmacy assistants were only available for only 2007 (83 pharmacy assistants), as the school of pharmacy assistants has not graduated any since 2007.[11] Also, an institution called the Academy of Health Sciences plays an important role in the initial training and continuing education of these cadres of personnel. Most assessments have reported a need for continuous training in drug quantification, procurement, inventory control, and rational drug use.

With regard to the workforce, according to the available resources, Sudan has about 5980 pharmacists and 2488 pharmacy assistants, mostly employed in the private sector and based in the capital. For example, 1542 pharmacists are employed in the public sector at the central and decentralized levels.[11] At the public health facility level, most activities are performed by pharmacy assistants, junior nurses, or other staff hired by health facilities to work in their pharmacies.

Regarding density, the number of pharmacists in Sudan is 1108, constituting 1.43% of the health workforce. Density per 1000 of the population is 0.034.[12] Pharmacy assistants show higher density in states with lower numbers of pharmacists because they carry some of pharmacists' responsibilities (Figures 7 and 8).

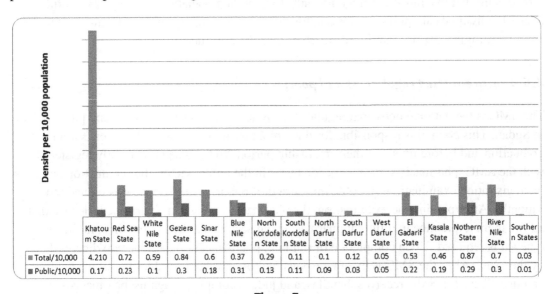

	Khatoum State	Red Sea State	White Nile State	Geziera State	Sinar State	Blue Nile State	North Kordofan State	South Kordofan State	North Darfur State	South Darfur State	West Darfur State	El Gadarif State	Kasala State	Nothern State	River Nile State	Southern States
Total/10,000	4.210	0.72	0.59	0.84	0.6	0.37	0.29	0.11	0.1	0.12	0.05	0.53	0.46	0.87	0.7	0.03
Public/10,000	0.17	0.23	0.1	0.3	0.18	0.31	0.13	0.11	0.09	0.03	0.05	0.22	0.19	0.29	0.3	0.01

Figure 7
Density of pharmacists per 10,000 populations in different states (2009). *Source: Assessment of human resources at the pharmaceutical sector.[11]*

The total number of actively employed pharmacists is estimated to be 4710. They are generally concentrated in the private sector (68%).[11] There were no data on the number of registered pharmacists who are not working (unemployed and inactive workforce). The distribution of pharmacists is as follows: 350 private wholesalers, 60 pharmaceutical manufacturers, 250 academia/teaching, 3 NGOs, 928 public sector, and 3129 private retail pharmacies.[11]

4.7 Pharmacy practice: private versus government

The data on the distribution of pharmacists between different sectors shed light on another fact: the number of pharmacists in the public sector is far lower than that of the private sector, even though it contradicts the goals of the country's 25-year pharmacy strategy. The ability of the pharmacy profession to provide patients with more support in using medicines and to make them more confident in the advice they are given depends entirely on the quality and quantity of pharmacy human resources (PHRs) available to do the job. PHRs in public sector are a critical component in the National Medicine Policy (NMP) and the 25-year pharmacy strategy. Implementation of the pharmacy strategy and achievement of its objectives depend upon people. It requires highly qualified and experienced professionals, including policymakers, pharmacists, doctors, pharmacy assistants, paramedical staff, economists, and researchers. The goals of the 25-year pharmacy strategy will not be achieved without increasing the number and quality of pharmacists working in the public sector. The brain drain will affect

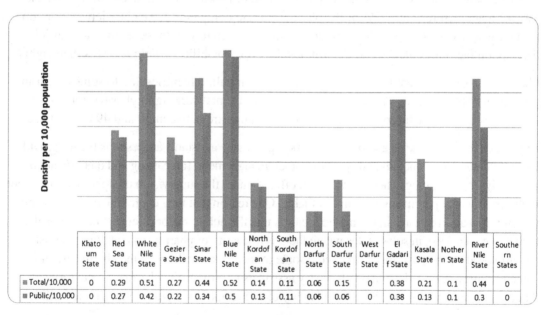

	Khato um State	Red Sea State	White Nile State	Gezier a State	Sinar State	Blue Nile State	North Kordof an State	South Kordof an State	North Darfur State	South Darfur State	West Darfur State	El Gadari f State	Kasala State	Nother n State	River Nile State	Southe rn States
Total/10,000	0	0.29	0.51	0.27	0.44	0.52	0.14	0.11	0.06	0.15	0	0.38	0.21	0.1	0.44	0
Public/10,000	0	0.27	0.42	0.22	0.34	0.5	0.13	0.11	0.06	0.06	0	0.38	0.13	0.1	0.3	0

Figure 8

Density of pharmacy assistants per 10,000 populations in different states (2009). *Source: Assessment of human resources at the pharmaceutical sector.*[11]

the pharmacists' key role in the implementation of NMP and 25-year pharmacy strategy. Pharmacists will implement the strategy only if they understand its rationale and objectives, are trained to do their jobs well, paid adequate wages, and motivated to maintain high standards. The lack of appropriate expertise has been a decisive factor in the failure of some countries to achieve the objectives of their national drug policies.

Also, it was observed that females constitute the majority of pharmacists in the public facilities, with majority of pharmacists falling into the 30–49 year age range, whereas males form the majority in pharmaceutical companies, with age of 25–49 years. The majority of pharmacists employed in private retail pharmacies were less than 30 years; those with manufacturers were aged 30–49 years.

Pharmacists in private retail pharmacies and public facilities are responsible for providing different services, including dispensing, stock management, forecasting, quantification, and compounding. In the pharmaceutical companies, they are responsible for stock management, forecasting and quantification, and promotion of the pharmaceuticals. At pharmaceutical manufacturers, they are mainly responsible for production, quality control, stock management, and forecasting and quantification. Manufacturers also offer the highest salary and other benefits for pharmacists, whereas the private retail pharmacies offer the lowest; this may explain the attrition of recently graduate pharmacists from the private retail pharmacies to the pharmaceutical companies and manufacturers. Also, working hours at pharmaceutical companies and manufacturers are less compared to public or private retail pharmacies. Moreover, 89% of manufacturers and 77% of the pharmaceutical companies have clear job description for pharmacists—something that further encourages them to join these sectors; a clear job description facilitates their work, determines their responsibilities, and preserves their rights.

Pharmacy assistants were found to be concentrated in public facilities and to some extent in private retail pharmacies. There are no pharmacy assistants working in pharmaceutical companies or manufacturers. Most pharmacy assistants are between 30 and 49 years of age.

At private retail pharmacies and public facilities, pharmacy assistants are responsible for providing different services, including dispensing, stock management, forecasting and quantification, and rarely, compounding. These services are offered under the supervision of a pharmacist, except in the areas where pharmacists are not available. One reason that may contribute to the concentration of pharmacy assistants in the public sector is that the public sector offers better salaries than the private one. Also, in some states where there is a scarcity of pharmacists, pharmacy assistants are employed by the government to handle some of the responsibilities of the pharmacist and some localities entirely depend on pharmacy assistants to provide the pharmaceutical services. Another possible reason may be the availability of a clear job description in the public facilities.

With the exception of the FMoH, the state's or locality's health authority, the private sector has a great advantage over public sector in that it has free authority to recruit pharmaceutical personnel.

Despite all benefits that the pharmaceutical companies used to offer, it appears that this has not stopped pharmacists' migration from this sector. This may be due to working for the same company in another country (especially for the multinational companies) or may be due to the temptations that are offered by foreign companies, especially in the Arab Gulf Region. On the other hand, manufacturers have the highest percent of facilities that have problems in filling pharmacist positions. This is often due to the scarcity of specialized personnel in the field of pharmaceutical manufacturing and technology.

Some pharmaceutical services are offered by health workers other than pharmacists and pharmacy assistants. In some areas where there is a dressing station or dispensary, the medical assistant, midwife, or even the doctor can carry a limited responsibility of dispensing, quantification, and even stock management of medicines, but all of this is done under the supervision of the district health authority or state pharmacy directorate. There is strong evidence that the civil service management system is a key factor in the retention of skilled pharmacists. The number of pharmacist jobs, salary scales, and other incentives schemes in the public sector is determined by the service affair authority in coordination with the Federal Ministry of Finance and Economic Planning. However, the incentive system was not flexible enough to cope with differences between health professionals and other civil servants, despite the fact that health professionals in hospitals tend to work in shifts and have to face different working conditions.[2] This happens even though the shortage of pharmacists at points of drug dispensing deprives the population of vital expertise in the management of medicine-related problems in both community and hospital settings.

In conclusion, the situation of human resources in the health sector in Sudan is not progressing, and has worsened further after the division of Sudan in 2011 into two independent nations: the Sudan and South Sudan. As a result of the secession of South Sudan, the government of the Sudan lost oil revenue and donor support. These losses negatively impacted Sudan's development and further weakened health systems, which included health worker shortages, a frequent mismatch between the skills that health workers had and those that were needed, and the maldistribution, migration, and poor productivity and retention of health workers.[20]

5. Pharmacy education

Pharmacy education started in 1964 with the establishment of the Faculty of Pharmacy at the University of Khartoum.[11] Presently, there are 15 pharmacy faculties with another two under construction. Of these 12, six faculties are governmental and six are private. From 1996 up to 2005, 10 other faculties were established. This expansion is in line with the reform in higher education throughout the Arab world.

The full-time teaching staff is estimated to be 250 in total for all 12 faculties.[11] All faculties offer the B.Sc. degree in Pharmacy. The length of the program is 45 months (5 years). Three of these faculties offer M.Sc. degrees in pharmacy. The mean program length for M.Sc. is

Table 3: Pharmacy education in Sudan

Name	Start	Ownership	Location	Website
University of Khartoum	1964	Government	Khartoum State, Khartoum	http://pharm.uofk.edu/en/
University of Gezira	1994	Government	Gezira State, Wad Medani	http://phs.uofg.edu.sd/en/
Omdurman Islamic University	–	Government	Khartoum State, Omdurman	http://oiu.edu.sd/en/#
University of Science and Technology	–	Private	Khartoum State, Omdurman	http://www.ust.edu.sd/fpha/
Ribat University	2001	Government	Khartoum State, Khartoum	http://ribat.edu.sd/ribat/eng
Ahfad University for Women	–	Private	Khartoum State, Omdurman	http://www.ahfad.net/index.php/school-of-pharmacy.html
National University	–	Private	Khartoum State, Khartoum	http://www.nu.edu.sd/details.php?linkid=7
Neelain University	2006	Government	Khartoum State, Khartoum	http://neelain.edu.sd/sites/colleges/4
Elrazi University	–	Private	Khartoum State, Khartoum	http://www.elraziuniv.net/ar/programs/ph.html
University of Medical Science Technology	–	Private	Khartoum State, Khartoum	http://www.umst-edu.com/Pharmacy.aspx
Khartoum College of Medical Sciences University	–	Private	Khartoum State, Khartoum	

about 30 months. The maximum annual enrollment and graduated students are not limited for research M.Sc. programs but are limited for taught M.Sc. programs. Only two of these faculties offer a Ph.D. degree in Pharmacy. The number enrolled or graduated is not limited. Only one faculty offers the pharmacy technologist diploma. It has started to graduate students, but this cadre has no clear job descriptions for either the public or private sector. There are five special schools that offer pharmacy assistant certificates. However, none of these schools have graduated any students since 2007.[11]

The highest continuing education program that is attended by pharmaceutical personnel is on the rational use of medicines (RUD). This is mainly because there was an active RUD unit at the DGoP–FMoH, which offers continuous on job training courses and workshops, especially for the pharmacists working at the public sector. The attended continuing education program depends upon the type of facility the personnel is working at and the nature of tasks he or she is responsible for (Table 3).

Since the establishment of the Faculty of Pharmacy at the University of Khartoum in 1964 up to 2003, the number of registered pharmacists with the SMC did not exceed 3000. From 2004 until 2009, this number doubled to exceed 7000 registered pharmacists.[11] This was due to the reform in higher education started in 1989 (widely known as Higher Education Revolution), which led to the expansion of pharmacy education and the opening of more than 10 new pharmacy faculties that started to graduate students at this period. Overall, only four faculties are sole public colleges of pharmacy: Khartoum, Gezira, Omdurman Islamic University, and Al-Neelain. The others either full private or semiprivate colleges, such as Rabat and Karrary; the latter used to be named as a private college with specific criteria. In Sudan, the Accreditation Board, Ministry of Higher Education and Scientific Research named colleges based on their types of intake (i.e., through payment or free affiliation).

The Pharmaceutical Annual Statistical Report 2007 showed that in 2006, the total enrollment capacity of the 12 faculties was actually greater than 1600 students. This high level of enrollment number was not accompanied by increases in the number of teaching staff as there has been no clear policy for the recruitment of academic staff. The large student intake and the small number of qualified staff may highly affect the student-to-staff ratio and consequently the quality of graduates.

6. Achievements in the pharmacy practice

One of the main factors that positively impacted pharmacy practice in Sudan, and facilitated and enhanced its achievements, is the reduction of the government deficit, which was as a consequence of the price liberalization and privatization strategy implemented in Sudan in recent years. Also, the approval of the investment law positively impacted many areas, among them health and pharmacy.

Implementation of these policies resulted in improvements in the availability of pharmacy supplies in the private sector. It also resulted in an increase in the number of retail distributers, medicine importers, and manufacturers. For example, the number of the pharmaceutical importing companies, local manufacturers, and community pharmacies increased from 77, 7 and 551, respectively, before the privatization policy to 283, 24, and 1422 in 2005.[21] Also, the number of registered medicines in Sudan showed a high increase, to nearly 3000 in 2005. The result is that the present situation of pharmacy services is far better than two decades ago.

In 2007, the government reviewed the structure of the DGoP and separated policy functions from regulatory functions. Now, functions are managed by two different bodies, which provides for a better focus on pharmacy practice issues; before this, the regulatory functions dominated the work of DGoP. Also, the Pharmacy Strategy for the Quarter Century 2005–2029 provides broad statements for establishing a good base for strong pharmacy practice role in PHC.

Another big achievement is the improvement in access to medicines as a consequence of the increase in the number of pharmacy outlets in both public and private sectors. However, the availability of medicines in the public sector remains a problem. CMS took a new promising approach to solve this problem, which focuses more on improving the distribution system to reach the periphery rather than bringing more medicines into the country. To improve access to good-quality medicines, especially at PHC facilities, CMS has launched a new model for unified supply system of medicines to the states and established a Medical Supply Fund (MSF) in each state, which is under the direct supervision of the state minister for health. The MSF is also responsible for the distribution of medicines that treat HIV/AIDS, TB, and malaria donated by the Global Fund (GFATM); and medicines that are dispensed free of charge during the first 24-hour in hospital outpatient clinics.

A great achievement was also attained in human resources development. During the last 10 years, the number of registered pharmacists increased to about 13,000 and number of undergraduate students increased to about 11,000. The number of specialized pharmacists doubled more than 15 times within a decade to reach more than 300. Main specialties include pharmaceutical services management and clinical pharmacy. These two specialties are now taught in the Sudan National Medical Specialization Board (fellowship in pharmacy services management) and University of Khartoum and Omdurman Islamic University (M.Sc. in Clinical Pharmacy).

In the field of pharmaceutical industry, a new policy was formulated to promote national pharmaceutical industry and attract foreign investment to this sector. According to this policy, foreign manufacturers who have interest in establishing a pharmaceutical production facility can enjoy fast-track registration; the accelerated stability study for 6 months will give them an expiration date of 1 year. They can also participate in the special tender for the local manufacturers. This policy is hoped to promote technology transfer and thereby assist in the development of the capacity of the national pharmaceutical manufacturers. It also hoped to contribute in the improvement in human resources in pharmaceutical technology by providing training opportunities for local workers. Finally it is hoped to reduce the reliance on imports and thereby contribute to managing foreign exchange flow.

7. Challenges in the pharmacy practice

Pharmacy practice in Sudan suffers from several inefficiencies. These include structural, financial, and human resources issues. However, in this section, authors present the main challenges faced by pharmacy practice development and progression in Sudan. Among those challenges are the following:

- The financial incentives to develop pharmaceutical services are very weak. Also, salaries of pharmacists are weak, something negatively affecting the quality of services.
- PHRs have different challenges from state to state and within same state. Most of these challenges are associated with the political commitment of the states' government and their ministers of health. Also, one of the main challenges adversely affecting public sector pharmacists is the severe underinvestment from the states as well as national funds.
- The practice is widely dominated, if not solely focused, on dispensing.

- There is a lack of control of drug promotion and advertisement and weak, if not total lack of, pharmacovigilance and drug information systems.
- There is a lack of enforcement of laws and regulations regarding the specification of pharmacy shops and professionals who work in community pharmacies and hospitals.
- A lot of effort is needed in the areas of inspections of pharmaceutical premises and assessment of pharmaceutical products for marketing authorization as these areas are still lagging behind. Also, the public supply chain is weak and suffers frequent out-of-stocks in the public health facilities.

8. Opportunities

- One of the objectives stated in the National Drug Policy is that "up-to-date pharmaceutical services in accordance with the concept of pharmaceutical care will be provided." This is in conjunction with the updated Act, which grants the NMPB full autonomy. The attendance of the first vice president at the first meeting of the NMPB represent a high political commitment toward pharmacy practice issues, which could highlight and solve challenges facing the profession.

9. Recommendations: way forward

- It is necessary to increase the awareness of the government about the importance of pharmacy services in the health care system in order to be convinced, and consequently committed, to put more resources to increase the number and quality of pharmaceutical personnel, and ultimately increase access to better pharmaceutical services.
- There is also an urgent need for the government to implement the provisions of the Medicines and Poisons Act 2009.

10. Conclusions

Improving the effectiveness of public pharmaceutical services could be accomplished by focusing and directing resources toward areas of need, reducing inequalities, and promoting better health. Also, it is essential to have clear incentives for pharmacists to control migration from the public sector.

11. Lessons learned/points to remember

- There is an urgent need for a strategy that critically responds to the current and future challenges in PHRs. Any approach that does not address job satisfaction is not expected to be successful.
- Strong advocacy should be directed toward achieving political awareness at federal and state levels. The introduction of a pharmaceutical care concept may be a good opportunity for reshaping the pharmacy services.

- Special care and consideration should be given to the devotion of public sector pharmacists, despite their low wages, and especially at difficult times they face during medicine supply shortages.
- A strategy considering the views of pharmacy professional associations, unions, universities, ministries of health, higher education, and all other stakeholders is needed to achieve pharmacists' job satisfaction.
- The discouraging salaries and incentive structures need to be addressed through the creation of new jobs and new incentive structures that support pharmacists over the course of their working lives.
- Inequalities in pharmaceutical services need to be addressed through a new redistribution of pharmacy workforces to reflect the pharmacy profession in Sudan.
- Raising awareness about the fundamental role of the pharmacist in building strategies for the provision of pharmaceutical care in both public and private sectors and the creation of national leadership is essential for the profession.
- Although the National Drug Policy and 25-year pharmacy strategy emphasize continuing pharmacy professional development, the issue is not being tackled yet.

References

1. Federal Ministry of Health, World Bank. *Sudan country status report (CSR) 2012*. 2012. Khartoum.
2. Central Bureau of Statistics (CBS). *Sudan in figures: 2005–2009*. Khartoum (Sudan): Central Bureau of Statistics; 2012.
3. Mohamed GK, Abdelrahman M, Abdeen MO. A prescription for improvement: a short survey to identify reasons behind public sector pharmacists' migration. *World Health Popul* 2006;**3**:77–100.
4. Federal Ministry of Health (FMoH) and the Central Bureau of Statistics (CBS). *Sudan household health survey (2010)*. 2011.
5. Federal Ministry of Health (FMoH) and the Central Bureau of Statistics (CBS). *Sudan household health survey (2006)*. 2007.
6. UNDP. *Status of MDGs in Sudan in 2012* [cited January 14, 2013]. Available from: http://www.sd.undp.org/m dg_fact.htm; 2012.
7. Bayoumi A. *The history of Sudan health services*. Nairobi: Kenya Literature Bureau; 1979.
8. Mustafa MS, Sara HM, Zahir AA. *Health system profile*. Sudan: Division of Health System and Services Development, Eastern Mediterranean Regional Office, WHO; 2005.
9. World Health Organization (WHO). *Sudan – pharmaceutical country profile* [cited March 20, 2011]. Available from: http://www.who.int/medicines/areas/coordination/sudan_pharmaceuticalprofile_december201 0.pdf; December 2010.
10. General Directorate of Pharmacy. *Federal Ministry of Health, General Directorate of Pharmacy, annual statistical report*. 2012.
11. Federal Ministry of Health. *Assessment of human resources at the pharmaceutical sector*. Federal Ministry of Health, Republic of Sudan in collaboration with World Health Organization; 2009.
12. *Procurement, contracting and disposal of surplus act*. Khartoum (Sudan): Ministry of Finance and National Economy; 2010.
13. African Union. Pharmaceutical manufacturing plan for Africa. In: *Third session of the African union conference of ministers of health; April 9–13, 2007; Johannesburg, South Africa*. 2007.
14. Mohamed GK. The impact of the pharmaceutical regulations on the quality of medicines on the Sudanese market: importers' perspective. *SJPH* 2007;**2**:157–67.

15. WHO. *Assessment of the national pharmaceutical sector level II health facilities survey.* [cited March 20, 2011]. Available from World Wide Web: http://apps.who.int/medicinedocs/documents/s19200en/s19200en.pdf; 2007 [accessed March 2011].

16. Aissatou Diack, Afthe. *Analysis of pharmaceutical sector policy, regulation and management.* Republic of Sudan. [cited May 18, 2013]. http://www.worldbank.org/en/topic/health/research/all?qterm=&lang_exact=English&teratopic_exact=Macroeconomics+and+Economic+Growth&os=20; 2011.

17. Mohamed GK, Yahia Y. Controlling medicine prices in Sudan: the challenge of the recently established medicines regulatory authority. *East Mediterr Health J* 2012;**18**(8):811–20.

18. Mohamed GK. *Accessibility of medicines and primary health care: the impact of the RDF in Khartoum State* [Ph.D. thesis]. Trent University; 2006.

19. National Fund for Health Insurance (NFHI). *Annual report. National fund for health insurance.* Khartoum (Sudan): Ministry of Social Welfare; 2002.

20. Badr E, Mohamed NA, Afzalc MM, Bile KM. Strengthening human resources for health through information, coordination and accountability mechanisms: the case of the Sudan. *Bull World Health Organ* 2013;**91**:868–73. [cited November 28, 2013] http://dx.doi.org/10.2471/BLT.13.118950.

21. *Federal Ministry of Health (FMoH). Annual statistical report, 2011.* Khartoum: Federal Ministry of Health, National Health Information Centre; 2011.

CHAPTER 17

Pharmacy Practice in Nigeria

Ahmed Awaisu, Shafiu Mohammed, Rabiu Yakubu

Chapter Outline

1. Introduction

This chapter provides a general overview of Nigeria's health care system, briefly highlights the indicators of healthcare quality, and broadly reviews the past, present, and future perspectives of pharmacy practice and education in Nigeria, including the challenges faced by the profession.

Pharmacy Practice in Developing Countries. http://dx.doi.org/10.1016/B978-0-12-801714-2.00017-4

Nigeria, the most populous country in Africa, has faced inadequate basic infrastructure for health, chronic shortages as well as migration of the existing health manpower resources, disparities in the rural-urban distribution of health workforce, proliferation of counterfeit drugs, wide distribution and handling of drugs by traders and vendors, and problems with the accessibility, availability, and affordability of medicines.[1–4] There is a global consensus that the highest attainable standard of health is a fundamental human right.[5] Pharmacy practice and education in general—as well as the availability, affordability, and accessibility of quality, safe, and effective essential medicines to the populace—are critical to the success of the healthcare delivery system.

This introductory section highlights the country background, health sector and system reforms, healthcare financing, statistics on morbidity and mortality, statistics on human capital and health workforce, and medicines expenditure and utilization in Nigeria.

1.1 Country background

Since the 1990s, pharmacy practice and education in Nigeria have changed considerably. The practice and education of the profession experienced a series of changes and processes that led to the current institutional structure in the Nigerian fabric. Nigeria became an independent nation in 1960 and a Federal Republic in 1963. The country has 36 states and a Federal Capital Territory, which are further subdivided into 774 Local Government Areas (LGAs). The states are clustered into six geopolitical zones; North-West, North-East, North-Central, South-West, South-East, and South-South according to ethnic homogeneity.[6] Nigeria is positioned between longitudes 80° east and latitude 100° north.[7] The country is located in West Africa (sub-Saharan Africa) and shares land borders with the Republic of Benin to the West, Cameroun to the East, Niger and Chad to the north, and the Atlantic Ocean to the South.

With a population of more than 150 million people in 2009, Nigeria is the most populous country in Africa.[7] The United Nations also estimated that 49.8% of Nigerians live in urban areas. Nigeria has 250 ethnic groups; the largest ethnic groups are Hausa, Yoruba, and Igbo.[6] In the past few years, the country had failed to incorporate population census figures in its planning, which made the Government's health planning unrealistic. According to the World Health Organization (WHO), the life expectancy at birth for both males and females was 54 years in 2009, the infant mortality per 1000 live births for both sexes was 88 in 2010, under-5 mortality per 1000 live births for both sexes was 143 in 2010, and the adult (between 15 and 60 years) mortality per 1000 population was 365 in 2009.[8]

Nigeria's major source of income is from the oil production. Despite attempts to focus on diversifying the economy, the country still highly depends on the oil and gas sector. The currency unit is the Nigerian Naira (₦), with fluctuating inflation compared to Euro (€) and US dollar ($) currencies. In the past few decades, the long-term military rule intertwined with corruption and mismanagement has hampered economic activities and growth in the country.

Despite the restoration of democracy and subsequent economic reforms, corruption and mismanagement are still prominent. According to the World Bank, Nigeria's Gross Domestic Product (GDP) per capita at purchasing power parity (PPP) in the year 2011 was US$2533, which is low compared to other low-middle income countries (LMICs).[9] The GDP in 2011 was estimated at an annual growth of 7% with a consumer price inflation of 11%.[9] These figures are mostly augmented due to the mono-economy of oil production, whereas other sectors of the economy such as health, education, agriculture, and power are in decline and poor conditions.

In Nigeria, the total health expenditure (THE) as a percentage of GDP was 6.1% in 2009, whereas the general government health expenditure (GGHE) as a percentage of THE in 2009 was 35.1%.[8] However, the GGHE as percentage of total government expenditure (TGE) was only 5.9% in 2009, whereas out-of-pocket (OOP) expenditure as a percentage of private health expenditure was one of the highest (95.6%) in the world.[8] The country's per capita total expenditure on health was low (US$136), and the per capita government expenditure on health was one of the lowest (US$48) in the world.[8]

1.2 Health care system in Nigeria

The health care delivery system in Nigeria is broadly divided into public and private sectors. The public sector is stratified into three levels of care: primary, secondary, and tertiary levels.[2] The tertiary level of care has full complement of 13 professional services—namely medical, pharmaceutical, nursing/midwifery, laboratory, optometric, radiography, physiotherapy, community health, health records, dental technology, dental therapy, chemistry, and analytical services.[10] The three levels of care are in alignment with the three-tier national system of government composed of the federal government, the state government, and the local government. The Federal Ministry of Health (FMoH) has the responsibility of developing policies, strategies, guidelines, plans, and programs that provide the overall direction of health care delivery in the country. Furthermore, the FMoH coordinates the provision of tertiary care services. State governments, through the State Ministries of Health (SMoH), are responsible for the provision of secondary health care services. The LGAs are largely responsible for primary health care services. However, the states and LGAs are supported in essential primary health care activities by Federal Government through the National Primary Health Care Development Agency, SURE-P; UN agencies such as WHO, Millennium Development Goals (MDGs), World Bank and United Nations Population Fund Agency (UNFPA); and other development partners such as the United States Agency for International Development (USAID) and United Kingdom Agency for International Development (DFID/UKaid).

Although the healthcare system is run concurrently, the autonomy of each tier of government has made the allocation of health resources inconsistent and the demarcation of responsibilities unclearly defined. Nonetheless, a two-way referral system linking the three levels of care has been an integral part of health sector reform encompassed in both the states and National Strategic Health Development Plans, of which the implementation is recording some successes. On the other hand, the private health sector is an enormous provider of health services, especially in urban areas. The quality of care provided by the private health sector in Nigeria is not well documented. However, a number of these private health facilities are believed to operate without proper licensure and accreditation from regulatory bodies.

Pharmacy practice as an integral part of health care system in Nigeria is categorized into four key areas of practice: the hospital pharmacy, retail/community pharmacy, pharmaceutical manufacturing, and the wholesale/importation of pharmaceutical products. The Pharmacists Council of Nigeria has set the benchmark for minimum levels of practice for quality assurance of pharmaceutical care based on these identified four key thematic areas.[11]

1.3 Health sector reform in Nigeria

The Millennium Development Goals (MDGs) are aimed at eradicating extreme poverty and hunger, reduce child mortality, improve maternal health, and combat HIV/AIDS, malaria, and other diseases orchestrated the need for health reforms in Nigeria and other LMICs. The Nigerian government established the Health Sector Reform Program (HSRP) in order to improve the performance of the health care system, so as to attain a better health status for the Nigerian population.[12] This change is compelled toward achieving the MDGs by the year 2015. Poor institutional arrangement and defective functional relationships have been the major constraints for the health sector and system.[13] The HSRP focused on strengthening the overall health system and its management, improving access and quality of health services, improving availability of health resources and their management, reducing the burden of diseases, improving the stewardship role of the government, and promoting effective collaboration and partnership within and outside the health sector.

As part of the HSRP, the National Health Insurance Scheme (NHIS) was launched in 1999. This scheme has become necessary in Nigeria due to inadequate provision of health facilities, the low income per person (US$310 in 1999), and the country's poor health indices.[14] In 2005, the scheme was implemented in the formal sector, especially at the federal level. This NHIS implementation was part of the health reform programs and strategies toward providing effective and efficient health care for all citizens, most especially for the poor and vulnerable people.[15]

Successive Nigerian governments therefore attempted to improve the health status of Nigerians through development of a uniform health plan framework, thereby putting in place nine indicators and targets toward achieving the MDGs and the Vision 20:2020. One of such major strides was the declaration by the President and 36 State Executive Governors of the establishment of National Strategic Health Development Plan (NSHDP). The NSHDP, a health sector component of Vision 20:2020, is a comprehensive reference document for

Table 1: National strategic health development plan key indicators and targets

Indicator	Baseline	Targets		
		2011	2013	2015
Life expectancy at birth	47 years	55 years	63 years	70 years
Under-5 mortality rate	157/1000 LBs (NDHS, 2008)	130/1000 LBs	103/1000 LBs	75/1000 LBs
Infant mortality rate	75 (NDHS, 2008)	60/1000 LBs	45/1000 LBs	30/1000 LBs
Proportion of 1 year olds immunized against measles	41.4 (NDHS, 2008)	60%	80%	95%
Prevalence of children under-5 years of age who are underweight	27.1 (NDHS, 2008)	24%	20%	17.90%
Percentage of children under 5 sleeping under insecticide-treated bed nets	5.5 (NDHS, 2008)	24%	42%	60%
Maternal mortality ratio	545/100,000 LBs (NDHS, 2008)	409/100,000 LBs	273/100,000 LBs	136/100,000 LBs
Adolescents birth rates	126/1000	114/1000	102/1000	90/1000
HIV prevalence among population aged 15–24 years	4.2% (ANC Sentinel survey)	3.2%	2.1%	1%

ANC, Antenatal Care; LB, live births; NDHS, National Demographic Health Survey.
Source: Adapted from FMoH.[16]

stakeholders at all levels in the health sector, toward delivery of shared results framework. Following the declaration of NSHDP and the State Strategic Health Development Plan in November 2009, the National Council on Health, the highest policy advisory body in Nigeria, in March 2010 approved the NSHDP 2010–2015. The NSHDP 2010–2015 is more comprehensive than the earlier versions; it is composed of eight goals or strategic priority areas, 33 strategic objectives, and 70 strategic interventions.[16] Some details are provided in Table 1. The development partner agencies would align and support implementation with close involvement of community-based organizations and the media.

Another giant stride by the government of Nigeria was the passage of the revised National Health Bill 2014 by the National Assembly, which aims to provide a framework for the regulation, development, and management of a National Health System and sets standards for rendering health services in the federation and other related matters.

1.4 Health financing system in Nigeria

Health care is funded in Nigeria through multiple sources, including budgetary allocations from the government at all levels (federal, state, and local), loans and grants, private sector contributions, and OUP expenses. During the past few decades, the value of private sector and OUP expenditure in financing the sector was not determined. Likewise, the real cost of health services still remained unknown because the system of National

Health Account (NHA) was at an infantile stage. Moreover, there were no reliable data on the combined federal, state, and LGA expenditures, nor on expenditures from private and donor sources. There was no broad-based health financing strategy, even with the planned commencement of NHIS.[17] Inadequacies of managerial accountability, health management information system, interministerial and state collaboration, and absence of good monitoring and evaluation all pose challenges to the country's health financing system. In recent years, Nigeria has started the estimation of NHA with technical and financial support from the WHO. The NHA serves as a tool for evidence-based decision-making in health policy, health financing, and health interventions. The WHO stated that it would devote efforts to building capacity to obtain health expenditure information, utilize relevant health financing and economic evidence to formulate plans and policies, and guide interventions for improving systems of health financing and social protection.[18]

Nigeria had consecutively two periods of NHA reports (1998–2002 and 2003–2005), but the third report has not been achieved. Despite the unavailability of data from some States, the second report (2003–2005) has led to the widening of the estimation to include the sub-National Health Accounts (SNHA) at the State levels. The two reports showed that the bulk of Nigeria's health spending was on curative care (average 70.23% in 1998–2002 and 74.10% in 2003–2005) of THEs, whereas preventive care (1.41% in 1998–2002 and 12.72% in 2003–2005) of THE was far-off second.[19,20] Households continued to be the major source of health financing, and the average household health expenditure (HHHE) was 64.25% in 1998–2002 and 68.45% in 2003–2005 of THE, which might have pushed people into catastrophic health expenditure. The burden that average HHHE contributed to State total health expenditure (STHE) was above 72% in 2003–2005, which was poor.[19,20]

A constant in health insurance expenditure was reported in the two reports with relatively 2% of THE.[20] Facilitating the extension of Social Health Insurance to the informal sector (70% of the population) might be an alternative means of financing to mitigate the catastrophic effects of high HHHE. The second report was incorporated into the National Strategic Health Development Plan (NSHDP 2010–2015). The plan has to be funded by the three tiers of government with the support of development partner agencies, estimated to cost ₦3.997 trillion over the 6-year period (Table 2). As part of Presidential Summit Declaration on Health, both federal and states governments are dedicated to achieving allocation and release of 15% of annual budget to the health sector by 2015.[21] The reports are also reflected in the "Nigerian Vision 20:2020" (First National Implementation Plan 2010–2013). Reporting of NHAs and SNHAs should become a periodic process and listed as routine work of health and health-related institutions geared toward evidence-based policy and decision making. Stepwise broadening of a coherent and consistent framework of the NHAs could help greatly in their institutionalization and applications.

Table 2: Estimated costs for the National Strategic Health Development Plan

Priority Area	₦	US$	Percent
Leadership and governance for health	27,587,202,750	183,914,685	0.69%
Health service delivery	1,946,257,153,350	12,975,047,689	48.68%
Human resources for health	1,664,676,299,550	11,097,841,997	41.64%
Financing for health	218,976,510,300	1,459,843,402	5.48%
National health information system	41,605,199,400	277,367,996	1.04%
Community participation and ownership	23,913,081,450	159,420,543	0.60%
Partnerships for health	25,502,477,700	170,016,518	0.64%
Research for health	49,448,161,050	329,654,407	1.24%
Sum	**3,997,966,085,850**	**26,653,107,239**	**100.00%**

Source: Adapted from FMoH.[16]

1.5 Health insurance scheme in Nigeria

A national health insurance scheme (NHIS) was introduced in 2005 to all federal establishments in Nigeria. It is intended that this scheme will provide financial protection and improve health care delivery and utilization of health services that is equitable and affordable to people by their contributions through risk pooling and purchasing of the services. Since its implementation, the scheme has led to a significant amount of additional financial resources allocated to the health sector.[6,22,23] Presently, the Federal Government and FMoH have agreed to allocate 25% of the health budget to the NHIS, out of the 4% of the federal budget allocated to the health sector.[23] However, the health insurance scheme is still at its nascent stage in the country and, therefore, is faced with numerous challenges and constraints. Problems reported by the NHIS from its annual reports were according to anecdotal evidence, such as insured-user complaints of poor attitude and behavior of health care providers operating in the health insurance scheme[24]; distortions within the referral system on the health providers' side, which hinders some of the objectives of the scheme[13,24]; complaints of delays and refusals to make payments to providers by some health management organizations (HMOs)[13,24]; and some providers' denying health care services to insured users on insubstantial or feeble excuses, while others charge additional fees on the pretext of noninclusion of the service in the benefit package.[13,24]

In Nigeria, the HMO model of operation creates a purchaser-provider split and the health insurers operate for profit or not for profit in the insurance scheme. HMOs according to the health insurance scheme in Nigeria are insurers who, vertically integrated in the scheme's revenue collection, pool and purchase healthcare services within a competitive framework. These HMOs are private organizations that coordinate all aspects of the delivery system and manage reimbursement to accredited health care providers (HCPs) within the system.[25] Furthermore, the HMOs have contract agreements with independently existing HCPs to provide health care services to their insured clients. In principle, a client can chose any HCP, and the HMO initiates a contract with the client's provider. In practice, these HCPs independently exist as either public or private health facilities, including hospitals and clinics. Presently, there are 62 HMOs in Nigeria licensed by the NHIS regulatory agency, which facilitates the interface between governmental organizations, health care providers related to delivery system, and eligible contributors.[26] These HMOs work with providers and insured clients under the supervision of the NHIS regulatory agency.

1.6 Vital health statistics in Nigeria

According to the WHO, the life expectancy at birth for both males and females was 54 years in 2009, the infant mortality per 1000 live births for both sexes was 88 in 2010, under-5 mortality per 1000 live births for both sexes was 143 in 2010, and the adult (between 15 and 60 years) mortality per 1000 population was 365 in 2009.[8] The age-adjusted adult mortality rates for women and men aged 15–49 years were 3.5 and 3.3 deaths per 1000 person-years of exposure, respectively (Table 3).[27] Furthermore, Nigeria has one of the highest maternal and childhood mortality rates per annum in the world. However, both infant and under-5 mortality

Table 3: Adult mortality rates and trends

Direct estimates of female and male mortality rates for the seven years preceding the survey, by five-year age groups: 2013 NDHS and 2008 NDHS				
	2013 NDHS			**2008 NDHS**
Age	**Deaths**	**Exposure Years**	**Mortality Rate[a]**	**Mortality Rate[a]**
Women				
15–19	198	84,788	2.3	3.3
20–24	263	93,675	2.8	3.4
25–29	311	87,756	3.6	4.3
30–34	261	73,521	3.6	6.2
35–39	232	52,655	4.4	5.2
40–44	155	32,414	4.8	6.3
45–49	93	18,292	5.1	6.3
15–49	1514	443,102	3.5[b]	4.7[b]
Men				
15–19	152	88,879	1.7	2.8
20–24	257	99,005	2.6	2.9
25–29	247	93,153	2.7	3.6
30–34	246	76,189	3.2	5.0
35–39	245	55,832	4.4	5.4
40–44	180	34,434	5.2	8.7
45–49	125	19,147	6.5	8.2
15–49	1452	466,639	3.3[b]	4.6[b]

[a]Expressed per 1000 population.
[b]Age-adjusted rate.
Source: NDHS.[27]

rates have declined by 26% and 31%, respectively, from 1998 to 2013.[27] Infant and under-5 mortality rates for 2008–2013 were 69 and 128 deaths per 1000 live births, respectively.[27] Maternal mortality ratio stands at 576 maternal deaths per 100,000 live births as reported in the 2013 NDHS[27]—a ratio that is not significantly different from the ratio reported in the 2008 NDHS. The high maternal mortality ratio may partly be attributed to sociocultural norms and gender inequalities; low educational status of women, health beliefs, traditional birth practices, early marriage, and lack of access to maternal health services. These are some of the indicators that impede the attainment of two of the MDGs (reduce child mortality and improve maternal health). Other health issues of public health significance include, but are not limited to, the high burden of communicable and waterborne diseases including malaria, tuberculosis, HIV/AIDS, and childhood diarrhea.

Health care financing is a crucial issue in the Nigerian health system; the country failed to achieve the Abuja Declaration target of 15% allocation to the health sector from the national budget and the MDG targets for public health sector spending. The reported expenditure on health in Nigeria is less than US$8 per capita, compared with US$34 recommended by the Commission of Microeconomics and Health. The inadequate funding at all levels of the health system is clearly reflected in the poor quality of resources and grossly impedes the development and performance of the system. On the other hand, the human resources for health in Nigeria are comparably higher than most sub-Saharan and other African countries. According to 2007 estimates, the pharmacist-population, physician-population, and nurse-population ratios were 9.3 per 100,000, 37 per 100,000, and 91 per 100,000, respectively.[28] In general, the distribution of health workforce is skewed to the urban areas, the Southern geopolitical zone, and tertiary care centers.[28] It is also worthwhile to note that in recent years there has been a high migration of health workforce from Nigeria to other developed countries including the UK, Ireland, USA, Australia, and Canada. The high attrition of health workforce could be attributed to the unfavorable compensation packages and working conditions, rendering young healthcare professionals to search for greener pastures in the developed world.

1.7 Summary of the current status of health sector in Nigeria

In general, the indicators and socioeconomic determinants of health as well as the Nigeria's health demography suggest that there were obvious necessities for health system reforms in Nigeria.[2,16] As described in the previous sections, during the past decade, the democratic dispensation and leadership in Nigeria has brought about some fortunes for the reformation of the health care system and increased access to health for the populace. The system has gradually undergone slow but steady transformations since the return of democracy in 1999 and there is a paradigm shift in the distribution and utilization of healthcare resources across different levels of the system. In 2004, there was a new policy, the Revised National Health Policy, which describes the goals, structure, strategy, and policy direction of the healthcare delivery system in Nigeria.[29] In a nutshell, the Government of Nigeria recognizes that to improve the health sector and the well-being of Nigerians, there would be a need for scale-up, strengthening the health systems including improved health sector financing, and strengthening the primary health care system. The reformation embarked has attempted to revamp the basic infrastructure and framework of the country's health care system. There has been emphasis on providing a continuum of effective health services delivery. Most recently, there was formulation of the National Strategic Health Development Plan (NSHDP) 2010–2015. This plan will serve as the overarching guidelines for all stakeholders to ensure transparency and reciprocal accountability in the healthcare delivery sector. The achievements so far cannot be without the significant input of international health and donor agencies such as WHO, UNICEF, World Bank, USAID, DFID/UKaid, Bill and Melinda Gates Foundation, NURHI, just to mention but a few. These organizations have played a significant role in the development and progression toward universal health coverage. Lastly, there are health system strategies and action frameworks in place towards the attainment of MDGs in Nigeria.

2. Pharmacy practice in Nigeria

This second segment of the chapter broadly reviews the regulation of pharmacy practice and education in Nigeria, pharmacy practice in key pharmaceutical subsectors, and medicine supply and distribution in Nigeria.

2.1 Regulation of pharmacy practice in Nigeria

Advancement of pharmacy practice is at the centerpiece of health system development in Nigeria. This could be traced to the metamorphosis undergone by pharmacy practice from pre-independence Nigeria to present day especially the milestones achieved over the last two decades under the Pharmacists Council of Nigeria (PCN), established in 1993. However, the advancement is faced with overwhelming challenges just like in most other African countries. Pharmacy practice and education are predominantly regulated by the PCN, which is the regulatory body charged with the control and responsibilities of (1) determining the standard of knowledge and skills for pharmacists and pharmacy technicians; (2) establishing and maintaining a register of persons qualified to practice as pharmacists and pharmacy technicians; and (3) regulation and inspection of pharmaceutical premises. In general, the Council sets the minimum standard for assurance of pharmaceutical care provided in pharmacies of health centers, community pharmacy including patent and proprietary medicine stores, wholesaling/distribution, importation, and manufacturing.[10] Other important regulatory agencies that are relevant to pharmacy in Nigeria are the National Agency for Food and Drug Administration and Control (NAFDAC) and the National Drug Law Enforcement Agency (NDLEA). While the former issues import license and inspects facilities to ensure compliance with current Good Manufacturing Practice (cGMP), the later enforced laws against the cultivation, processing, sales, trafficking, and use of illegal drugs including narcotics.

2.2 Pharmacy education in Nigeria

Pharmacy education in Nigeria has undergone a modest transformation from a science-based curriculum to a blended science- and practice-based curriculum. The first bachelor of pharmacy degree program was started at Obafemi Awolowo University, Ile-Ife in 1964, followed by Ahmadu Bello University Zaria in 1968. Today, there are 17 accredited faculties of pharmacy in Nigeria, 15 within public universities, and two within private universities.[10] There were also 20 Schools of Health Technology training pharmacy technicians and pharmacy assistants as at 2007.[30] Since the 1990s, the faculties of pharmacy offer a 5-year baccalaureate (BPharm) degree program. The content of pharmacy curricula varies across schools, but in general the schools widely use traditional curricula of pharmaceutics, pharmacognosy, medicinal chemistry, pharmacology, with clinical pharmacy and practice becoming a commonplace.

A pharmacy graduate must complete a 1-year mandatory internship training at an accredited center before being licensed to practice. Upon completion of the internship, the provisionally registered pharmacist must apply to the PCN for full registration (i.e., a practicing license) as a pharmaceutical chemist. The practicing license has to be renewed annually. In an effort to encourage lifelong learning endeavor and to keep up to date with the rapidly changing pharmaceutical knowledge, pharmacists in Nigeria are required to undertake a three-year cycle Mandatory Continuing Professional Development Program (MCPD) for recertification.[31] The MCPD program is intended to update the knowledge, skills, and enhance the continued competence of pharmacists, to enable them keep abreast of advancements in pharmacy and to enhance their skills in the process of providing pharmaceutical care. Schools of pharmacy also have varying graduate degree programs, including pharmacy practice-related courses.

The process of improving pharmacy education began in 1994 when the Federal Ministry of Health through the PCN sponsored the Deans of Faculties of Pharmacy on a study tour of pharmacy schools in the United Kingdom and the United States.[32] This led to the recommendation that pharmacy practice in Nigeria should be more patient-focused. New courses including pharmaceutical care, pharmacoeconomics, pharmacogenetics, pathology, clinical toxicology, biostatics, and research methods were introduced in the curriculum. Another major transformation in pharmacy education is the introduction of a 6-year doctor of pharmacy (PharmD) degree program, which has already commenced in the University of Benin.

2.3 Pharmacy practice in key pharmaceutical subsectors

The pharmaceutical sector in Nigeria mainly comprises four key areas of practice: the pharmaceutical manufacturing, the hospital pharmacy, the retail/community pharmacy, and the wholesale/importation of pharmaceutical products. The minimum service package for each key area is described in four-part compendium for pharmaceutical care in Nigeria.[11]

Nevertheless, there are pharmacists who work with nongovernmental organizations and a few with higher academic degrees have joined the pharmacy academy. As of 2008, there were 13,199 pharmacists in Nigeria.[28]

One of the major challenges in the sector is the scarcity of pharmacists due to inadequate remuneration packages and unfavorable working conditions, with the majority working in urban areas. The 13,199 registered pharmacists in Nigeria are unevenly distributed across geopolitical zones and rural vs. urban areas.[28] In Nigeria, pharmacy practice still focuses on traditional drug dispensing and distribution, while transformation toward patient-centered care is uncommon. Although changes are happening at different paces in different subsectors of pharmacy practice, drug regulations generally exist but are not been strictly enforced. Also, distribution and handling of drugs by traders and vendors (nonpharmacists, who lack a pharmacy background) is a commonplace.

2.3.1 Pharmacy practice in the manufacturing subsector

The first major boost in the pharmaceutical sector came up with the launching of the maiden National Drug Policy (NDP) in 1990 as one of the key components of National Health Policy. The policy goals are to make sustainably available adequate quantities of safe, qualitative, efficacious and affordable medicines to Nigerians, to ensure rational use and simulate increased local production of such essential medicines.[33] The launching of NDP in 1990 marked the beginning of a new era for increasing access and achieving sustainable availability of quality and affordable drugs in the Nigerian healthcare system, especially sourcing through local manufacturing. One of the objectives of the policy was to encourage local production of drugs and research into local production of raw materials.[33] The four-part compendium describes the minimum standards required for good and effective professional practice in the manufacturing subsector. It also describes services rendered such as drug production, distribution, quality control/assurance, professional seminars, clinical presentations, production of drug monographs, research and development, and contract manufacturing.[11]

The efforts of the Presidential Committee on Pharmaceutical Sector Reform (PCPSR), inaugurated in 2003, in reviewing and implementing the policy have improved the local manufacturing of drugs. The membership of Pharmaceutical Manufacturing Group of Manufacturers Association of Nigeria (PMG-MAN) has increased from 20 at inception of the association in 1983 to 74 registered members but an overall total of 159 local manufacturers in 2013.[10] During a January 2012 meeting of PMG-MAN organized by CHAI and Partnership for Transforming Health System II (PATHS2) with stakeholders from across PATHS2 five focal States, the chairman of PMG-MAN narrated that the annual turnover of the manufacturing sub-sector was about US$2.5 billion. In spite of this relative progress been recorded in the sub-sector, he reported only about 35% of drug needs of the Nigerians was so far met. Apart from favorable policy, the manufacturers have been supported with the Federal Government grant to boost their output. On the other hand, both

NAFDAC and PCN are keeping up with their responsibilities of regulating licensing and practice in the subsector and ensure compliance with best practices. Hitherto, as of 2012, only Swiss Pharma Nigeria Limited had achieved full certification of current Good Manufacturing Practice (cGMP) of WHO in the country, while host of others were at various stages of this certification process. However, by October 2014, three additional pharmaceutical manufacturers (Evans Medical Plc, May & Baker Plc, and Chi Pharmaceutical Ltd) were also certified by WHO and could participate in international bidding/tender in accordance with the WHO cGMP.[34] One of the advantages of achieving WHO cGMP certification is to accord pharmaceutical companies the opportunities to promote their products in international markets, in addition to guarantee of quality of the products. The National Association of Industrial Pharmacists seeks to support its members to achieve greater heights in professional development.

The research and innovation for new drug products is an area that is yet to make impressive performance. This is in spite of National Institute for Pharmaceutical Research and Development (NIPRD) established in 1989. Underfunding of research in public universities and virtual nonexistence of such research grants in the Nigerian private sector continue to retard significant progress across the pharmaceutical sector. The cause of major stagnant decline in the industry and technology sector is mainly due to poor performance in the energy and power sector of the country. This contributed to massive importation of medicines into Nigeria from Asian countries, including China and India.

2.3.2 Hospital pharmacy practice

The practice of pharmacy in the health facilities dates back to the pre-independence era that mainly focused on drug compounding and dispensing. The predominant functions of hospital pharmacies were compounding, procurement, dispensing, and drug information in some hospitals.[1] Today, hospital pharmacy could be categorized based on the level of health care comprising of primary, secondary, and tertiary healthcare pharmacies.[11] This categorization took into consideration organizational structure, size and quality of operations, complement of human resources, and scale of operations, among others, informing the type of services and level of minimum standards prescribed for each level in the PCN's publication, the four-part compendium of minimum standards. Drug dispensing in the public sector varies with the type of facility. For instance, in dispensaries and primary health care facilities, medicines are prescribed and dispensed by community health extension workers or staff nurses who manage these type of facilities, while in secondary and tertiary health facilities, pharmacists are usually solely responsible for dispensing functions. On the other hand, there is no clear separation between prescribing and dispensing functions in private facilities, and majority of private clinics dispense medicines in their health facilities. Although by law pharmacies and licensed drug outlets could only provide prescription-only medicines (POMs) against a valid prescription, poor enforcement by the responsible authority meant patients could still buy them without a valid prescription.[1] With these revelations, one would assume that there is huge chaos and there are dire needs to sanitize the pharmaceutical sector in Nigeria, particularly in the importation, manufacture, sale, and distribution of medicines.

Since the 1990s, hospital pharmacy practice has undergone a transformation from being a largely product-oriented practice to more patient-focused pharmaceutical care. This was not by accident, as the pharmacy curriculum continues to evolve to reflect current strategies across the globe. The first giant step was the introduction of clinical pharmacy courses in the curriculum in the late 1980s, followed by the recent introduction of PharmD degree programs in some universities. Nevertheless, there are still challenges facing patient-oriented hospital pharmacy practice. These include (but are not limited to) inadequate health manpower resources, inadequate professional development of pharmacists, pharmacists' resistance to change, and physicians' resistance due to perception of role enroachment.[1]

Pharmaceutical care services with a focus on rational drug use and pharmacovigilance (adverse drug reactions reporting), among other services rendered, have been implemented in hospital pharmacy practice. Various policies with a direct impact on health service delivery were developed at the federal level and have also been adopted and implemented at the state level. The policy documents include the National Drug Policy (revised, 2005), Standard Treatment Guidelines (2008), Pharmacovigilance Policy (2012), and Essential Medicine List (revised, 2012).

However, cognitive clinical pharmacy services, such as pharmacokinetic consult services and therapeutic drug monitoring, renal dosing adjustment services, total parenteral nutrition, intravenous (IV) admixture programs, and direct patient care activities, including clinical rounds with healthcare team members, are not commonly available. Hospital practice is still far from witnessing specialized clinical pharmacy services, such as pharmacist-managed anticoagulation or heart failure clinics.

2.3.3 Retail pharmacy practice

The retail pharmacy, also known as the community pharmacy, is the pharmaceutical service that is most accessible and closest to the general public. The four-part compendium highlights the required organizational specifications and sets minimum standards of practice for community pharmacy practice. The responsibilities that are commonplace include logistics and supply chain management, filling of prescriptions and over-the-counter (OTC) drugs, and patient counselling and education. A community pharmacy premises has to be registered under the name of a superintendent pharmacist, who shall be the director. The PCN and NAFDAC regulate and control community pharmacy practice, of which implementation of the regulations and best practices are also supported by Association of Community Pharmacists of Nigeria (ACPN). In Nigeria, it is interesting to note that there are no chain pharmacies, rather all community pharmacies are independent. The number of these retail outlets are grossly inadequate and are concentrated in urban areas (cities), with over 50% in Nigeria's biggest commercial city of Lagos.

Unfortunately, the dearth of qualified and registered pharmacists, especially in the rural areas, has resulted in the continuity of an old unprofessional practice in which nonpharmacists are allowed to market and sell simple medicinal remedies under a Patent and Proprietary Medicine Vendor (PPMV) license.[11] These medicine vendors are simply people who can read and write; they are licenced based on guidelines having very limited provisions, largely for selling OTC drugs. The vendor stores, unlike pharmacies, are found in every nook and corner of the country and promote access to drugs, especially to rural communities. In spite of the overwhelming combined efforts of regulatory bodies comprising of PCN, NAFDAC, and the NDLEA, there are wide abuse and unwholesome practices, including the supply of a range of prescription medicines including narcotic agents. There is also proliferation and distribution of fake and counterfeit medicines by the vendors and others, who in some cases illegally rebranded into wholesaling, importation, or even manufacturing. The vendors operate under Nigerian Association of Patent and Proprietary Medicine Dealers (NAPPMED). As part of the efforts to sanitize drug distribution in Nigeria, the PCN has approved during its 36th Council meeting in May 2014, giving preference for licensed pharmacy technicians to operate PPMV outlets/shops.

2.3.4 Wholesale and importation of pharmaceutical products

PCN (2008) described pharmaceutical importation as a duly registered business for the importation of pharmaceutical products from a foreign country and distribution in Nigeria by a licensed pharmacist or corporate body. The importation and distribution go hand-in-hand and form an interface between manufacturers and retailing by health facilities, community pharmacies, and PPMV shops. The importation is to fill existing gaps due to the low manufacturing capacity of local manufacturers, while wholesaling largely serves as the main distribution hub of drugs for hospitals and retail outlets.

The four-part compendium described the organization of importation and the minimum standards set by the PCN. Sequel to this, Mora (2014) reported that all imported drugs with the exception of orphan drugs that require only NAFDAC permit must be registered with NAFDAC, and business premises registered by the PCN.[10] The importer must also comply with rules and regulations set by the Nigeria Custom Services and Nigerian Port Authority among others. The importers and wholesalers must comply with good distribution practice to ensure that drugs, medical consumables, and related substances maintain their potency throughout the period of importation and distribution.

With the view of encouraging local manufacture of drugs, the Federal Government of Nigeria developed an importation prohibition list comprising of 17 drugs.[11] This is also in line with provision of existing National Drug Policy. The Association of Pharmaceutical Importers of Nigeria, having 165 importing companies as registered members, seeks to promote good practices and better opportunities. Subsequently, the overall efforts of the regulatory agencies at least over the last decade have impacted meaningfully in sanitizing the channel of drug distribution and reducing unwholesome practices in the pharmaceutical sector.

2.4 *Medicine supply and drug distribution system in Nigeria*

The drug distribution channel in the country is the source for the supply of medicines dispensed by service providers to consumers at all levels of health care, public and private. At the apex of the distribution channel are the pharmaceutical manufacturers and importers, while the pharmacies/dispensaries and medicine shops are closest to the patrons. In the public sector, the Central Medical Store system plays the central role for drug distribution, making bulk procurement and serving as a source for re-ordering essential medicines by public health facilities. This hub of public drug supply is mainly financed by governments, which is inadequate to guarantee the sustained availability of essential medicines in public health facilities.[35] Generally, public procurement methods used in the country are mainly open tender (through contractors) and direct procurement. These methods most often suffer from poor supplier lead time due to delays in payments and late order placement, which leads to stock-outs of essential medicines in the supply chain. Nonetheless, drug supply management systems operated by a few of the states in the federation have advanced to more organized and financially more autonomous drug management agencies. These states operate the WHO model of Drug Revolving Fund (DRF) scheme, mainly initiated and supported by development partners with the DFID/UKaid in the forefront. The DRF, which is one of the strategies for implementing the National Drug Policy, aimed to improve access and uninterrupted availability of quality and affordable essential medicines to generality of Nigerians.[33] Most of the agencies operating the DRF scheme conduct national competitive tender to outsource supplies of essential medicines based on National Procurement Guidelines, State Due Process procedures and incorporating international best practices. The tertiary health institutions have been ahead in domesticating and implementing the DRF model. For the private sector, medical sale representatives of pharmaceutical companies supply medicines to private hospitals, clinics, pharmacy stores, and sometimes directly to patent medicine vendors and local market dealers.

In spite of various strategies adopted by past and present governments of Nigeria over the last two decades to sanitize and streamline the drug distribution system in the country, the drug distribution channel has remained uncoordinated.[36] This dysfunctional and often chaotic drug distribution system persistently threatens the Nigerian health care system and put the health of the public at risk. Substandard and counterfeit medicines pass through the system mostly undetected by law enforcement officials, and continue to impact negatively on consumers, thereby exposing them to dangerous health hazards. Sales of drugs in the open marketplaces by unqualified persons is a common everyday practice. Indeed, Nigeria and most African countries, parts of Asia, and Latin America are where more than 30% of medicines on sale may either contain wrong, low, or no drug content as claimed on the product label.[37] The question is how do less-privileged people and the poor ensure they are getting safe, effective, and good-quality medicines/drugs in the country.

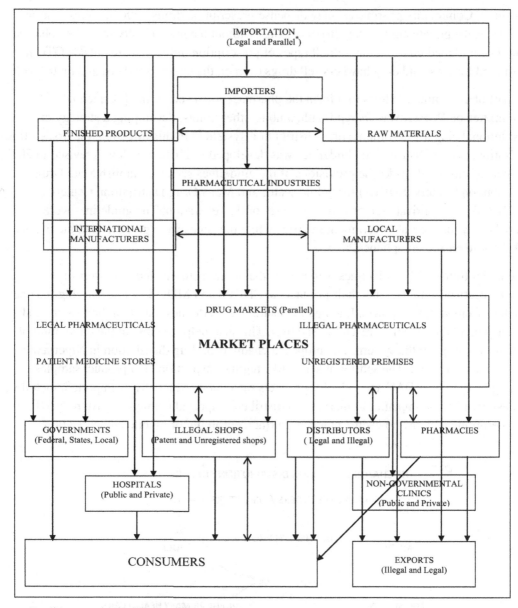

*Parallel = unregulated or illegal means and routes.

Figure 1: A schematic view of a chaotic drug distribution pattern in Nigeria.
Source: Adapted from Abdulrazaq.[38]

Sources of medicines to patients in Nigeria include private community pharmacies, public hospital pharmacies, private health clinics, licensed proprietary medicine vendors (PPMVs), and nonlicensed medicine sellers (Figure 1). The weaknesses in the drug distribution system and the pharmaceutical sectors have rendered it easy for several unethical and dangerous practices. Community pharmacies may dispense prescription drugs without a prescription. Similarly, the private clinics may dispense drugs without having a legally registered pharmacy unit, licensed medicine vendors sell all types of prescription drugs that are outside OTC list permitted by laws, and drug hawkers sell drugs even on the streets, markets, and motor parks.

As part of government efforts to reform the pharmaceutical sector, the Presidential Committee on PCPSR was charged with, among other things, developing a strategy on institutionalizing a well-ordered drug distribution system.[36] In this direction, the first edition of National Drug Distribution Guidelines was developed in 2010, which was revised in 2012. As part of this giant stride, the provisions of the guidelines seek to establish State Drug Distribution Centers (SDDCs) for public sector and Mega Drug Distribution Centers (MDDCs) for the private sector in all the states of the federation. The guidelines were launched by the federal government in 2013, while the states were given a deadline of June 30, 2014 to ensure compliance.

The major thrust of the guidelines is to ensure that manufacturers and importers of pharmaceuticals only channel their products to SDDCs and MDDCs while starving the open markets from getting supplies. It aimed to ensure that medicines maintain their safety and potency up to the time they reach the end user. This also helps to combat the circulation of counterfeit drugs in the system. The proposed channels of drug distribution in Nigeria are presented in Figure 2. The setting of standards, regular inspection, and product samples testing by both NAFDAC and PCN for products manufactured locally or imported, including licensing of local companies to market and distribute imported medicines have reduced counterfeiting and unwholesome practice. Further, enforcing of mobile authentication

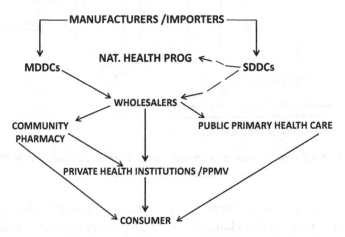

Figure 2: National Drug Distribution Guidelines' drug distribution channel.
Source: FMoH.[36]

services (MAS) code by NAFDAC in 2014 to guarantee the authenticity of antimalarial and antibiotic products through Short Mobile Service is yielding results.

2.5 Pricing and drug advertising

According to a 2004 National Medicines Price Survey in Nigeria, medicines in Nigeria cost as much as 2–64 times their international reference prices, which is a cause of great concern.[4] The study documented a wide variability in prices of the same medicines between facilities, sectors, and different types of the same product. Postulated factors that could be responsible for these exorbitant prices include a lack of stringent regulations on drug distribution and handling, lack of reliable and sustainable means for proper drug procurement in the public sector, and high and inconsistent profit margins by drug importers due to a lack of stringent national medicine pricing policies. Hence, there are certainly urgent needs to adequately address the factors responsible for the exorbitant medication prices.[4]

The findings of the price survey stimulated the government of Nigeria to revise the national drug policy in 2005. This action was applauded in 2008 WHO and Health Action International (HAI) report on the findings of over 50 surveys conducted around the globe pertaining to measuring medicine prices, availability, affordability, and price components accessibility.[39] Other efforts toward streamlining and reducing medicine prices in the country were achieved through collaborations with UN agencies and international development partners.

It is obvious that the prices of some essential medicines, especially those used in the treatment of priority diseases, are controlled to some extent due to availability of either free or subsidized drugs supported by partners. For instance, contraceptive pills are obtained for free through support by UNFPA and partners including DFID and Planned Parenthood Federation of Nigeria. Similarly, the World Bank through Malaria Booster Project and Clinton Health Access Initiative (CHAI) provides antimalarial drugs either for free or at subsidized prices. One of the strategies in the drug policy document is the establishment of Drug Revolving Fund (DRF) scheme at all levels of health care in Nigeria. In this direction, almost one decade of partnership between DFID/UKaid and three northern States of Jigawa, Kaduna, and Kano has resulted in low prices of medicines in over 1352 DRF operating health facilities—as much as between 50% and 63% less expensive than the same brands of similar medicines sold by private pharmacies.[40]

3. Current developments in pharmacy practice in Nigeria

As experts on drugs, today's pharmacists' contribution to healthcare in Nigeria is currently taking on new dimensions to support patients in their use of medicine and likewise form an integral part of clinical decision-making across various specialties. Through the emergence of pharmaceutical care and collaborative drug therapy management in Nigeria, pharmacists have started engaging in patient-centered care together with other health professionals as a team. This is stimulating a high demand for pharmacists, particularly in the hospitals, research institutions, academic institutions, and international nongovernmental organizations.[32]

Recently, the ACPN has been calling on the Federal Government to ensure effective implementation of the newly launched Nigerian National Pharmacovigilance Policy and National Drug Distribution Guidelines. To ensure strict adherence to these guidelines, there is a need for the Nigerian government to use statutory regulatory bodies empowered by law, and also make funds available for pharmacists to participate effectively in the drug distribution system from the main source down to the end user. These would ensure that all medicines/drugs in the national drug distribution system are safe, efficacious, effective, affordable, and of good quality.

Attempts have been made to develop and implement PharmD degree programs in many pharmacy schools in Nigeria, but not much success has been achieved to date. This is because of human resource constraints, limited expertise, and cost implications to establish such programs in these institutions in Nigeria. To date, a PharmD degree program is only available in two universities (University of Benin and University of Ibadan), still with implementation challenges. Despite the support of the national regulatory agency of the profession (PCN), the idea of a PharmD program in the country is still in its nascent state.

4. Achievements in pharmacy practice in Nigeria

According to our findings and experiences, we would like to highlight five major achievements on pharmacy practice and education in Nigeria during the past 20 years.

First, the conservative role of community pharmacists as healthcare professionals who primarily sell and dispense drug prescriptions written by doctors has changed considerably. Since the 1990s, community pharmacists have been offering clinical services, aside from their dispensing role, which is leading to greater integration with other healthcare teams. These clinical services offered by community pharmacists include treatment for minor ailments, health promotion, and disease prevention including screening services, vital signs measurements and monitoring, support for self-care, and medicine management support for physicians.

Second, pharmaceutical care has been recognized as a new concept and practice philosophy for the pharmacy profession in Nigeria. However, it is still not widely operational in most practice settings. Mutual understanding of the roles and coordination of healthcare among pharmacists and physicians would significantly improve patient care outcomes and should be promoted in the health care workplaces.[32] In the hospital or clinical settings, a multidisciplinary team approach to health care provision would provide ample prospects and possibilities for teamwork among health care professionals that is geared towards achieving improved health outcomes. Clinical pharmacy as a patient-centered approach relating to pharmaceutical care continues to prepare the future pharmacists to play significant roles in the health care system.

Third, from the pharmaceutical industry perspective, there is an increasing number and turnover of local manufacturers, which may result in improved availability and access to quality drugs.

Fourth, there are improvements in the regulations pertaining to manufacture, importation, wholesaling, and overall distribution of pharmaceutical products. NAFDAC and PCN have played a significant role in sanitizing the subsector.

Finally, the last two decades have seen achievements in pharmacy practice and public health through the contribution of logistics and supply chain management of health commodity to the achievement of MDGs, Vision 20:2020. Partners and UN agencies, FMoH, and SMoH have played important roles through the development and implementation of policies, regulations, guidelines, and programs that have impacted positively on pharmacy practice in general.

5. Challenges in pharmacy practice

There are challenges relating to pharmacy practice and education in Nigeria. The country's pharmaceutical sector is a complex one and various players and actors have taken advantage of its weaknesses and disorganization. It is therefore imperative to conduct more research in order to identify ways forward.

The dysfunctional medicine supply system relating to drug distribution in the country has been a major concern in ensuring safe, efficacious, and good-quality essential medicines. Transportation of drugs via roads and poor storage facilities mainly contribute to enormous losses of drug potencies before they get to the end users. Furthermore, the absence of a well-functioning drug management information system in both the public and private pharmaceutical sectors, which would effectively coordinate medicine supply management in the country, poses a great challenge to the system. Quacks or unqualified individuals and corporate bodies are engaged in the distribution and sales of drugs, thereby cementing the chaotic drug distribution system in Nigeria. Many unregistered pharmaceutical premises, patent medicine stores, and individuals, including politicians and local businessmen, are engaged in drug business under the existing poorly regulated and corrupt medicine distribution system.[32,41] These illicit activities in the pharmaceutical sector and the entire health system must be put to a halt by enacting stringent laws, policies, and regulations in the country to protect the lives of the populace.

In Nigeria, the advancement of pharmacy education and practice is faced with several challenging factors, including a low level of appropriate academic manpower, disparity within the pharmacy profession, inadequate remuneration of professionals in public service, limited faculties of pharmacy, low numbers of pharmacy technicians to assist pharmacists in dispensing functions, and enforcement of areas of specialization for pharmacists in hospital and community practice.[32,41] We cannot ignore the fact that the practice of hospital and community pharmacies in the country has suffered major impediments from numerous factors, including poor staffing, poor infrastructure, inefficient coordination of activities, failure of hospital and community pharmacists to adopt new changes, and the continuous resistance of most physicians against patient-oriented pharmaceutical services.[32]

Inadequate human resources relating to the pharmacy profession is a major challenge in the country. There is scarce distribution of pharmacists and registered pharmaceutical premises in comparison with Nigeria's population and vast land mass. Available data for 2008 indicated that the number of registered pharmacists per 100,000 population varies from less than 1–40 in different states of the country.[32] Furthermore, most pharmacists and pharmaceutical premises are concentrated within cities, and they are virtually absent in rural areas and smaller hospitals/clinics. Expanding the pharmacists' labor force to effectively match the country's healthcare system and expected demand is urgently needed, but may also be a long way to come.

6. Basic statistics of some essential pharmacy infrastructure in Nigeria

In this section, we attempt to provide some basic statistics about the rank and quality of pharmacy infrastructure in Nigeria in relation to education, practice, and manufacturing. There is no official ranking of top pharmaceutical companies having a share in the market, top pharmaceutical manufacturers (indigenous, foreign, or multinational), and top colleges of pharmacy. However, we provide some basic information and statistics that may serve as a guide in assessing quality. We believe accreditation of academic institutions by credible accreditation agencies is a measure of quality. Similarly, further certification of pharmaceutical companies by WHO apart from by NAFDAC is an index and advanced seal of quality assurance that also gives the manufacturers opportunities to participate in international biddings. Below is a list of accredited pharmacy schools and WHO-certified pharmaceutical manufacturers in Nigeria (Tables 4 and 5).

7. Recommendations: ways forward

To promote mutual understanding between pharmacists and other health care professionals, there is a need to promote interprofessional education and collaborative care through joint training, seminars, fora, and clinical meetings at various levels, which aim at harnessing the mutual integration and respect of health professionals into the healthcare processes to benefit patients and the health system. Through this window of opportunity, the PharmD program and the pharmaceutical care practice in Nigeria can be fully integrated into the healthcare system, and patients would have the most benefits relating to desired health outcomes. Again, matters related to overprescription, adverse drug reactions, and pharmacovigilance can be traced, and

Table 4: List of accredited faculties of pharmacy/pharmaceutical sciences in Nigeria

Institution	Type	Year
Obafemi Awolowo University	Public	1963
Ahmadu Bello University, Zaria	Public	1968
University of Nigeria, Nsukka	Public	1968
University of Benin	Public	1970
University of Lagos	Public	1980
University of Ibadan	Public	1980
University of Jos	Public	1986
University of Uyo	Public	1998
Olabisi Onabanjo University	Public	2000
Niger Delta University	Public	2009
University of Maiduguri	Public	2010
Nnamdi Azikwe University	Public	2011
Usmanu Danfodiyo University	Public	No evidence
Kaduna State University	Public	No evidence
University of Port Harcourt	Public	No evidence
Delta State University	Public	No evidence
Madonna University	Private	2009
Igbinedion University	Private	2011

Source: Olurinola[41] and Mora.[42]

Table 5: An overview of pharmaceutical companies in Nigeria

List of WHO Certified Pharmaceutical Manufacturers in Nigeria	
Company	**Type**
Swiss Pharma (Swipha) Nigeria Ltd	Indigenous
Evans Medical Plc	Indigenous
May & Baker Nigeria Plc	Indigenous
Chi Pharmaceuticals Ltd	Indigenous
Source: May & Baker[43] and Obi.[34]	
List of Pharmaceutical Companies in the Stock Exchange Market in Nigeria	
Institution	**Type**
May & Baker Nigeria Plc	Indigenous
Fidson Healthcare Plc	Indigenous
Evans Medical Plc	Indigenous
Glaxo Smithkline Consumer Nig. Plc	-
Neimeth International Pharmaceuticals Plc	–
Source: The Nigerian Stock Exchange.[44]	
List of Some Renowned Pharmaceutical Companies in Nigeria[a]	
Company	**Type**
GlaxoSmithKline (GSK)	Multinational
Novartis	Multinational
Pfizer	Multinational
Roche	Multinational
Sanofi	Multinational

[a]This list is by no means a ranking of the companies and it is neither exhaustive nor complete.

future interventions can be developed. There is a need for more studies to identify the factors that affect dissemination and use of treatment guidelines in the country.

Apart from focusing on mainly clinical services, the potential for pharmacists to be involved in public health intervention programs in Nigeria geared toward effecting dramatic improvements in people's health remains largely untapped. With an advent of rising noncommunicable diseases in developing countries such as Nigeria, pharmacists can lower costs of medicines and improve health by helping patients to manage chronic conditions including cancer, hypertension, and diabetes. Therefore, "public health pharmacy" is another potential area to prepare pharmacists for public health roles.

The findings call for strategies to intensify drug regulatory activities and be proactive to current global trends in pharmacy education and practice to meet future societal challenges and demands in the country. We suggest for appropriate channels to ensure the regular availability of safe, affordable, efficacious, and good-quality essential medicines in both the public and private sectors of the healthcare system in Nigeria. To tackle the problems of poor governance and administrative failures related to medicine supply management in Nigeria, there is a need for major reforms through the use of public–private partnerships under the supervision of an independent regulatory agency in the pharmaceutical sector to assure the effectiveness, efficiency, and compliance of standards in the system.

Improved access to essential medicines, especially to the most vulnerable people and the underprivileged, is recognized as one of the main identities of the performance of healthcare delivery system of any country, including Nigeria. However, fully implementing the current National Drug Policy, which provides policy direction to the country, is inadequate to ensure efficient attainment of the desired core objectives relating to improvement and functionality of the pharmaceutical sector. A clarion call to appraise this implementation of the National Drug Policy and review the current condition is necessary in an attempt to improve accessibility, availability, affordability, and utilization of essential medicines in the country.

8. Conclusions

Despite considerable progress in pharmacy education and practice over the last two decades, implementation of stringent regulations, chaotic drug distribution system, professional complacency and conservatism, extrinsic system failure, and inadequate human resource for health remain challenging problems in Nigeria's pharmaceutical sector and the entire healthcare system. Holistic and coherent pharmaceutical sector and system management has not been effectively addressed and efficiently utilized in Nigeria, resulting in huge unmet needs in the health system.

In the future, progressivity in developmental growth in Nigeria could augment rapid extension of pharmacy education and practice related to the increasing number of pharmacy graduates and pharmacists, development and use of information and technology system, expansion of clinical and nonclinical services offered by pharmacists, and engagement in applied and field research activities. The pharmaceutical sector and entire healthcare system, of which pharmacy practice and education is a part, would certainly benefit by providing a greater safeguard through active regulations, including the fight against counterfeit and substandard drugs and institutionalizing a more effective regulatory system in Nigeria.

9. Lessons learned

In recent years, pharmacy practice and education in Nigeria have changed considerably, with achievements and challenges that demand attention.

Another important lesson derived from this chapter is that there is a huge gap in the area of applied and field research, and policy and implementation research activities on pharmacy practice, which remain untouched by academic pharmacists and pharmacy practitioners in Nigeria. Evidence-based information for policymaking and implementation might assist in advancing the pharmacy profession and practice in the country.

In Nigeria, despite the presence of pharmaceutical regulatory and inspection agencies at federal and state levels, the drug distribution system has remained uncoordinated in the last three decades. This situation has posed a great challenge to both the pharmaceutical sector and the entire health system with substandard, adulterated, and fake drugs in circulation, which is detrimental to the consumers and not in the interest of the healthcare delivery system.

Opportunities exist in the manufacturing subsector for sourcing raw materials locally and enhancing the production capacity of the local manufacturers toward meeting the demand of increasing Nigerian population and beyond, which at present is far below average. This subsector is part of the nation's industrial revolution drive under the Vision 20:2020.

Relating to pharmacy education in Nigeria, the PharmD degree program is still at its infantile stage of development in universities. Again, pharmaceutical care has only recently been recognized as a practice philosophy for the pharmacy profession in Nigeria, but it is still not widely operational in most practice settings.

References

1. Alo A. Pharmacy in Nigeria. *Am J Health-Syst Pharm* 2006;**63**:670–3.
2. Asuzu MC. The necessity for a health system reform in Nigeria. *J Community Med Prim Health Care* 2004;**16**(1):1–3.
3. Africa Health Workforce Observatory (AHWO). *Human resources for health country profile: Nigeria.* [cited March 28, 2014]. Geneva: Global Health Workforce Alliance and World Health Organization. Available from: http://www.unfpa.org/sowmy/resources/docs/library/R050_AHWO_2008_Nigeria_HRHProfile.pdf.
4. Federal Ministry of Health in collaboration WHO, EU & HAI. *Medicine prices in Nigeria – prices people pay for drugs.* Abuja: Federal Ministry of Health; 2006.

5. Backman G, Hunt P, Khosla R, Jaramillo-Strouss C, Fikre BM, Rumble C, et al. Health systems and the right to health: an assessment of 194 countries. *Lancet* 2008;**372**:2047–85.

6. Federal Government of Nigeria. *Annual abstract of statistics*. Abuja (Nigeria): National Bureau of Statistics; 2009.

7. United Nations - Nigeria: United Nations statistics division. [cited October 11, 2012]. Available from: http://data.un.org/CountryProfile.aspx?crName=NIGERIA; 2010.

8. World Health Organization. *World health statistics: country health system fact sheet*. Geneva (Switzerland); 2012.

9. World Bank - Nigeria: World development indicators. Washington, DC. [cited November 11, 2012]. Available from: http://databank.worldbank.org/ddp/html-jsp/QuickViewReport.jsp?RowAxis=WDI; 2011.

10. Mora AT. *The lizard shape: model in drug distribution in Nigeria*. Zaria: Woodpecker Communication Services; 2014.

11. Pharmacists Council of Nigeria. *The 4-part compendium of minimum standards for the assurance of pharmaceutical care in Nigeria*; 2009.

12. Federal Ministry of Health. *Health sector reform document: final version*. Abuja (Nigeria); 2005.

13. National Health Insurance Scheme - Nigeria. *National health insurance scheme annual report*; 2006.

14. Okonkwo A. Abuja Nigeria set to launch health insurance scheme. *Lancet* 2001;**358**(9276):131.

15. McIntyre D. *Learning from experience: health care financing in low and middle income countries*. Geneva: Global forum for health research; 2007.

16. Federal Ministry of Health. *National strategic health development plan (NSHDP) 2010–2015*. Abuja (Nigeria). [cited March 7, 2012]. Available from: http://www.health.gov.ng/doc/NSHDP.pdf.

17. Federal Ministry of Health Nigeria in collaboration with World Health Organization. *National drug policy*. First Revision. Abuja: Federal Ministry of Health; 2005.

18. World Health Organization. *National health accounts*. Geneva (Switzerland): World Health Organization; 2006.

19. Soyibo A, Lawanson O, Olaniyan L. *National health accounts of Nigeria, 1998–2002*. Final report submitted to World Health Organization, Geneva (Switzerland); 2005.

20. Soyibo A, Olaniyan O, Lawanson AO. *National health accounts of Nigeria, 2003–2005: incorporating sub-national health accounts of states*. Main report submitted to Federal Ministry of Health; 2009.

21. Federal Government of Nigeria. *Annual health report 2011*; 2011.

22. Lagomarsino G, Garabrant A, Adyas A, Muga R, Otoo N. Moving towards universal health coverage: health insurance reforms in nine developing countries in Africa and Asia. *Lancet* 2012;**380**(9845):933–43.

23. National Health Insurance Scheme. *Strategic plan of operations 2008–2010*. Abuja (Nigeria): NHIS; 2008.

24. National Health Insurance Scheme. *National health insurance scheme official report*. Abuja (Nigeria): NHIS; 2008.

25. Awosika L. Health insurance and managed care in Nigeria. *Ann Ib Postgrad Med* 2007;**3**(2):40–51.

26. Joint Learning Network. *Nigeria: national health insurance system*. [cited March 07, 2012]. Available from: http://www.jointlearningnetwork.org/content/nigeria.

27. National Population Commission. *Nigeria demographic and health survey, 2013*. Abuja (Nigeria): National Population Commission; 2013.

28. Africa Health Workforce Observatory. Human resources for health country profile: Nigeria: (Geneva: Global Health Workforce Alliance and World Health Organization). [cited December 26, 2014]. Available from: http://www.unfpa.org/sowmy/resources/docs/library/R050_AHWO_2008_Nigeria _HRHProfile.pdf; 2008.

29. National Population Commission. *Nigeria demographic and health survey 2008 (2008 NDHS)*; 2009.

30. Pharmacists Council of Nigeria. *List of accredited faculties of pharmacy in Nigeria universities*. [cited March 28, 2014]. Available from: http://pcn.gov.ng/Universities%20Accredited%20for%20Pharmacy%20Programme%20in%20Nigeria.htm.

31. Pharmacists Council of Nigeria. *Mandatory continuing pharmacists development program*. [cited March 28, 2014]. Available from: http://pcn.gov.ng/MCPD%20Programme.htm.

32. Erah P. The PharmD program: prospects and challenges in Nigeria. *Niger J Pharm Res* 2011;**9**(1).

33. Federal Ministry of Health - Nigeria. *National drug policy*; 2005.

34. Obi P. *WHO approves more Nigerian pharmaceutical companies* [database on the Internet]. This Day Live [cited December 26, 2014]. Available from: http://www.thisdaylive.com/articles/who-approves-more-nigerian-pharmaceutical-companies/191442/#.VR025SDc794.mailto.

35. Mohammed S, Magaji M, Lawal G, Masoud M. Medicine supply management in Nigeria: a case study of ministry of health, Kaduna state. *Niger J Pharm Sci* 2008;**6**(2):114.

36. Federal Ministry of Health. *National Drug Distribution guidelines*. 2nd ed; 2012.

37. *Counterfeit drugs kill. IMPACT brochure* [database on the Internet]. World Health Organization. [cited December 26, 2014]. Available from: http://www.who.int/impact/en; 2008.

38. Abdulrazaq A. *Pharmacy Jurisprudence II. Lecture note 400 level students*. Zaria (Nigeria): Ahmadu Bello University; 2013.

39. World Health Organization/Health Action International. *Measuring drugs prices, affordability and price components*. WHO/PSM/PAR/2008.3. 2nd ed. Switzerland: World Health Organization/Health Action International; 2008.

40. Partnership for Transforming Health Systems Phase II. *Innovation service delivery solutions for improved survival of women and children in Northern Nigeria*; 2015.

41. Olurinola PF. *The pharmacy profession: a focus on Nigeria*. Zaria: Onis Excel Publishing; 2003.

42. Mora AT. *The contributions of students and alumni associations: towards promoting pharmacy education and practice in Nigeria*. Zaria: Woodpecker Communication Services; 2014.

43. May & Baker. *WHO certifies May & Baker Nigeria Plc on cGMP* [database on the Internet]. May-Baker.com. [cited December 26, 2014]. Available from: http://www.may-baker.com/images/helix/slide/WHO_Certifies_MAY.pdf; 2014.

44. The Nigerian Stock Exchange. *Market data: company listing* [database on the Internet]. nse.com.ng. [cited April 04, 2015]. Available from: www.nse.com.ng/Pages/index.aspx; 2015.

Appendix

List of Some Abbreviations and Acronyms

ACPN	Association of Community Pharmacists of Nigeria
AIPN	Association of Industrial Pharmacists of Nigeria
ALPS	Association of Lady Pharmacists
B.Pharm	Bachelor of Pharmacy
CBOs	Community-based Organizations
CP	Community Pharmacist
DFID	Department for International Development
FMoH	Federal Ministry of Health
HCPs	Health Care Providers
HMOs	Health Management Organizations
HSRP	Health Sector Reform Program
ICT	Information Communication Technology
LGA	Local Government Area
LMICs	Low–Middle Income Countries
MDGs	Millennium Development Goals
NAFDAC	National Agency for Food and Drug Administration and Control
NAGPP	National Association of General Practice Pharmacists
NAHAP	National Association of Hospital and Administrative Pharmacists
NAPA	National Association of Pharmacists in Academia
₦	Nigerian Naira (the local currency in Nigeria)
NEEDS	National Economic Empowerment Development Strategy
NHIS	National Health Insurance Scheme
NIPRD	National Institute for Pharmaceutical Research and Development

OOP	Out-of-Pocket
OTC	Over the Counter
PANS	Pharmaceutical Association of Nigerian Students
PCN	Pharmacists Council of Nigeria
PCPSR	Presidential Committee on Pharmaceutical Sector Reform
PSN	Pharmaceutical Society of Nigeria
UKaid	United Kingdom Agency for International Development
UNFPA	United Nations Population Fund Agency
USAID	United States Agency for International Development
US$	United States Dollar
WHO	World Health Organization

CHAPTER 18

Pharmacy Practice in Burkina Faso

Sybil Nana Ama Ossei-Agyeman-Yeboah

Chapter Outline

Pharmacy Practice in Developing Countries. http://dx.doi.org/10.1016/B978-0-12-801714-2.00018-6
371

1. Country background

Located in the heart of West Africa, Burkina Faso covers an area of 274,000 km². Its population was estimated at 15,730,977 inhabitants in 2011. According to the general census of population and housing (GCPH) of 2006, the population is characterized by its youth (46% of residents are under 15 years), its high growth rate (3.1%), and the predominance of women (51.7% of the population), which results in a relative strength of 93 men for every 100 women. The country is divided into 13 administrative regions, 45 provinces, and 351 municipalities.

Burkina Faso is ranked among the heavily indebted poor countries. The socioeconomic characteristics of the country in 2013 are presented as a gross domestic product (GDP) per capita equal to 225,259 FCFA, rate of real GDP growth 8.0%, Human Development Index 0.334, total population living below the poverty line 43.9%, incidence of poverty in urban areas 19.9%, and incidence of poverty in rural areas 50.7% (Source Statistical Yearbook 2013).

The literacy level of the population remains low in Burkina Faso. According to the 2006 GCPH, it appears that among persons aged 10 years and older, only 26% are able to read and write in the national or foreign language Table 1. In 2010, the gross enrollment rate was 74.8% at the primary and 29.7% at the secondary school level (Table 1).

Table 1: Other indicators from the 2006 GCPH (Institut national de statistique et de la démographie, Burkina Faso, 2006)[1]

Annual Growth Rate (%)	Crude Birth Rate (per 1000)	Overall General Fertility Rate Corrected (per 1000)	Total Fertility Rate	Crude Mortality Rate (per 1000)	Life Expectancy at Birth (Years)	Quotient of Child Mortality (per 1000)
3.1	45.8	202.2	6.2	11.8	56.7	141.9

2. Vital health statistics

Health information is a tool that informs and directs governments, decision-makers, and managers of programs to support the structures in the health system technically and financially so as to achieve the best outcome. The utilization of correct and evidence-based results aids in best decision-making, the development of strategic frameworks, and the creation of value logic models that are fair and easily understood by all stakeholders. This is what the information from the various tiers of the health sector and system in Burkina Faso seems to provide (Table 2)[14].

2.1 Statistics on morbidity and mortality

The key statistical indicators are morbidity rate, which in 2007 was 8.4%; mortality rate, 11.8% in 2006; and maternal mortality rate, between 566 and 307 deaths per 100,000 live births in 2006. This rate is still far from the 142 deaths referred to in 2015 as part of the Millennium Development Goals (MDGs). The neonatal mortality rate is 31% and the infant mortality rate is 81%. More than half of infant deaths occur during the neonatal period. Most indicators of service delivery have increased since 2005[7,21].

3. Overview of health care system

It is the responsibility of any government to invest in the health care system and ensure that funds and resources such as personnel, equipment, clinical materials, medicines, and other medical products are available to deliver the appropriate services and product acquisition. A major reorganization of how local health and care teams work together and new initiatives, such as offering new support and career advice, are equally essential, covering existing staff, overhead, and other costs currently funded in the country by the National Health System. Better care could lead to fewer people "falling through the cracks" of services. Identifying the gaps and addressing them to ensure effective health care delivery is what is expected of all low- and middle-income countries to strive to achieve.

Table 2: Performance indicators highlighted by data from the Health Statistical Yearbook 2013 (Annuairestatistiques 2013)

Indicator	Level in 2013
Rate of births attended by skilled personnel	80.5
Couple years of protection (CYP) (%)	17.4
Number of new contacts per capita per year for children under 5 years	1.7
Cesarean section rate among births expected (%)	2.1
Prevalence of underweight children under 5 years (%)	21.0
Lethality of malaria in pregnant women (%)	0.6
Lethality of severe malaria in children less than 5 months (%)	2.4
Immunization coverage	99
Proportion (%) of people living with AIDS, justifiable antiretroviral (ARV) treatment, and on ARV treatment	87.1
Intrahospital mortality (CHU/CHR, CMA) per 1000	68.4

The Ministry of Health in Burkina Faso has three levels of administrative structure; the central level consists of central and related structures organized around the office of the Minister and the General Secretariat, the intermediate level includes 13 regional health directorates, and the peripheral level consists of health districts that are operational entities, a most decentralized national health system. In 2013, 63 of 70 health districts were operational.

Public health care facilities are organized within these three hierarchies to provide primary, secondary, and tertiary care. The first hierarchy corresponds to the health district, which comprises two levels. The first level of care is the health and social promotion centers (HSPCs), which numbered 1606 in 2013. The second level of care is the medical center with surgical antenna (MCA). This is the health facility reference center in the district. In 2013 there were 45 functional MCAs and 11 regional hospitals, which served as references to the MCAs. The third level consists of three teaching hospitals; these are the highest level of reference.

In addition to the health facilities of the Ministry of Health, there are other public health structures such as military health services and the health services of the National Social Security Fund pertaining respectively to the Ministry of Defense and Ministry of Social Security.

In addition to public structures, Burkina Faso has private clinics concentrated in the cities of Ouagadougou and Bobo-Dioulasso. In 2013, there existed 398 private care structures.

In 2013, the theoretical average radius of distance between the health care facilities (including private) was 6.5 km, with a ratio of one HSPC per 9759 capita. The number of private pharmacies and drugstores was 693 in 2013.

3.1 Human resources

The human resource capacity is vital in the development and sustainability of any enterprise. The human resource quality and quantity determine the strength, competence, and capability of the institution to deliver its mandate, mission, and vision and thus provide the reasons the organization, leadership, and employees perform their roles and responsibilities to promote integrity, accountability, compliance, and innovation. I would quote from Agnes Soucat, the AfDB's Director for Human Development, from her book, "The Labor Market for Health Workers in Africa: A New Look at the Crisis." She said "The global community needs to change its traditional approach to health workforce in a fundamental way. It is critical to adopt a comprehensive labor market approach to understand the market forces influencing both the supply and demand of health workforce. This is particularly important to Africa with high disease burden and low density of health workforce" (http://elibrary.worldbank.org/doi/book/10.1596/978-0-8213-9555-4)[17].

Would not this statement apply to the health workforce in Burkina Faso as well? The answer is YES.

As of 2013, the situational status of health personnel in the public health facilities was 787 physicians, 33 dentists, 207 pharmacists, and 8427 nurses. Training of health professionals was ensured at the national level by the University of Ouagadougou for pharmacists and physicians and the National School of Public Health for nurses. On average, 25 pharmacists are trained annually at the University of Ouagadougou.

A human resources development plan was developed in 2010. This plan aims to improve the performance of the health system by making available to the sector skilled human resources, motivated and in sufficient number[3].

4. Medicine supply system and medicines use issues

The medicine supply system has been carefully aligned to handle the challenges facing the Economic Community of West Africa States (ECOWAS), taking into consideration the disease burden and cross-border issues and the high incidence of priority diseases such as HIV/AIDS, malaria, tuberculosis, infectious diseases, neglected tropical diseases, and noncommunicable and communicable diseases. Other challenges include the fight against counterfeit and illicit trade in medicines, the utilization of the World Trade Organization (WTO) Agreement on Trade-Related Aspects of Intellectual Property Rights (TRIPS) flexibilities provisions on pharmaceutical products, pharmacovigilance, medicine regulation and quality control of medicines, and the strengthening of the pharmaceutical production of medicines. West Africa is highly dependent on imported pharmaceuticals and medical products, ranging from 70 to 98% across the region, and locally produced medicines, ranging from 0 to 30%.

In general, there exists a pharmaceutical distribution system across the ECOWAS region. In the private sector, the distribution system is largely poorly organized and disjointed. There are several unauthorized intermediaries involved in pharmaceutical distribution. This poses a great challenge in conducting audit trails of imported or locally manufactured products from the point of supply to the ultimate consumer. The environmental and climatic conditions under which pharmaceutical products are stored negatively influences product availability, security, the final price, and in turn accessibility. Across the region, the distribution of medicines is based in the public sector as the Central Medical Stores and the Essential Medicines Procurement Agency (Céntralé d'Achat des Médicaments Essentiéls et Génériqués; CAMEG); however, distribution is much better organized and managed through the national procurement agencies. Global initiatives support these national procurement agencies to ensure access to essential medicines such as antiretrovirals (ARVs), artesunate combination therapies (ACTs), and anti-tuberculosis medicines (retrieved from the ECOWAS Regional Pharmaceutical Plan[16]).

The case of human immunodeficiency virus (HIV) is a clear example: Africa is the home of nearly 70% of the 34 million people living with HIV globally, and yet it imports more than 80% of its antiretroviral drugs. The HIV/AIDS response acts as a pathfinder to catalyze progress in Africa across health care and can be leveraged to support Africa to enhance pharmaceutical security for tuberculosis (TB), malaria, and other health challenges (retrieved from the Joint United Nations Program on HIV/AIDS (2012))[22]. Today, there is a real opportunity for West Africa to develop its pharmaceuticals sector, both to enhance medicine supply security and to advance industrial development. Interventions made by way of policy and guidelines development, building capacities, support for ECOWAS member states in the provision of stock security of ARV therapies to treat people living with HIV/AIDS, and establishment of pharmacovigilance centers and centers of excellence of quality control laboratories. Equal support has been given to some pharmaceutical manufacturing companies in the region by means of enhancing their facilities to increase the production of essential medicines, which is one of the key objectives of the West Africa Health Organization (WAHO) to strategically intervene for easier and early access to essential medicines (retrieved from the ECOWAS Regional Pharmaceutical Plan[16]).

Health systems rely on the continuous availability of safe, affordable pharmaceuticals of assured quality. Results from surveys done between 2001 and 2007 by the United Nations (2008) indicate that the availability of essential medicines in developing countries averages at 35% in the public sector and 63% in the private sector. The World Health Organization (WHO) (2004) estimates that almost 2 billion people lack regular access to essential medicines, and addressing this gap could save up to 10 million lives every year. Poor access and irrational use of pharmaceuticals influence the performance of health systems and ultimately affect health outcomes.

On the supply side, however, ECOWAS countries have very little production capacity, and hence almost all of the region's medicines are imported from India, China, and other countries. There is concern in some quarters that the low margins in antiretroviral and other essential medicines manufacturing for Africa may cause Indian manufacturers to shift their capacity away from African medicine volumes toward higher-margin products and markets, creating a real urgency for the region to develop its own supply system. It has, indeed, created an awakening in the region to boost its production of medicines to meet demands and save the life of the population (retrieved from the ECOWAS Regional Pharmaceutical Plan[16]).

Burkina Faso, like most West African member states, finds itself in this dilemma and has to strategically find ways to improve the supply chain systems managed by both the public and the private sectors.

4.1 Medicine supply and distribution

According to the provisions of Arreté No. 2001-0250/MS/CAB of 21/11/2001, regulating the distribution of products in the pharmaceutical sector, the distribution of products under a pharmaceutical monopoly for fee or for free is the exclusive responsibility of the pharmaceutical distribution or wholesale structures and pharmacies and drugstores duly authorized by the Ministry of Health.

Purchasing (and import), storage, and wholesale distribution of medicines are handled by wholesale distributors, which are the only structures authorized by the code of public health. Currently, seven wholesale distributors are authorized in Burkina Faso.

Burkina Faso has a public and private procurement and distribution system for pharmaceuticals with clear links between the two systems.

The Ministry of Health of Burkina Faso has established a system for the supply of essential medicines in the public sector, which is based on CAMEG and its 10 regional sales offices and district distribution warehouses (DDWs) with a system of cost recovery of pharmaceuticals.

CAMEG ensures imports and supply to DDWs, which in turn supply the essential medicines stores of health facilities. The supply of specific projects and programs of the Ministry of Health and hospitals is also realized via CAMEG. Vaccine supply is provided by the Directorate of Prevention through Vaccination in collaboration with UNICEF and CAMEG.

The private supply system works through private wholesalers that supply pharmacies and private medical stores, and the importation of narcotics is exclusively reserved for the Ministry of Health, which is empowered to give them in return for payment or free to hospitals.

A map of medicine and other health product supply and distribution systems in Burkina Faso is presented in the diagram in Figure 1.

4.2 Medicines in the market and medicine use issues

The business hours of pharmacies are fixed and regulated by the National Order of Pharmacists.

The opening hours of pharmacies are fixed and regulated by the National Order of Pharmacists. Besides the mandated period of operation, pharmacies provide 24 hours per week services. The opening hours of pharmacies in Burkina Faso are between 8:00am to 12:30pm and 15:30pm to 20:00pm from Monday to Friday; and on Saturday from 8:00am to 12:00pm.

Medicines available on the market are categorized into groups defined by the Public Health Code (Articles 209–212). These categories are proprietary medicines (pharmaceutical specialties), generic medicines (generic in brand name and generic in international nonproprietary name), magisterial preparations, officinal preparations, homeopathic medicines, and drugs from traditional medicines.

According to the Public Health Code, the issuance to the public following the regimen of poisonous substances (List I, List II, and list of narcotics) medicines are conditional upon presentation of a prescription issued by an authorized prescriber.

According to the terms of the Public Health Code, any renewal of specialties containing active substances included in List I (such as amoxicillin) is prohibited unless expressly stated

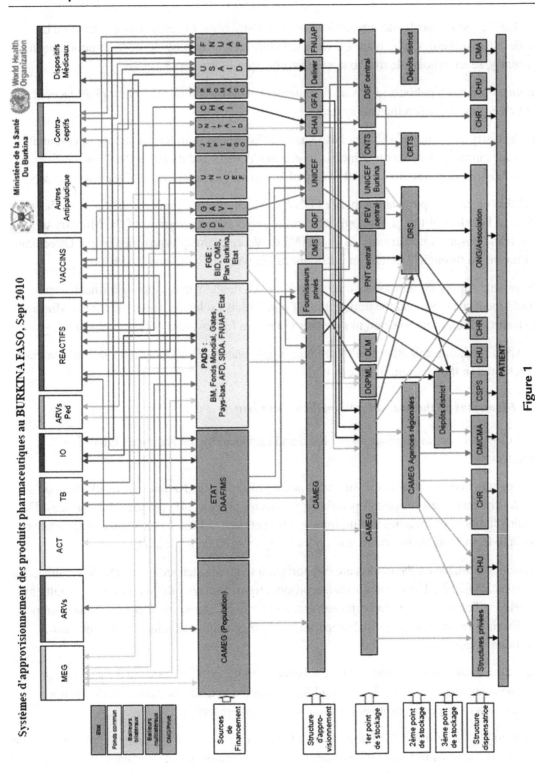

Figure 1

Map of medicine supply and distribution systems in Burkina Faso.[2]

otherwise by the prescriber. However, even in this case, the term of prescription shall not exceed 12 months, except for medicines for the treatment of chronic diseases. For specialties containing active substances included in List II, unless otherwise stated by the prescriber "Do not renew," the patient may obtain upon request a reissue[15]. However, the limitation period obeys the rule of a maximum of 12 months.

Other than medicines, items sold in pharmacies include medical products such as sterile or nonsterile medical devices, medical devices for in vitro diagnostics, cosmetics, special food commodities, and optical products.

Medicine distribution in Burkina Faso is provided by a chain of pharmaceutical facilities. Section 183 of the Public Health Code states: "It is forbidden for any person, even a pharmacist provided with a Diploma of Pharmacy, to display or distribute any form of medicine on the public highway, in the fairs, or in the markets."

Order No. 2001-0250/MS/CAB of 21/11/2001 relating to the distribution of health products under the monopoly of pharmacists states: "distribution and wholesale delivery of medicinal products whether paid or free is solely under the exclusive competence of pharmaceutical companies, the pharmacies and drugstores duly authorized by the Minister of Health."

In Burkina Faso,[11] there is no insurance system for medicines. Only private insurance exists (private companies, associations, and mutual). Patients purchase their own medicines by direct payment. The patients finance more than 37% of the total procurement budget for medicines and other health products. However, medicines for priority diseases are subsidized, such as ACTs, medicines of obstetric and neonatal emergency, and kits for sexually transmitted infections. Other medicines are issued free, such as medical products to manage epidemics, vaccines of the Expanded Program on Immunization, TB vaccines, and ARVs. Tables 3 and 4 list the 20 most important drugs in terms of spending and use.

These 20 best-selling medicines represent 40.21% of total sales in financial value. Five treatment groups comprise the 20 best sellers in terms of financial volume; they are antibiotics, antimalarials, antipyretics, antispasmodics, and intravenous solutions (Figures 2 and 3).

The five therapeutic groups of the 20 top-selling medicines in term of quantity are nonsteroidal anti-inflammatories, antibiotics, antiparasitics including antimalarials, antihistamines, and vitamins.

5. Overview of pharmacy practice and key pharmaceutical sectors

ECOWAS has set its goal to have a harmonized and functioning pharmaceutical sector within its member states in accordance with nationally and internationally recognized policies and standards. Such initiatives incorporate all critical areas and the various relevant institutions to make their contribution to improving public health in the regions for which they are

Table 3: The 20 most important drugs in terms of spending in 2013 (Ministère de la santé, Décembre 2013)

No.	Designation	Form	National sales (FCFA)
1	Amoxicillin 500 mg gel, blister	Capsule	731 948 978.13
2	Quinine sulfate 300 mg cp, blister	Tablet	624 327 706.16
3	Paracetamol 500 mg cp, blister	Tablet	364 252 030.97
4	Cotrimoxazole 240 mg/5 ml, 60 ml syrup	Syrup	359 156 443.17
5	Artesunate + amodiaquine (270 + 100) mg cp FDC adult	Tablet	341 917 712.3
6	Isotonic glucose solution 5%, 500 ml injectable	Injectable	321 433 991.22
7	Cotrimoxazole 480 mg cp, blister	Tablet	293 261 072.05
8	Artesunate 25 mg + amodiaquine 50 mg/5 ml, 60 ml susp. buv.	Syrup	252 837 665.68
9	Quinine resorcin 400 mg/4 ml, 4 ml injectable	Injectable	241 148 633.3
10	Phloroglucinol 80 mg cp, blister	Tablet	233 410 329.5
11	Paracetamol 120 mg/5 ml, 100 ml syrup	Syrup	233 314 301.97
12	Amoxicillin 250 mg/5 ml, 60 ml syrup	Syrup	218 364 360.64
13	Erythromycin 500 mg cp, blister	Tablet	196 017 004.8
14	Ibuprofen 400 mg cp, blister	Tablet	175 807 437.21
15	Ampicillin 1 g injectable	Injectable	175 418 500.37
16	Butylscopolamine 10 mg cp, blister	Tablet	150 766 751.2
17	Acetyl salicylate of lysine 900 mg injectable	Injectable	141 254 385.16
18	Artesunate + amodiaquine, adolescent	Tablet	139 856 574.7
19	Ceftriaxone 1 g injectable	Injectable	126 978 397
20	Isotonic glucose solution 5%, 250 ml injectable	Injectable	114 957 216
	Total value of 20 best-selling drugs		**5 436 429 491.63**

Table 4: The 20 most important medicines in terms of use (Profil pharmaceutique du Burkina Faso, Organisation Mondiale de la Santé, 2012)[11]

No.	Designation	Form	National Quantity (Unit)
1	Paracetamol 500 mg cp, blister	Tablet	105 063 217
2	Cotrimoxazole 480 mg cp, blister	Tablet	38 888 804
3	Amoxicillin 500 mg gel, blister	Capsule	28 827 394
4	Ibuprofen 400 mg cp, blister	Capsule	24 930 596
5	Chlorpheniramine maleate 4 mg cp, blister	Tablet	21 682 092
6	Diclofenac 50 mg cp, blister	Tablet	19 538 721
7	Quinine sulfate 300 mg cp, blister	Tablet	17 182 991
8	Metronidazole 250 mg cp, blister	Tablet	15 081 847
9	Acetylsalicylic acid and ferric + folic acid (200 + 0.4) mg, blister	Tablet	10 912 029
10	Aluminum hydroxide 500 mg cp, blister	Tablet	9 490 047
11	Phenobarbital 100 mg	Tablet	8 266 425
12	Butyl scopolamine 10 mg cp, blister	Tablet	8 148 133
13	Ciprofloxacin 500 mg cp, blister	Tablet	7 357 215
14	Multivitamin 10 mg cp, blister	Tablet	5 430 913
15	Erythromycin 500 mg cp, blister	Tablet	4 777 862
16	Acetylsalicylic acid 500 mg cp, blister	Tablet	4 552 645
17	Penicillin V 250 mg	Tablet	3 973 141
18	Phloroglucinol 80 mg cp, blister	Tablet	3 662 632
19	Furosemide 200 mg	Tablet	3 182 137
20	Mebendazole 100 mg cp, blister	Tablet	3 000 014

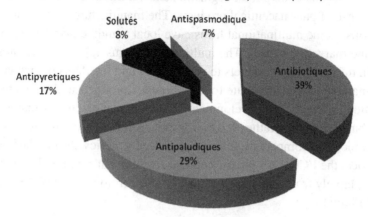

Répartition des 20 médicaments les plus vendus en valeur
financiere en fonction des groupes thérapeutiques

Figure 2
Distribution of 20 best-selling medicines in financial value according to the treatment group
(Ministère de la santé, Décembre 2013).

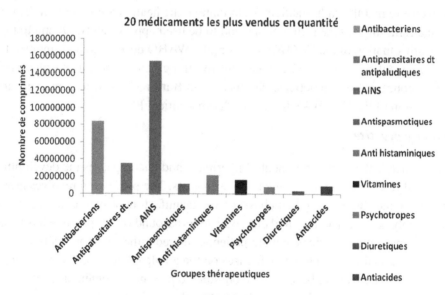

Figure 3
The 20 most important medicines in terms of use according to the treatment group (Ministère de la
santé, Décembre 2013).

responsible and will contribute to West Africa truly becoming self-sufficient in the provision of health care.

The pharmaceutical sector and system comprises the pharmacists and pharmacy technicians within the Ministry of Health (MOH), hospitals and clinics, training and academic institutions, manufacturers, distributors, wholesalers, retail pharmacies, procurement units, medicines regulatory authorities, and quality control laboratories as well as the policies, guidelines, and legislative frameworks that underpin the regulation and control of the manufacture, distribution, sale, and rational use of pharmaceutical products. The manufacturers are either local or multinational firms. Some multinational firms have local manufacturing units, but most have only scientific and marketing offices. The multinational firms appoint distributors of their products, who in turn sell these products to wholesalers and retailers countrywide. The multinationals manufacture or distribute for sale branded products and compete in the market through innovation, research, and development. The local manufacturers may or may not have appointed distributors, but they rather sell their products directly to wholesalers, retailers, hospitals, and clinics and compete by selling low-priced generics. As in other regions of sub-Saharan Africa, the ECOWAS pharmaceutical sector is characterized by net imports of pharmaceuticals, largely from India and China (retrieved from the ECOWAS Regional Pharmaceutical Plan[16]).

Burkina Faso has not been any different in finding solutions to address the challenges the country faces in the acquisition of essential medicines. The country has gone through the history of developing its pharmaceutical sector, improving systems to attend to best pharmacy practices to ensure that the right medicines circulate in the health care system in the right quality, at the right time, to the right people, and to be used appropriately. Owing to the common health situation in the ECOWAS region, the WAHO developed a harmonized regional pharmaceutical plan to address the gaps by strengthening the various pharmaceutical sectors and encouraging best practices. Pharmacists in Burkina Faso were key in ensuring the coming to fruition of the ECOWAS Regional Pharmaceutical Plan.

5.1 Pharmacy practice

Pharmacy practice is the core component of pharmacy and encompasses the development of the professional roles and responsibilities of pharmacists. The profession revolves around people and medicines, with special emphasis on the manufacture of medicines and their regulation, supply, appropriate use, and effects. The turnaround of the practice has been for it to provide pharmaceutical services that are patient-centered rather than product-centered. Such move toward patient-oriented care focuses on the amalgamated teamwork among health workers intended to deliver the best practice possible to patients. Efficient and effective pharmacy practice necessitates the comprehension of the public health situation within which the practice of pharmacy is acknowledged and that the provisions of the needs of the users of pharmaceutical services are much appreciated. Taylor and Harding[19] postulated that "pharmacy practice provides a background to the social context of pharmacy including: the development of pharmacy practice, international dimension of pharmacy practice, health, illness and medicines use, professional practice, meeting the pharmaceutical care needs of specific populations, measuring regulating medicines use, research methods, evaluation, audit and clinical governance."

5.2 Historical background on the pharmaceutical sector in Burkina Faso

Before the 1960s, the national pharmaceutical supply system was organized around the supply pharmacy named "Pharmapro," which was a state enterprise responsible for the supply of health products. In the same year, Pharmapro changed its name and became "Pharmacie Nationale," a public administrative institution with powers to ensure the supply of medicines in the country.

In 1975, the Directorate of Pharmacy Services was created and attached to the General Directorate of Public Health with integration of its attributions of pharmaceutical regulatory functions, in addition to the pharmaceutical supply.

Since subscribing to the Alma-Ata Declaration in September 1978, Burkina Faso has embarked on a reform of its health system, resolutely opting for building a health system based on the principles of primary health care.

By adopting the national document to strengthen primary health care according to the approach of the Bamako Initiative, the government resolutely turned toward the essential generic medicines. This option resulted in enacting regulations on medicinal taxes and customs duties exemptions and the creation of CAMEG in 1992.

In 1994, pharmacies, which were previously state property, were liberalized and reassigned to the private pharmacy sector. To provide a coherent framework for the pharmaceutical sector, the first national pharmaceutical policy was developed and adopted in 1996.

Burkina Faso reformed the hospital system with the adoption of Hospital Law 034/98/AN of May 18, 1998. The government adopted, in September 2000, a national health policy and, in July 2001, a national plan for health development for the period 2001-2010.

In 2002, the Pharmacy Directorate of Health was transformed into the General Directorate of Pharmacy, Medicines, and Laboratory (GDPML), which is directly linked to the office of the Secretary General of Health.

After the final evaluation of the national plan for health development 2001–2010, carried out in October 2010, the MOH invested in a review process of the national health policy and development of a new national plan for health development. The process led to the adoption of these two documents respectively in July and August 2011[4,6].

The review of the first national pharmaceutical policy adopted in 1996 was necessary to integrate new priorities in terms of health development, such as the MDGs, and to take into account the evolution of the health context, such as the utilization of the WTO TRIPS flexibilities provisions on pharmaceutical products, the circulation of counterfeit and illicit medicines, pharmacovigilance, and access to medicines for nontransmissible diseases.

The revision process began in 2009 and continued until 2012 by the adoption of the national pharmaceutical policy and the operational plan including a pharmaceutical strategic plan for the period 2012–2016[9,10].

6. Medicine- and pharmacy-related regulations, policies, and ethics

Ensuring the provision of quality and low-priced pharmaceuticals to the population is a complicated undertaking, ranging from the identification and selection of medicines to the procurement and quality assurance of medicines circulating on the market. The oversight responsibility lies in the hands of the pharmacists and the national medicine regulatory authorities. National registration of medicines is one way to ensure the quality, safety, and efficacy of essential medicines being provided to the population. To achieve that, an autonomous, robust regulatory system that is enduring, sustainable, competitive, and managed in an integrated manner needs to be established in each nation in the region. However, registration of medicines can be cumbersome, requiring a lot of information from applicants. As a result it is sometimes difficult to get pharmaceutical companies to cooperate fully in the registration process, as the cost may outweigh the benefits.

In Burkina Faso, the GDPML plays a key role in the regulatory oversight in ensuring that medicines circulating in the country are of assured quality. The national pharmaceutical policies adopted in 2012 address the inspection of pharmaceutical premises, medicine registration, quality control evaluation of dossiers, and ethical issues.

The health system as described previously is based on the National Health Policy and National Health Development Plan. Also, "Health Foresight 2030" is the health vision of Burkina Faso[5].

Burkina Faso adopted its new national pharmacy policy document, Decree No. 2012-910/PRES/PM/MS/MEF/MICA/MRSI, on November 26, 2012 and the pharmaceutical strategic plan 2012–2016, Decree No. 2012-966/PRES/PM/MS/MEF/MICA/MRSI, on December 13, 2012.

The Burkina Faso medicine regulatory system was developed by the GDPML, which manages all regulatory functions with the exception of the inspection unit, which is managed by the Technical Inspector of Health Services (TIHS). The quality control of medicines is well managed by the National Public Health Laboratory. These are all public institutions whose statuses are defined by law. In 2010, a framework for dialog between these different stakeholders was set up by the GDPML; they meet quarterly but are not formal.

The promotion and advertising of medicines are regulated by Order No. 2010-244/PRES/PM/MS of May 20, 2010 and Order No. 2010-291/MS/CAB of October 1, 2010. The committee in charge of this regulation was created by Order No. 2013-69 of March 13, 2013, which also defines its powers, composition, and functioning. The working tools of the committee consist of the guidelines laid down in Decision No. 10/2010/CM/WAEMU.

The Public Health Code in Article 247 provides that "Advertising of medicinal products shall be authorized by the medical, pharmacy and nursing staff when it is within the health ministry." The main regulatory requirements are that only those medicines for which marketing authorization has been obtained can be advertised, advertising of medicinal products to the general public is prohibited in the member states of the West African Economic Monetary Union (WAEMU), and that advertising to health professionals for an authorized product, as well as advertising campaigns for public health programs, is subject to prior authorization by the National Medicines Regulatory Authority (ies)(NMRA) authority.

The exercise of the profession of a medical advertiser is governed by Order No. 2010-290/MS/CAB of October 1, 2010 and the conditions of opening and operating of a branch of medical promotion by Order No. 2010-288/MS/CAB of October 1, 2010.

Most of medicines regulatory functions such as registration, the licensing of pharmaceutical facilities, pharmaceutical information, pharmacovigilance, and the control of publicity are managed by the GDPML. It shares the regulatory inspection and authorization of clinical trials respectively with the TIHS and the CNBE.

6.1 Medicine registration

Several national and community regulations govern the approval of health products in Burkina Faso. These include Regulation and Decision No. 06/2010/CM/WAEMU relating to procedures and guidelines for registration of pharmaceuticals for human use, Order No. 2013-537/MS/CAB of May 31, 2013 relating to the regulation of medical devices and medical devices for in vitro diagnostics, and Order No. 2003-341/MS/SG/GDPML of December 24, 2003 relating to the conditions of registration of traditional medicines in Burkina Faso[12].

The GDPML has a National Committee and Committee of Experts for medicine approval. Experts are subject to a declaration of conflict of interest and a commitment to confidentiality. It is also equipped with software for the registration process.

Approval of modern medicines (specialty and generic), drugs from traditional medicines, medical supplies, and medical biology reagents is attributed to the Director of Regulation and Pharmaceutical Licenses, an operational branch of the GDPML.

6.2 Medicine pricing

The selling prices of essential generic medicines under International Nonproprietary Name (INN) at various levels of the chain of distribution of medicine in the public sector are jointly administered annually by the MOH and the Ministry of Trade. Indeed, for essential generic medicines from CAMEG a joint order of the MOH and the Ministry of Trade fixes annually the selling price to the public of essential generic medicines. These selling prices are applicable to health facilities in the public and nonprofit private sectors but also to private pharmaceutical facilities (pharmacies or drugstores) that obtain medicines from CAMEG.

For brand name health products, the prices have been liberalized since June 1994 and are determined by the mechanisms of supply and demand, without a regulating mechanism. Thus, although these medicines are exempt from customs duty and value-added tax, their cost is much higher than that of the generics. Indeed, the margin wholesalers charge varies from 19.0 to 23.5% for generic to specialties, while a margin of 32.0% is applied in the pharmacies.

CAMEG makes available nearly 500 generic essential medicines to public health facilities and private pharmacies.

A 2009 study on prices and affordability of medicines shows that originator specialties are on average 5.6 times more expensive than their generic equivalents in the pharmacies of Burkina Faso[13].

6.3 Pharmaceutical inspection

The GDPML has a pharmaceutical inspection service (PIS) attached to the Directorate General. The PIS is responsible for conducting inspections of pharmaceutical facilities. There is unfortunately a legal mandate, as for any inspection operation; there must be a warrant from the TIHS. There are also no legal provisions for the appointment of inspectors and the definition of their power. The PIS has a general inspection procedure, standardized tools such as guidelines developed by the West African Economic Monetary Union (WAEMU), and inspection grids, sheets, and forms.

Three pharmacist inspectors and one pharmacy technician work in this service. Inspectors do not have the adequate power or delegated authority necessary to carry out their tasks. They have the skills to carry out the inspection of pharmaceutical activities, laboratories, and clinical trial sites. These skills deserve to be extended to the inspection of manufacturers of Active Pharmaceutical Ingredients (APIs) and quality control laboratories.

6.4 Authorization of pharmaceutical facilities

The authorization of pharmaceutical companies is regulated by Order No. 0068/MS/CAB of February 22, 2000 relating to the opening and operating conditions of a pharmaceutical company for sales or wholesale distribution, Order No. 0069/MS/CAB of February 22, 2000 relating to the opening and operating conditions of a pharmaceutical manufacturer, Order No. 2010-359/MS/CAB of October 27, 2010 relating to the setup conditions of a private pharmacy, and Order No. 2010-360/MS/CAB of October 27, 2010 relating to the opening and operating conditions of a private pharmacy.

Management of applications to open a pharmaceutical facility is transparent, with an annual publication of the list of applicants and the establishment of maps of available sites.

Management of a pharmacy is a private matter and dispensing of medicines and other pharmaceutical deeds is under the sole responsibility of the pharmacist, who must be the owner of the pharmacy. The pharmacy must be managed by an authorized pharmacist who personally operates it. The operation of a pharmacy is incompatible with the exercise of another profession.

Owing to the personal exercise of the profession, which is a provision of the Public Health Code, each pharmacist may have only one pharmacy. The establishment of a new pharmacy follows progression according to the proportion of the population using the following criteria: one pharmacy per 10,000 inhabitants per administrative entity in cities with more than 500,000 inhabitants, one pharmacy per 20,000 inhabitants per administrative entity in cities in which the number of inhabitants is between 250,000 and 500,000, and one pharmacy per 30,000 inhabitants for communities of fewer than 250,000.

The minimum distance between pharmacies is 500 m, measured as the crow flies and certified by a qualified geometrician. However, in certain commercial areas of cities, this distance can be scaled down, but cannot be less than 300 m.

The GDPML has a written procedure for the licensing process, expert committees, and a national commission for the processing of applications.

7. Core pharmacy practices

Even though modern trends in practice have increased over time due to the evolution of scientific responses to emerging health demands, the core pharmacy practices have remained at the hospital, community, and institutional pharmacy levels, such as prescription orders and order entry, compounding and dispensing, sterile products and large-volume parenterals, record-keeping, patient interviewing and counseling, patient profiles and medical records, prescription benefit programs and reimbursement, legal requirements and regulatory issues, communication with patients and other health professionals, and inventory control and purchasing. The main purpose has been to provide patient care in cooperation with patients, prescribers, and other members of an interprofessional health care team based upon sound therapeutic principles and evidence-based data.

7.1 Hospital practice

Taking into account the relevant legal, ethical, social, cultural, economic, and professional issues; emerging technologies; and evolving biomedical, pharmaceutical, social, behavioral, administrative, and clinical sciences that may influence therapeutic outcomes, the shift to higher and more demanding care has expanded pharmaceutical practice. Modern trends in patient management and rational use of medicines require a stringent health care system and resource support to personnel to promote health, provide access, and coordinate safe, accurate, and time-sensitive medication distribution and to improve therapeutic outcomes of medication use.[18]

In all public hospitals in Burkina Faso (CHU, CHR, and CMA), at least two pharmacists are recruited by the government to manage the hospital pharmacy services and the biomedical analysis laboratory services. As of this writing, it is estimated at about 75 pharmacists are practicing in public hospitals in Burkina Faso.

The activities of pharmacists in hospital pharmacy services are similar in some respects to those of pharmacists in private pharmacies, but there are some differences. The main responsibilities of hospital pharmacists, among others, are the management of medical products, including medicines and medical devices; the management of sterilization and hospital hygiene activities; overseeing the clinical pharmacy activities; the management of hospital preparations; pharmacovigilance services; and the promotion of the rational use of medicines.

The main responsibilities of pharmacists practicing in the medical biology analysis laboratory services of hospitals and other public health care facilities are the coordination and/or implementation of biomedical analysis, the validation of biomedical analysis results, and to ensure reactovigilance and materiovigilance.

7.2 Industrial pharmacy

Industrial pharmacy is a discipline that includes manufacturing, development and formulation, marketing, and distribution of drug products, including quality assurance of these activities. This broad research area relates to various functions in the pharmaceutical industry. Research in industrial pharmacy and pharmaceutical technology are collaborative components of the pharmaceutical industry, which focus on addressing issues such as product formulation, characterization of medicines, and efficiency of manufacturing processes. The industry is licensed by the establishment of a marketing authorization, through procedures of current good manufacturing practices and evaluation of good clinical practices and good laboratories practices in the consenting countries. The national medicine regulatory authorities in each country have overarching regulatory responsibility on the pharmaceutical industry to ensure effective and efficient operation of their affairs, by providing high-quality, safe, and efficacious medicines.

The production of modern medicines including generic medicines existed in Burkina Faso in the past. However, pharmaceutical manufacturing units established in the 1990s that were viable were closed in the 2000s, owing to various difficulties. There were also units of production of medicines from traditional medicines, of which some products were promoted by the MOH. These have been integrated into the national essential medicines and distribution list in the public health system.

Aware that the local production of medicines is an important opportunity for economic growth and for the consolidation of local expertise, the government has committed to a national pharmaceutical policy, to implement incentive provisions to allow the emergence of local pharmaceutical production.

The first specific objective of the pharmaceutical policy is to "increase the local pharmaceutical production to meet 25% of domestic demand for essential health commodities." The measures specified in the national pharmaceutical policy are exemption from any customs fee; the import of equipment, materials, and pharmaceutical inputs used exclusively in the production of medicines and other health products for all pharmaceutical manufacturing units legally established in Burkina Faso; and taking necessary measures to ensure that imported medicines are no longer entitled to any exemption from customs duties if domestic production of one or more equivalents of the product is approved and meets more than 75% of the national demand.

The registration fees applicable to finished products and pharmaceutical inputs manufactured in Burkina Faso have been set at a maximum rate of 25% of the expected pricing for similar products if imported.

Exemption is given, in the context of public procurement, to any pharmaceutical production unit legally established in Burkina Faso, to ensure that qualified and locally manufactured drugs are considered only if their sale price does not exceed 15% those of their imported counterparts.

It should be noted, however, that the application of these measures is not yet effective.

7.3 Community pharmacy practice

At the peripheral level, the pharmacist practices in the regional directorates of health and sanitary districts. The number of pharmacists at the peripheral level was estimated at 90 in 2013.

The main duties of a pharmacist in the regional directorates of health and sanitary districts are participation in monitoring the implementation of health programs; management and dispensing of medicines, equipment, and biomedical devices; promotion of traditional medicine; supervision of management and use of drugs at the peripheral level; and training and information sharing about medications.

7.4 Public health practice and health promotion

In the promotion of health improvement, wellness, and disease prevention, it is very relevant to incorporate the patients, communities, at-risk populations, and the members of an interprofessional team of health care providers, which are expected to enable growth in achieving professional competency. Therefore, regardless of the point of service, pharmacy practice should be at its best. The main goal is to provide patient-centered care and add value to life.

In addition to medicine, public health initiatives "emphasize the prevention of disease and the health needs of the population as a whole." Even though the pharmacists who practice in hospitals and health systems play vital roles in maintaining and promoting public health, they need to have an expanded responsibility to participate in international, national, regional, and institutional efforts to promote public health and to integrate the goals of those initiatives into their practice. "Furthermore, health-system pharmacists have a responsibility to work with public health planners to ensure their involvement in public health policy decision-making and in the planning, development, and implementation of public health efforts" (www.ashp.org/DocLibrary/BestPractices/SpecificStPubHlth.aspx)[20].

The four traditional areas of public health practice are health administration and policy, health education, biostatistics, and epidemiology. The pharmacist plays key roles in the deposit of documents, program descriptions, and the realm of prevention. Efforts aimed at disease surveillance, infectious disease control, immunization, chronic disease maintenance, and disease-related data management, which provide an ample and readily available source of information, are also important for the pharmacist to exhibit his or her capability. Health care research and quality information on evidence-based clinical practice, clinical preventive services, and quality measurement of health care cannot be overlooked.

At the national level, the pharmacist's role is in the ministries of health, serving as a team player in making major policies for public health priorities and strategies and the main provider of health information on medicines and relevant health attributes. The pharmacist is found in a range of advisory groups, task forces, and planning committees whose output shapes the public health agenda. He or she also provides input and direction for national legislative bodies to address, legislate, and provide funding (www.ashp.org/DocLibrary/BestPractices/SpecificStPubHlth.aspx)[20].

In Burkina Faso the main contributions of pharmacists to the regional directorates of health and sanitary districts are participation in monitoring the implementation of health programs; management and dispensing of medicines, equipment, and biomedical devices; promotion of traditional medicine; supervision of management and use of drugs at the peripheral level; and providing training and information on medication.

8. Special pharmacy-related services and activities

8.1 Drug information specialists and centers

Burkina Faso has a Center for Documentation and Information on Medicines (CDIM), which publishes the *Letter of the CDIM*, which is a pharmacotherapeutic newsletter to the attention of health professionals and even the general public. This bulletin is distributed internationally and is posted on partner sites of such agencies as the Regional Office for Africa. The CDIM is linked to the GDPML and is directed by a pharmacist.

8.2 Traditional and herbal medicines

The practice of traditional medicine has become legal in Burkina Faso since the adoption of Law No. 23/94/ADP of May 18, 1994[8] relating to the public health code. The texts for implementation of this law concern the activities of traditional healers and the market authorization of medicinal products derived from traditional medicines.

The practice of traditional medicine is subject to obtaining a license issued by the Minister in Charge of Health. Traditional healers have a code of ethics that sets out their rights and duties.

Traditional medicines are entitled to registration in the national nomenclature. In 2013, there were 35 medicinal products derived from traditional medicines listed in the nomenclature.

There are two types of production of herbal medicines: artisanal and semi-industrial production.

The first is mainly the work of traditional healers, and medicinal products are essentially of the first and second grades.

Semi-industrial production is ensured by four major producers of herbal medicines. The main producers of herbal medicines are Phytosalus and Gamet in Ouagadougou, Phytofla in Banfora, and Kunnawolo in Bobo Dioulasso.

To date, six traditional medicines have been registered on the national list of essential medicines.

In addition, the Department of Traditional Medicine Research of the Health Sciences Institute develops lines of research to document the traditional medicine and pharmacopoeia and to promote the rational use of medicinal plants and herbal medicines produced following good manufacturing practices.

The quality control of medicinal products derived from traditional medicines is generally performed on raw materials and mainly concerns microbiological and physicochemical aspects. Standardization and formulation tests are carried out in collaboration with the University of Ouagadougou.

8.3 Research in pharmacy practice

In Burkina Faso, research on health is currently performed by universities and health research centers. The main activities of research are preclinical and clinical studies on herbal medicine, vaccines, malaria, and HIV treatment protocols. The existing technical platform allows botanical, phytochemical, pharmacological, and toxicological studies necessary for isolation and identification of a molecule of therapeutic interest. This is how research institutions have focused on the involvement of traditional medicine in the treatment of priority diseases and produced nationally and internationally recognized results. In this respect, the most significant advances have been in malnutrition, malaria, and HIV/AIDS. Orphan diseases are not forgotten with the development of FACA, a drug used in the prevention of sickle cell crises.

At the MOH, institutions that have research as a main mission are distinguished (Center Muraz, National Center for Research and Training on Malaria, Center for Health Research of Nouna). Some health facilities also have research as part of their duties (National Public Health Laboratory, university hospitals, regional hospitals, medical centers with surgical antennas).

Other institutions that perform research are universities, on the one hand, and on the other hand, the departments of the National Center for Scientific Research and Technology, such as the Institute for Research in Health Sciences.

These structures have international expertise and are involved in national and international multicenter research on topics including vaccines and HIV/AIDS. Examples include the following few clinical trials: pharmacovigilance of *Spirulina*; study of the interactions between *Spirulina* and HIV/AIDS medicines among PLHIV in Ouagadougou, Burkina Faso; evaluation of virological failure and resistance to ARVs in HIV-positive patients treated in national programs and structures in Burkina Faso, Cameroon, Côte d'Ivoire, Senegal, Thailand, Togo, and Vietnam; evaluation of three strategies of second-line antiretroviral therapy in Africa (Dakar, Bobo-Dioulasso, Yaoundé); protocol for the prevention and monitoring of the emergence of drug resistance of HIV to ARV and system factors of antiretroviral therapy in Burkina Faso; vaccine trial of RTS S, a malaria vaccine from GlaxoSmithKline laboratories to study in a clinical research center in Nanoro, Burkina Faso; an essay on an anti-HIV vaccine that has already received a favorable opinion of the Ethics Committee for Research.

Some operational research is being conducted on the practice of pharmacy, including, but not limited to, an evaluation of personal exercise and the quality of dispensing of medicines in pharmacies; evaluation of the quality of the delivery of antimalarial drugs in pharmacies; realization of the mapping of medicine supply and distribution systems in Burkina Faso; evaluation of the national drug regulatory system; evaluation of the implementation of drug regulation on special import of pharmaceuticals; evaluation of the implementation of drug regulation on clinical trials; study on the structure of prices and availability of medicines in Burkina Faso; current situation of magisterial and hospital preparations in university hospitals; current situation of magisterial and officinal preparations in pharmacies of Burkina Faso; evaluation of the impact of control actions on trends in the illicit drug market.

The legal framework for clinical research regulation in Burkina Faso is materialized by the following: the establishment of a comprehensive regulation (ethical and technical approval provisions for clinical trials); an effective ethics review of clinical trials by the ethics committee to examine the various protocols of research on human beings was created and in operation since 2000; an effective regulatory oversight of clinical trials by the GDPML and the 2011 establishment of the National Technical Committee for examining applications for authorization of clinical trials; inspection of clinical trials by the PIS of the GDPML.

9. Pharmacy education

Most of the training curricula in the ECOWAS region's universities have been tailored to suit both traditional and modern trends of pharmaceutical developments. Areas such as regulatory affairs, pharmaceutical technology and innovation, drug formulation and development, traditional medicines, and clinical studies have been strengthened. Attention has been paid to the regional harmonization of educational curricula at the undergraduate, postgraduate, and pharmacy technician levels, which would lead to the education of qualified personnel to improve the quality of pharmacy practice in the region. These specialized areas and even more in the pipeline will strengthen and increase the human resources needs.

The pharmacist is trained and educated to acquire a wide spectrum of the diverse facets of the pharmaceutical sciences. Of fundamental importance is that the educated professional is developed to become a scholar practitioner with satisfactory skills, knowledge, and inspiration to provide significant, essential, and valuable services. It is expected that the pharmacist is trained to embrace general and specialized knowledge: general, because without it one is too narrow a specialist, and specialized, because it equips one with the faculty for accurate judgment in the practice of the profession. These take into consideration a wide range of scientific, professional, and managerial functions that best serve the pharmaceutical needs of the community and the nation. It is therefore obligatory on the pharmacist to possess sufficient adaptability to meet the demands of a rapidly changing health care delivery system.

The new paradigm shift in pharmacy practice has been structured to improve capability and educational results. The minimum standards lead to the degree of Bachelor of Pharmacy (B'Pharm), and the enhanced program known as the Doctorate of Pharmacy (PharmD), in addition to the focus on pharmaceutical care, highlights patient-oriented care.

Modernization of the pharmacy practice exhibits skills and competencies in evidence-based clinical practice, policy issues, quality assurance in pharmaceutical services, pharmacovigilance, emerging disease patterns, pharmacoeconomic analyses, management of health care teams, use of information and communication technology, information management, interpersonal communications, medicinal products testing and quantification, adaptation approaches against the impact of climate change on medicinal plants and herbs, research, and instruction.

The courses are designed to give the students a good grounding in the main disciplines of pharmacy, including pharmaceutics, pharmaceutical technology, industrial pharmacy, pharmaceutical and medicinal chemistry, pharmacognosy, pharmaceutical microbiology, pharmacy management, pharmacology and toxicology, hospital pharmacy, pharmacy jurisprudence and ethics, clinical clerkship, procurement and logistics management, medicines regulation, and pharmaceutical services. Graduates are expected to be well equipped for professional practice.

Burkina Faso, like most of the French-speaking West African countries and some English-speaking countries, for example Ghana, has moved from the B'Pharm to the PharmD program.

Pharmaceutical studies last at least six years. They are taught in the unit of training research in health sciences and conducted in three cycles, each comprising two years. The seventh year is generally reserved for the preparation and defense of a thesis accompanied by a state diploma of Doctor of Pharmacy.

9.1 The postgraduate pharmacy education and Continuing Professional Development (CPD)

Burkina Faso has several public and private universities, some of which have faculties or institutes for training of general and specialized medical personnel. However, only the University of Ouagadougou provides training for pharmacists.

The University of Ouagadougou and University Bobo-Dioulasso offer specialized training at the master level to pharmacists and other health professionals: in pharmacology, toxicology, pharmaceuticals, chemical protective analyses, medical biology, and parasitology.

In terms of international postgraduate education, many courses lasting from 2 to 4 weeks and leading to the award of interuniversity diplomas are organized in these universities in partnership with the National Health Ministry, foreign countries, and international organizations such as the WHO.

In this respect may be mentioned the following IUDs housed in universities or not and which see the participation of more than 40 nationals from more than 15 African countries and national and international trainers:

- The Interuniversity diplomas (IUD) on the overall care of people affected by HIV/AIDS organized for more than 10 years at the University of Ouagadougou;
- The IUD on medicine supply management organized since 2011 at the University of Ouagadougou;
- The IUD on vaccinology, organized since 2011 at the Polytechnic University of Bobo-Dioulasso.

In Burkina Faso there are no board, certificate, or licensure examinations. Conditions of practice are he or she should be (1) a graduate in Pharmacy or have a certificate recognized and considered equivalent by the government of Burkina Faso; (2) of Burkinabe nationality or a national of an ECOWAS member state; and (3) registered in the national order of Pharmacists of Burkina Faso.

For holders of foreign pharmacy degrees, practicing in Burkina Faso is limited to two situations: Burkinabe with a degree obtained abroad, if a graduate with a diploma of Doctor of Pharmacy or having a certificate recognized and considered equivalent by the government of Burkina Faso, or non-Burkinabe, the same condition applies if from an ECOWAS country or a country with a reciprocal agreement with Burkina Faso.

It is expected that the opening of training courses for specialists in the pharmaceutical sector at the University of Ouagadougou in the academic year 2014–2015 for the training of health professionals will allow an increase in national pharmaceutical expertise.

The implementation of this specialized training was conducted in conjunction with the MOH through a training plan aimed at correcting imbalances between the supply and demand of personnel. It is also provided for the establishment of a permanent forum for consultation between the Ministry of Higher Education and the MOH for the continuous adaptation of training to fulfill the real needs of the MOH.

In this context, the MOH has recruited 104 physicians and pharmacists for specializations in Burkina Faso and 16 for specializations outside the country.

10. Achievements in pharmacy practice

Achievements in pharmacy practice are enormous, in all disciplines of the profession at the local, national, and international levels. These achievements were made possible by breaking through the challenges encountered and taking advantage of the strengths and available opportunities to overcome the weaknesses and threats.

In Burkina Faso, the SWOT analysis of the practice of pharmacy shows how well they have been able to handle the health care system. Even though there are still some setbacks to be addressed, there seems to be light at the end of the tunnel.

10.1 Strengths

There is the existence of an operational mechanism of collaboration within the GDPML and other entities that perform pharmaceutical regulatory functions, the existence of a formalized framework within the GDPML and national professional associations in the pharmaceutical field. The GDPML has a good capacity in terms of drug registration. Drug registration is strongly regulated by national and regional laws. A transparency mechanism, which addresses interest conflicts and confidential declarations, has been put in place and procedures, guidelines, and software for drug registration are available. A national commission and two expert committees have also been established for dossier assessment.

The expertise is appropriate for dossier assessment, and a system of pharmacovigilance of health products was establish in 2011 and managed by GDPML. The system for regulation and monitoring of clinical trials, administrative authorization, ethical approval, and inspection of clinical trials and pharmaceutical inspection is currently managed by the GDPML and directly linked to the Director General. The function of pharmaceutical licensing including market authorization for pharmaceutical and traditional medicines is regulated as well by the GDPML, except for imports and distribution of medical biology products. There is also a framework for hospital pharmacy activities and regulation for the destruction of expired and substandard health products.

The administration of the selling price of essential generic drugs under their INN at various levels of the medicine distribution chain is controlled as well as the adoption and implementation of the regulation procedure on the publicity of health products. The financial autonomy of CAMEG is acquired and its status allows the reinvestment of the earnings on the investments and the sale of essential generic drugs at relatively affordable prices compared to the private sector. A formal operational consultative framework to monitor the use of ACTs, pharmaceutical inputs in the fight against HIV/AIDS, reproductive health products, and TB treatments exists. This framework is an effective model for coordinating medicine supply. A National Essential Medicines List at the level of the health care system is reviewed regularly and is a reference for the subregional sector owing to its composition and the fact that it incorporates improved traditional medicines. There is a national therapeutic formulary and standardized strategy for diagnosis and treatment of priority diseases for the first level of the health system. The public health sector is relatively well endowed with pharmacists even though more staff is needed.

10.2 Opportunities

The government of Burkina Faso has demonstrated a strong political will and commitment to improving the pharmaceutical sector, and other developing and financial partners and stakeholders have equally shown such commitment to the growth of the pharmaceutical sector. The GDPML was designated a Center of Excellence of the WAEMU for the registration of health products and was also designated a Center of Excellence of New Partnership for Africa Development (NEPAD) for the authorization and monitoring of clinical trials.

10.3 Policies

The national health policies, national health development plan, and national pharmaceutical policies were adopted in 2012, as well as the pharmaceutical strategic plan in 2012–2016.

10.4 Needs and expectations of the community

The best possible access to health products that are of good quality, safe, and efficacious should be distributed throughout the country by an effective supply chain system at a cost adapted to the purchasing power of the population, which will contribute to their well-being.

11. Challenges

Pharmacists are important members of the health care team; they therefore have a very crucial role to play to uplift the image of their chosen profession. They face many challenges that have to be dealt with in this modern time: issues of workload, managerial skills, good inter-personal relationships, balancing customer and organizational needs, good communication skills, and patient and staff charters. A flourishing trade in counterfeit and illicit medicines and a lack of political will to invest in its fight, a lack of appropriate infrastructure, weak governance, and corruption in the health system impede effective medicine regulatory functions and access to funds, and there is a shortage of relevant personnel. Outdated health policies and poor access to relevant technologies are more challenges. In addition they must deal with a low level of human resource capacity and changes or reversals that have drawback effects on investment plans to strengthen the pharmaceutical sector.

11.1 Weaknesses

The status of the GDPML does not fit into the real national medicine regulatory authority, with regard to financial and managerial autonomy; instances of discipline of the national regulation of pharmacists of Burkina Faso are not functional, the business climate is unfavorable to the growth of investment in the pharmaceutical sector, and the inspection capacity of the GDPML is limited. The inspection service of the GDPML has no legal mandate, as for any inspection operation there must be a warrant from the TIHS. There are also no legal provisions for the appointment of inspectors or the definition of their power. The swearing-in of inspectors also appears as an essential factor in strengthening the legitimacy and authority of pharmaceutical inspectors.

The national quality control laboratory has limited capacity to control the quality of medicines, but it is hoped it will improve in due time. It does not yet have all the international certifications in medicine control, including the WHO prequalification, nor the International Standard Organization 17025 certification. The possibilities of the application of TRIP flexibilities agreements, including the use of compulsory licenses, have still not been taken into account by the national regulatory authority and the government. The registration of certain product features such as medical gases and special foods has not been considered and their premarketing quality control is not systematized.

There is a lack of a sustainable financing system of quality control in postmarket surveillance, and the technical expertise in the detection of counterfeit products is insufficient at all levels of the pharmaceutical supply chain. Illicit trade and counterfeit health products are persistent, and the reporting of adverse effects of pharmaceuticals still remains low. The number of qualified human resources and quantity of materials and financial resources for pharmacovigilance are still insufficient. The risk of losing the quality of essential generic medicines with respect to poor storage conditions at district and hospital medicine stores is high.

Access to generic medicines for the treatment of chronic and nontransmissible diseases is insufficient and the cost of specialty medicines to manage pathologies in the private sector is very high. Inequality in the geographical distribution of private pharmacies, mostly concentrated in urban areas, and the persistence of customs taxes for raw materials are not favorable for the development of local production of medicines, and prescriptions in INN are not effective in the private sector and remain lower in public hospitals.

The lack of standardized therapeutic protocols, medicines commodities, and individual nominative dispensation in the hospitals leads to the irrational use of medicines; the right of substitution of a generic medicine for the brand name specialty is statutorily usable by the pharmacist but its application remains relatively low. Inadequate investments in research and development, inadequate human resource capacity, poor remunerations (which poses a brain drain), and porosity of borders equally affect the pharmacy practice.

11.2 Threats

The circulation of substandard, falsified, falsely labeled, and counterfeit and illicit health products; increased resistance to many treatments; inadequate health care budgets; dependence on donated medicines; dependence on imports for medicine supply; and international financial crises aggravation are great threats to the practice of pharmacy and health care delivery in Burkina Faso.

12. Recommendations/way forward

Coordination of all medicine regulatory functions by only one entity, accreditation and/or prequalification of the national public health laboratory, the development of a system of health risk sharing in collaboration with the collectivities are necessary to improve the financial accessibility of essential medicines as well as increasing the pharmaceutical local production to cover at least 25% of the national needs in essential medicines.

Improvement of the availability and access to health products, development and capacity building of human resources, and reinforcement of pharmaceutical cooperation on regional and international levels are essential components of an effective development of the pharmaceutical sector.

13. Conclusion

The practice of pharmacy in the overall pharmaceutical sector in Burkina Faso has been focused on providing the best outcomes to improve the health care system by delivery of high-quality, safe, and efficacious medicines and services to the population. These have not come about without challenges and difficulties. Inadequate human response capacity development, insufficient infrastructure and equipment, inadequate health information system, and poor telecommunication and networking as well as operational autonomy have been the major problems. But the important aspect of it all is that the core pharmacy best practices have been put in place to ensure a high level of medicine delivery and accessibility of medicines to the population, even though the services could be improved to compete with international standards.

14. Lessons learned

The current work enlightened me by providing better understanding of the practice of pharmacy in Burkina Faso. A few issues to be highlighted are that:

1. The health sector identified its shortcomings in the pharmaceutical sector and quickly, within 9 years, made drastic changes to improve the various competences and capacity developments as well as systems improvement.
2. Lots of policies, legal/legislations, and regulations were developed to enforce and strengthen the practice of pharmacy and improve access to quality essential medicines.
3. Teamwork among the pharmacists was evident because of the limited number of staff available to fulfill various tasks.
4. What was noted was the pharmaceutical monopoly in the procurement and supply chain system in both the public and the private sectors. There was not enough competition and that could affect pricing and quality of medicines in circulation.
5. In addition there is dedication and determination to address the challenges with little available resources.

Acknowledgment

I acknowledge Dr. Djenebou Lamizana ALADE, a pharmacist currently in private community practice, who was the Director of Quality Control of medicines and cosmetics at the National Laboratory for Public Health, Ouagadougou, and Dr. Josias Gérard Boumbéwendin Yameogo, Head of the Technical Support Service, General Directorate of Pharmacy, Medicines, and Laboratories, Ministry of Health, Burkina Faso, for their enormous support in verifying the authenticity of the information researched.

References

1. *Recensement général de la population et de l'habitation (RGPH)*. Burkina Faso: Institut national de statistique et de la démographie; 2006.
2. *Cartographie des systèmes d'approvisionnement et de distribution des médicaments et autres produits de sante au Burkina Faso*. Direction générale de la Pharmacie, du médicament et des laboratoires (DGPML), Ministère de la santé; December 2010.
3. *Stratégie de croissance accélérée et de développement durable (SCADD), 2010 Stratégie de croissance accélérée et de développement durable (SCADD) 2011–2015*. Gouvernement du Burkina Faso; September 2010.
4. *Plan national de développement sanitaire 2011–2020*. Ministère de la santé du Burkina Faso; 2011.
5. *Prospective santé 2030*. Ministère de la santé du Burkina Faso; 2011.

6. *Politique nationale de santé*. Ministère de la santé du Burkina Faso; 2011.

7. Enquête Démographique et de Santé (EDS). Institut National de la Statistique et de la Démographie; April 2012.

8. Loi N°23/94/ADP du 18 mai 1994 portant code de la santé publique du Burkina Faso.

9. *Plan stratégique pharmaceutique*. Ministère de la santé du Burkina Faso; December 2012.

10. *Politique pharmaceutique nationale*. Ministère de la santé du Burkina Faso; November 2012.

11. *Profil pharmaceutique du Burkina Faso*. Organisation Mondiale de la Santé; 2012.

12. *Recueil des textes réglementaires du secteur pharmaceutique au Burkina Faso*. Direction générale de la Pharmacie, du médicament et des laboratoires, Ministère de la santé (DGPML); 2013.

13. *Statistiques d'importation des médicaments au Burkina Faso*. Direction générale de la Pharmacie, du médicament et des laboratoires, Ministère de la santé; December 2013.

14. *Annuaire statistiques 2013*. Ministère de la santé du Burkina Faso; May 2014.

15. Liste nationale des médicaments et consommables essentiels (LNMCE). Ministère de la santé du Burkina Faso, Edition 2014.

16. *ECOWAS regional pharmaceutical plan*. 2015. WAHO/XVI.AHM/2015/Res-04/d.

17. Soucat A, Scheffler R, Ghebreyesus TA. *The labor market for health workers in Africa: a new look at the crisis*. 2013. ISBN: 978-0-8213-9555-4. e-ISBN:978-0-8213-9558-Retrieved from: http://elibrary.worldbank.org/doi/book/10.1596/978-0-8213-9555-4.

18. American Pharmaceutical Association Academy of Students of pharmacy/American Association of Colleges of Pharmacy Council of Deans (APhA-ASP/AACP-COD). *Task force on professionalism*. June 26, 1994. Retrieved from: www.acp.edu/files/6913/9508/4984/CPPE_Manual_2014.pdf.

19. Taylor KMG, Harding G. *Pharmacy practice*. 2010. Retrieved from: www.alibris.com/Pharmacy-Practice-Kevin-Taylor-M-D/book/7984070.

20. ASHP Statement on the Role of Health-System Pharmacists in Public Health. Medication Therapy and Patient Care: Specific Practice Areas–*Statements*. p. 324–328. Retrieved from: www.ashp.org/DocLibrary/BestPractices/SpecificStPubHlth.aspx.

21. Burkina Faso Demographic and Health Survey. *Global Health Data Exchange*; 2003. http://ghdx.healthdata.org/record/burkina-faso-demographic-and-health survey.

22. AIDS - UNICEF: Joint United Nations Programme on HIV/AIDS (UNAIDS) … with efforts to address tuberculosis, malaria and other…enhancing pharmaceutical security for other health. (2012). www.unicef.org/aids/files/aids__togetherwewillendaids_en.pdf.

Pharmacy Practice in Latin America

CHAPTER 19

Pharmacy Practice in Chile

Patricia Acuna

Chapter Outline

Pharmacy Practice in Developing Countries. http://dx.doi.org/10.1016/B978-0-12-801714-2.00019-8

1. Geographic, social, and demographic background

Talking of pharmacy in Chile draws attention to a permanent state of development in accordance with the changes in a profession struggling to win a prestigious place in society. Over time, many men and women have contributed to giving a definite personality to the pharmacy practice and set it in a place of advance among Latin American countries.

The Chilean geographical boundaries have imposed on Chile limited resources compared to developed countries.

Chile is located in the World Health Organization's (WHO's) Americas Region[5]. It has an area of 756,102.4 km² and an Antarctic claim (Chilean Antarctic Territory) of 1,250,257.6 km². Its perimeter is 12,774 km.

The surface of Chile (American, Antarctic, and insular) is 2,006,096 km², without considering its territorial sea, its Exclusive Economic Zone, and the continental shelf.

1.1 Limits

Chile borders Peru to the north, across the Line of Concord, and Argentina and Bolivia to the east (Figure 1). It extends south to the South Pole and west to the Pacific Ocean, including the Exclusive Economic Zone of 200 nautical miles. Limit distances are as follows:

    Chile–Argentina limit, 8542 km;
    Chile–Bolivia limit, 860 km;
    Chile–Peru boundary, 171 km;
    Chilean sea coastline, 6435 km.

Figure 1

Chile: geographical location.[a]*Source:* http://www.ine.cl/canales/menu/publicaciones/calendario_de_publicaciones/pdf/COMPENDIO_2013.pdf.[b]

[a]Data: National Institute of Statistics 2013.

[b]All maps included in the National Institute of Statistics, Compendium 2013, have been approved by Special Resolution No. 280 of 9 July 2012 by the National Directorate of Borders and Boundaries Department, Ministry of Foreign Affairs. Edition and circulation of maps that refer or relate to the limits and boundaries of Chile do not compromise in any way the State of Chile, according to Art. 2, letter "g," of DFL No. 83 of 1979, Ministry of Foreign Affairs.

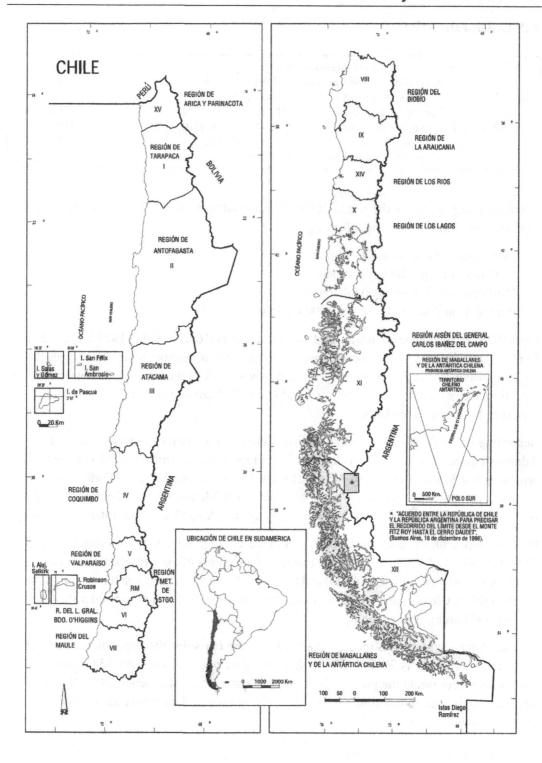

CHILE

REGIÓN DE
ARICA Y PARINACOTA
XV

REGIÓN DE
TARAPACÁ
I

REGIÓN DE
ANTOFAGASTA
II

I. San Félix
I. San
Ambrosio

I. Salas
y Gómez

I. de Pascua

0   20 Km.

REGIÓN DE
ATACAMA
III

REGIÓN DE
COQUIMBO
IV

REGIÓN DE
VALPARAÍSO
V

I. Alej.
Selkirk

I. Robinson
Crusoe

RM

REGIÓN
MET.
DE
STGO.

R. DEL L. GRAL.
BDO. O'HIGGINS
VI

REGIÓN DEL
MAULE
VII

PERÚ

BOLIVIA

ARGENTINA

OCÉANO PACÍFICO

MAR CHILENO

UBICACIÓN DE CHILE EN SUDAMERICA

0   1000   2000 Km

VIII

IX

XIV

X

XI

XII

REGIÓN DEL
BIOBÍO

REGIÓN DE
LA ARAUCANÍA

REGIÓN DE LOS RÍOS

REGIÓN DE LOS LAGOS

REGIÓN AISÉN DEL GENERAL
CARLOS IBAÑEZ DEL CAMPO

REGIÓN DE MAGALLANES
Y DE LA ANTÁRTICA CHILENA
PROVINCIA ANTÁRTICA CHILENA

TERRITORIO
CHILENO
ANTÁRTICO

0   500 Km.   POLO SUR

★ "ACUERDO ENTRE LA REPÚBLICA DE CHILE
Y LA REPÚBLICA ARGENTINA PARA PRECISAR
EL RECORRIDO DEL LÍMITE DESDE EL MONTE
FITZ ROY HASTA EL CERRO DAUDET".
(Buenos Aires, 16 de diciembre de 1998).

REGIÓN DE MAGALLANES
Y DE LA ANTÁRTICA CHILENA

100   50   0   100   200 Km.

Islas Diego
Ramírez

OCÉANO PACÍFICO

MAR CHILENO

ARGENTINA

1.2 General statistics[c]

Total population (2013)	17,620,000
Gross national income per capita (PPP Intl $, 2013)	21,030
Life expectancy at birth, M/F (years, 2012)	77/83
Probability of dying under 5 years (per 1000 live births, 2012)	Not available
Probability of dying between 15 and 60 years M/F (per 1000 population, 2012)	110/56
Total expenditure on health per capita (Intl $, 2012)	1606
Total expenditure on health as % of GDP (2012)	7.2

Population projections for the period 2010–2015 according to the National Institute of Statistics (INE) in 2013 are the following:

- Life expectancy at birth, 79.1 years;
- Birth rate, 14.5 per 1000 inhabitants;
- Mortality rate, 5.9 per 1000 inhabitants;
- Rate of natural increase, 8.6 per 1000 inhabitants.

Until 1930 the main population was rural. In 1875 it reached 65.1% and in 1920 it reached 53.6%. In a 1940 census count the situation is reversed, and according to the 2002 census the rural population (2,026,322 people) represented only 13.40% of the total population. Projections for 2013 indicate a total of 2,274,481 rural and 15,282,334 urban; that is, only 13.0% corresponds to a rural population.

According to the Administrative and Political Division System of Government and Administration, the country is divided into 15 regions, which in turn are subdivided into 54 provinces and 346 municipalities. As of 2013, the 15 regions are Arica and Parinacota, Tarapaca, Antofagasta, Atacama, Coquimbo, Valparaiso, Metropolitan, O'Higgins, Maule, Bio-Bio, La Araucania, Los Rios, Los Lagos, Aysen, and Magallanes and Antarctic Territory.

In accordance with its economy, Chile is part of the group of high annual income countries (WHO, 2014).[6] In 2010, the country became the 31st member of the Organization for Economic Cooperation and Development (OECD) and the first in South America to join this organization. For the OECD, Chile's membership is a major milestone in its mission to build a stronger, cleaner, and fairer global economy.

Considering its autonomous income, the Chilean state classifies the population in quintiles. Each quintile represents 20% of households ranked by per capita household income: the first quintile represents the poorest 20% and the last quintile the richest 20%. Social stratification is used to determine the poverty and misery of the country among other considerations.

[c]Source: http://www.who.int/countries/chl/en/.

Table 1: Chile: poor and homeless profile 1990–2011

Year	Poor (%)	Homeless (%)
1990	38.4	12.8
1996	23.1	5.8
2000	20.5	5.7
2003	18.7	4.7
2006	13.7	3.2
2009	15.1	3.7
2011	14.4	2.8

According to a report by the OECD (March 2014) Chile is the fourth of the 34 member countries with a higher proportion of poor. Specifically, 18% of the population has an income below 50% of the average, and it is one of the countries with more income inequality between rich and poor. However, the rate of poor population was reduced by more than one percentage point between 2007 and 2010. According to data, poverty has declined steadily since 1990, from nearly 40% to 14% in 2011 (Table 1).[1]

Regarding birth and death rates between 1990 and 2011, it is possible to say that the Chilean population is getting older and births are declining. The following birth and mortality rates have been recorded by the INE in 2013:

Year	Births	Deaths
1990	292,146	78,434
2000	248,893	78,814
2011	247,358	94,985

Chilean health profile indicators are shown in Table 2.

2. History of pharmacy in Chile

2.1 Pre-Columbian medicine and pharmacy[2]

The history of pharmacy in Chile is a sum of wills and personal efforts and initiatives of pharmacists who had to reconcile and balance technical aspects with the commercial function of the pharmacy practice.

As in the rest of the American countries, the Chilean history of pharmacy has a before and after the arrival of Christopher Columbus to America. In the pre-Columbian era, the original inhabitants could be divided into two main ethnic groups: the Atacamenia and the Mapuche. Both groups faced their relationship to the environment with a magical–religious concept, which allowed them to find satisfactory answers to questions regarding their existence.

The Atacamenian people, belonging to the Andean cultures, applied an ecological worldview in which diseases were understood as the result of an imbalance with the world around them. Disease was seen as a mood of sadness and general decay and the most common source was, therefore, "the theft or loss of the soul." The Mapuches owned a very different worldview from the rest of the indigenous people of the Americas. However, the ritual and therapeutic way in which they approached the health–disease relationship was very similar to that of other tribal groups. It was based on the action of an intermediary who possessed a magical or religious power to apply various therapeutic resources from nature. The main character in Mapuche medicine is the Machi, and the therapeutic and magical ritual is called "machitún," which is carried out to remove evil spirits from the body and soul. The magical–religious function of the Machi differs from the empirical function of the healer, in that the latter possesses extensive knowledge and experience about medicinal herbs and, therefore, can treat diseases of natural causes. Mapuche medicine counts on over 200 herbs, bushes, and trees, which provide them

Table 2: Chilean health profile according to the World Health Organization 2012[d]

		Country	Regional Average	Global Average
General	Total population (thousands)	17,465		
	Population living in urban areas (%)	89	80	53
	Gross national income per capita (PPP Intl $)	21,310	27,457	12,018
	Total fertility rate (per woman)	1.8	2.1	2.5
	Life expectancy at birth (years), both male and female	80	76	70
Mortality and morbidity	Life expectancy at age 60 (years), both male and female	24	22	20
	Healthy life expectancy at birth (both sexes)	70	67	62
	Under 5 years mortality rate (per 1000 live births) (both sexes)	9	15	48
	Adult mortality rate Male	110	161	187
	(probability of dying Female	56	89	124
	between 15 and 60 years per 1000 inhabitants)			
	Maternal mortality ratio[a] (per 100,000 live births)	22	68	210
	Prevalence of HIV (per 100,000 population)	222	315	511
	Prevalence of tuberculosis (per 100,000 population)	21	40	69

[a]Data refer to 2013.
Source: WHO; Chile: Health Profile, 2012.

[d]Data refer to 2013.

Table 3: Mapuche medicinal plants frequently used in Chile today

Scientific Name	Common Name	Part of the Plant	Use
Apium australe	Celery	Leaves and roots	Blood purification and rheumatism
Buddleja globosa	Orange-ball tree	Leaves	Infusions to treat ulcers Poultices for bruises
Peumus boldus	Boldo	Leaves	Hepatic problems
Polygonum sanguinaria	Sanguinaria	Leaves	Gallstones
Solanum crispum	Natri	Leaves	Fever
Allium sativum	Garlic	Bulbs	Antiseptic and antihelminthic properties Tincture: hypotensive
Matricaria chamomilla	Chamomile	Flowers	Antispasmodic External use: anti-inflammatory, healing
Persea americana	Avocado	Leaves	Infusion: stomach and menstrual discomfort
Plantago lanceolata	Llanten	Leaves	Anticancer Wound wash

Source: Historia de una profesion. Colegio Químico Farmacéutico y Bioquímico de Chile A.G. Santiago, Chile, 2002.

with seeds, bark, leaves, and flowers for medicinal purposes; all of them are used to this day (Table 3). The medicinal properties attributed to plants have an empirical basis.

2.2 Spanish Chile: fifteenth–eighteenth centuries[3]

Pharmacy in Spanish America was ruled by an institution created by the Catholic monarchy in the late fifteenth century called the "Protomedicato." In Chile it was officially established in 1566 and depended on Lima, Peru, until 1786. Some of its responsibilities were the management of teaching, examination, and accreditation of candidates for new physicians and apothecaries. The "Protophysician" was entitled by the governor and was periodically evaluated by examiners. After the country's independence from Spain (nineteenth century) the Protomedicato joined the Faculty of Medicine at the University of Chile.

The first 59 years after the founding of Santiago (capital city), up to the year 1600, were marked by the conquest of the territory and its expansion into the south, with a fierce reaction from the Mapuche people. The first hospital in Santiago was the Virgin of Relief and although the exact date of its founding is not known, it already existed in 1554. It is important to note that the first public apothecary, Diego Cifontes, worked in this hospital.

During the seventeenth century (colonial period) the city of Santiago was just a village with no more than 700 Spaniards and 2000 indigenous people. Regarding pharmacy practice it can be inferred that public apothecaries were not in high demand. However, famines and calamities and five epidemics of smallpox that killed a quarter of the population of Santiago stimulated progress. In this scenario, the Jesuits played an important role in the development of pharmacy in Chile and their contribution of European knowledge allowed them to gain importance in the rising Chilean community. In the first half of the eighteenth century the situation did not change much from the previous century. However, during the reign of Charles the Third in Spain Jesuits were expulsed from all Hispanic domains. More than 350 Jesuit priests abandoned Chile in 1767, among them, and after 22 years of service, was Brother Joseph Zeitler, a well-renowned apothecary.

2.3 Pharmacists in the nineteenth century[3]

The beginning of the nineteenth century in Chile was marked by what would be its independence from the kingdom of Spain. It was a time of change and among the first reforms was that of the health sciences, including pharmacy and essential aspects of professional practice in particular. At the same time, pharmacy education had a preponderant significance since it was seen as the way to provide educated citizens to the emerging nation.

The nineteenth century apothecary in Chile consisted of room for selling recipes and specific medicines, a recipe room for pharmaceutical preparation, and a medical consultation room.

2.4 The pharmaceutical industry in Chile[3]

Foreign pharmacists who arrived in the country were characterized by their order, perseverance, responsibility, and self-discipline, which allowed the Chilean pharmacy to become more methodical, scientific, and neat. Many of these immigrants settled in the city of Valparaiso, which led to smaller labs and drugstores that would become the future pharmaceutical industry.

The first pharmacist–businessman was the Italian citizen and professor of pharmacy Antonio Puccio, who sought national and international expansion. Germans also stimulated the development of the emerging pharmaceutical industry in the country. Laboratories Chile was the first laboratory in the country that, over time, would play a role of great significance in Chilean public health. This laboratory, although the most significant, is only one of many others that arose in the country in the first half of the twentieth century, driven by the advancement of research and science and the need to respond to public health needs.

2.5 Pharmacy in Chile in the twentieth century[3]

In the first two decades of the twentieth century, health was not the only problem facing the country. The health professionals were aware of this situation and the urgent need to improve conditions.

At the beginning of the twentieth century the diffuse image of the apothecary/pharmacist of the nineteenth century gave way to another one, clearly defined. Modernization of the Chilean pharmacy and scientific advances in chemistry, as well as the predominance of the master recipe that was tightly bound to doctors and pharmacists, along with the significant role played by outstanding pharmacists, favored the social identity of the "pharmaceutical chemists."[e] Thus, in 1942, by Law No. 7,205, a major milestone in the pharmacy profession history was achieved: the creation of the Chilean Pharmaceutical Association. This organization continues developing its work on behalf of the profession, supported by the rule of law and based on its terms of public policy. Among its many achievements, two have been particularly important. The first is its contribution to the Law of National Drug Formulary, issued in 1969. Nine years later, the Chilean experience was used by the WHO to model its policy of essential drugs under generic names addressed to all countries of the "third world." The second achievement has to do with its involvement in the promulgation of Presidential Decree No. 773 amending the Bylaw of Pharmacies, Drugstores, and Other Authorized Bodies and introducing improvements in the pharmacy practice for pharmacists and pharmacy technicians.

Another noteworthy initiative undertaken by the Chilean Pharmaceutical Association was the foundation of the Academy of Pharmaceutical Sciences of Chile, as a body to stimulate progress and development of pharmaceutical sciences and the pharmacy profession. It was modeled after the Royal Academy of Pharmacy of Spain and initial affiliates were Chilean pharmacists and professors that at the time of its creation were appointed as members of the Spanish Academy.

3. The Chilean health system[4]

The Chilean health system consists of public and the private contributions.[f] The public health system consists of a social health insurance administered by the National Health Fund (FONASA). The insurance operates on the basis of a sharing scheme, which is financed with a single payment of 7% of the taxable income of policyholder and resources from general taxes in the nation. The benefits provided by this scheme are the same for all members, regardless of the amount of the insurance prima and the size of the family covered. The private health system consists of Preventive Health Institutions (ISAPRES) and individual health producers. ISAPRES operate as a health insurance system based on agreed individual contracts with policyholders, and the granted benefits depend directly on the amount of the premium being paid. Private health care providers include hospitals, clinics, and independent professionals serving both the insured persons belonging to the ISAPRE and the contributors to the public system (Figure 2).

Both active and passive workers are required to contribute 7% of their taxable income to the health system, with a maximum of UF4921 monthly.[g] This payment can be made to FONASA

---

[e]From now on called "pharmacists."

[f]Available at http://www.previsionsocial.gob.cl/subprev/?page_id=7229.

[g]The Unit de Foment (UF) is not money, and represents the indexation of the Chilean peso (CLP) in line with inflation, so it is variable. As of 31 January 2015, the UF was worth CLP24,557.15, equivalent to approximately US$39.04.

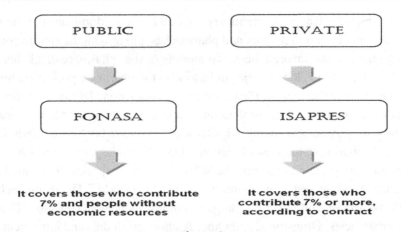

Figure 2
The Chilean health care system.

or to an ISAPRE. The worker may pay an additional amount over 7% to gain more benefits. Contributors who are part of FONASA can choose between two modes of health care: institutional (closed care) and free election (open care). In the first mode contributors receive their benefits in either hospitals or primary health care institutions. In the second case, contributors get their services from private providers. The homeless are part of the public health care system.

The institutional mode requires a copayment, which varies according to the income level of the contributor. Homeless beneficiaries and those whose income is below a certain level, as well as noncontributors to the public system, are excluded from the copayment. The first group has medicine coverage.

3.1 The Chilean Institute of Public Health[20]

The Institute of Public Health (ISP) is the national scientific and technical institution developing reference, surveillance, and control functions. It depends on the Chilean Ministry of Health for approval of its policies, rules, and general administrative plans and for monitoring their implementation. However, it has autonomous operation, legal personality, and its own assets. Regarding operational aspects, it is organized in six departments: (1) National Agency for Medicines (ANAMED), (2) Biomedical Laboratory, (3) Environmental Health, (4) Occupational Health, (5) Scientific, and (6) Administration and Finance (Figure 3).

Other units answering directly to the Head of the ISP are Occupational Health & Environmental Protection, Legal Advice, Quality, Internal Audit, Strategic Planning and Management Control, Audit, Communications, and Institutional Image.

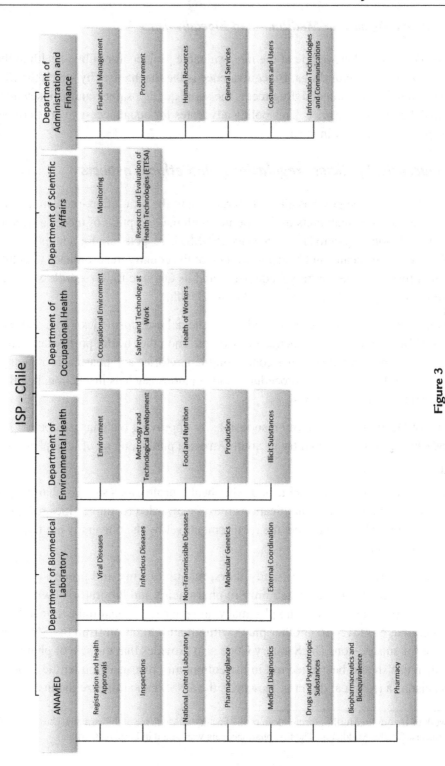

Figure 3
National Institute of Public Health of Chile: organizational structure.

3.2 The National Agency for Medicines and Bioequivalence[20]

The ANAMED of the ISP drove one of the most valuable projects for public health in the country, the bioequivalence of drugs. Bioequivalence is the mechanism by which the ISP certifies that a generic or a branded drug meets the same quality, safety, and efficacy attributes as the original, but at a lower price. This policy advocates for equal access to drugs of better quality, benefiting those most in need.

4. Pharmaceutical policies, regulations, and ethical aspects

In Chile, the Sanitary Code governs all matters relating to the promotion, protection, and recovery of health of the inhabitants of the country with the exception of those subject to other laws. The National System Health Service (SNSS) is responsible for addressing all matters related to public health and hygienic welfare of the country in accordance with the Constitution of the State, the Sanitary Code itself, and its Organic Law, regardless of the responsibilities and rights of the Ministry of Public Health.[8]

The IV Book refers to pharmaceuticals, food for medicinal use, cosmetics, food, and medical devices. The V Book refers to the practice of medicine and other health professions, and the VI Book describes the regulatory issues concerning laboratories and pharmacies, among others. Last, the IX Book relates to procedures and penalties, such as inspection, health proceedings, and sanitation penalties.

The Ministry of Health is the authority responsible for approving the pharmacopeia governing the country. Chile was the first country in South America publishing an official pharmacopeia in 1886.[h]

With respect to the practice of medicine and other health professions such as pharmacy and dentistry, the Code indicates that qualifications must be awarded by universities recognized by the State of Chile. Those who meet the requirements set by the university are legally entitled to practice their profession.

Regarding laboratories, pharmacies, and others, manufacturing and processing of pharmaceutical products are permitted only in pharmacies and laboratories with the corresponding authorization. Thus, no pharmacy and pharmaceutical industry can be installed, operated, or moved to another place without authorization from the SNSS, which is responsible for supervision. The Sanitary Code also provides that the sale of pharmaceuticals for human use should be carried out in the community pharmacy under the supervision of a pharmacist as a technical director. However, the SNSS can authorize the installation and

---

[h]It was the work of Dr Adolfo Murillo, former dean of the Faculty of Medicine and Pharmacy, University of Chile, and the pharmacist Charles Middleton. The first pharmacopeia was edited in Leipzig, Germany.

operation of drugstores (other than community pharmacies) for dispensing pharmaceuticals of low complexity (over-the-counter (OTC) drugs) run by a pharmacy technician. The SNSS can also authorize the operation of medicine cabinets for dispensing or sale of drugs and first aid items according to health regulations. These cabinets can be placed in clinics, maternities, nursing homes, mining camps, spas, medical centers, military barracks, and ships. Instead, drugstores and pharmaceutical laboratories, medicinal foods, cosmetics, and hygiene products should be technically managed by a pharmacist. On the other hand, the processing of raw materials and drugs of biological origin obtained by biological processes can be carried out under the technical direction of a biochemist, a physician–microbiologist, or a veterinary surgeon.

As for pharmaceuticals, these can be sold to the public only by prescription, except those determined by regulation.

4.1 National Drug Policy[9]

The National Drug Policy of Chile (Resolution No. 1248 of the Ministry of Health published in August 1996) replaced the one in existence since 1985. This new policy defined the drug as primary for social good health, proposing equitable access to essential medicines, ensuring an efficient use of resources for drugs, and promoting rational drug use (RDU) and quality assurance standards. Its strategic guidelines were based on the updated list of the National Drug Formulary and the National Drugs and Cosmetics Registration System, to encourage the manufacturing of high-quality medicines—effective and safe—and the import of biological products and vaccines to meet therapeutic coverage in major diseases. Furthermore, the existence of a national system of quality control, registration and sale of pharmaceuticals, medicinal foods, and cosmetics ensures transparency, efficiency, and quality of the system.

In relation to marketing, the proposal was looking after the achievement of international agreements on the control of illicit use of narcotic drugs and psychotropics and the strengthening of professional responsibility in drug prescribing, in terms of compliance with the conditions of sale and authenticity of the prescription. The pharmacist would play an important role in dispensing and in the maintenance of medical indications under the marketing conditions of the drugs. Other issues raised in this resolution were strengthening the role of the public sector in purchasing drugs and advertising restrictions for drugs, since until then drug publicity had not favored RDU.

Finally, the training of health professionals would support the importance of medicines in health care and would facilitate the pharmacist as an active member of health teams. Regarding research, the proposal integrated all aspects related to medicines and ensured compliance with international agreements on human experimentation.

In summary, seven lines of action with the character of warranty reflected in technical standards and other legal instruments were considered in the context of health reform by the National Drug Policy in 1995:

1. Access to and availability of drugs
2. Quality of drugs
3. Rational drug use
4. New role of pharmacy and the pharmacist
5. Implementation, development, and evaluation of drug policy
6. Scientific and technological research
7. Training of human resources

However, the need to update the National Drug Policy led to a new health reform in 2002. Since drugs are an important part of out-of-pocket spending in Chilean homes, in 2000 the government had already adapted this policy to the so-called Regime of Explicit Health Guarantees to "ensure timely and equitable access of the population to drugs."[6] Finally, the new National Drug Policy was approved by Resolution No. 515/2004. At that time, the private drug spending expressed in units sold was as follows: 39.4% generic, 38.5% branded generics, and 22.1% brand name drugs. In the private sector, brand name drugs were the main contribution to the total market (43.3%), while generics accounted for only 7.7%. Drug coverage was represented as 87.3% of out-of-pocket expense, while self-medication amounted to 50% of consumption, mainly by pharmacy retail, of which 37% of the pharmacies belong to three big chains controlling 90% of the private market. Moreover, important shortcomings such as gaps in access and availability of drugs in the National Drug Formulary, failures in the supply of medicines in the public sector, weakening of health programs in terms of administration, and shortage of professional resources in the pharmacy network were identified.

Against this background, the update of the National Drug Policy was intended to "ensure availability and access to essential medicines in the National Formulary to the entire population, efficiency and guaranteed quality, safe and affordable and rational drug use to maximize health benefits to the people and control the expenditure they represent" in order to reduce inequities in access, timeliness, and quality of health care.

The results of the National Health Survey 2009–2010 revealed the importance of chronic nontransmissable diseases in shaping the country's epidemiological profile. Also, a change in the demographic pyramid was seen, with a growing elderly population. According to drug consumption, it became clear that about half of the Chilean population was consuming any medication, with an average of two drugs per person.[10]

In relation to total consumption per household, Chile is one of the countries with the largest out-of-pocket health expenditure in the OECD (4.6% vs 3% on average).[9] Drugs are the main component of this spending, affecting more the households in the lowest income quintiles (Figure 4).[11]

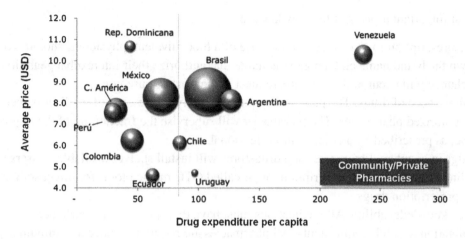

Figure 4

Average price of drugs vs drug expenditure in pharmacies in various Latin American countries. The size of the bubble reflects the population of each country. Values are expressed in terms of output prices of a pharmaceutical laboratory. *Source: IMS Midas–IMS Consulting.*

Considering that people whose income is below a set level have drug coverage delivered through the public health network, the hypotheses in relation to the designated out-of-pocket expense were as follows:

1. It corresponds to a self-medication consolidated at the private pharmacy (community pharmacy).
2. It is the result of the purchase of medicines that should be bought through the public network but are purchased in the private sector.
3. They are prescriptions corresponding either to private medical attention or to the Free-Choice Mode of FONASA, for which there is no drug coverage in the public network.

To correct and regulate the failures of the drug market, the so-called "Drug Law" underwent parliamentary debate between 2010 and 2014. The health status of pharmacy and the role of public institutions regarding medicines were some of the targeted issues under discussion.

4.2 A new drug law

On 24 February 2014, a new drug law came into force. This new law defines the pharmacy as a health center and medicines as essential goods for health and not as a commodity.

The new National Drug Law has three pillars: (1) access, (2) product quality, and (3) price. Its enactment led to a modification of the Sanitary Code in terms of the regulation of pharmacy and medicines.

The most important aspects of the new law are:

- The prescription form changes. In the case of a bioequivalent, physicians should write down the brand name and the generic name that authorize their interexchangeability. The exchange will occur at the patient's request at the time of purchase.
- Unitary dose of drugs. The patient may purchase only the amount of medication needed in authorized pharmacies. The pharmacist will supervise the fractioning of the required dose, as prescribed by a competent professional.
- Drugs in counters. Pharmacies and drugstores will install shelves available to users for selling drugs without a prescription, or so-called OTC medications, for direct selling of nonprescription drugs.
- Price knowledgeability. All medications must have their price on the package.
- Obligation to sell bioequivalents. All pharmacies are required to have a minimum supply of bioequivalent products for sale if the customer demands.
- Mobile pharmacies and drugstores can be installed in places such as small towns and neighborhoods where there are no pharmacies.
- Prohibition of fees associated with certain products.
- Purchase abroad. This empowers the national supplying warehouse (CENABAST)[i] to provisionally register drugs or products in case of shortage, emergency, or inaccessibility.
- Advertising of prescription drugs in mass media is prohibited.

4.3 The new molecules in Chile[15]

According to international estimates 32–36 new molecules come annually onto the global drug market. Eventually, a proportion of these enter local markets owing to restrictions imposed by regulatory agencies. In Chile the entity in charge of registering medicines, including new molecules, is the ISP. According to its records 33 new molecules were approved in 2013 (Figure 5), just six more molecules than in the United States, where 27 new molecules of 36 applications (75%) were approved in the same year.[16]

As of April 2014, eight applications for new molecule approval had been presented to the ISP at a constant rate of two per month. However, there is a significant gap relative to the world market, which is about 2 years ahead. Note that although the ISP has detailed information about the effectiveness and safety of new molecules owing to the registration process itself, this entity has no evidence on health technology assessment, either nationally or internationally. This includes evidence of cost effectiveness, expected demand for the new molecule in the Chilean health care system, and other specific considerations that can be addressed only through an evaluation process not yet systematized in our country.

---

[i]Acronym corresponding to the name of the organization in Spanish: Central Nacional de Abastecimiento.

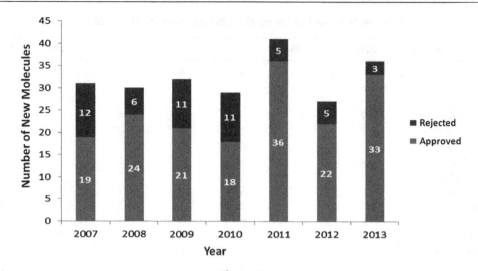

Figure 5
Approved and rejected new molecules in Chile from 2007 through 2013. *Source: Subdepartment of Registration and Health Authorizations, ANAMED, ISP, 2013.*

The ISP has registered new molecules accepted in Chile from the year 2007 onward. During the period 2007–2013 the new molecules approved for marketing according to the ATC (Anatomical, Therapeutic, and Chemical) Classification System mainly belong to the central nervous system, cardiovascular, oncology, and metabolic categories. The group of anticancer drugs has shown the greatest development in recent years, reaching 11 new molecules in 2013 (Table 4).

The new molecules have been classified by the Pharmacoeconomics Unit of the School of Public Health, University of Chile, in collaboration with the ISP and from legal sources, as follows:

- Orphan drugs: Any drug for the diagnosis, prevention, or treatment of a rare disease appropriately declared as such. Additionally, any drug considered the only option available on the market to treat a specific medical condition is considered an orphan drug.
- "First-in-class": Molecules that show a new and unique mechanism of action for treating a disease. This classification is an indicator of the innovative nature of the new molecule.
- "Me too": Molecules chemically similar or showing the same mechanism of action as another molecule already registered.
- High-cost medication (MAC): Expensive drugs used for the treatment of infrequently existing diseases (expensive).[j]

---

[j]FONASA. Definicion Modificada de Medicamentos de Alto Costo según FONASA. In: Report New Molecules in Chile. Sub-Department of Studies and Scientific Department ETESA, ISP, January–April 2014. Available at: http://www.fonasa.cl/wps/wcm/connect/internet/sa-general/asegurados/plan+de+salud/programas+especiales/med icamentos+de+alto+costo/medicamentos+de+alto+costo.

Table 4: New molecules on the Chilean market: 2007–2013

Therapeutic Class	2007	2008	2009	2010	2011	2012	2013
Oncology	4	5	6	4	10	3	11
Central nervous system	4	3	2	2	5	3	2
Cardiovascular	2	2	4	2	5	4	2
Metabolic	0	3	1	2	4	2	3
Endocrine	2	2	0	1	2	2	2
Antiviral	2	2	1	0	0	2	4
Diabetes	1	0	1	0	1	2	5
Antibiotic	0	2	1	3	1	1	0
Gastrointestinal	0	0	1	1	3	1	0
Genitourinary	0	0	0	3	1	0	1
Respiratory	0	1	1	0	1	0	2
Ophthalmic	1	0	1	0	2	1	0
Antifungal	2	0	1	0	0	0	0
Musculoskeletal	0	2	0	0	0	1	0
Hematology	0	1	1	0	0	0	0
Radiology	0	0	0	0	0	0	1
Dermatology	0	0	0	0	1	0	0
Phototherapy	1	0	0	0	0	0	0
Antihelminthic	0	1	0	0	0	0	0
Total	19	24	21	18	36	22	33

Source: Subdepartment of Registration and Sanitary Authorizations. ANAMED, ISP, 2013.

Considering the profile of new molecules registered in the period 2007–2013, about 25% were orphan drugs; more than 30% were classified as "First-in-class," indicating the innovative character of the new drugs entering the country; about 70% corresponded to the "Me too" group, and approximately 20% belong to the MAC category (Figure 6).

With respect to therapeutics, in 2013 the ISP reported a total of 21 new molecules, mostly for cancer therapies, followed by antiretroviral drugs, antidiabetic drugs, and drugs used for the central nervous system and metabolic diseases (Table 5).

In 2014, ANAMED and ETESA started a registration database of new molecules and their pharmacoeconomic profiles. This was done to provide timely information to the appropriate authority on the expected demand for these drugs, the health technology assessment processes occurring in other countries, and their estimated international price. Thus, between January and April 2014 there were eight applications for registration: four corresponding to orphan drugs and "First-in-class," one of them being a "unique on the drug market" type (ocriplasmin—Jetrea® for ophthalmic use); two nonorphan drugs corresponding to the "Me too" group; and two nonorphan drugs that were "First-in-class." Of these, more than 60% were antineoplastic and immunosuppressive molecules (Table 6).

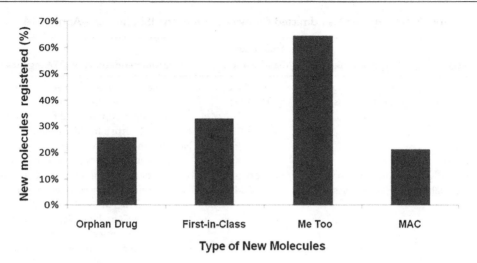

Figure 6

New molecules registered in the period 2007–2013 according to classification. *Source: Subdepartment of Registration and Health Authorizations, ANAMED, ISP, 2013.*

Table 5: New molecules entering the pharmaceutical market in Chile in 2013

Active Ingredient	Brand Name	Therapeutic Area	Disease
Bendamustine hydrochloride	Ribomustin®	Oncology	Chronic lymphocytic leukemia
Regorafenib	Stivarga®	Oncology	Colorectal cancer Gastrointestinal stromal tumors
Degarelix acetate	Firmagon®	Oncology	Prostatic cancer
Axitinib	Inlyta®	Oncology	Renal cell carcinoma
Vemurafenib	Zelboraf®	Oncology	Melanoma
Crizotinib	Xalkori®	Oncology	Non-small-cell lung cancer
Afatinib	Giotrif®	Oncology	Non-small-cell lung cancer
Pertuzumab	Perjeta®	Oncology	Breast cancer
Taliglucerase alfa	Uplyso®	Metabolic	Gaucher's disease type I
Idusurfase	Elaprase®	Metabolic	Hunter's disease
Pasireotide	Signifor®	Endocrine	Cushing's disease
Insulin aspart 30%	Ryzodeg 70/30®	Diabetes	Diabetes
Lixisenatide	Lyxumia®	Diabetes	Diabetes
Dapagliflozin	Forxiga®	Diabetes	Diabetes
Rilpivirine hydrochloride	Edurant®	Antiviral	Human immunodeficiency virus (HIV)
Emtricitabine + Rilpivirine hydrochloride	Complera®	Antiviral	Human immunodeficiency virus (HIV)
Gadobutrol	Gadovist®	Radiological diagnosis	Magnetic resonance imaging (contrast enhancement)
Promestriene	Colpotrophine®	Genitourinary tract	Vaginal trophic disorders
Teriflunomide	Aubagio®	Central nervous system	Multiple sclerosis
Fampridine	Fampyra®	Central nervous system	Multiple sclerosis
Apixaban	Eliquis®	Cardiovascular	Thromboembolism

Source: Subdepartment of Registration and Health Authorizations, Department of Scientific Affairs, ANAMED, ISP, 2013.

Table 6: New molecules admitted for evaluation of the ISP, January–April 2014

Drug	Type of Drug	Therapeutic Classification	Recommendations of HTA Agencies
Jetrea® (ocriplasmin)	Orphan drug "First-in-class"	Ophthalmic (S01XA22)	NICE: Recommended for use in the English health system. SMC: Not recommended for use in the Scottish health system. Health Canada: Recommended for use as a treatment for vitreous-macular traction.
Lemtrada® (alemtuzumab)	Orphan drug "First-in-class"	Antineoplastic (L01XC04)	NICE: In development, although the committee has no willingness to recommend it. SMC: In development. Health Canada: In development. FDA: Approval rejected. Does not demonstrate that benefits are greater than adverse effects.
Cosentyx® (secukinumab)	Nonorphan drug "First-in-class"	Immunosuppressive (L04AC10)	Without information
Erivedge® (vismodegib)	Nonorphan drug "First-in-class"	Antineoplastic (L01XX43)	AWMSG: Not authorized because necessary documents were not submitted. Thus, it cannot be accepted or prescribed by the Wales health system.
Mekinist® (trametinib)	Orphan drug "First-in-class"	Antineoplastic (L01XE25)	NICE: Indicates that it is not appropriate to include an appraisal as monotherapy. Is developing an appraisal as a combination therapy. Health Canada: It was approved as a monotherapy and combination therapy. Among the reasons for acceptance shows only risk/benefit analysis and clinical effectiveness study. FDA and TGA: Both have approved as monotherapy and combination therapy.
CIMAher® (nimotuzumab)	Orphan drug for the treatment of gliomas "First-in-class"	Antineoplastic monoclonal antibody	NICE: Making an appraisal for the treatment of pancreatic cancer, but the manufacturer has not indicated that CIMAher® is indicated for such treatment. EMA: Has rejected the marketing application for the treatment of gliomas in adults and children.
Tachyben® (urapidil)	Nonorphan drug "Me Too"	Antihypertensive (C02CA06)	Without information
Fenticonazole (generic)	Nonorphan drug "Me Too"	Antifungal (G01AF12) (D01AC12)	Without information

HTA, Health Technology Assessment; AWMSG, All Wales Medicines Strategy Group (Wales); EMA, European Medicines Agency (Europe); FDA, Food and Drug Administration (USA); NICE, National Institute for Health and Care Excellence (England and Wales); SMC, Scottish Medicines Consortium (Scotland); TGA, Therapeutic Goods Administration (Australia).
Source: Subdepartment of Registration and Health Authorizations, Department of Scientific Affairs, ANAMED, ISP, 2013.

5. Drug use issues in Chile

5.1 The Chilean pharmaceutical market[12]

The National Center for Pharmacoeconomics (CENAFAR), under the ISP, is the unit for the study and monitoring of the pharmaceutical market.

The morphology of the pharmaceutical market in Chile can be described on three levels: production, distribution, and dispensing of pharmaceuticals. According to the ANAMED, in the year 2013, there were 29 laboratories producing drugs, five conditional pharmaceutical laboratories, and 219 companies or individuals registered for importing drugs into Chile. Distribution of drugs may be carried out by public or private distributors. The public supplier is CENABAST and it is responsible for buying drugs and medical supplies for the local public health care network.

Dispensing of drugs is divided into the dispensation granted in hospitals and clinics of the public system and marketing by private pharmacies. Concerning the latter, more than 90% of the sales in this market are due to three main pharmacy chains (Cruz Verde, FASA Chile, and SalcoBrand).[k] According to official statistics in October 2013 there were 2719 pharmacies established in Chile. Of these, 1303 are in the Metropolitan Region (47.9%), 283 in the Valparaiso Region (10.4%), and 267 (9.9%) in the Bio-Bio Region, which together represent 68% of all pharmacies in the country (Table 7).

Table 7: Pharmacies in Chile by region, October 2013

Region	Number of Pharmacies
Arica y Parinacota	27
Tarapacá	50
Antofagasta	79
Atacama	45
Coquimbo	92
Valparaiso	283
Metropolitan	1303
O'Higgins	134
Maule	164
Bio-Bio	267
Araucania	99
Los Rios	44
Los Lagos	102
Aysen	9
Magallanes	21
Total nation	2719

Source: Department of Pharmaceutical Policies and Medical Professions, Ministry of Health.

[k]Two other pharmacy chains are also in Chile: Carmen, and Belen and Mendoza.

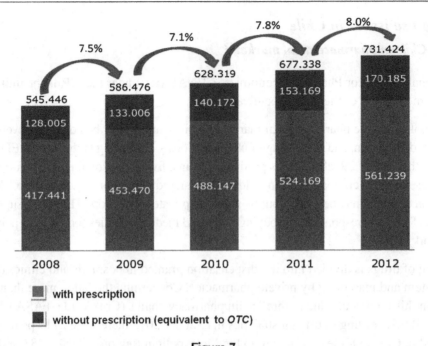

Figure 7

Drug market behavior in Latin America from 2008 to 2012. *Source: Report Ministry of Economics. In: Data Base IMS Chile, 2013.*

Likewise, according to data provided by Vasallo[1] in 2010 on the pharmaceutical market, Chile is relatively small in the Latin American context, occupying 2.6%, far below the leaders: According to a report by the Ministry of Economics of Chile, the largest top three Retail Pharmacy Chains have presented a sales growth on drugs between 7% and 8% per year since 2008. (Figure 7). Of this total, 76.7% is accounted for by drugs that require a prescription and the remaining 23.3% were direct-selling drugs.

Four types of pharmaceutical products coexist in the Chilean market:[13]

1. OTC drugs, which can be freely purchased by the patient;
2. Ethical or prescription drugs that do not require stock control;
3. Ethical drugs requiring stock control (inventory) (e.g. psyhotropic); and
4. Special imported drugs, usually purchased directly by health centers and whose use is limited to hospitals and health centers.

In terms of their marketing in pharmacies, four drugs are distinguished:

1. Generic: includes drugs sold under the name of the active ingredient that has proven therapeutic equivalence.
2. Brand: those produced by the laboratory that owns the patent.

---

[1]Vasallo, C. 2010. In: El mercado de medicamentos en Chile, 2013. These results correspond to a consultancy made by the Ministry of Health in 2010.

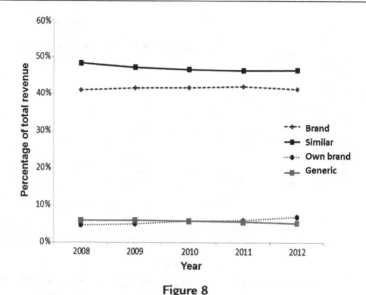

Figure 8
Drug market share by type of marketing in terms of percentage of the total revenue. *Source: Report "The Pharmaceutical Market in Chile," Ministry of Economics, 2013.*

3. Related: those drugs marketed under a name other than the active principle.
4. From own brand: those produced by the same laboratories belonging to the pharmacy itself.

According to Vassallo, one of the most important factors underlying the major changes in the pharmaceutical market in Chile since 1995 is the emergence of three pharmacy chains in the late 1990s. Today they represent over 90% of the retail pharmaceutical market. This structure has allowed them to exert a great bargaining power and, therefore, to have the ability to manage drug prices. At the same time, agreements between these pharmaceutical chains and department stores have also allowed people to access credit. At the beginning of the twenty-first century, competition between chains caused a significant drop in prices of drugs that adversely affected their own profits. Subsequently, drug prices increased progressively. One of the reasons that explained this behavior was collusion between pharmacy chains, which has been recently confirmed by the Chilean courts.

As was mentioned, a report from the Ministry of Economics showed that similar drugs accounted for 46.5% of 2012 revenues of pharmacies, followed by branded pharmaceuticals (41%), pharmacies' own branded drugs (7%), and generics (5.3%). An analysis carried out between 2008 and 2012 showed that the proportion of sales by brand was maintained, similar drugs went down between 1 and 2%, own brand increased by 2.3%, and generics decreased by 0.6% (Figure 8).

The same distribution was observed by units sold in 2012 and shows the high consumption of similar drugs (38.6%) versus 28.5% for generics, 20.6% for brands, and 12.3% for own pharmacy brands (Figure 9).

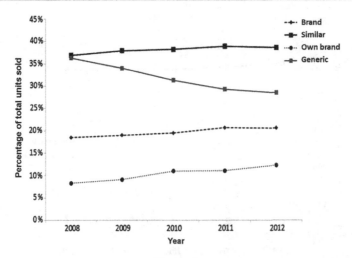

Figure 9

Drug market share by type of marketing in terms of percentage of total units sold. *Source: Report "The Pharmaceutical Market in Chile," Ministry of Economics, 2013.*

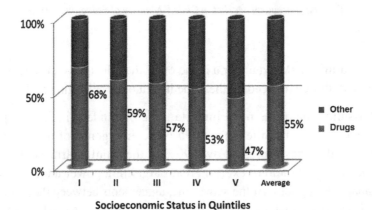

Figure 10

Relationship between percentage of total out-of-pocket health expenditure and socioeconomic status: 2009–2010. *Source: National Health Survey (2009–2010), Ministry of Health. In: CENAFAR, 2013.*

Regarding the population's total expenditure on health in 2009–2010, 55% was due to drugs, with a gradient disfavoring the poorest, at approximately 68% (Figure 10). Moreover, the CASEN[m] National Survey revealed that 33% of patients buy all the medicines prescribed.

---

[m]Survey conducted by the government of Chile since 1985, characterized by measuring the socioeconomic conditions of households in the country in terms of access to health, education, work, and housing conditions. This survey provides data such as the poverty and indigence of the population and income distribution, among others. The design allows for guidance of new projects and making changes to remuneration schemes of benefits to improve targeting those selected. Universities, academic institutions, and other entities are also users of the information provided by the CASEN survey.

In terms of drug prices, Chile does not have a policy of price regulation concerning the private sector or retail. The Chilean market displays a large dispersion, and the differences can be as high as 6533%. In the public system, although CENABAST is the entity in charge of buying medicines and medical supplies, it is far from managing all public purchases.

In Chile, drug consumption is mainly determined by the patients' needs and the choice made by health professional prescribers. However, the pharmaceutical market has imperfections, which determine relative importance of other factors, such as:

- Prescriber's information regarding the supply of drugs on the market;
- Therapeutic equivalence and relative prices;
- Effect of the pharmacist and the pharmacy technician on the patient's final election of a certain drug;
- Marketing exercised by the pharmaceutical industry on physicians and the patients themselves;
- Loyalty to established brands.

In Chile there is insufficient information on drug use. The available data correspond to results from the National Health Survey 2009–2010 mainly based on self-report of respondents and on the diagnosis and analysis of the CASEN survey applied in 2009. In summary, it can be concluded that:

- Women have a prevalence of at least one drug compared to men, adjusted for age (64% vs 40.7%, $p < 0.001$).
- The average of drugs consumed is 1.4 with an asymmetric distribution and consumption values of up to 16 drugs.
- The prevalence of consumption increases significantly with age.
- The prevalence of polypharmacy (consumption of five or more drugs) was estimated at 8.2%.
- Less educated and lower income groups consume more drugs (62.4% vs 48.4 and 55.5% in the medium- and high-level socioeconomic groups, respectively).
- The average number of drugs consumed did not differ between rural and urban area, although according to geographical distribution the Region of Antofagasta in northern Chile (Region I) reports increased consumption of at least one drug (73.8%). This value is significantly higher than the Metropolitan Region (55.3%) (Figure 11).

Regarding the prevalence of consumption by type of drug, 22.7% of the population reported consuming analgesics, 13.3% antihypertensive agents of the renin–angiotensin–aldosterone axis, and 8.3% anti-inflammatory and antirheumatic agents (Table 8).

In relation to the prevalence of acute and chronic use of drugs as chemical type in the general population, the most consumed drug was acetylsalicylic acid followed by paracetamol and enalapril. Regarding the chronic use of drugs (1 month or more) the list is quite similar; the first one is acetylsalicylic acid, followed by enalapril and paracetamol (Table 9).

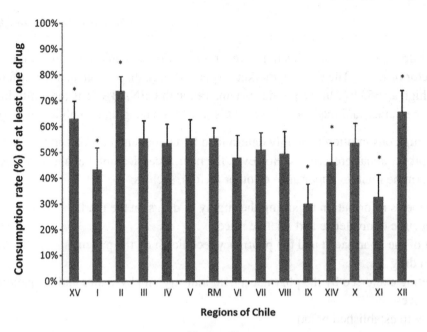

Figure 11

Prevalence of at least one drug consumed. RM, Metropolitan Region. *p < 0.05 compared to prevalence in the Metropolitan Region. *Source: Margozzini P, Olea R, Passi A. Deferred Report No. 2 ENS 2009–2010. In: Report New Molecules in Chile. Subdepartment of Studies and Scientific Department ETESA, ISP, January–April 2014.*

Table 8: Prevalence and 95% confidence intervals of the 20 most commonly used types of drugs by the Chilean population

Type	Prevalence (%)	Confidence Interval (%)
Analgesics	22.7	20.8–24.7
Agents acting on the renin–angiotensin–aldosterone axis	13.3	11.9–14.9
Anti-inflammatory and antirheumatic	8.3	7.2–9.5
Sex hormones and modulators of the genital system	8.0	6.8–9.4
Psychoanaleptics	7.8	6.7–9.2
Agents for treating disorders caused by acids	6.5	5.6–7.6
Diuretics	6.1	5.2–7.1
Drugs used in diabetes	5.9	5.0–7.0
Lipid-lowering agents	5.3	4.3–6.4
Beta-blockers	5.1	4.2–6.1
Psycholeptics	4.6	3.7–5.8
Systemic antihistamines	3.9	3.2–4.8
Vitamins	3.7	3.0–4.6
Calcium channel blockers	3.6	2.9–4.4
Antiepileptic	3.2	2.4–4.3
Mineral supplements	3.1	2.4–3.9
Thyroid therapy	2.9	2.3–3.6
Systemic antibiotics	2.1	1.5–2.9
Drugs for obstructive airway diseases	1.9	1.3–2.7
Drugs for functional diseases of the stomach and intestine	1.7	1.1–2.4

Source: Margozzini P, Olea R, Passi A. Deferred Report No. 2 ENS 2009–2010. In: Report New Molecules in Chile. Subdepartment of Studies and Scientific Department ETESA, ISP, January–April 2014.

Table 9: Prevalence (and 95% confidence interval) of consumption of the 20 active substances most consumed by the Chilean population according to self-report of the ENS 2009–2010, global use and chronic use only (1 month or more)

	Acute and Chronic Use		Chronic Use	
	Active Ingredient	**Prevalence (CI 95%)**	**Active Ingredient**	**Prevalence (CI 95%)**
1	Acetylsalicylic acid	12.0 (10.5–13.6)	Acetylsalicylic acid	10.4 (9.2–11.7)
2	Paracetamol	10.2 (8.9–11.8)	Enalapril	8.6 (7.5–9.9)
3	Enalapril	9.1 (7.9–10.4)	Paracetamol	7.5 (6.4–8.7)
4	Ethinylestradiol	6.5 (5.4–7.8)	Ethinylestradiol	6.4 (5.3–7.6)
5	Metformin	5.0 (4.1–6.0)	Metformin	4.8 (3.9–5.8)
6	Hydrochlorothiazide	4.8 (4.0–5.7)	Hydrochlorothiazide	4.6 (3.8–5.5)
7	Omeprazole	3.8 (3.1–4.7)	Omeprazole	3.6 (2.9–4.4)
8	Ibuprofen	3.8 (3.1–4.7)	Losartan	3.5 (2.8–4.4)
9	Losartan	3.6 (2.9–4.5)	Levonorgestrel	3.4 (2.6–4.5)
10	Levonorgestrel	3.5 (2.7–4.5)	Atorvastatin	2.8 (2.1–3.7)
11	Atorvastatin	2.9 (2.2–3.8)	Atenolol	2.7 (2.0–3.5)
12	Atenolol	2.8 (2.2–3.7)	Levothyroxine sodium	2.6 (2.0–3.4)
13	Levothyroxine sodium	2.8 (2.2–3.5)	Ibuprofen	2.5 (1.9–3.2)
14	Caffeine	2.8 (2.1–3.7)	Caffeine	2.3 (1.7–3.1)
15	Calcium carbonate	2.3 (1.7–3.0)	Nifedipine	2.2 (1.7–2.8)
16	Metamizole sodium	2.2 (1.7–3.0)	Glibenclamide	2.0 (1.5–2.7)
17	Nifedipine	2.2 (1.7–2.8)	Clonazepam	2.0 (1.3–2.9)
18	Glibenclamide	2.1 (1.6–2.7)	Calcium carbonate	1.8 (1.3–2.5)
19	Clonazepam	2.1 (1.5–3.1)	Metamizole sodium	1.8 (1.3–2.5)
20	Chlorpheniramine maleate	2.0 (1.5–2.7)	Chlorpheniramine maleate	1.7 (1.2–2.3)

Source: Margozzini P, Olea R, Passi A. Deferred Report No. 2 ENS 2009–2010. In: Report New Molecules in Chile. Subdepartment of Studies and Scientific Department ETESA, ISP, January–April 2014.

5.2 Rational and responsible drug use

The WHO states that governments should ensure RDU in terms that "Patients should receive appropriate drugs and doses for an appropriate time and at the lowest cost for them and the community, according to their clinical needs and individual situation."

In connection with the WHO guidelines, Chile has a National Drug Policy, which includes rational use and responsible medication in order to: "Ensure the availability and access to effective, safe and affordable essential medicines in the National Formulary to the entire population, so that its rational use leads to maximize benefits both to the people's health and the expenditure control they represent."

However, the current drug market situation does not meet the assumptions outlined above. Currently, people perceive the pharmacy market as being very competitive and it should be more transparent and closer to them because of its vital importance for the population.

Furthermore, the availability of drugs under current conditions is against some of the goals of the Public Health Policies, as the provision of drugs is limited or scarce in several communes. Thus, modifications incorporated into the actual Drug Law extend the places to purchase drugs in accordance with health regulations.

The National Survey of Rational Drug Use carried out by the Ministry of Health in 2011 showed that 71% of the population purchases drugs in pharmacies and drugstores. The remaining 29% of the population do so in unauthorized kiosks, public markets, and street trading, which do not meet sanitary requirements and supply the country's poorest population. Therefore, 3 of 10 Chileans buy drugs in places that are not specifically authorized. Usually, these are commonly used drugs without prescription, but others do need it.[7,14]

The new Drug Law approved in 2014 authorizes the sale of direct-sale drugs or those without prescription (OTC) in groceries, mini-markets, convenience stores at gas stations, and supermarkets, which may have extended operating hours and are widely distributed throughout the country. These places must meet the health conditions and regulations established by the Ministry of Health. Enforcement and punishment of these places will be made by the ISP. The objective is to bring the availability of low-risk drugs to the population and promote responsible citizenship care.

Direct-selling drugs must be submitted in packages containing the necessary therapeutic indication on the outside to facilitate the decision to purchase and ensure adequate administration. In addition, packages must have labels for verifying whether the contents have been handled. Direct-selling drugs must be available on shelves or racks that allow direct access for purchasing in a special area designed exclusively for this purpose, so as to allow adequate preservation and storage. Implementation of security measures to prevent easy reach by children must be taken.

Data from the ISP show that in January 2013 the number of direct-selling medicines authorized in the country was 2431, representing 15.8% of registered products. Also, 23.3% of the value and 36.9% of the units corresponded to drugs sold over the counter, while 76.7% of revenues and 63.1% of the units were prescription drugs (Table 10).

Table 10: Types of drugs registered by the ISP, in January 2013, and market share and sales units of drugs in 2012

Products Registered by ISP	Number of Units	Percentage (%)	Market Share (%)	Market Share in Units (%)
Direct selling (without prescription)	2431	15.8	23.3	36.9
Dispensed with prescription	12,837	83.3	76.7	63.1
Exclusive to hospitals and clinics	143	0.9	–	–
Total	15,411	100	100	100

Source: ISP, 2013. In: Bulletin "Pharmacies and Poverty in Chile," Ministry of Economics, 2013.

5.3 Spending on drugs

Drugs registered in Chile are divided into 266 therapeutic classes. The first five represent 20.5% of total pharmacy sales and the top 20 account for almost 50% of market sales.

The female contraceptive hormone is a therapeutic class that generated more revenues for the three major pharmacy chains in 2012, with 6.4% of sales, followed by nonnarcotic analgesics with 3.9%, antirheumatics with 3.8%, antidepressants with 3.4%, and dermatological products with 3.1%. All of these products require prescription with the exception of dermatologicals representing 11.7% of direct sale products.

Other products sold in pharmacies without prescription showing a significant percentage of sales of direct-selling drugs are emollients and skin protectors with 11.6%, nonnarcotic analgesics with 9.8%, and antiflu medication with 5.1%.

Drug spending in the Chile will continue as economic development increases. Currently, it has an expense of US$82 per capita, while in Europe spending reaches US$261 per capita and in the United States US$1042 per capita. In comparison to Latin American countries, Chile's expenditure on drugs is lower than that in Argentina, Brazil, and Venezuela (Figure 12).

The top 20 medicines by therapeutic class based on expenditure and utilization are listed in Tables 11–13.

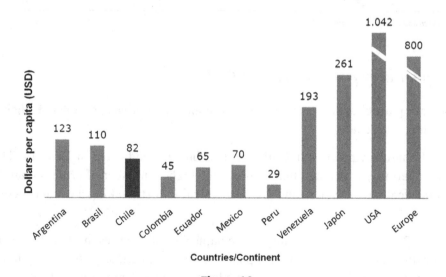

Figure 12
2012 per capita values for drug expenditure in U.S. dollars. *Source: IMS Health, World Review, Cartagena 2012.*

Table 11: The 20 most commercialized drugs in 2011 and 2012: total market share (net sales in CL pesos)

	Therapeutic Class	Market Share 2011 (%)	Market Share 2012 (%)
1	Contraceptive hormones	6.2	6.4
2	Nonnarcotic analgesics, antipyretic drugs	4.1	3.9
3	Nonsteroidal antirheumatics	3.8	3.8
4	Antidepressants and balancing drugs	3.5	3.4
5	Other dermatological products	2.7	3.1
6	Pediatric food	3.0	3.1
7	Emollients and protectors	2.9	3.0
8	Antiflu excipients (anti-inflammatory)	2.5	2.5
9	Antiepileptics	2.5	2.4
10	Antiulcer drugs	1.9	1.8
11	Antihistamines	1.9	1.7
12	Cholesterol and triglyceride regulators	1.8	1.7
13	Antidiabetics, biguanides	1.5	1.7
14	Broad-spectrum penicillins	1.6	1.5
15	Angiotensin II antagonists (combined–hypertension)	1.5	1.5
16	Other muscle and skeletal products	1.4	1.4
17	Antipsychotics	1.4	1.3
18	Antivirals (HIV)	1.1	1.3
19	Products against erectile dysfunction	1.2	1.2
20	Multivitamins with minerals	1.1	1.1
	Subtotal 20 most important drugs	47.2	47.5
	Other	52.8	52.5
	Total	100	100

Source: IMS Health and Ministry of Health, 2012.

6. Core pharmacy practice areas in Chile

Core pharmacy practice areas are manufacturing, community/private, hospital, medicine promotion/drug companies.

The areas of pharmacy practice in Chile are distributed as indicated in Table 14. The community pharmacy is the area that employs the highest number of professionals (65%), with both the health care system and pharmaceutical industry taking a distant second place.

In January 2012 the information existing on the number of pharmacies in Chile, both allopathic and homeopathic (both of them require a pharmacist), and pharmacies belonging to the health care system, whether pharmacies or medicine cabinets from primary health care centers, was as follows: 2507 allopathic pharmacies, 155 homeopathic pharmacies, 5300

Table 12: The 20 most commercialized prescription drugs in 2011 and 2012 (net sales in CL pesos)

	Therapeutic Class	Market Share 2011 (%)	Market Share 2012 (%)
1	Contraceptive hormones	8.0	8.3
2	Nonsteroidal antirheumatics	4.5	4.4
3	Antidepressants and balancing drugs	4.5	4.4
4	Antiepileptics	3.2	3.1
5	Pediatric food	2.8	2.8
6	Antiulcer drugs	2.4	2.3
7	Antihistamines	2.4	2.3
8	Cholesterol and triglyceride regulators	2.3	2.2
9	Antidiabetics, biguanides	2.0	2.2
10	Nonnarcotic analgesics, antipyretic drugs	2.1	2.2
11	Broad-spectrum penicillins	2.0	1.9
12	Angiotensin II antagonist (combined–hypertension)	1.9	1.9
13	Antipsychotics	1.8	1.7
14	Antiflu excipients (anti-inflammatory)	1.6	1.7
15	Antivirals (HIV)	1.5	1.7
16	Products against erectile dysfunction	1.5	1.5
17	Other muscle and skeletal products	1.5	1.5
18	Angiotensin II antagonists (only active principle)	1.4	1.4
19	Antitussives	1.4	1.3
20	Beta-blockers (only active principle)	1.2	1.2
	Subtotal 20 most important drugs	49.8	50.0
	Other	50.2	50.0
	Total	100	100

Source: IMS Health and Ministry of Health, 2012.

pharmacists working in community pharmacies,[n] and 220 working in health care pharmacies.[o]

6.1 Community pharmacy practice

From the beginning of the twenty-first century the institution of pharmacy practice in Chile has been clearly influenced by the economic logic implemented in the early 1980s. The clearest effect was the uncertainty of drug policy and, as said before, the phenomenon of the concentration of the ownership of pharmacies in large consortia with the top three being Cruz Verde, FASA Chile, and SalcoBrand.

[n]The calculated number of pharmacists corresponds to an average of two professionals per location. This number may be overestimated considering the vices and bad practices that occur in the area of community/private pharmacy.
[o]Source: Department of Pharmaceutical Policies and Medical Professions, ISP, April 2012.

Table 13: The 20 most commercialized nonprescription direct-selling drugs in 2011 and 2012 (net sales in CL pesos)

	Therapeutic Class	Market Share 2011 (%)	Market Share 2012 (%)
1	Other dermatological products	10.2	11.7
2	Emollients and protectors	11.4	11.6
3	Nonnarcotic analgesics, antipyretic drugs	11.0	9.8
4	Antiflu excipients (anti-inflammatory)	5.3	5.1
5	Antiobesity food	3.6	4.4
6	Stomatology	4.3	4.1
7	Pediatric food	3.7	3.8
8	Expectorants	4.0	3.8
9	Antacids, antiflatulents	3.4	3.0
10	Laxatives	2.9	2.8
11	Multivitamins with minerals	2.5	2.8
12	Platelet aggregation inhibitors	2.7	2.5
13	Healing	2.3	2.3
14	Tonics (diverse syrups)	2.0	2.3
15	Decongestants (pharynx)	2.2	2.2
16	Antirheumatic and topical analgesics	1.7	1.7
17	Pregnancy and ovulation tests	1.5	1.5
18	Other nontherapeutic products	1.6	1.5
19	Nonsteroidal antirheumatics	1.5	1.5
20	Dermatological antifungals	1.6	1.4
	Subtotal 20 most important drugs	79.4	79.9
	Other	20.6	20.1
	Total	100	100

Source: IMS Health and Ministry of Health, 2012.

Table 14: Main areas of pharmacy practice in Chile

Areas of Pharmacy Practice	Percentage
Community/private pharmacy	65
Health care	15
Pharmaceutical industry	15
Cosmetic industry	2
Regulatory affairs and other	3
Total	100

6.2 Poverty rate and number of community pharmacies[17]

The 2013 Report of the Ministry of Economics describes the relationship between the number of pharmacies and the regional poverty rate. Data were obtained from the CASEN survey of 2011, demographics from the INE, 2013, and administrative records of the Ministry of Health (the number of pharmacies by region in January 2013). The relationship between poverty and regional inhabitants per pharmacy is shown in Figure 13.

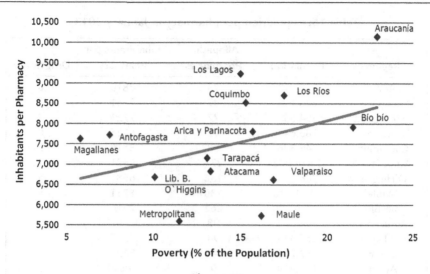

Figure 13
Poverty and regional inhabitants per pharmacy relationship in Chile: 2013. *Source: Bulletin "Relationship between number of pharmacies and poverty," Department of Studies, Ministry of Economics, 2013.*

Other conclusions obtained are the following:

- The more poverty, the more inhabitants per pharmacy. The correlation between the poverty rate and the number of inhabitants per pharmacy in a region is 0.4. That is, there are fewer pharmacies among the poorest population groups.
- The higher the income, the fewer inhabitants per pharmacy. The correlation between per capita income of households and the number of pharmacies per capita is −0.4. That is, there are fewer pharmacies in population groups with lower incomes.
- Poor regions have fewer pharmacies. The Region of La Araucania has 10,147 inhabitants per pharmacy and Bio-Bio 7916. Both regions have a poverty rate above 20%. The national average is 6603 inhabitants per pharmacy.
- The extreme regions have fewer pharmacies than the rest of the country. The Region of Aysen (south) has 11,911 inhabitants per pharmacy and Arica-Parinacota (north) 7810 inhabitants per pharmacy.
- Forty-eight percent of pharmacies are found in the Metropolitan Region. Of 2659 pharmacies nationwide, 1264 are located in the metropolitan area.
- Ninety-six communes[p] in the country do not have a pharmacy. Among them, 18 are situated in the region of Bio-Bio, 14 in Araucania, and 12 in Los Lagos.
- Chile is under the Latin American average. In 2008 Chile had 9438 inhabitants per pharmacy, whereas in Latin America the average was 3427.

Note that as reported by the Ministry of Economics (2013) revenue of pharmacies grew by 34.1% in 5 years. In 2008, sales were 545.446 million Chilean pesos and in 2012, 731.424 million pesos.

---

[p]A commune comprises a small city and its surroundings.

Table 15: Population per pharmacy in January 2013

Region	Population	Allopathic Pharmacies	Inhabitants per Pharmacy	Drugstores[a]
Arica	179,623	23	7810	0
Tarapaca	336,115	47	7151	1
Antofagasta	594,553	77	7721	4
Atacama	286,643	42	6825	0
Coquimbo	749,376	88	8516	5
Valparaiso	1,814,072	274	6621	1
O'Higgins	908,559	136	6681	4
Maule	1,031,618	180	5731	5
Bio-Bio	2,074,086	262	7916	5
Araucania	994,374	98	10,147	14
Los Lagos	867,344	94	9227	5
Los Rios	382,713	44	8698	3
Aysen	107,919	9	11,991	3
Magallanes	160,169	21	7627	2
Metropolitan	7,069,647	1264	5593	2
Total country	17,556,811	2659	6603	54

[a]As said before, other than community pharmacies.
Source: Bulletin "The Market for Medicines in Chile," Ministry of Economics, 2013.

According to records of the Ministry of Economics, in January 2013 there were 2659 allopathic or traditional pharmacies, and 1264 (48% of the total number) were located in the Metropolitan Region; of those, close to 1100 were in the capital city of Santiago. It is noteworthy that within the city there is a high level of displacement of the inhabitants, so most pharmacies are open during the daytime, and a very few are on duty or have an urgency service at nighttime. The number of pharmacies by region, as well as the regional population projected for 2013, and the number of inhabitants per pharmacy are shown in Table 15.

6.3 Municipalities without a pharmacy

The country has 96 municipalities that do not have pharmacy, mainly located in remote areas with low population. Of these, 27 have a pharmaceutical warehouse, and therefore, 69 do not have any property that has drugs for the population.

Pharmacies are usually located in large urban centers and market not only drugs but also other products. There are regions where all pharmacies are in the regional capital city, while other municipalities in the region do not have pharmacies and drugstores. In the southern regions, where there are several outlying towns and sparse population, the number of communes (municipalities) without pharmacies is high. In some cases, drugstores supply the entire population of the commune. Thus, the poorest, most remote, and least populated areas are

Table 16: Municipalities without pharmacy or drugstore by region of the country, 2013

Region	Number of Municipalities (Communes)	Municipalities without a Pharmacy	Percentage without a Pharmacy (%)	Municipalities without a Pharmacy and a Drugstore	Percentage without a Pharmacy and a Drugstore (%)	Poverty Index
Arica	4	3	75	3	75	15.7
Tarapaca	7	3	43	3	43	13.1
Antofagasta	9	3	33	2	22	7.5
Atacama	9	2	22	2	22	13.3
Coquimbo	15	6	40	4	27	15.3
Valparaíso	38	4	11	4	11	16.9
O'Higgins	33	9	27	8	24	10.1
Maule	30	3	10	2	7	16.2
Bio-Bio	54	18	33	16	30	21.5
Araucania	32	14	44	4	13	22.9
Los Lagos	12	1	8	1	8	15.0
Los Rios	30	12	40	8	27	17.5
Aysen	10	7	70	4	40	9.8
Magallanes	11	8	73	5	45	5.8
Metropolitan	52	3	6	3	6	11.5
Total country	346	96	28	69	20	14.4

Source: Bulletin "The Market for Medicines in Chile," Ministry of Economics, 2013.

lacking a vital health service. This can be explained because both the regulations and the structure of the pharmaceutical market were developed in the mid-1980s and are not relevant to the current conditions and needs of the population.

Table 16 shows the numbers of municipalities that have no pharmacy/drugstores by region and the regional poverty rate. It is observed that in the poorest regions a greater number of municipalities do not have a pharmacy or even at least a drugstore.

6.4 Community pharmacies in Chile compared to other Latin American countries

According to data from 2008, Chile has 9438 inhabitants per pharmacy; this is a poor indicator compared to Latin American countries. It is followed far behind by Venezuela, with 5449 inhabitants per pharmacy. Although by 2013 the number of pharmacies had increased, the relationship remains below those of other countries in the region (Table 17).

Based on 3427 inhabitants per pharmacy in Latin America one may say that Chile is far from a level that could be considered adequate. Note that in developed countries the number of inhabitants per pharmacy is even lower, and therefore, there is a wide gap to overcome. According to data reported by the Chilean Ministry of Health in 2013 there were 2400 inhabitants per pharmacy in Spain and 1100 in the United States.

Table 17: Number of pharmacies and population in Latin America: 2008

Country	Number of Pharmacies	Population (Thousands)	Inhabitants per Pharmacy
Chile	1798	16,970	9438
Venezuela	5246	28,583	5449
Dominican Republic	1980	10,090	5096
Central America	8686	39,500	4548
Peru	8287	29,165	3519
Mexico	31,398	109,610	3491
Bolivia	2867	9863	3440
Paraguay	1861	6349	3412
Brazil	58,232	193,734	3327
Argentina	12,979	40,276	3103
Uruguay	1250	3361	2689
Colombia	19,068	45,660	2395
Ecuador	5915	13,625	2303
Total Latin America	159,567	546,786	3427

Source: Ministry of Health, 2008.

6.5 Health care and hospital pharmacy practice[18]

As said before, the health care system in Chile is both public and private. Health facilities are diverse and widely distributed throughout the country. The following data were provided by the INE for 2013 (Table 18).

Pharmacy practice at the health care and hospital level is concerned with serving the people in their pharmaceutical needs, through the selection, preparation, acquisition, monitoring, and dispensing of drugs; providing drug information; and other activities aimed at achieving appropriate use, safe and cost-effective medicines, and health products that benefit patients seen in the hospital and its sphere of influence.

Even though in the early 1970s Chile was a leader in Latin America regarding clinical pharmacy, it was only at the beginning of the 1990s that pharmaceutical care acquired an important role in pharmacy practice, and the pharmacy curriculum started to move from a scientific-drug-centered pharmacist to a patient-centered profession. Yet, even though there has been important movement forward, when looking back at pharmacy practice in the Chilean health care system, there is still a lot to work to do now and in the near future, considering the new Drug Law approved in 2014.

Pharmacy practice in the health care system can be divided into that of the hospital pharmacy and primary health care. The total number of pharmacists in both hospitals and primary health care is not well known. However, according to the Ministry of Health, the number of pharmacists belonging to the National Health Services System (SNSS) between 2007 and 2011 has shown a moderate increment.[q] However, these numbers are very low compared to other health care professionals such as physicians, nurses, dentists, and midwives, among others (Table 19).

[q]National Institute of Statistics: Statistics Compendium 2013.

Table 18: Health facilities by grade of complexity and subsector (public/private) 2007–2011

	Year				
	2007	2008	2009	2010	2011
Total public and private health facilities	2386	2543	2464	2607	2594
Total public facilities	2197	2351	2288	2423	2489
National Health Services System (SNSS)	2183	2337	2272	2400	2477
Total hospitals SNSS	205	212	210	208	201
Hospitals (according to complexity)[a]					
High complexity	60	61	61	61	62
Medium complexity	23	23	23	23	26
Low complexity	99	99	99	99	99
Hospitals with agreement of collaboration	23	29	27	25	14
Total ambulatory health care centers (including municipal)	1978	2125	2062	2192	2276
Ambulatory health care centers of specialties	10	15	16	16	23
Primary health care centers	798	945	880	1012	1092
Rural health services	1170	1165	1166	1164	1161
Other public hospitals	14	14	16	23	12
Total private facilities	182	192	176	184	105
Employers mutuality hospitals	42	40	40	37	17
Private hospitals and clinics[b]	147	152	136	147	88
Total hospital beds	37,797	38,011	38,314	34,829	36,110
Beds in SNSS facilities	27,363	27,182	27,143	25,273	25,594
Beds in others public hospitals	2805	3064	3102	2789	3463
Beds in private facilities	7629	7765	8069	6767	7053
Availability of beds per 1000 inhabitants	2	2	2	2	2

[a]The Supreme Decree No. 140 of 2004 defines the classification of hospitals belonging to the public health care network according to their complexity (Law No. 19,937).
[b]Excluding homes, nursing homes, and similar. Including private hospitals and not-for-profit, the no longer existing ISAPRES, and agency administrators considered in Law No. 16,744.

Table 19: Numbers of some health care professionals in the SNSS between 2007 and 2011

Year	Pharmacists and Biochemists[a]	Physicians	Nurses	Midwives	Dentists	Dietitians
2007	420	16,165	7686	3987	3033	1601
2008	475	17,185	8002	4476	3.439	2037
2009	542	15,432	10,330	5481	4086	2768
2010	570	14,713	9859	4560	3659	1.996
2011	644	15,052	9601	4568	3874	1974

[a]Includes clinical chemistry laboratories; either pharmacists or biochemists are technical directors of the laboratories.

The distribution of pharmacists across the country is shown in Table 20.

Some important concepts about health care pharmacy practice are the following:

- Distribution and logistics
  - Receiving drugs

Table 20: Number of pharmacists in the SNSS by region: 2011

Region	2011
Arica and Parinacota	7
Tarapaca	10
Antofagasta	32
Atacama	10
Coquimbo	18
Valparaiso	76
O'Higgins	14
Maule	37
Bio-Bio	137
La Araucania	38
Los Rios	16
Los Lagos	26
Aysen	4
Magallanes	9
Metropolitan	210
Total	644

- • Goods in transit
- • Storage and distribution
- Dispensing
  - • Normal dispensing system
  - • Dispensing systems
  - • Presence of master formulas
- Clinical pharmacy

Pharmacological validation of prescriptions, drug monitoring and follow-up until discharge from the pharmacotherapy of hospitalized patients and at the primary health care system.

The National Corporation of Pharmaceutical Specialties Certification (CONACEF)[19] is the national agency responsible for carrying out the certification of particular pharmacy practice areas, in particular clinical chemistry and pharmacy practice in the health care system (hospital pharmacists and primary health care pharmacists). Its role is to accredit that training and pharmacy practice experience to allow the pharmacist to be considered as a specialist.

CONACEF is an autonomous body and most institutions involved in pharmacy practice and education are represented, that is, faculties of pharmacy of Chilean universities, the Chilean Academy of Pharmaceutical Sciences, the Chilean Society of Health Care Pharmacists (SCHFA), the Chilean Society of Clinical and Forensic Laboratory, and the Association of Pharmacists of Chile AG, which guarantees its independence and authority in their decisions. Certification is a voluntary process; however, it gives official recognition of special training in designated specialty areas.

Specific requirements for certification of specialists in health care pharmacy by CONACEF are:

Certification of a pharmaceutical chemist (pharmacist) awarded by a Chilean university and/ or foreign institution legalized, validated, and/or recognized in Chile.

At least 9 years of experience in pharmacy health care.

Proof of having completed a specialist training program in pharmacy health care of at least 1500 h certified by a Chilean university, considering drug management, drug information, management of sterile areas (oncology and parenteral nutrition), pharmaceutical care, pharmacoeconomics, pharmacoepidemiological formulation, and evaluation of projects and drug delivery systems. Online courses may have a differentiated score if the committee agrees.

In the case of graduate programs and degrees obtained abroad, the Certification Committee will evaluate the background and determine if they may be considered in the application.

Proof of at least 1500 h of training courses, seminars, workshops, or seminars in the pharmacy health care area within a maximum period of 9 years. These training activities should relate to pharmaceutical administration, drug information, sterile handling areas (oncology and parenteral nutrition), pharmaceutical care, pharmacoeconomics, pharmacoepidemiology, and drug dispensing systems.

An accredited training period postqualification equivalent to an academic year dedicated to the pharmacy health care area, in formal continuing education programs considering pharmaceutical management information, drug management in sterile areas (oncology and parenteral nutrition), pharmaceutical care, pharmacoeconomics, pharmacoepidemiology, formulation and projects evaluation, and drug dispensing systems.

It is important to highlight that both the Chilean Society of Health Care Pharmacists and its chapter of primary health care pharmacists[r] are very active professionally and are playing an important role relative to the new Drug Law.

6.6 Pharmacy education

6.6.1 Historical background of pharmacy education

The first "class" of pharmacy at the National Institute was founded on 28 February 1833. This institution did not have university status but its goal was to deliver "a methodical instruction of useful and necessary science." Its first chairman was José Vicente Bustillos, Professor of Organic Chemistry and Pharmacy.

At the end of the nineteenth century and after 90 years of independence, despite favorable circumstances arising from the exploitation of natural resources such as coal and silver, the shipping

---

[r]More information about their goals and activities is found at http://www.schfa.cl.

traffic through the Strait of Magellan, and the beginning of the nitrate boom, Chile had not managed to consolidate an economic, political, and social environment that allowed a balanced development. However, the economic and social flourishing of Chile attracted an immigrant flow of people with a good level of education. The city of Valparaiso hosted German pharmacists arriving in the 1850s who had studied chemistry and pharmacy and were imbued with the scientific spirit prevailing in Europe. These "new Chileans" transformed colonial pharmacy in a gradual but profound way into real laboratories where scientific and commercial research was carried out.

The forward thinking of the wealthy middle classes that characterized the Chilean society in the second half of the nineteenth century allowed in 1899 the first graduation of a woman pharmacist with a college degree, Maria Griselda Hinojosa Flores. This was an early recognition in the profession of equal rights for women.

Since the mid-nineteenth century the University of Chile has been the center of thinking for public and private action in the country. Proposals to improve the academic education as well as policies and procedures to be taken to give rise to social medicine emerged from health professionals who were turning to intense political activity.

Thus, various legal modifications separated the pharmacy school from medicine. In 1911, the School of Chemistry and Pharmacy within the Faculty of Medicine of the University of Chile was founded, and various changes in the years 1928, 1931, and 1936 prepared the way for the foundation of the first Faculty of Chemistry and Pharmacy in 1945. In 1917 a new university was founded in the city of Concepción (center south) without support or supervision of the state. Owing to the pharmaceutical progress in academia one of the first four courses that initiated their activities in 1919 in the recently created University of Concepción was Chemistry and Pharmacy. One year later (1920) this course would join the Faculty of Science.

In Chile, the history of the study of pharmacy is mainly linked to faculties of science or chemistry, which explains the strong basic science component that prevails in the pharmacy curriculum today. In fact, all pharmacy curricula are of chemistry and pharmacy and the professionals are called "pharmaceutical chemists."

6.7 Pharmacy education in 2015

As of this writing, there are 10 chemistry and pharmacy schools (Table 21).

Today's selection of chemistry and pharmacy students to enter the university is through a national test.

Some of the common characteristics of the chemistry and pharmacy curricula are:

- Generalist
- All curricula are defined as scientific and professional

Table 21: Faculties or Schools of Chemistry and Pharmacy in Chile as of February 2015

University	Category (Public/Private)	Foundation (Year)	Accreditation Status	Region
U. de Chile	Public	1911[b]	Yes	Metropolitan
U. de Concepcion	Private[a]	1919	Yes	Bio-Bio
U. de Valparaiso	Public	1972	Yes	Valparaiso
Pontificia U. Catolica	Private[a]	1987	Yes	Metropolitan
U. Austral de Chile	Private[a]	1994	On self-evaluation	Los Rios
U. Arturo Prat	Public	2000	Yes	Tarapaca
U. Catolica del Norte	Private[a]	2000	Yes	Antofagasta
U. Andres Bello	Private	1999	Yes	Metropolitan and Valparaiso
U. San Sebastian	Private	2000	Yes	Metropolitan and Bio-Bio
U. de Santiago	Public	2013	No[c]	Metropolitan

[a]Private universities that receive state contributions to the budget.
[b]First Class of Pharmacy at the National Institute, 1833.
[c]Recently founded.

- Once curricular requirements are accomplished the pharmacist is legally enabled to practice in community pharmacy, hospital pharmacy and health care system, pharmaceutical and cosmetics industries, regulatory entities, universities, and clinical laboratories, among other practice possibilities
- Duration of studies is 5–6 years depending on the particular school.

Although pharmacy schools may define their own pharmacist professional profile to support the pharmacy curriculum (most of them are defined by competencies), the National Accreditation Commission has defined it as:

> "Health Professional, specialist in drugs and other biologically active substances with solid knowledge in biological and chemical sciences with particular emphasis on pharmaceutical sciences, able to participate in actions related to the drug and its application to the individual in order to promote rational drug use and participate in the promotion of public health and improvement of the quality of life."[s]

7. Conclusions

In summary, the market for drugs is relevant in our country for the therapeutic needs of the population. During 2012, the three major pharmacy chains comprised around 95% of the market with sales of over US$1500 million just on drugs. Based on the analysis, a reform of

[s]National Accreditation Commission 1998. Available at: http://www.cnachile.cl/Criterios%20de%20carreras/quimi cayfarmacia.pdf.

the marketing system of direct sales drugs (OTC) is justified to easily provide them to the general public, improve education and awareness of responsible medication, and avoid health risks when not accomplished by the current regulations.

In addition, the health authority has a complete guideline to identify risks and implications of the various types of drugs. According to the ISP, direct-selling drugs correspond to 15.8% and prescription to 84.2% of the total.

Currently, the new Drug Law will allow families to compare by type of drug being marketed (brand, similar, own brand, and generic) and freely choose, especially those behind the counter requiring interaction with pharmacy technicians.[1] It is also necessary to consider that 29% of the population acquires drugs in public markets and other places without any sanitary care.

The most important issues of the National Drug Law, which amends the Sanitary Code, are:

- Prescription drugs by generic drug name guarantee transparency for users
- Dispensation by unit dose instead of more medication than required
- Quality
- Bioequivalence
- Restructuring of CENABAST
- New role of the pharmacist regarding the population's health; particularly important is the role of the health care pharmacist at different levels, either public or private
- Redefinition of the concept of "pharmacy"
- Strengthens the role of the Health Authority
- Sanctions on perverse incentives to increase sales

Some laws associated with the National Drug Law to date:

- National Drug Law, which amends the Health Code (Books IV and VI)
- Opening of sales of nonprescription drugs
- Establishment of the ANAMED

The new role of the pharmacist as individual or as an active member of the health care team is the biggest challenge the pharmacy profession is facing today in Chile. Pharmacotherapy monitoring, identification of adverse drug reactions, and patient education on knowledge and proper use of medications are some of the tasks pharmacy schools have considered in their new curricula. Competencies needed for a pharmacist whose professional goal was the drug but is now focused on the patient are challenges that have been faced since the late twentieth century. Pharmacists are directly involved in ensuring the population has access to safe, effective, high-quality, and low-cost drugs. The results regarding this "brand new pharmacist" will be seen more clearly in the coming years, as this requires not only an educational approach but also a governmental and political one related to the implementation and adjustment of the new public health policies.

---

[1] In Chile the role of the pharmacy technician is much more like that of a salesman.

Thus, from my perspective some of the challenges for the pharmacist and pharmacy practice in Chile as a member country of the OECD in the coming years are those of promoting the development of public policies to improve the quality of life of the population and are the following:

7.1 Access to medication

It has been suggested that the failure that occurs in Chile today in relation to access to medicines is a problem of the private sector, and that the three major pharmacy chains are part of the problem, and they are. However, this sector accounts for less than 30% of the population. Over 70% of the Chilean population is registered in the public system (FONASA), so that the state must ensure this access through the primary health care. However, it is this group of the population facing the greatest difficulties in accessing medications in a timely, safe, and efficient manner. Since 2014, the National Drug Fund has guaranteed a stock of medicines to the population suffering the three chronic nontransmissible diseases of higher prevalence in Chile (over 5 million): hypertension, type 2 diabetes, and hyperlipidemia. It is expected that others, such as epilepsy and arthritis, will be included in the near future.

7.2 Drug law, choice of medication for economic reasons, and bioequivalence

This aspect is closely linked to the certification of bioequivalence for a certain drug in comparison to the original. Interchangeability refers to the ability of a pharmacist to replace a brand for a generic that is equivalent in effect, that is, bioequivalent, if the prescription indicates. However, for this exchange to be effective requires a policy to ensure the existence of certified bioequivalent products and the required stock. To achieve this goal bioequivalence must be evaluated by independent laboratories only and drug production must be properly planned by the pharmaceutical industries to efficiently meet the needs of the population.

While bioequivalence certification represents for our country a breakthrough in drug policy, its implementation has weaknesses that must be resolved to have a real impact on the health of the population. A policy of this nature should prioritize essential medicines in the National Formulary (Decree No. 466 of 1984), that is, those that are the basis for the drugs used in Chilean public facilities. However, at present it is the pharmaceutical companies themselves who set the priorities for the selection of which drugs on the list of the Ministry of Health will be certified as bioequivalent by the ISP. Moreover, they themselves are responsible for carrying out the certification process of selected products.

Yet, according to data provided by the ISP on 13 January 2015, since 2009 this entity has certified a total of 573 bioequivalent drugs corresponding to 108 active principles belonging to the national drug arsenal. In this aspect, the ISP permanently monitors the existence of these products in pharmacies, to ensure the user has the option to exchange it and access to an effective and quality-certified treatment.

7.3 Widening the sale market for drugs

Regarding the counter medications, there is a misconception among the public when calling OTC medications those displayed in special counters of free access. From the technical point of view, there is a difference between a policy of OTC and the condition of direct sales we have today. In the first case, when a drug is declared OTC, restrictions are imposed on the presentations available for sale to the public to minimize potential damage to the health of those who consume it. At the same time, an OTC policy considers an education program on the use of medicines to reduce the risk of damage to the population. This is a task in which the pharmacist must work directly with the health authority and, therefore, is of great importance in the practice of pharmacy, especially because as a country we have a well-known history and "tradition" of self-medication.

The present condition of direct sales in pharmacies does not establish any of the above considerations. So far, pharmacies count on the presence of a pharmacist the patient can consult if necessary (Sanitary Code). What will happen in the markets and other places selling nonprescription drugs in the near future? The existence of an OTC policy and its proper implementation can ensure that the counter medications are effective and secure for people, and the goal of reducing congestion at health systems for minor illness will be achieved.

It is important to note that the issue of access to medicines is unrelated or less solved with OTC drug access concerns and should be guaranteed for those drugs that have an impact on public health, which is not the case for those of direct sale.

References

1. Barozet E, Fierro J. *Medium class in Chile, 1990–2011: some social and political implications.* Konrad Adenauer Stiftung; December 2011. [Chilean Office].
2. *Historia de una profesión.* Santiago de Chile: Colegio Químico Farmacéutico y Bioquímico de Chile A.G; 2002.
3. *Historia de la Farmacia en Chile.* Santiago de Chile: Colegio Químico Farmacéutico y Bioquímico de Chile A.G; 2008.
4. *Basic indicators on health.* Chile: Department of Statistics and Information on Health, DEIS; 2013. Chilean Ministry of Health.
5. World Health Organization (WHO). *Chile health profile*; 2012.
6. World Health Organization (WHO). *World health statistics: regional and income groupings.* 2014. Sub secretariat of Social Prevision. Government of Chile. Available from: http://www.previsionsocial.gob.cl/subprev/?page_id=7229.
7. National Accreditation Commission (CNA). Evaluation Criteria for Chemistry and Pharmacy Curricula. 1998. Available from: http://www.cnachile.cl/Criterios%20de%20carreras/quimicayfarmacia.pdf.
8. Sanitary Code. Decree-Law No. 725 *Chil Official J* January 31, 1968.
9. Ministerio de Salud. *Política Nacional de Medicamentos en la Reforma de Salud.* Resolución Exenta N° 515 Chile: Ministerio de Salud. 2004. p. 31.
10. Ministerio de Salud; *Encuesta ENS Chile 2009–2010.* Capitulo V - Resultados [Internet] 2010. pp. 10–35. Available from: http://epi.minsal.cl/wp-content/uploads/2012/07/Informe-ENS-2009-2010.-CAP-5_FINALv1 julioccepi.pdf.

11. Subsecretaria de Salud Publica. *Estudio Nacional sobre Satisfaccion y Gasto en Salud.* Informe de resultados. Santiago de Chile; 2005. p. 159.
12. *Drugs in Chile: Revision de la evidencia del mercado nacional de fármacos.* Centro Nacional de Farmacoeconomia (CENAFAR), Insituto de Salud Publica de Chile; 2013. pp. 4–18. Available from: http://www.ispch.cl/sites/default/files/EstudioMedicamentos-22012014A.pdf.
13. *The Drug market in Chile.* División de Estudios. Ministerio de Economia de Chile; Abril, 2013. pp. 3–5.
14. León Vargas E, Martínez Becerra A. *2011El mercado farmacéutico: necesidades. Colección Ideas.* Septiembre, 2011. Año 12 N° 122.
15. *Report new molecules in Chile January–April 2014.* Sub-Department of Studies and Scientific Department ETESA, ISP; 2014.
16. IMS IfHI. *The global use of medicines: outlook through 2016.* July 2012. Available from: http://www.ispch.cl/sites/default/files/NM%20Enero-Abril%202014-07102014A.pdf.
17. *Relación entre Cantidad de Farmacias y Pobreza.* Division de Estudios, Ministerio de Economia, Fomento y Turismo; Marzo 2013.
18. National Institute of Statistics (INE). *Statistics compendium.* 2013. Available from: http://www.ine.cl/canales/menu/publicaciones/calendario_de_publicaciones/pdf/COMPENDIO_2013.pdf.
19. CONACEF.Fromhttp://schfa.cl/wp-content/uploads/2012/07/CONACEF-FCIA.ASISTENCIAL-CONVOCATORIA.-MC.M.P..pdf.
20. Home Web page of the Chilean Institute of Public Health: http://www.ispch.cl

CHAPTER 20

Comparative Analysis and Conclusion

Mohamed Izham Mohamed Ibrahim, Ahmed Ibrahim Fathelrahman,
Albert I. Wertheimer

Chapter Outline

1. Introduction

Nowadays, people across the globe are living longer, particularly because of positive development of the health care system in many parts of the world, technology advancement, new cost-effective medicines, better lifestyles, better understanding of diseases, various research discoveries, and better trained health care personnel. Population structure in most countries is generally showing fewer children and larger elderly populations. Life expectancy generally in many countries has reached the mid-80s, while the life expectancy in some low-income countries can be below 60. As the population ages, it will experience more chronic diseases and consume more medicines. The world population in 2013 was 7.125 billion, with an annual change of 1.2%.[18] It is estimated that developing countries accounted for 97% of this growth because of the dual effects of high birth rates and young populations.[8]

Of the world population, 60% of it is located in Asia, 15.5% in Africa, and around 8.6% in Latin America and the Caribbean.[20] Nevertheless, several of these countries have low incomes, high economic vulnerability, and poor human development indicators.[23] From time to time, some developing countries suffer from additional burdens such as disease epidemics, war, and natural hazards (e.g., earthquake and tsunami). All these challenges contribute to higher demands for a good health care system, competent health providers, and high-quality facilities. At times, these must stretch to meet the changing needs of the society. A pharmacy workforce is in great demand for society owing to the nature of its work, knowledge, skills, and competency to face these challenges. Thus, the practice of pharmacy and its workforce should be prepared according to the needs and the demands of the country.

In 1993, the International Pharmaceutical Federation (FIP) first adopted the guidelines for good pharmacy practice (GPP). Then in 1997, the World Health Organization (WHO) endorsed the revised version, followed by the approval of the FIP council.[10] Later in 2011, both the FIP and the WHO adopted an undated version of GPP. The WHO[29] in addition produced guidelines in relation to community and hospital practice. GPP is defined as "the practice of pharmacy that responds to the needs of the people who use the pharmacists' services to provide optimal, evidence-based care. To support this practice it is essential that there should be an established national framework of quality standards and guidelines." It supports pharmacy practice to "contribute to health improvement and to help patients with health problems to make the best use of their medicines." How far since 1993 (after more than 2 decades) has pharmacy practice in the developing countries improved and responded to the proposal?

In 2000, the United Nations established the Millennium Development Goals (MDGs), which represent eight major public health and humanitarian agenda based on a declaration and a commitment among all United Nations member states and a group of international organizations and include three purely public health-related goals, namely, reducing child mortality, improving maternal health, and combating HIV/AIDS, malaria, and other diseases.[22,25] However, all of the MDGs are having an impact on public health directly or indirectly. Fifteen years later, how far are we from meeting the United Nations MDGs? Pharmacists and medicines are important elements to meet these goals. This chapter will analyze and summarize several characteristics of pharmacy practice of the 19 countries included in the book. The analysis is done by referring to the GPP guidelines[32] and based on a few other recommendations from other studies.

The improvement in the quality and responsible use of medicines in society is very much dependent on the overall quality of the health care and pharmaceutical system; effective medicine policies, regulations, and guidelines; and education quality and training of health care professionals, for example, knowledge and competency of the pharmacists.

The aims of this chapter are to critically analyze the status of the 19 countries in terms of the practice of pharmacy in each country and to compare between them. The objectives are to find, via comparisons, which countries are practicing well based on satisfying community needs and making use of resources and to identify the gaps (present situations vs. recommended conditions) and recommending the way forward.

It is hoped that the findings of such analyses could provide the reader with good information about the practice in the 19 countries. The authors have no intention of generalizing the findings to other developing countries, but the findings would provide a good insight since the experiences of the countries included would certainly benefit other countries having similar or comparable backgrounds and situations.

2. How was the analysis done?

First, countries were divided into categories based on the World Bank list of countries by income classifications, that is, gross national income (GNI) per capita.[33] Accordingly, four lists of developing countries were established: low income (poorest), lower middle income, upper middle income, and high income (wealthiest).

Second, a list of variables was used to compare the pharmacy practice, policy and regulation, and education and training aspects. Important statistics, that is, country population, gross domestic product (GDP), overall life expectancy, and the number of pharmacists per 10,000 of population ratio for the 19 countries were also included. We would expect that a reasonable number of accepted practices in each country, under the pharmacy practice, policy and regulation, and education and training criteria, should exist. Therefore, a score of "1" was given for a "Yes, or positive practice," while "0" was given to a "No, or negative practice," answer. This was decided arbitrarily to assist in the comparison. As for the number of pharmacists per 10,000 population ratio, the WHO recommendation of 1:2000 was adopted (=5:10,000). The total score was then calculated for each country (maximum score of positive practice is 14; the higher the score, the better is the practice). Performance was then compared to see how well a country was doing generally and compared to other countries of similar wealth.

For this analysis, we adopted the definition of pharmacists and pharmacies used by the FIP[11]:

Pharmacist: A professional who in accordance with the local legal provisions and definitions may provide pharmacy services (in the community, hospital, academia, research, industry, etc.) in the country.

Pharmacies: Premises that, in accordance with the local legal provisions and definitions, may operate as a facility in the provision of pharmacy services in the community or hospital setting.

Data were then tabulated. The data were gathered from various sources, including the chapters in this book. The information then was shared with the authors from each country for validation. Data were analyzed descriptively (i.e., frequency (%), mean (SD), and median (IQR)) using IBM SPSS Statistics® version 22.

3. Findings and discussion

The World Bank classification was used to categorize the 19 countries.[33] As of July 1, 2013, the World Bank classified the income by GNI per capita as indicated in Table 1. Almost half of the countries ($n = 9$; 47.4%) are categorized as lower middle-income countries.

Table 1: Country economies by per-capita GNI in 2012

UN Category Based on Income	Income Bracket	Country
Low income	$1035 or less	Burkina Faso, Nepal
Lower middle income	$1036 to $4085	Egypt, India, Indonesia, Nigeria, Pakistan, Palestine, Sri Lanka, Sudan, Yemen
Upper middle income	$4086 to $12,615	China, Iraq, Jordan, Malaysia, Thailand
High income	$12,616 or more	Chile, Qatar, Saudi Arabia

Source: Ref. 31.

Table 2: Developing countries by region and income status

Region	Country	Income Status	Country That Is Least Developed
Asia (*n* = 8)			
Eastern Asia	China	Upper middle income	
Southeastern Asia	Thailand	Upper middle income	
Southeastern Asia	Malaysia	Upper middle income	
Southeastern Asia	Indonesia	Lower middle income	
Southern Asia	Pakistan	Lower middle income	
Southern Asia	Sri Lanka	Lower middle income	
Southern Asia	India	Lower middle income	
Southern Asia	Nepal	Low income	Least developed (as of November 2013)
Middle East (*n* = 6)			
Western Asia	Qatar	High income	
Western Asia	Saudi Arabia	High income	
Western Asia	Jordan	Upper middle income	
Western Asia	Iraq	Upper middle income	
Western Asia	Palestine	Lower middle income	
Western Asia	Yemen	Lower middle income	Least developed (as of November 2013)
Africa (*n* = 4)			
Northern Africa	Sudan	Lower middle income	Least developed (as of November 2013)
Northern Africa	Egypt	Lower middle income	
Western Africa	Nigeria	Lower middle income	
Western Africa	Burkina Faso	Low income	Least developed (as of November 2013)
Latin America (*n* = 1)			
South America	Chile	High income	

Source: Ref. 31.

In Table 2, the countries are classified into income status and associated with geographical location. There are four countries that are categorized as the least developed, that is, Nepal, Yemen, Burkina Faso, and Sudan; two in the African region; one in Asia; and one in the Middle East.

The profiles for each country were further reviewed and the criteria of pharmacy practice, regulation and policy, and education and training were analyzed (Tables 3–6).

Table 3: Criteria in low income countries

Criteria for Comparison	Country	
	Burkina Faso	Nepal
Country Background		
Population[b]	18,365,123 (2014)	30,986,975 (2014)
GDP per capita ($, ppp)[b]	1700 (2014 est.)	2400 (2014 est.)
Life expectancy (years)[b]	54.78	67.19
Number of licensed pharmacists (per 10,000 of population)	409 (0.2)	1200[a] (0.387)
Practice Criteria		
Is selling medicines outside of pharmacies allowed?	No	No
What is the popular area of practice?	Community pharmacy	Pharmaceutical industry
Any unique services?	None	None
How are controlled substances handled?	Only with prescription	Only with prescription
Is CE for pharmacists required?	Yes	No
Are there enough pharmacists to cover the community needs?	No	No
Does practice match available resources?	No	No
Are e-health technologies used in pharmacy practice?	No	No
Policy and Regulation		
Is state licensure required to practice?	Yes	Yes
Is a non-pharmacy degree holder allowed to operate a retail pharmacy without a pharmacist?	Yes (but under the license of a pharmacist)	Yes
Must a pharmacy shop have a registered/ licensed pharmacist present to operate?	Yes	Yes (owing to the lack of pharmacists license is given to pharmacy assistants)
Are there location requirements for opening a community pharmacy?	Yes	No
Is there regulation to handle controlled substances?	Yes	Yes
Does a national drug policy exist?	Yes	Yes
Score	9/14	7/14

[a]FIP[11,28].
[b]Central Intelligence Agency[9].
PPP, purchasing power parity

The analysis of the background of countries showed that the median average (IQR) of the populations is 30,986,975.0 (18,365,123.0–177,155,754.0), with the highest in India (1,355,692,576.0) and the lowest in Qatar (2,123,160.0). Qatar is different compared with other countries because only close to one-third of the population are Qataris. Data on life expectancy showed that the median average (IQR) is 73.5 years (67.1–75.0), with the highest in Chile and Qatar (78.4 years) and the lowest in Nigeria (52.6 years). Qatar has the highest GDP per capita (US$144,400.00), while Burkina Faso has the lowest (US$1700.00); the

Table 4: Criteria in lower middle income countries

Criteria for Comparison	Egypt	India	Indonesia	Nigeria	Pakistan	Sri Lanka	Sudan	Yemen[f]	Palestine
				Country Background					
Population[b]	86,895,099	1,236,344,631	253,609,643	177,155,754	196,174,380	21,866,445	35,482,233	26,052,966	4,548,000[d]
GDP per capita ($, ppp)[b]	11,100	5800	10,200	6100	4700	10,400	4500	3900	2465.10[e]
Life expectancy (years)[b]	73.45	67.8	72.17	52.62	67.05	76.35	63.32	64.83	75.01
Number of licensed pharmacists (per 10,000 of population)	150,000[a] (17.3)	680,482[a] (5.5)	46,336 (1.8)	15,377[a] (0.9)	12,000[a] (0.6)	7237[c] (NA)	7685 (2.2)	4309 (1.7)	4048 (8.9)
				Practice Criteria					
Is selling medicines outside of pharmacies allowed?	Yes (only limited OTC items are allowed)	Yes	Yes (only for limited items)	Yes	Yes (only some OTC items are available at grocery stores)	Yes	Yes (only limited OTC items are allowed)	Yes	No
What is the popular area of practice?	Community pharmacy	Pharmaceutical industry	Community pharmacy	Pharmaceutical industry	Pharmaceutical industry	Community pharmacy	Community pharmacy	Community pharmacy	Community pharmacy
Any unique services?	None	Drug and poison information center	None	None	None	None	None	None	Poison control and drug information
How are controlled substances handled?	Law, prescription, recording	Law, prescription	Law, prescription, recording	Law, prescription, recording	Law and prescription record and registers at pharmacies	Law, need prescription	Law, prescription, recording	Law, prescription, recording	Law, prescription, recording, supervision and field inspection
Is CE required?	No (not for renewal of registration)	No (not for renewal of registration)	Yes	Yes (for renewal of registration)	No (not for renewal of registration)	No (not for renewal of registration)	No (not for renewal of registration)	No (not for renewal of registration)	No (not for renewal of registration)
Are there enough pharmacists to cover the community needs?	No	No	No	No	No	No	No	No	Yes
Does practice match available resources?	No	No	Yes (but limited)	No	No	No	No	No	No

					Policy and Regulation					
Are e-health technologies used in pharmacy practice?	No	No	No	No	No	No	No	No	No	No
Is state licensure required to practice?	Yes	Yes	Yes	Yes	Yes	Yes	Yes	Yes	Yes	Yes
Is a non-pharmacy degree holder allowed to operate a retail pharmacy without a pharmacist?	No	Yes	No	No	Yes	No	Yes	No	No (allowed only in drugstore)	No
Are there policies that well regulate practice?	Yes (but not sufficient)	Yes (but not sufficient)	Yes	Yes	Yes (but not sufficient)	Yes	Yes	Yes	Yes (but not sufficient)	Yes
Must a pharmacy shop have a registered/licensed pharmacist present to operate?	Yes	Yes	Yes	Yes	No	Yes	No	Yes	Yes	Yes
Are there location requirements for opening a community pharmacy?	Yes	No	Yes	Yes	No	Yes	No	Yes	Yes	Yes
Is there regulation to handle controlled substances?	Yes	Yes	Yes	Yes	Yes	Yes	Yes	Yes	Yes	Yes
Is there regulation on selling medicines outside of pharmacies?	Yes	Yes	Yes	Yes	Yes	Yes	Yes	Yes	Yes	Yes
Does a national drug policy exist?	No	Yes	Yes	Yes	Yes	Yes	Yes	Yes	Yes	No
Score	9/14	10/14	11/14	10/14	6/14	11/14	7/14	9/14	9/14	11/14

a FIP[11].

b Central Intelligence Agency[9].

c WHO. The Pharmaceutical Sector Country Profile Survey of Sri Lanka; majority are nonpharmacists with diploma degree and data for 2010[30].

d Population Pyramids of the World from 1950 to 2100 http://populationpyramid.net/state-of-palestine/2015/[16].

e Palestine: GDP=http://www.tradingeconomics.com/palestine/gdp-per-capita-ppp[21].

f Ministry of Public Health & Population of Yemen[14].

Table 5: Criteria in upper middle income countries

Criteria for Comparison	Country				
	China	Iraq	Jordan	Malaysia	Thailand
Country Background					
Population[b]	1,355,692,576	32,585,692	7,930,491	30,073,353	67,741,401
GDP per capita ($, ppp)[b]	12,900	14,100	11,900	24,500	14,400
Life expectancy (years)[b]	75.15	71.42	74.1	74.52	74.18
Number of licensed pharmacist (per 10,000 of population)	200,000[a] (1.5)	11,857 (3.6)	13,840[a] (17.5)	10,077[a] (3.4)	28,272[a] (4.2)
Practice Criteria					
Is selling medicines outside of pharmacies allowed?	Yes (only OTC)	No	Yes (only paracetamol)	Yes (only OTC)	Yes
What is the popular area of practice?	Hospital pharmacy	Community pharmacy	Pharmaceutical industry	Hospital pharmacy	Hospital pharmacy
Any unique services?	Pharmaceutical care	None	None	Medication therapy adherence interventions	Smoking cessation and medication therapy management
How are controlled substances handled?	Law; prescription item; recording	Law; prescription item; recording	Law; prescription item; recording	Law; prescription item; recording	Law; prescription item; recording
Is CE required?	No	No	Yes	No	No
Are there enough pharmacists to cover the community needs?	No	No	Yes	No	No
Does practice match available resources?	No	No	Yes (to a certain extent)	Yes (to a certain extent)	No
Are e-health technologies used in pharmacy practice?	Yes (to a certain extent)	No	Yes (to a certain extent)	Yes (to a certain extent)	Yes (to a certain extent)
Policy and Regulation					
Is state licensure is required to practice?	Yes	Yes	Yes	Yes	Yes
Is a non-pharmacy degree holder allowed to operate a retail pharmacy without a pharmacist?	No	No	No	No	Yes (for type 2 drugstore)
Must a pharmacy shop have a registered/licensed pharmacist present to operate?	Yes	Yes	Yes	Yes	Yes (for type 1 drugstore)

Table 5: Criteria in upper middle income countries—cont'd

Criteria for Comparison	Country				
	China	Iraq	Jordan	Malaysia	Thailand
Are there location requirements for opening a community pharmacy?	No	Yes	Yes	No	No
Is there regulation to handle controlled substances?	Yes	Yes	Yes	Yes	Yes
Is there regulation on selling medicines outside of pharmacies?	Yes	Yes	Yes	Yes	Yes
Does a national drug policy exist?	Yes	Yes	No	Yes	Yes
Score	9/14	9/14	12/14	10/14	8/14

[a]FIP[11].
[b]Central Intelligence Agency[9].

median average was US$10,400.00 (US$4500.00–14,400.00). The number of pharmacists per 10,000 population ratio showed that the median average (IQR) is 2.8 (0.8–5.5); Jordan has the highest ratio (17.5), which achieved the WHO recommendation, while Burkina Faso has the lowest ratio (0.2). Based on the WHO recommendation for developing countries (1:2000), we need a minimum of five pharmacists per 10,000 population.

More detailed analyses indicated that five (26%) countries do not allow selling of medicines outside of pharmacies. Others allow selling of only limited medicines, that is, over-the-counter (OTC) items such as paracetamol. The most popular area of practice is community pharmacy ($n=10$; 53%), followed by hospital pharmacy ($n=5$; 26%) and the pharmaceutical industry ($n=5$; 26%). The majority of the countries do not have any unique service in the pharmacy practice ($n=12$; 63%).

All countries have laws that regulate controlled substances, for example, psychotropic medications; they can be dispensed only with prescription. In some countries, pharmacists are required to record the transaction of these medications, for example, procurement and dispensing. About the requirement for continuing education (CE), pharmacists in 13 (68%) countries are not required to do their CE; a few are required, but in only one country are pharmacists required to attend CE for their renewal of registration.

The review also looked at resources. Regarding the adequacy of pharmacists to cover the community needs, 17 (90%) countries do not have enough pharmacists, while only two (10%) countries are fine. We further checked whether the practice is matching the available resources; in 14 (74%) countries it is not, while the rest of the countries are satisfactory, but to a certain extent. In addition, we also looked at if e-health technologies are used in

Table 6: Criteria in high income countries

Criteria for Comparison	Country		
	Chile	Saudi Arabia	Qatar
Country Background			
Population[b]	17,363,894	27,345,986	2,123,160
GDP per capita ($, ppp)[b]	23,200	52,800	144,400
Life expectancy (years)[b]	78.44	74.82	78.38
Number of licensed pharmacists (per 10,000 of population)	644 (0.4)	14,928[a] (5.5)	998 (4.7)
Practice Criteria			
Is selling medicines outside of pharmacies allowed?	Yes (with authorization)	No	Yes (only limited items)
What is the popular area of practice?	Community pharmacy	Community/ hospital pharmacy	Hospital pharmacy
Any unique services?	None	Medication therapy management	Anticoagulation clinic in hospital
How are controlled substances handled?	Law, prescription, recording	Law, prescription, recording	Law, prescription, recording
Is CE required?	No	Yes	No
Are there enough pharmacists to cover the community needs?	No	No	No
Does practice match available resources?	No	Yes (to a certain extent)	Yes
Are e-health technologies used in pharmacy practice?	No	Yes (to a certain extent)	Yes (to a certain extent in the hospitals)
Policy and Regulation			
Is state licensure required to practice?	Yes	Yes	Yes
Is a non-pharmacy degree holder allowed to operate a retail pharmacy without a pharmacist?	No	No	No
Must a pharmacy shop have a registered/ licensed pharmacist present to operate?	No	Yes	Yes
Are there location requirements for opening a community pharmacy?	No	Yes	Yes
Is there regulation to handle controlled substances?	Yes	Yes	Yes
Is there regulation on selling medicines outside of pharmacies?	Yes	Yes	Yes
Does a national drug policy exist?	Yes	Yes	No
Score	6/14	14/14	10/14

[a]FIP[11].

[b]Central Intelligence Agency[9].

pharmacy practice; countries' authors confirmed that six (32%) countries use e-health technologies to a certain extent and others do not.

In addition, we reviewed pharmaceutical policy and regulation. The first question was if state licensure is required to practice. All countries have laws that require pharmacists to have a license to practice. Next, we checked if a non-pharmacy degree holder is allowed to operate a retail pharmacy. Only four (21%) countries allow, and two (10%) countries allow non-pharmacy degree holders to operate a drugstore (different from a pharmacy). Others do not allow it. For if a pharmacy shop must have a registered/licensed pharmacist present to operate, only three (16%) countries do not require it, while others ($n = 16$; 84%) do impose such requirement. In countries where there is a lack of pharmacists, either licenses are given to pharmacy assistants or retail pharmacies are operated illegally by a nonpharmacist. Around 42% ($n = 8$) of the countries put a requirement on the location for opening a community pharmacy, while others allow pharmacies to be operated anywhere. All countries have regulations on handling controlled substances. Only four (21%) countries are without a national medicines (drug) policy.

When scores were assigned to positive practices in countries (maximum of 14), the findings showed that the mean score (SD) was 9.3 (1.9). It ranged from 6.0 to 14.0. Countries in the low-income category had a mean score (SD) of 8.0 (1.4), followed by lower middle-income countries (9.1 ± 1.7), upper middle-income countries (9.6 ± 1.5), and high-income countries (10.0 ± 4.0). There was a clear upward trend; the higher the income category, the higher the mean score, which indicates more positive practices.

A national medicines policy is an initiative to bring about better health outcomes for the society. The findings indicated that generally many countries have a national medicines policy and pharmaceutical acts and regulations. The problems in many of these countries are weaknesses in enforcement, the lack of motivated and dedicated authorities to carry out their duties and responsibilities. In developing countries with low income, salaries of employees are low. People have to struggle for a living and this is vulnerable to corruption. The lack of human resources and low salary, in addition to ineffective policies and regulations and lack of punitive action, could be the factors that contribute to a poor pharmaceutical sector in a country. There is a high possibility that substandard and counterfeit drugs will penetrate the pharmaceutical market and affect people's health. There is also the likelihood of distribution of illegal Western medicines.

There are countries like Nepal and Sri Lanka, which earlier had few or no colleges of pharmacy, that had opened the door to allowing non-pharmacy graduates with few or no qualifications to operate a retail pharmacy or drugstore. In other situations, with a lack of enforcement, in countries like Yemen, Pakistan, and Burkina Faso, community pharmacies are operated by nonpharmacists. The possibility of controlled medicines that can be bought easily without prescription is high. In a country like Malaysia, where there is no dispensing separation between general practitioners and community pharmacists, community pharmacists do sell prescription items illegally, for example, antibiotics without a prescription.[2,3] Lack of ethical practices and professionalism plus the conditions explained above makes the pharmaceutical sector weak and places the society at risk.

Even though the aspect of laws in regard to medicine price control was not reviewed in this chapter, in many of the developing countries, prices of medicines are not effectively controlled. In countries like Yemen, medicine availability and affordability are a major concern. These problems could cause the penetration of counterfeit medicines into the country and the possibility of illegal supply of Western medicines with low prices. No country is immune from this problem. In China, India, Nepal, Qatar, Egypt, and Pakistan, for example, there are mechanisms to control medicine prices. In Nepal, prices are controlled only on limited items; it is not comprehensive. In another example, the Qatar Supreme Council of Health, which applied an open market policy in the past, issued a new price schedule in the late 2014 with new wholesale and retail rates for various drugs. This means that consumers should pay the same price for an item when filling a prescription throughout the pharmacies in Qatar. The government of Egypt implements an active national medicines price monitoring system for retail prices. It is mandated that retail medicine price information should be publicly accessible. On the other hand, Chile does not have a policy of price regulation concerning the private or retail sector. In Malaysia, the phenomenon called "price wars" brings a negative impact on the pharmacy profession through an unhealthy business competition among community pharmacies through the undercutting of the price of medicines. Even if a country has a mechanism to control medicine prices, what does it matter if the policy and regulations are not enforced? In addition, we should study the impact of price controls on the health of the public and the economy of the country.

In many of the developing countries, issues of medicine production, procurement, and consumption are critical. Some countries do not have adequate local manufacturers to produce generic medicines; domestic medicine production is not sufficient for the country. Medicines have to be imported for local consumption. When medicine prices are not well regulated, and medicines need to be imported, plus an ineffective generic medicines policy, public out-of-pocket expenditures for health and medicines will be high. Countries do need an effective and efficient pharmaceutical financing scheme, which offers significant potential to reduce the burden of disease and poverty. Many countries face problems of inadequate supply, unavailability, inaccessibility, and unaffordability of essential medicines for the general public. Ill health and poverty are closely associated. For many of the developing countries, ineffective financing systems have placed a high burden on the poor people.

In terms of the procurement process, countries are facing problems with transparency during the tender process, lack of clear criteria when selecting suppliers, limited quality testing for products, lack of qualified personnel for inventory management, and inefficiency in the medication quantification process. Furthermore, many of the developing countries have little or no information technology system.

A strong, competent, and experienced government is crucial for ensuring better health for the society. Several developing countries including, but not limited to, Iraq, Yemen, Palestine, and Nepal are facing economic instability, war and political crisis, lack of leadership, and poor management of the government sectors. Another factor is the availability of quality local academic institutions such as in Sri Lanka and Nepal, which should produce quality health-related graduates who would fill positions in various health care sectors. Academic institutions are supposed to prepare a well-designed curriculum and ensure graduates are equipped for the roles and responsibilities they have to perform in various pharmacy settings. Several countries have inadequate local public pharmacy colleges. If they exist, these public colleges, such as in Sudan and Yemen, suffer from lack of quality curriculum and program; they still have traditional curricula and are not up to date. They will also suffer from lack of a competent faculty. Available private colleges in most cases will focus on profit generation for survival, with a lack of emphasis on competency in the academic program, quality of the graduates, and the research component. In some countries, a degree in pharmacy needs to be obtained abroad because of the limitations mentioned above (e.g., Sri Lanka). Countries with poor resources would not be able to send many candidates to fulfill the human resource needs of the countries. Another challenge facing the health care sector is the migration of pharmacists to other countries for a better position, salary, and living conditions (e.g., India and Sudan). In some countries, due to the lack of pharmacists and imbalances in the distribution between the rural and the urban areas, the government needs to relax its regulations and allow non-pharmacy degree holders to operate a pharmacy or drugstore. Countries with a weak system and lack of enforcement are vulnerable to the illegal establishment of drugstores/pharmacies or illegal operators running a drugstore/pharmacy, especially in rural areas. Such environment is susceptible to irrational use of medicines and low-quality medicines including substandard and counterfeit medicines. This again will put the people at risk, especially in a society with a high number of people with low education and poor health literacy.

4. Gaps and Challenges

A gap analysis is a technique for identifying needed improvements by comparing the current environment and current processes against an envisioned future state, that is, the gap between the current practice and the desired practice.[1] It will be desirable if countries with a low score in the criteria, that is, poor practice standards, benchmark countries with a high score, that is, better practice standards, within the same category of economy, environment, or geographical type.

As mentioned by the WHO[29] the mission of pharmacy practice is "to provide medications and other health care products and services and to help people and society to make the best use of them."

The findings above clearly indicate that there is much to be done by countries to improve the pharmacy practice in order to fulfill the needs of the society; some have to do much more in the way of improvement than others. It is true that one cannot "compare an apple with an orange." It is definitely unfair to compare a low-income country with a developed country. But, it is fine if a country could learn, adopt, and adapt a set of best practices from others. According to Babar et al.[7] GPP could be achieved by promoting the rational use of medicines. As defined by the WHO[26] rational use of medicines means "patients receive medications appropriate to their clinical needs, in doses that meet their own individual requirements, for an adequate period of time, and at the lowest cost to them and their community." Medicine use includes the steps from marketing of the medicine until it is used by individuals. The medication use process thus includes the following activities: procurement, prescribing, preparation, dispensing, administration, and monitoring.[13] The quality use of medicines is very much dependent on pharmacists, other players in the health care system, and the system of the health sector. The cost of health care in developing countries can be unnecessarily high if an efficient system and process are not in place. A GPP needs the power of a quality system and process. It is the duty and responsibility of pharmacists to ensure that the service they provide to the society is up to the standard, that is, of appropriate quality.

It is indicated that the pharmacy practice in the 19 countries varies from country to country and, as mentioned by the authors even within their country, the conditions of practice may vary between areas, for example, rural versus urban, due to the lack of resources and infrastructure.

The GPP guidelines are a good approach for pharmacists and pharmacy organizations in countries to implement pharmaceutical care.[27,29] In fulfilling the responsibilities and requirements of GPP and pharmaceutical care, there are a few aspects that pharmacists and pharmacy organizations need to consider to gauge the gaps in practice and between countries:

1. Professionalism—How far is the professionalism factor built in the pharmacy practice?
2. Decision-making—Are pharmacists the main players and key decision-makers in matters related to medicine use?
3. Health care team—Are pharmacists key players on the health care team? And how is the pharmacist's relationship with other members of the health care team?
4. Patient information—Do pharmacists have access to patient information, that is, medication profile, in order to perform effective pharmaceutical care?
5. Academic programs—Does the country have adequate pharmacy colleges? And what is the quality of the pharmacy program and the credentials of the faculty members in the pharmacy colleges?
6. CE—Do pharmacists have the opportunity to upgrade or improve their knowledge, skill, and competency throughout their career?
7. Standard of practice—Does the country has a minimum standard of practice in all pharmacy settings?
8. Scholarly activity—How far is the pharmacy practice research? How many publications in quality journals? And what is the impact on pharmacy practice and pharmaceutical policy?

Regarding research and publications, even though not much was discussed in this book, in general, there is a great disparity in publications from developing countries, which accounts for over 80% of the world population.[15,24] Only around 10% of research is done in the developing countries.[19] Most of the research is in the developed world, while people in the developing countries have the most health suffering.

To look into the gaps between countries specifically, based on a simple developed scoring system, the findings showed that Chile, Pakistan, Nepal, Sri Lanka, and Thailand are below the median average, while Saudi Arabia and Jordan are on the high side; the others are considered moderate. It shows that around 90% of the countries have missing important practices. For example, Chile has only 6/14 practices compared to Saudi Arabia, which has 14/14. The number of pharmacists in all countries, except Jordan, Saudi Arabia, Palestine, Egypt, and India, is below the required figure as suggested by the WHO. Most of the countries do allow medicines to be sold outside the pharmacy premises. Six countries do allow nonpharmacists to handle and sell medicines and operate drugstores. The majority of the countries do require a registered/licensed pharmacist to present and practice in the pharmacy. In general, many countries have a medicines policy and regulation to control medicine use in the society, yet several of the practice conditions are not satisfied. Two huge challenges are corruption and vested interests not wanting change.

There is a big gap in terms of hospital pharmacy practice and special services between countries. Hospital pharmacy practice is more popular in Thailand, China, Malaysia, Saudi Arabia, and Qatar. It is interesting to know that all these countries are at the upper tier of the developing economy. Hospital pharmacy practices in these countries are somewhat advanced. Services like pharmaceutical care, medication therapy management, patient counseling, discharge counseling, home visits, adverse drug reaction reporting, anticoagulation clinic, and therapeutic drug monitoring are provided by pharmacists in the hospital. Community pharmacy practice, on the other hand, is more popular in countries coming under low income and lower middle income categories. Services provided in the community pharmacy generally are still traditional, are more distributive, and lack clinical and patient-oriented services.

This chapter also highlights several other gaps, which have been mentioned in earlier chapters: uneven distribution of pharmacies; inequality in allocation of resources; more traditional services versus nontraditional services; low salary, poor compensation, and unattractive benefits for pharmacists; inadequate training and CE programs for professional development of pharmacists; inadequate number and quality of pharmacy colleges; insufficient production of medicines for local consumption and having to rely on imported medicines; lack of an effective drug regulatory system; failure to implement and enforce policy and regulations; issues with medicine adequacy, availability, accessibility, affordability; and little or no minimum standard of pharmacy practice.

According to Babar and Scahill[6] barriers to effective pharmacy practice could be linked to the country's health systems (macro level), level and quality of services provided by community pharmacies (meso level), and education, training, and professional factors (micro level). The gaps mentioned above and the facts stated by the country authors clearly indicate that the countries included in this book do suffer from ineffective pharmacy practice due to these factors, that is, under the three levels. Pharmacists and pharmacy organizations do need to strategize, plan, and work toward overcoming these barriers.

Research findings could contribute to further development of pharmacy practice in the countries. Quality research demands good understanding of research methodology, steps and processes, and access to information and quality data. Parts of the significant challenges for developing countries are the absence of information and quality data. These will jeopardize the research quality and hinder acceptance by journals. For example, research findings in developing countries do not provide quality data allowing one to determine whether national drug policies improve medicine use because of poor study design.[17] Local pharmacy and health journals also suffer from quality issues, for example, attracting members of the editorial board, reviewers, financial support, and quality articles.

5. Way forward

Brodie[34] has mentioned that pharmacists must identify the boundaries of duty and responsibilities and he encouraged the practice of pharmacy to move toward the patient and fulfill the needs of the society. In 1980, the American Public Health Association recognized pharmacy as a profession with major responsibilities for public health.[5] In addition, the FIP and the WHO reemphasized the importance of the role of pharmacists through their GPP guidelines. The different stakeholders related to pharmacy and health in the countries should revisit the various guidelines and recommendations. Albanese and Rouse[4] in their article "Scope of contemporary pharmacy practice: roles, responsibilities, and functions of pharmacists and pharmacy technicians" concluded that the evolution of health care and pharmacy practice has created excellent opportunities for pharmacists to serve the society beyond the traditional roles.

There is room for pharmacists to conduct quality studies to evaluate the status of pharmacy practice and the overall pharmaceutical sector in the country. We need to build more evidence-based information and research for developing and commissioning quality pharmacy practice, as studies and evidence are lacking or old. Effort is critically needed to narrow the gap of practice within a country, for example, rural and urban settings[12]; between developing countries; and if possible between developing and developed countries.

Pharmacy education in each developing country should be directed toward addressing local needs and making use of the available opportunities. For example, in the countries where hospital pharmacy is more popular (i.e., most of pharmacists' jobs/working opportunities are hospital based), pharmacy curriculum should be clinically based to allow for producing pharmacists with good clinical knowledge and competencies. In countries where community pharmacy is the most popular setting for practice, there may be more focus on the pharmacy curricula in public health education as community pharmacies are a good setting for wellness and health promotion programs such as caring for chronically ill patients, vaccination, and smoking cessation. On the other hand, where the pharmaceutical industry is the popular form of practice, there is a need for strengthening the traditional pharmacy education. In countries with a rich and long history of herbal and traditional medicines, there is a need for conducting pharmaceutical research in this area searching for evidence that supports the accumulated knowledge and cultures.

Here are a few recommendations that could be considered especially by pharmacists and pharmacy organizations in developing countries to improve the pharmaceutical sector condition:

- Conduct a gap analysis (decide on the goals, benchmark the current state, analyze the gap, compile the report, then plan to address the gaps, taking into consideration the output from Strengths Weaknesses Opportunities Threats (SWOT) analysis).
- Examine guidelines and best practices from most advanced countries such as the United States, Canada, Sweden, the Netherlands, Australia, and Germany.
- Develop and strengthen the national medicines policy.
- Ensure an essential medicines list exists and benefits the society.
- Ensure an effective drug regulatory system exists, which would ensure the quality of medicines in the country.
- Review the quality of pharmacy education and build a competence-based education that focuses on patient care, systems management, and public health.[4]
- Build a quality CE program and progressively implement compulsory CE points for registration renewal of pharmacists.
- Strengthen the research capacity in the area of pharmacy practice.

6. Conclusion

The pressure on the whole health care system worldwide will continue and there is no escape for the pharmaceutical sector of a country. The pain of the pressure is felt more by the low- and middle-income countries. An effective pharmacy practice is supposed to ensure responsible and quality use of medicines from all angles. The countries' chapters and the analyses demonstrated in this chapter clearly indicate that for many countries, gaps, barriers, and challenges to effective pharmacy practice still exist. The role of pharmacists still has a long way to go. In summary, further work and effort in the developing countries are warranted to bring the pharmacy practice and profession to another level and standard.

References

1. AHRQ. *AHRQ quality indicators toolkit.* http://www.ahrq.gov/professionals/systems/hospital/qitoolkit/d5-gapanalysis.pdf [accessed 29.05.15].
2. Alamin Hassan MAA, Ibrahim MIM, Mohamed Azmi AH. Dispensing practices of general practitioners and community pharmacists in Malaysia – a pilot study. *J Pharm Pract Res* 2013;**43**:187–9.
3. Alamin Hassan MAA, Ibrahim MIM, Mohamed Azmi AH. Do professional practices among Malaysian private healthcare providers differ? A comparative study using simulated patients. *J Clin Diagn Res* 2013;**7**:2912–6.
4. Albanese NP, Rouse MJ. Scope of contemporary pharmacy practice: roles, responsibilities, and functions of pharmacists and pharmacy technicians. *J Am Pharm Assoc* 2010;**50**:e35–69.
5. American Public Health Association. Policy statements adopted by the governing council. The role of the pharmacist in public health. *Am J Public Health* 1981;**71**:213–6.
6. Babar ZU, Scahill S. Barriers to effective pharmacy practice in low- and middle-income countries. *Integr Pharm Res Pract* 2014;**3**:25–7.
7. Babar ZU, Vaughan C, Scahill S. Pharmacy practice: Is the gap between the North and South widening? *South Med Rev* 2012;**5**(1):1–2.
8. Haub Carl. *Fact sheet: world population trends.* 2012. http://www.prb.org/Publications/Datasheets/2012/world-population-data-sheet/fact-sheet-world-population.aspx.
9. Central Intelligence Agency. *The world factbook.* https://www.cia.gov/library/publications/the-world-factbook/rankorder/rankorderguide.html [accessed 20.03.15].
10. FIP (International Pharmaceutical Federation). *Good pharmacy practice in developing countries: recommendations for step-wise implementation.* The Hague (Netherlands). http://www.fip.org/files/fip/Statements/GPP%20recommendations.pdf [accessed 15.02.15].
11. FIP (International Pharmaceutical Federation). *Workforce report. Developing the healthcare workforce of the future.* 2012. The Hague (Netherland).
12. FIP (International Pharmaceutical Federation). *Global pharmacy workforce and migration report.* 2009. The Hague (Netherland).
13. Ninno Mark A, Ninno Sharon Davis. Quality improvement and the medication use process. In: Malone Patrick M, Kier Karen L, Stanovich John E, editors. *Drug information: a guide for pharmacists.* USA: McGraw-Hill Education, LLC; 2012.
14. Ministry of Public Health & Population of Yemen. *Yemen pharmaceutical country profile.* http://www.who.int/medicines/areas/coordination/YemenPSCP_Narrative2012-12-16Final.pdf [accessed 10.04.15].
15. Patel V, Kim YR. Contribution of low- and middle-income countries to research published in leading general psychiatry journals, 2002–2004. *Br J Psychiatry* January 2007;**190**:77–8.
16. Wulf MD. Population Pyramids of the World from 1950 to 2100. http://populationpyramid.net/state-of-palestine/2015.
17. Ratanawijitrasin S, Soumerai SB, Weerasuriya K. Do national medicinal drug policies and essential drug programs improve drug use? A review of experiences in developing countries. *Soc Sci Med* 2001;**53**(7):831–44.
18. Schlesinger R. *The 2014 US and world populations.* US News & World Report; 2013. http://www.usnews.com/opinion/blogs/robert-schlesinger/2013/12/31/us-population-2014-317-million-and-71-billion-in-the-world [accessed 29.03.15].
19. Smith R. Publishing research from developing countries. *Stat Med* 2002;**21**(19):2869–77.
20. Population Reference Bureau. *World population by region: world population data sheet 2014.* http://www.worldometers.info/world-population/#region [accessed 06.04.15].
21. Trading Economics. *Palestine GDP per capita PPP.* http://www.tradingeconomics.com/palestine/gdp-per-capita-ppp [accessed 10.04.15].
22. United Nations. *Millennium development goals and beyond 2015.* http://www.un.org/millenniumgoals/bkgd.shtml [accessed 02.02.15].
23. United Nations Population Division. *World population prospects: the 2010 revision, medium variant.* 2011.

24. Vetter N. Research publication in developing countries. *J Public Health Med* 2003;**25**(3):189.
25. Wage J, Banerji R, Campbell O, et al. The millennium development goals: a cross-sectoral analysis and principles for goal setting after 2015. *The Lancet* 2010;**376**:991–1023.
26. WHO. http://apps.who.int/medicinedocs/en/d/Jh3011e/1.html; 1985 [accessed 25.05.15].
27. WHO and FIP. *Developing pharmacy practice – a focus on patient care*. 2006. Geneva (Switzerland).
28. WHO. *Global health observatory data repository. Pharmaceutical personnel.* http://apps.who.int/gho/data/view.main.PHARMS [accessed 15.05.15].
29. WHO. *Good pharmacy practice in community and hospital pharmacy settings*. Geneva; 1996.
30. WHO. The pharmaceutical sector country profile survey of Sri Lanka. http://www.who.int/medicines/areas/coordination/Sri_Lanka_PSCPQuestionnaire.pdf [accessed 05.05.15].
31. World Bank. *World development indicators: size of the economy*. 2014.
32. FIP/WHO. Good pharmacy practice. Joint FIP/WHO guidelines on good pharmacy practice: standards for quality of pharmacy services. World Health Organization. http://whqlibdoc.who.int/trs/WHO_TRS_961_eng.pdf
33. World Bank. New country classifications. http:// data.worldbank.org/news/new-country-classifications-2015
34. Brodie CD. *Pharmacy's societal purpose. Am J Hosp Pharm* 1981;**38**:1893–6.

Index

Printed in the United States
By Bookmasters